Handbook of
WOMEN'S SEXUAL
AND
REPRODUCTIVE HEALTH

ISSUES IN WOMEN'S HEALTH

Series Editors: Ralph J. DiClemente and Gina M. Wingood
Emory University
Rollins School of Public Health
Atlanta, Georgia

HANDBOOK OF WOMEN'S SEXUAL AND REPRODUCTIVE HEALTH
Gina M. Wingood and Ralph J. DiClemente

INTIMATE PARTNER VIOLENCE
Societal, Medical, Legal, and Individual Responses
Sana Loue

Handbook of
WOMEN'S SEXUAL
AND
REPRODUCTIVE HEALTH

Edited by

Gina M. Wingood, ScD, MPH

Emory University
Atlanta, Georgia

and

Ralph J. DiClemente, PhD

Emory University
Atlanta, Georgia

KLUWER ACADEMIC / PLENUM PUBLISHERS
New York, Boston, Dordrecht, London, Moscow

Library of Congress Cataloging-in-Publication Data

Handbook of women's sexual and reproductive health/edited by Gina M. Wingood and
Ralph J. DiClemente.
        p.   ; cm. — (Issues in women's health)
    Includes bibliographical references and index.
    ISBN 0-306-46651-1
        1. Reproductive health—Handbooks, manuals, etc.   2. Women—Health and
hygiene—Handbooks, manuals, etc.   3. Women—Sexual behavior—Handbooks, manuals,
etc. I. Wingood, Gina M., 1963– II. DiClemente, Ralph J.   III. Issues in women's health
(Kluwer Academic Publishers)

RG103 .H27 2002
618—dc21

2001053919

ISBN 0-306-46651-1

©2002 Kluwer Academic / Plenum Publishers, New York
233 Spring Street, New York, New York 10013

http://www.wkap.nl/

10 9 8 7 6 5 4 3 2 1

A C.I.P. record for this book is available from the Library of Congress

Printed in the United States of America

Our parents educated us and their love sustains us,
Our scholarship stimulates us,
Our relationship enlightens us,
Our friends and colleagues support us,

We dedicate this book to all in our lives

Contributors

Hortensia Amaro, Ph.D. • Department of Social and Behavioral Sciences, Boston University School of Public Health, Boston, Massachusetts 02118

Sevgi O. Aral, Ph.D. • Division of STD Prevention, Centers for Disease Control and Prevention, Atlanta, Georgia 30333

Nancy E. Avis, Ph.D. • Department of Public Health Sciences, Wake Forest University School of Medicine, Winston-Salem, North Carolina 27157

Amida Ayala, Ph.D. • Department of Psychiatry and Biobehavioral Sciences, University of California at Los Angles, Los Angeles, California 90024-1759

Jeanne Brooks-Gunn, Ph.D. • Institute for Child Psychology, Child Development, and Education, Teachers College, Columbia University, New York, New York 10027

Jane D. Brown, Ph.D. • School of Journalism and Mass Communication, University of North Carolina at Chapel Hill, Chapel Hill, North Carolina 27599-3365

Kathleen M. Cardona, MPH. • Department of Population and Family Health Sciences, Johns Hopkins School of Hygiene and Public Health, Baltimore, Maryland 21205

Jennifer Vargas Carmona • Department of Psychiatry and Biobehavioral Sciences, University of California at Los Angeles, Los Angeles, California 90024-1759

Thomas F. Cash, Ph.D. • Department of Psychology, Old Dominion University, Norfolk, Virginia 23529-0267

Dorothy Chin, Ph.D. • Department of Psychiatry and Biobehavioral Sciences, University of California at Los Angeles, Los Angeles, California 90024-1759

Kerith Jane Conron, MPH. • Department of Social and Behavioral Sciences, Boston University School of Public Health, Boston, Massachusetts 02118

Sybil Crawford, Ph.D. • University of Massachusetts Medical School, Worcester, Massachusetts 01655

Richard A. Crosby, Ph.D. • Department of Behavioral Sciences and Health Education, Rollins School of Public Health, Emory University, Atlanta, Georgia 30322

Ralph J. DiClemente, Ph.D. • Department of Behavioral Sciences and Health Education, Rollins School of Public Health, Emory University, Atlanta, Georgia 30322

Kirk Elifson, Ph.D. • Department of Behavioral Sciences and Health Education, Rollins School of Public Health, Emory University, Atlanta, Georgia 30322

Anne Foster-Rosales, M.D. • Department of Obstetrics, Gynecology, and Reproductive Sciences, University of California, San Francisco, California 94143-0744

Pamina M. Gorbach, MHS, Dr.PH. • Graduate School of Public Health, San Diego State University, San Diego, California 92182-4162

Julia A. Graber, Ph.D. • Department of Psychology, University of Florida, Gainesville, Florida 32611

Catherine B. Johannes, Ph.D. • Epidemiology Division, Ingenix Pharmaceutical Services, Newton, Massachsuetts 02462

Edward O. Laumann, Ph.D. • Department of Sociology, University of Chicago, Chicago, Illinois 60637

Sandra L. Leiblum, Ph.D. • Department of Psychiatry, Robert Wood Johnson University of Medicine and Dentistry, Piscataway, New Jersey 08855

Tamra Burns Loeb, Ph.D. • Department of Psychiatry and Biobehavioral Sciences, University of California at Los Angeles, Los Angeles, California 90024-1759

Sana Loue, J.D., Ph.D., MPH. • Department of Epidemiology and Biostatistics, School of Medicine, Case Western Reserve University, Cleveland, Ohio 44109-1998

Jenna W. Mahay, M.A. • Department of Sociology, University of Chicago, Chicago, Illinois 60637

Joan H. Marks, M.A. • Human Genetics Program, Sarah Lawrence College, Bronxville, New York 10708

Colleen M. McBride, M.A., Ph.D. • Duke University Comprehensive Cancer Center, Durham, North Carolina 27710

Donna Hubbard McCree, Ph.D., MPH, R.Ph. • Centers for Disease Control and Prevention, National Center for HIV, STD, and TB Prevention, Atlanta, Georgia 30333

Kim S. Miller, Ph.D. • Division of HIV/AIDS Prevention, Centers for Disease Control and Prevention, Atlanta, Georgia 30333

Mary H. Miller, Ph.D. • St. Vincent's Hospital, New York, New York 10010

Melinda L. Morgan, MSW, Ph.D. • Department of Psychiatry, UCLA Neuropsychiatric Institute and Hospital, Los Angeles, California 90095

Amanda M. Navarro, B.A. • Department of Social and Behavioral Sciences, Boston University School of Public Health, Boston, Massachusetts 02118

Anita Raj, Ph.D. • Department of Social and Behavioral Sciences, Boston University School of Public Health, Boston, Massachusetts 02118

Andrea J. Rapkin, M.D. • Department of Obstetrics and Gynecology, Center for the Health Sciences, UCLA School of Medicine, Los Angeles, California 90095-1740

Debbie Saslow, Ph.D. • American Cancer Society, Atlanta, Georgia 30329

Delia Scholes, Ph.D. • Group Health Cooperative of Puget Sound Center for Health Studies, Seattle, Washington 98101-1448

Catlainn Sionéan, Ph.D. • Centers for Disease Control and Prevention, National Center for HIV, STD, and TB Prevention, Atlanta, Georgia 30333

Robert A. Smith, Ph.D. • American Cancer Society, Atlanta, Georgia 30329

Claire E. Sterk, Ph.D. • Department of Behavioral Sciences and Health Education, Rollins

School of Public Health, Emory University, Atlanta, Georgia 30322

Susannah R. Stern, Ph.D. • Communications Department, Boston College, Chestnut Hill, Massachusetts 02467

Felicia H. Stewart, M.D. • Department of Obstetrics, Gynecology, and Reproductive Sciences, University of California, San Francisco, California 94143-0744

Katherine P. Theall, MPH. • Department of Behavioral Sciences and Health Education, Rollins School of Public Health, Emory University, Atlanta, Georgia 30322

Andrea Tone, Ph.D. • School of History, Technology and Society, Georgia Institute of Technology, Atlanta, Georgia 30322-0345

Nina Williams, Psy.D. • Highland Park, New Jersey 08904

Michael Windle, Ph.D. • Department of Psychology, University of Alabama at Birmingham, Birmingham, Alabama 35294-1170

Rebecca C. Windle, MSW. • Department of Psychology, University of Alabama at Birmingham, Birmingham, Alabama 35294-1170

Gina M. Wingood, Sc.D., MPH. • Department of Behavioral Sciences and Health Education, Rollins School of Public Health, Emory University, Atlanta, Georgia 30322

Gail E. Wyatt, Ph.D. • Department of Psychiatry and Biobehavioral Sciences, University of California at Los Angeles, Los Angeles, California 90024-1759

Laurie Schwab Zabin, Ph.D. • Department of Population and Family Health Sciences, Johns Hopkins School of Hygiene and Public Health, Baltimore, Maryland 21205

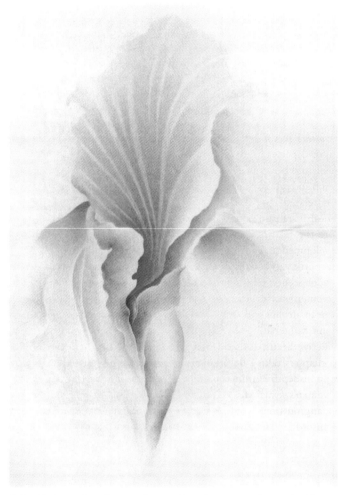

"The Moonflower" (by Christina Camphausen. Source: Camphausen, R. C. (1996). *The Yoni: Sacred Symbol of Female Creative Power* (p. 66). Rochester, VT: Inner Traditions International. Reprinted with permission.) The flowering of the Yoni (a Sanskrit word that translates to "womb," "origin," and "source," and more specifically, "vulva") is captured by this drawing. Several cultures believe that during menstruation, the flowering of the Yoni is a special time for women, a time during which women should be valued and honored.

Preface

The *Handbook of Women's Sexual and Reproductive Health* provides an in-depth examination of the epidemiology, social, and behavioral correlates, effective intervention and prevention strategies, and health polices related to women's sexual and reproductive health. The first nine chapters of this text explore the relationships between how historical, developmental, and social structures such as media portrayals of women, family rearing of female adolescents, religious beliefs, gendered norms, women's sociocultural experiences, and exposure to alcohol and drugs serve to increase women's vulnerability to adverse sexual and reproductive health consequences.

The next 10 chapters take a life-span approach to provide an in-depth examination into a diverse array of women's sexual and reproductive health issues ranging from women's body image and eating disorders, HIV/AIDS, breast and cervical cancers, pregnancy, and menopause. Each of these chapters examines effective prevention programs aimed at reducing women's risk of acquiring an adverse sexual and reproductive health condition. Additionally, these chapters review effective intervention strategies that are designed to help women cope and live with these conditions. While this text is empirically-based, it also integrates narratives, such as those of women who are living with breast cancer, chronic pelvic pain, HIV/AIDS, sexual dysfunction, and sexual abuse, and women who are discontent with their body image. Each chapter concludes by addressing health policy implications for each sexual and reproductive health condition.

The last four chapters examine the ethical and legal issues confronted in women's sexual and reproductive health. This handbook is designed to motivate scientists, policymakers, and practitioners to intervene on the gender-based social norms, social relations, and social systems, such as the media, and religious institutions and family systems. Moreover, it is hoped that this handbook will help generate greater scientific discourse, reduce the stigma, and validate the importance of women's sexual and reproductive health.

The *Handbook on Women's Sexual and Reproductive Health* is for anyone interested in having access to the cutting-edge knowledge of research in this area. The aim of the handbook is to alert our readers in a useful and intellectually stimulating manner to the wealth and most current information regarding the epidemiology, psychosocial influences, and prevention strategies with respect to women's sexual and reproductive health. The handbook uses a multidisciplinary perspective, bringing together historians, anthropologists, psychologists, sociologists, epidemiologists, public health researchers, genetic counselors, attorneys, demographers, journalists, social workers, nurses, and physicians. As such, these individuals, as well as women's health advocates, students, and practitioners can benefit greatly from this text.

The *Handbook on Women's Sexual and Reproductive Health* explores the realities of female adolescents' and women's sexual lives; considering some of the statistics:

- Nearly, 25% of 14–15-year-old; 39% of 16-year-old, and 52% of 17-year-old girls have had intercourse; and by age 19, 77% of girls will have engaged in sexual intercourse.

- According to one study, 61% of women suffering from chronic pelvic pain do not have a diagnosis. Another study reported that almost 40% of women reported chronic pelvic pain persisting for more than six months at some point in their lives.
- A woman who has unprotected sex with an infected partner just once has a 1% chance of contracting HIV, a 30% chance of contracting genital herpes, and a 50% chance of contracting gonorrhea.
- In a national survey, 48% of American women reported being dissatisfied with their overall appearance. Further, 13% of early adolescent girls and 18% of middle and late adolescent girls report having binged and purged.
- Approximately 10.2% of women nationally are infertile.
- It is estimated that 1 in 8 women will be diagnosed with breast cancer in her lifetime and 1 in 30 will die from the disease. Excluding skin cancers, invasive breast cancer is the most frequently diagnosed malignancy among U.S. women, accounting for nearly 1 in 3 new cancer diagnoses.
- Only 165 of the nearly 14,000 sexual references, innuendos, and jokes the average teenager views on television per year dealt with topics such as birth control, abstinence, or STDs. Exposure to sexually explicit media has been associated with engaging in unprotected sex and having multiple sexual partners.
- Approximately half of the women who use illicit drugs are of childbearing age. Several states include drug exposure *in utero* in their child abuse and neglect laws.
- According to a recent national survey 43% of American women reported some type of sexual problem and 1 out of every 3 women reported being uninterested in sex.
- Overall, it has been estimated that 25% of all young women experience a pregnancy

by age 18, and half will become pregnant by age 21.

- Limited parental monitoring is associated with a range of adverse sexual outcomes, including acquiring STDs, having unprotected sex, and having multiple partners. Further, more than a third of African-American and European-American women and almost half of Latinas reported interfamilial sexual abuse.
- Nearly 1 in 3 African-American, European-American, and Latina women report at least one incident of sexual abuse prior to age 18. History of child sexual abuse is associated with engaging in early first intercourse, having more sexual partners, having a greater number of unintended pregnancies, and acquiring STDs, including HIV infection.
- Nearly 34% of women reported using alcohol in the last 12 months, and 8.4% meet the clinical diagnostic criteria for an alcohol disorder. Alcohol use by women has been associated with breast cancer, sexual dysfunction, risky sexual behavior, and sexual victimization.
- Presently, HIV is estimated to be the most prevalent sexually transmitted infection in the United States, with 15% of all sexually active adults in the United States infected. Acquisition of this infection is highly predictive of the development of cervical cancer.

While we have attempted to be comprehensive within the space limitations of this text, we are aware of important health conditions that were not included. We hope that we will be able to address these conditions in future editions of this handbook. At its heart, this text is about the science of prevention. As such, the *Handbook of Women's Sexual and Reproductive Health* provides in-depth analysis of effective prevention strategies related to women's sexual and reproductive health. Our intent is to improve the science of prevention related to women's sexual and reproductive health, and in this same light we hope to improve the quality of women's lives.

Acknowledgments

We are deeply indebted to Ms. Linda Brockman, B.A., our Editorial Assistant at Emory University for her relentless dedication, her attention to detail with every chapter, and her masterful editorial skills that have allowed us to shape this handbook into the text that we wanted it to be.

Also, of great importance, we express our enormous gratitude to Ms. Mariclaire Cloutier at Kluwer Academic / Plenum Publishers for her indispensable assistance throughout the editorial process and for making this a pleasant and rewarding experience. We have benefitted greatly from the assistance of Teresa Krauss in the final preparation of this manuscript.

We want to thank all of the women and men in our families—our grandparents, parents, siblings, and in-laws who have given us the historical inspiration, motivation, and support to write this handbook. Our familial interactions have allowed us to gain a deeper understanding of the generational, social, relational, and cultural influences on women's sexuality. We are blessed as a result of this experience.

This handbook would have been impossible without the research support received from the National Institute of Mental Health (NIMH), National Institutes of Health. The support of Drs. Willo Pequegnat and Ellen Stover have allowed us to explore, ask, and answer so many questions about women's sexual and reproductive health within the context of HIV prevention.

Further, we want to thank all of the contributors to the handbook. It is really through their hard work, dedication, and commitment that his handbook has come to fruition. We have had the privilege of working with many outstanding scientists in the diverse fields which encompass women's sexual and reproductive health. We have benefitted enormously through their collaboration.

Finally, we want to express our sincere appreciation to the women that we have enountered in our research who have helped shape our world and who have given us a better understanding of the social complexities and realities that affect women's sexual and reproductive health.

Contents

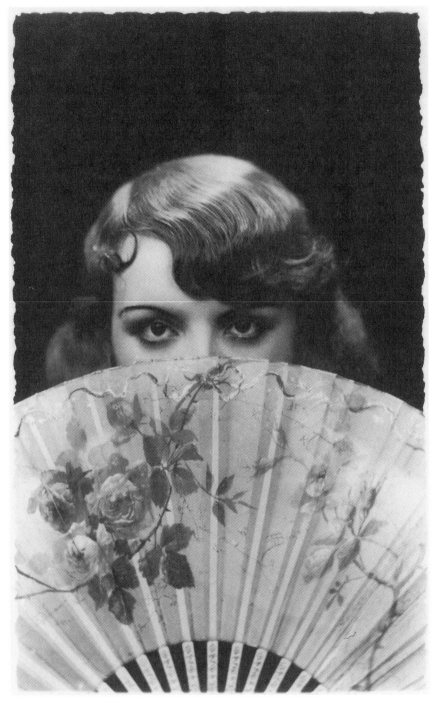

"Woman with Fan," by anonymous photographer, c. 1920, silver gelatin print (KI-DC: 12585). (Reproduced with permission of the Kinsey Institute for Research in Sex, Gender, and Reproduction.) Inspired by silent movie publicity stills, this image emphasizes the model's seductive gaze. The partial obscuring of her face by the fan also capitalizes on the tension between concealing and revealing part of the body to enhance the sense of intrigue. This image represents the more open attitude towards sexuality that developed among some segements of American society in the years following World War I.

I

Historical, Social, and Developmental Influences in Women's Sexual and Reproductive Health

1

Women's Sexual and Reproductive Health: An Overview

GINA M. WINGOOD, CATLAINN SIONÉAN,
and DONNA HUBBARD MCCREE

WHY WOMEN'S SEXUAL AND REPRODUCTIVE HEALTH?

Since the 1970s women's health has gained greater recognition as a discipline. Historically, women's health research and policy have been defined by reproductive health issues. However, outside of women's reproductive health, the field of women's sexual and reproductive health has received less attention and is at a point where there is a need for a comprehensive reference covering a wide variety of topics. Further, such a handbook needs to integrate the authoritative works of distinguished physicians, social scientists, and public health scientists who conduct research in women's sexual health.

The *Handbook of Women's Sexual and Reproductive Health* uses a multidisciplinary perspec-

GINA M. WINGOOD • Department of Behavioral Sciences and Health Education, Rollins School of Public Health, Emory University, Atlanta, Georgia 30322. CATLAINN SIONÉAN and DONNA HUBBARD MCCREE • Centers for Disease Control and Prevention, National Center for HIV, STD and TB Prevention, Division of STD Prevention, Atlanta, Georgia 30333.

Handbook of Women's Sexual and Reproductive Health, edited by Wingood and DiClemente. Kluwer Academic / Plenum Publishers, New York, 2002.

tive, bringing together historians, anthropologists, sociologists, public health researchers, nurses, and physicians. The chapters represent a confluence of perspectives from the leading medical, behavioral, and social scientists engaged in clinical practice and research related to women's sexual and reproductive health. Such disciplinary integration is necessary as women's sexual and reproductive health depends on a complex interplay of biological, psychological, and social factors.

It is important to focus on women's sexual and reproductive health for a variety of reasons. First, sexual health conditions, such as breast cancer and HIV/AIDS, are some of the leading causes of mortality among women. HIV/AIDS, for instance, is the leading cause of death among African-American women 18–44 years of age. Second, many sexual conditions, such as chronic pain and cervical cancer, are unique to women and receive limited attention. Third, other sexual and reproductive health conditions, such as pregnancy and menopause, are the most prevalent health conditions affecting women. Fourth, the imbalance of power inherent in many sexual relationships may uniquely impact women's sexual health, particularly with respect to sexual abuse, and women's lack of power over condom use, which may increase their vulnerability for exposure to HIV and STDs. Fifth, in our culture young girls turn into women, yet how they define themselves as sexual beings and what our culture tells them about being female are factors that also impact their sexual and reproductive health. Therefore, examining the developmental, sociocultural, and historical influences on women's sexual health is critical. Sixth, in our culture little value is given to women's sexual desire, and stigma is often associated with discussing women's sexuality. These factors make it difficult to address women's sexual health conditions, such as sexual dysfunction, and distort the importance of issues such as a woman's body image. Seventh, women's health care utilization is often related to sexual and reproductive issues, such as birth control and screenings for cancer of the breast or reproductive tract. Eighth, it is imperative to keep abreast of the legal and ethical issues affecting women's sexual and reproductive health, including those having a well-established history, such as abortion, as well as newly evolving fields, such as genetic counseling and testing.

DEFINING SEXUAL AND REPRODUCTIVE HEALTH

Sexual health is a nebulous term and difficult to define because it can refer to physical as well as social facets of human interaction (Alexander & LaRosa, 1998). Some scientists refer to the psychosocial, cultural, and emotional relationships that women form with other individuals as women's sexual health. Other scientists refer to women's sexual health as designing programs to prevent women from acquiring sexually acquired conditions, such as HIV and sexually transmitted infections. Sexual health can also be defined as enhancing women's ability to cope with sexual and reproductive health conditions, such as breast and cervical cancer, sexual dysfunction, pelvic pain, menopause, and sexual abuse. Many scientists define women's sexual health more narrowly as reproductive health. Other researchers explore women's sex-

ual health to understand women's self-concept and appearance such as that associated with their body image. In this handbook we embrace the various definitions used to describe women's sexual health. Further, we examine traditional reproductive health issues, such as pregnancy and contraceptive and reproductive technologies. Understanding sexual and reproductive health requires a multifaceted examination of psychosocial, emotional, and medical aspects of women's sexuality.

DOMAINS OF WOMEN'S SEXUAL AND REPRODUCTIVE HEALTH

The chapters in the *Handbook of Women's Sexual and Reproductive Health* have been organized to encompass three domains. The first domain addresses developmental, sociocultural, historical, and behavioral influences. The influences discussed in this domain may indirectly or directly increase women's risk for certain sexual and reproductive health conditions. Moreover, examining social conditions, social structures, and behavioral factors on women's sexual and reproductive health helps us understand how women's sexual experiences are perceived and addressed. The second domain addresses sexual and reproductive health conditions prevalent among women over the life span. This domain allows us to examine some of the sexual and reproductive health conditions and ways to alleviate the symptoms associated with these conditions. The third domain examines legal/ ethical and technological aspects of women's sexual and reproductive health.

Historical, Developmental, Social, and Behavioral Influences Affecting Women's Sexual and Reproductive Health

The chapters in the first domain of this handbook describe current research regarding historical, developmental, social, and behavioral influences on women's sexual and reproductive health. While sexual and reproductive behaviors may appear to be largely determined by characteristics of individuals, or even couples, Tone, in Chapter 2, discusses how they are also influenced by long-standing historical and sociopolitical factors. Graber and Brooks-Gunn in Chapter 3 discuss sexual and reproductive health in relation to adolescent females' sexual development. Amaro and colleagues in Chapter 5 inform us of how cultural beliefs, social norms, and social economic conditions shape women's sexual and reproductive health. Social structures are highly influential in understanding women's sexual and reproductive health. Social structures such as religiosity are examined by Mahay and Laumann in Chapter 4, Brown and Stern in Chapter 6 discuss the influence of the media on women's sexual and reproductive health, and Crosby and Miller in Chapter 7 explore familial influences that affect women's sexual and reproductive health. In addition to social influences, behavioral influences have a strong impact on women's sexual health. Thus, in Chapter 9 Windle and Windle examine the role of alcohol use, and in Chapter 8, Theall, Sterk and Elifson focus on the role of drug use on women's sexual and reproductive health.

Epidemiologic, Psychological, Prevention, and Policy Issues Affecting Women's Sexual and Reproductive Health

The second domain essential to understanding women's sexual and reproductive health concerns the sexual health conditions that are a part of many women's lives. Each chapter in this domain (1) addresses a certain sexual health condition, (2) provides an epidemiologic overview of the condition, (3) examines social and behavioral correlates of this condition, (4) discusses effective primary prevention strategies, (5) reviews effective secondary prevention efforts aimed at ameliorating the condition, (6) uses case vignettes to illustrate women living with this health condition, and (7) reviews health policy issues relevant to this condition.

In the first chapter of this domain, Cash,

in Chapter 10, enhances our understanding of women's self-concept by discussing women's body image and eating disorders. Wyatt and colleagues in Chapter 11 provide an in-depth examination of sexual abuse and its impact on women's sexual health. Compelling research on pelvic pain is provided by Rapkin and Morgan in Chapter 12, and stimulating work on sexual dysfunction is elaborated on by Williams and Leiblum in Chapter 16. Zabin and Cordona in Chapter 13 inform us of the latest advances in pregnancy prevention. Sexually acquired conditions such as STDs (Aral and Gorbach) and human immunodeficiency virus (Wingood and DiClemente) have become increasingly prevalent among women and are discussed in Chapters 14 and 15, respectively. Insightful chapters on cervical and breast cancer are, respectively, provided by McBride and Scholes (Chapter 17) and Smith (Chapter 18). Avis, Crawford, and Johannes in Chapter 19 keep us abreast of the most recent literature on menopause.

All of the chapters in this domain are designed to enhance our knowledge of the prevalence, incidence, and epidemiologic trends of sexual health conditions, provide an in-depth examination of effective primary and secondary prevention strategies, inform us of the impact of these conditions on women's lives, and enhance our awareness of the health policy issues, such as the cost effectiveness of primary and secondary prevention strategies impacting womens' sexual and reproductive health.

Technological and Ethical Influences Affecting Women's Sexual and Reproductive Health

The third domain on technological and ethical influences affecting women's sexual health integrates the works of attorneys, anthropologists, genetic counselors, physicians, and psychologists. In Chapter 20, Rosales and Stewart review the rapid advances made in contraceptive technology. Marks and Miller's chapter on reproductive health technologies (Chapter 21) explores the advances made in this exciting field and discusses the risks and benefits associated with many of these procedures. Loue in Chapter 22 explores the long-standing and newly formed ethical and legal principles inherent in women's sexual and reproductive health. The legal tenets and statutes illustrate the demands placed upon many women in the areas of sexual and reproductive health. Finally, DiClemente and Wingood in Chapter 23 urge us to consider new options in examining women's sexual reproductive health.

DIVERSITY AND WOMEN'S SEXUAL AND REPRODUCTIVE HEALTH

This handbook utilizes a life-span approach. The life-span approach provides the opportunity to examine in-depth sexual and reproductive health conditions that are of particular relevance for different developmental stages. For example, during childhood and adolescence, parents and mass media are particularly important influences on the development of sexual attitudes and behaviors that may affect the risk for pregnancy or STDs. Many sexual and reproductive health conditions such as pelvic pain and sexual dysfunction may develop or persist across various stages of the life course, while other conditions, such as breast cancer, are typically experienced in mid-to-late adulthood. Sexual and reproductive issues are integral to women's lives and remain of critical importance to women's health and well-being at each stage in the life course.

Of particular relevance to the diversity of women's sexual and reproductive health is the influence of race/ethnicity, culture, and social class (Zierler *et al.*, 2000). These fundamental social statuses intersect with gender to influence and organize women's sexuality and reproduction. Their relevance for women's sexual and reproductive health is described in all chapters and is highlighted in chapters by Mahay and

Laumann and by Amaro *et al.* Moreover, acknowledging the diverse sexual relationships that women form is critical. Amaro *et al.* also highlight the sexual and reproductive health concerns of women who have sex with women.

CONCLUSION

The chapters in the *Handbook of Women's Sexual and Reproductive Health* are intended to stimulate thinking about women's sexual and reproductive health. Moreover, we hope that the following chapters will encourage new options and new directions for research on women's sexual and reproductive health (Wingood & DiClemente, 2000). Given the diversity of women, we have emphasized the social influences that can increase women's susceptibility to sexual and reproductive health conditions. Also, we believe that only by hearing the words and voices of women living with these conditions can we truly appreciate their impact on women's lives. Thus, we highlight women's stories when discussing sexual and reproductive health conditions. Further, we hope that this handbook will reduce the stigma associated with women's sexual and reproductive health conditions and provide a greater opportunity for scientific discourse in the area.

REFERENCES

Alexander, L. L., & LaRosa, J. H. (1998). Sexual health. In L. L. Alexander & J. H. LaRosa (Eds.), *New dimensions in women's health* (pp. 182–215). Boston: Jones and Barlett.
Wingood, G. M., & DiClemente, R. J. (2000). Application of the theory of gender and power to examine HIV-related exposures, risk factors, and effective interventions for women. *Health Education & Behavior, 27,* 539–565.
Zierler, S., Krieger, N., Tang, Y., Coady, W., Siegfried, E., DeMaria, A., & Auerbach, J. (2000). Economic deprivation and AIDS incidence in Massachusetts. *American Journal of Public Health, 90,* 1064–1073.

2

Historical Influences on Women's Sexual and Reproductive Health

ANDREA TONE

INTRODUCTION

To understand contemporary debates over women's sexual and reproductive health in American society, we must first look to the past. Since the beginning of time, perceptions of female sexuality have shaped medical practices, public policy, legal rights, technology, and the contours of women's everyday experiences. To answer a battery of questions—Why are most contraceptives for women? Why are abortions stigmatized decades after the Supreme Court declared them legal?—we need to understand the complex history that has defined our modern age. Unlocking the past, familiarizing ourselves with the powerful political and social forces that have affected women's sexual and reproductive health over time, we equip ourselves with the knowledge we need to begin the long task of challenging the present and changing the future.

ANDREA TONE • School of History, Technology, and Society, Georgia Institute of Technology, Atlanta, Georgia 30332-0345.

Handbook of Women's Sexual and Reproductive Health, edited by Wingood and DiClemente. Kluwer Academic / Plenum Publishers, New York, 2002.

EARLY VIEWS OF FEMALE SEXUALITY

Colonial Attitudes

At its founding, the United States was a country that championed maternal sexuality, the belief that women ought, and were meant, to have children. The view that sex could be unrelated to childbearing—that it could be, for example, "just for fun"—was taboo. Most Americans viewed women's procreative role as biologically and religiously preordained, a mandate from nature and God and the very "essence" of all that defined a woman (D'Emilio and Freedman, 1989). Women were expected to bear children from marriage to menopause, and consistently high fertility rates from the eighteenth through the early nineteenth centuries suggest that most did. On average, married women bore between five and seven children. Economic and political imperatives buttressed cultural and religious ideas about women's reproductive role. With high infant mortality and low life expectancy rates the norm in all states, frequent procreation promised needed laborers and a steady stream of settlers to populate new frontiers.

Women and men were expected to procreate, but only within the confines of marriage.

Those who transgressed this code, which reinforced the primacy of matrimonial, reproductive sex, were punished. In the colonial era, fornication, adultery, bastardy, sodomy, and bestiality were all crimes, crimes against God and crimes against society and social order. Especially in Puritan New England, colonists saw little distinction between the two. Communities were charged with the task of policing sexual behavior and bringing violators before church or court. In 1670, for example, the Quarterly Court of Salem, Massachusetts, fined a man and his wife for fornication before marriage, a sexual coupling that resulted in a telltale "prenuptial" pregnancy. In 1702, Hannah Dickens of Kent County, Delaware, got 21 lashes for bearing "one bastard male child" (Friedman, 1993). Hierarchical authority sought to suppress illegitimate sexuality, but it did not always succeed. Colonial courts handled thousands of fornication cases, suggesting that the threat of painful or humiliating punishments did not prevent many colonists from defining sexuality on their own terms.

Public vs. Private Passion

By the nineteenth century, Americans had been given more latitude with which to express their own brand of sexuality, at least in private. The Victorian era is often portrayed as the height of American prudery, a time of widespread sexual repression. As is often the case, however, historical reality confounds stereotype. Throughout the nineteenth century, public policy reflected far more interest in suppressing public sexual misconduct than clandestine illicit acts. Hence, prostitutes who strutted their wares on busy commercial streets were a problem. Fornication in the privacy of a bedroom, however, was not. This distinction between public and private would have been anathema to Puritans, who strived to unmask and eradicate *concealed* sin. But by the early nineteenth century America was a young republic comprised, according to the political ethos of the day, of women and men who were virtuous and self-disciplined. If this bold new experiment in democracy were to succeed, they must be trusted to take the honorable path without the watchful eye of the government guiding them (Friedman, 1993).

Prostitution

But if legislators and law enforcers increasingly turned a blind eye to what transpired in the privacy of the bedroom, most states and municipalities adopted measures to reign in excessive, and egregiously public, passion. Female prostitutes, women who sold sexual services for money, were primary targets of the Victorian crackdown on public indecency. Prostitution had existed since colonial times, but by the mid-nineteenth century it had become especially visible in the country's burgeoning urban centers. One social reformer estimated that there were over 6000 prostitutes in New York City in the late 1850s, one for every 64 men (D'Emilio and Freedman, 1989; Gilfoyle, 1992). Many prostitutes were working-class and immigrant women whose regular income was insufficient to care for their needs. Others were, in the parlance of the times, "fallen women"— women whose social reputation and prospects had been "ruined" by seduction or rape. Because Victorian society lionized female purity as the bedrock of public virtue, women who deviated from sexual norms that trumpeted chastity before marriage and fidelity within it paid a heavy price for their experimentation. Barred from decent employment and the social respectability that came with a proper marriage, these female outcasts often gravitated to prostitution, one of the few trades available to them (Gilfoyle, 1992).

Antiprostitution groups in the nineteenth century found their biggest following among middle-class, Protestant women. Cast as social guardians of virtue and morality, these women had much to lose from the existence of prostitution, which, in uncoupling sex and marriage, threatened to undermine their traditional claim to maternal authority. To preserve their role and the social power they exercised as guardians of virtue, antiprostitution reformers declared nonmarital sexuality immoral and proclaimed sex's chief function to be the generation of offspring. (Many of these women also opposed abortion and birth control for the same reason.) Female reformers were not indifferent to prostitutes' plight; many emphasized the urban evils and sexual double standard that victimized women. Reformers' rhetoric often portrayed men as aggressively lecherous and overpowering to a young, unwitting woman. To protect impressionable women from deceptive men, the Women's Christian Temperance Union, the largest female organization in the late nineteenth century, along with numerous social purity groups, campaigned successfully for the passage of age-of-consent legislation. These laws, passed by 29 states between 1886 and 1895, raised the age at which women could consent to intercourse, which in some states had been as low as 10 (Odem, 1995; D'Emilio and Freedman, 1989).

Still, prostitution thrived. The depiction of male lust as an irrepressible and uncontrollable force encouraged many Americans to resign themselves to its existence. In 1870, the city of St. Louis, Missouri, adopted the nation's first system of regulated prostitution. A political victory for St. Louis doctors, the system required prostitutes to have weekly medical checkups. Doctors issued health certificates to women determined to be disease free. Rescinded in 1874, the St. Louis experiment had attempted to balance men's ostensibly "natural" sexual drive with the community health risks it imposed, particularly the transmission of venereal diseases, incurable in the days before antibiotics. By 1900, most cities had carved out "red-light districts" in working-class parts of town. These districts were a compromise. They permitted prostitution and brothels to exist as long as they were "hidden" in neighborhoods where affluent residents were not obligated to work or live. In New Orleans, the Common Council went so far as to adopt a municipal ordinance that specified the boundaries of the red-light district by street name (Friedman, 1993). Regular payments to the police enabled brothels operating within the agreed-upon boundaries to function with impunity.

FERTILITY CONTROL

Abortion

A woman's right to control her fertility was another subject of heated debate in the nineteenth century. Under British common law (laws derived from court decisions rather than explicit legislative enactment), abortion before quickening was legal until the mid-nineteenth century. Quickening referred to the time during pregnancy, usually in the fourth or fifth month, when a woman first detected fetal movement. At a time when pregnancy tests and ultrasound technology were centuries away, quickening was the only evidence a woman had that she was pregnant. A missed menstrual period was not considered an automatic indication of pregnancy. It could also be a sign of a dangerous medical disorder—a blockage that, left unattended, could jeopardize a woman's health. Accordingly, women's efforts to restore "natural menses" before quickening were culturally sanctioned and completely legal. The most common abortion was the ingestion of an abortifacient, a potion that induced miscarriage by irritating or poisoning the body; recipes for abortifacient brews of aloes, pennyroyal, and especially savin (extracted from juniper bushes that grew wild in North America) occupied a prominent place in traditional American folk medicine. Less frequently performed were mechanical abortions that attempted direct fetal expulsion through the insertion of an instrument (Tone, 1997).

Between 1821 and 1841, ten states enacted measures criminalizing abortion, making it a statutory offense for the first time in American history. Generally these laws sought to protect women from poisonous abortifacients and dangerous procedures performed by "unscrupulous" practitioners. Hence, the state of Connecticut, the first to regulate abortion, punished abortion providers but not women having abortions. And in deference to the quickening tradition, Connecticut's 1821 abortion statute made only premeditated attempts to "procure the miscarriage of any woman, then being quick with child" a crime. By the mid-nineteenth century, abortion laws had become more inclusive and severe, as new proponents of abortion legislation, especially licensed doctors, lobbied for more restrictive measures.

Organized in 1847, the American Medical Association (AMA) had become the leading proponent of abortion statutes by the late 1850s. The AMA opposed abortions for several reasons. First, mounting scientific evidence had convinced doctors that gestation (the evolution of fetal development from fertilization to birth) was a continuous process, one substantially more complicated than that allowed by the quickening distinction. If fetal life predated fetal movement, then an abortion before quickening, many doctors argued, was wrong. Second, physicians wanted medical control over female reproduction. To assert their standing as men of science in an open medical market, licensed physicians discredited and distanced themselves from homeopaths, midwives, and other "quacks" who frequently performed abortions. Tellingly, the abortion laws the AMA helped pass in the late nineteenth century typically provided therapeutic exemption clauses that permitted abortion when the mother's life was in danger. But only professional doctors were authorized to make this determination or to perform medically indicated abortions. The new restrictions, in short, made abortion a doctor's prerogative rather than a woman's choice. Third, abortion rates rose rapidly in the 1840s and 1850s as the practice became more commercialized and growing numbers of married, white, native-born, affluent Protestant women had them.

An estimated 20% of all pregnancies between 1840 and 1870 ended in abortion (Mohr, 1978; Reagan, 1991). Like prostitution, this trend threatened traditional gender roles, allowing the freedom to have sex without consequence. Some contemporaries worried that abortion would incite sexual indulgence; others averred that because it was "unnatural" for women to be childless, abortion would wreak physiological, emotional, and mental havoc on women's health. Doctors chimed in this chorus,

and in 1864 the AMA established an annual prize for the best essay written to educate women about the "criminality and physical evils of forced abortion" (Tone, 1997). Criminality was indeed of mounting concern for women. By 1900, abortion restrictions in every state punished women who had abortions at any point during pregnancy.

Contraception

By the dawn of the twentieth century, birth control had likewise been banned. Contraceptives were neither an American nor a modern invention, but before rubber vulcanization technology was applied to their manufacture in the 1840s, most women and men used natural methods. Prolonged lactation, periodic abstinence, and *coitus interruptus* (male withdrawal) had long been practiced by women and men wishing to avoid pregnancy (Brodie, 1994). By the 1860s, these traditional methods had been supplemented by a cornucopia of devices—rubber and animal membrane condoms, douching syringes, vaginal pessaries, suppositories and solutions, among others—commonly advertised in newspapers and circulars and sold in local drugstores and through the mails. Hence, like abortion and prostitution, birth control had become both more commercialized and visible. In 1873, at the urging of antivice crusader Anthony Comstock, Congress passed the first law to clamp down on this thriving and highly visible trade. Comstock was a devout Protestant who feared that the escalating public traffic in sexual vice—which included contraceptives but also abortifacients, pornography, and the sensationalist pulp press—was corroding the nation's morals and corrupting its youth. The 1873 statute, commonly called the Comstock Act, was an antiobscenity law. It classified as obscene a wide array of goods, including all physical instruments, visual images, and written materials pertaining to birth control, and prohibited their interstate distribution and sale. Supporting the federal initiative, individual states passed similar anticontraceptive measures, called mini-Comstock acts, that forbade the advertisement, manufacture, or purchase of birth control within state lines. Connecticut's 1879 law was the most extreme; it forbade the actual use of contraceptives by state residents. It would not be overturned until 1965, the year of the Supreme Court's landmark decision in *Griswold v. Connecticut* (Tone, 1997).

The new laws did not eradicate contraceptives. Birth rates continued to plummet in the late nineteenth century, dropping from 7.04 children to 3.56 for white women between 1800 and 1900 (Gordon, 1977). By 1900, only France had a lower birth rate in the Western world. The decline in family size was not exclusive to whites; in the 1880s the fertility rates of African-American women began an even sharper decline. Still, the new laws took their toll on women's sexual health and reproductive autonomy. Restrictions pushed birth control underground, beyond regulatory reach. Contraceptives became less accessible and more expensive. In addition, by classifying birth control as obscene, the new restrictions thwarted efforts to treat it as a serious and integral component of public health. The scientific community was prevented from undertaking badly needed research to test, standardize, and develop safe and effective methods. When women used black-market birth control, they took their health and the law into their own hands.

Margaret Sanger

Appalled by this contemptible state of affairs, Margaret Sanger sought direct and immediate reform. Born Margaret Higgins in 1879, she studied nursing in White Plains, New York, before marrying artist and architect William Sanger, with whom she had three children. In 1911 Margaret Sanger and her family moved to Manhattan where she became active in leftist politics. Working as an obstetrical nurse among the poor of the Lower East Side, she became increasingly concerned about the lack of sex education among working-class and immigrant women. Defying the law, she publicly championed the need for universal access to affordable and effective birth control. By

1912 she had made a name for herself as a sex education lecturer, and in 1914 she published *The Woman Rebel*, a journal in which she demanded legal birth control and full women's rights. The June 1914 issue first used the term *birth control*. When the journal was censored by the U.S. Post Office, Sanger flaunted the law again by writing the pamphlet "Family Limitation," a practical home guide to contraception.

An outspoken critic of abortion, Sanger saw contraception as key to both women's emancipation and the elimination of poverty. Dismayed by medical inertia (until 1937, the AMA did not consider dispensing contraception to be a valid medical service), she and her sister opened the first birth control clinic, in Brooklyn, on October 16, 1916, where they taught women how to use condoms, suppositories, and cervical caps. As she would throughout her life, Sanger favored female methods, because they gave women full control over pregnancy prevention. Entrusting men with this responsibility, she feared, kept women vulnerable and dependent. The Brooklyn clinic helped almost 500 needy women before it was shut down by the police 10 days after it opened. The raid provided Sanger with an opportunity to test the legality of New York's antiobscenity law under which she had been arrested. In 1918, as the result of Sanger's challenge, a New York appellate court ruled that birth control was legal when prescribed by physicians to prevent diseases, including gonorrhea, syphilis, and life-threatening pregnancies. Finally, birth control had earned a modicum of legitimacy as a public health measure. Sanger made the most of the court's ruling and, in 1923, opened in New York under medical supervision the first permanent birth control clinic in the United States.

Sanger's actions had been motivated by a sincere desire to bring birth control to those she believed needed it most, the poor. She argued that a desire to escape poverty and its concomitant psychological degradation would motivate women and men to use contraceptives. Unlike many of her contemporaries, she believed that indigence, criminality, and mental diseases were by-products of a bad environment, not bad genes. "Children who are underfed, undernourished, crowded into badly ventilated and unsanitary houses and chronically hungry cannot be expected to attain the mental development of children upon whom every advantage of intelligent and scientific care is bestowed," she proclaimed (McCann, 1994). Still, Sanger embraced some of the core tenets of the eugenics movement, which at this time was gaining support among a wide spectrum of scientists and policymakers. She condoned the sterilization of the "unfit" and the use of birth control to "better" the human race. "Birth control," she stated emphatically in 1920, "is nothing more or less than the facilitation of the process of weeding out the unfit [and] of preventing the birth of defectives" (McCann, 1994).

Eugenics

Eugenics framed arguments for and against reproductive autonomy in late nineteenth- and twentieth-century America. The term was first coined in 1883 in England by Sir Francis Galton, a cousin of Charles Darwin. It described a new applied science based on the supposition that intellectual, physical, and behavior traits are inherited. Its objective was human perfection, its method selective breeding. According to Galton, eugenics was "the science of improving stock [by giving to] the more suitable races or strains of blood a chance of prevailing speedily over the less suitable" (Tone, 2001).

In the United States, eugenicists fell into two distinct intellectual camps. Both were elitist and racist and identified differential fertility rates among socioeconomic groups as a public problem. Those who embraced positive eugenics demanded more children from "fit" Americans. Adherents of this camp included President Theodore Roosevelt. Like many Progressives, he condemned the use of birth control by "selfish" middle-class and upper-class women as "race suicide." He worried that high birth rates among foreigners and the poor would swamp the country with "incompetence" and drain America of its hearty, superior, pioneer stock. He argued that native-born, white, afflu-

ent women who practiced fertility control were forsaking their natural duties as women and as citizens. "Exactly as the measure of our regard for the soldier who does his [full] duty in battle is the measure of our scorn for the coward who flees," he wrote in 1911, "so the measure of our respect for the true wife and mother is the measure of our scorn and contemptuous abhorrence for the wife who refused to be a mother" (Tone, 1997).

While Roosevelt hoped to inspire affluent Anglo-Saxon women to bear more children, advocates of negative eugenics adopted a more pernicious approach. They sought to suppress, through coercion if necessary, the procreation of unfit groups. By the 1920s, scores of scientists had come to believe that a host of human traits, including insanity, blindness, deafness, "feeble-mindedness," criminality, epilepsy, and low intelligence were inherited. The only way to prevent the transmission of these "defects" across generations, they argued, was to force those who suffered from them not to reproduce. Eugenicists assigned distinctive traits to specific ethnic and racial groups. Americans of Anglo-Saxon descent were considered the smartest and tidiest and the least likely to harbor defective genes. In contrast, Serbs were slovenly, Italians predisposed to crimes of personal violence, and African-Americans were, according to one 1926 tract, "germinally lacking in the higher development of intelligence" (Tone, 1997).

Eugenics and Sterilization

Negative eugenicists supported compulsory sterilization to prevent the procreation of unfit persons. The first sterilization surgery was performed by Dr. Harry C. Sharp in 1890 on an Indiana inmate who had complained of an uncontrollable urge to masturbate. After the vasectomy, Sharp published his findings, which he claimed cured the inmate of his "pathological desire." Subsequent research has shown that vasectomies do not effect sexual drive and that the desire to masturbate—either by a man or a woman—is neither a physiological nor psychological problem. But Sharp was captive to the prejudices of his time, and like many contemporaries insisted that sexual deviance was of biological origin. Sharp performed over 450 vasectomies on inmates and lobbied the Indiana legislature to pass the first eugenic law mandating the coerced sterilization of unfit persons, which it did in 1907 (Tone, 2001).

Other states followed suit, and soon women and men were being sterilized en masse against their will. In 1927, a dramatic court case, *Buck v. Bell*, tested the legitimacy of these laws. The case involved the reproductive autonomy of Carrie Buck, a single, white, pregnant Virginia woman who had been committed to the Virginia Colony for Epileptics and Feeble Minded in Lynchburg, Virginia. In 1924 the Virginia legislature had passed a eugenics statute that legalized the coerced sterilization of "socially inadequate persons." Carrie's status as the "daughter of an imbecile" and her pregnancy (which she insisted was the result of rape) supplied the primary evidence substantiating the charge of mental ineptitude. Doctors at the asylum sought her sterilization; she resisted. The case made its way to the Supreme Court, which was charged with the task of answering several pressing philosophical questions. Did the Virginia law unfairly suppress civil liberties in the name of public health? Did it give doctors too much power? The court's answer to these questions was an unequivocal no. Writing for the majority, Justice Oliver Wendell Holmes likened sexual sterilization to compulsory vaccination. "It is better for all the world, if instead of waiting to execute degenerate offspring for crime, or let them starve for their imbecility, society can prevent those who are manifestly unfit from continuing their kind. The principle that sustains compulsory vaccination is broad enough to cover cutting the Fallopian tubes.... Three generations of imbeciles are enough." Buck was sterilized on October 19, 1927, a few months after the Supreme Court's ruling (Tone, 1997).

The court's decision encouraged other states to adopt similar legislation. By 1932 twenty-six states had passed laws permitting the forced sterilization of individuals considered feebleminded, retarded, delinquent, or otherwise "unfit." By 1937, almost 28,000 people had been sterilized. Most (16,000) were women. The court's decision also had international consequences. The Virginia act served as the model for the drafting of Germany's Hereditary Health Law in 1933. During the Nuremberg trials following World War II, Nazi war criminals cited *Buck v. Bell* to justify the forced sterilization of 2 million Germans.

Germany's eugenics experiment dampened American enthusiasm for coercive sterilization, but it did not eradicate sterilization abuse altogether. In the postwar decades, poor women and women of color who received welfare payments were threatened by state officials and doctors. In some cases, women were told that if they did not get sterilized, their welfare assistance would be terminated (Solinger, 1992). In others, doctors required sterilization as a precondition for delivering a mother's child. Additionally, poor women pressured to consent to tubal ligation performed in teaching hospitals often found themselves regaining consciousness only to discover that they had been given a total hysterectomy, a more dangerous and invasive operation that generated added revenue for the hospital and gave medical residents extra "training" at women's expense (Roberts, 1997).

In 1973 a shocking incident exposed the extent of sterilization abuse in this country. Two sisters, aged 14 and 12, were enrolled in what their mother believed was a federally funded clinical study of a new contraceptive, the injectable drug Depo-Provera. The family of eight lived in Montgomery, Alabama, and survived through government relief payments and seasonal employment as farmhands. Unknown to the mother, who could not read or write, the Food and Drug Administration had ceased clinical trials of Depo-Provera (fearing that the drug was still too dangerous) shortly before she had marked the consent form with an "X." Instead of receiving injections, the girls were sterilized. A subsequent investigation conducted by the Southern Poverty Law Center found that 100,000 to 150,000 poor women and girls, half of whom were black, had been sterilized under federally funded programs. In 1978, the Department of Health, Education, and Welfare revised its rules to regulate sterilizations performed on women receiving federal funds such as Medicaid and Aid to Families with Dependent Children (Roberts, 1997). Even today, however, sterilization is frequently heralded as a valid remedy for curbing population growth, poverty, and a host of social problems.

THE SEXUAL WOMAN

As eugenicists sought to limit women's procreative potential, others were beginning to explore a related but neglected topic: women's sexual pleasure. In the early twentieth century, Sigmund Freud had described the sexual urge as a constitutive force of human nature, overturning social purists' depiction of female sexual desire as weaker and more underdeveloped than men's. Still, popular understanding of what constituted "natural" female sexuality was shaped by prescriptive literature, which distinguished between legitimate and illegitimate female sexual expression in ways that reflected conventional gender norms. For example, the 1947 bestseller, *Modern Woman: The Lost Sex*, insisted that the more educated a woman is, the greater the chance there is of sexual disorder. Disorder was evidenced in a desire for education, employment, and a small family.

Kinsey Study

Against this backdrop, Alfred Charles Kinsey's *Sexual Behavior in the Human Female*, published in 1953, was nothing short of revolutionary. A sequel to a 1948 volume on male sexuality, the book sought to transcend moralistic declarations by documenting women's everyday sexual experiences, the truth behind the myths. When Kinsey was a professor of zoology at Indiana University, he became interested in the scientific study of human sexuality after teaching a course on marriage and the family to undergraduate students in the late 1930s. Dis-

appointed by the absence of nonmoralistic data on sexual behavior, he and a small research team began to compile sexual case histories of men and women, over 11,000 of whom were interviewed for the two books. What Kinsey discovered was that far from being monolithic, "normal" female sexuality occupied a wide spectrum of behavior. Three-fifths of female interviewees masturbated regularly—a stinging rebuke of both lingering assertions of female sexual passivity and Freud's suggestion that female orgasm could only be accomplished with a man. Kinsey's study showed that women were far more self-sufficient in achieving sexual satisfaction. It also demonstrated that 90% of American women had engaged in petting and that half had engaged in premarital intercourse. At a time when pundits were routinely condemning or denying nonmarital female sexuality, Kinsey's findings raised intriguing questions about the chasm separating prescriptive ideal and routine practice. It also encouraged further research by establishing the scientific legitimacy of female sexuality as a topic of investigation.

Betty Friedan and *The Feminine Mystique*

Kinsey's study helped launch the sexual revolution, which saw its fullest expression in the 1960s and which challenged decades old assumptions about women's sexual, procreative, and social roles. The confluence of several historical events helped give this revolution steam. One was the publication in 1963 of Betty Friedan's *The Feminine Mystique*, which became for many women the principal handbook of the feminist movement. A 1942 graduate of Smith College, Friedan worked in New York as a journalist covering labor issues and civil rights before marrying war veteran Carl Friedan in 1947. Following societal expectations, she quit her job, moved to the suburb of Queens, and raised three children. At the time, the media promoted what Friedan would call "the feminine mystique," a postwar ideology that celebrated the naturalness of female domesticity and gender difference.

Only a few years earlier, during World

War II, the government's "Rosie the Riveter" campaign had told women that it was their patriotic duty to be wage earners. Women had heeded the government's call: over 6 million joined the workforce during the war, 2 million in heavy industry jobs that had traditionally been denied women. But once the war ended, women were urged to go "back to the kitchen"; in 1946 alone, 4 million were fired. The media did its part to ease the transition. Television shows such as "Ozzie and Harriet" profiled supportive self-sacrificing female wives and mothers as the norm. Advertisements and reports on television and in magazines encouraged women to believe that they could achieve full psychological fulfillment by buying the right bleach or luncheon meats. Magazines romanticized an image of women as apolitical entities satisfied by a life centered on the kitchen, shopping, the laundry room, babies, and the home. Single women, women who wished to remain childless, or to have a career or education were portrayed as psychologically imbalanced, a diagnosis instrumental to the phenomenal growth of the tranquilizer industry in the 1950s.

The postwar ideal clashed with the reality of women's experiences. The typical woman was supposed to be a stay-at-home mom, but in 1952 two million more wives were at work than at the peak of wartime production (Coontz, 1992). In addition, non-wage-earning mothers like Friedan found that domestic life was not always fulfilling. For her fifteenth Smith college class reunion, Friedan surveyed the satisfactions and frustrations of 200 women graduates of the class of 1942. From there she went on to interview suburban housewives across the country. A striking pattern emerged. Women confessed to Friedan their overwhelming doubts, dissatisfactions, and resentment with domestic life. They found that conforming to the image of the feminine mystique was a goal whose unattainability made them feel guilty, anxious, and inadequate.

In *The Feminine Mystique*, Friedan labeled this schizophrenic split the "problem that has no name," and reassured female readers that they need not experience their despair and frus-

trations alone. It was okay, Friedan wrote, for women to want something more out of life than diapers, dinners, and dirty floors. Friedan also addressed the question of women's sexual satisfaction. Alarmed by the media's depiction of the typical American woman as a procreative "sex-seeker," she warned that women's apparent hunger for sex and children often stemmed from boredom. In a society that routinely characterized female careers and female childlessness as abnormal, women had few legitimate outlets for self-expression. By overemphasizing the value of female physicality, Friedan warned, the media nurtured the belief that women were incapable of being more than sexual objects. *The Feminine Mystique* was an instant bestseller that elicited thousands of appreciative letters from women around the globe. Thrust in the media spotlight, Friedan became a spokesperson for the women's liberation movement. In 1966 she founded the National Organization for Women, which remains today one of the most important feminist organizations and political lobbying groups in the United States.

Helen Gurley Brown

While Friedan and other feminists discussed the larger meanings and political dangers of the sexual objectification of women, other women saw things differently. One was Helen Gurley Brown. Brown believed that American society was still mired in old and repressive stereotypes about female prudery and women's proper place. In 1962 the 40-year-old married, advertising executive published *Sex and the Single Girl*, which, like *The Feminine Mystique*, became an overnight sensation. Brown glamorized the newly liberated single woman who had come to symbolize the sexual revolution. She portrayed positively what used to be called "spinsterhood" and encouraged single women to flaunt their sexual prowess and to have intercourse freely. Rather than being a stepping stone to marriage, premarital sexuality should be enjoyed in its own right. The success of her book brought Brown the editorship of the magazine *Cosmopolitan*, a publication that had started out in 1886 as a reputable family magazine. Like many periodicals of the early 1960s, *Cosmopolitan* had suffered a circulation decline brought on by competition from television. To reverse the magazine's fortunes, Brown transformed it into a sassy, sexually forthright publication that discussed what, at the time, television would not: orgasms, impotence, and strategies for seducing men. Some feminists immediately denounced the magazine's preoccupation with female beauty and its predatory "how-to-catch-a-man" message. In 1968, dozens of feminists boycotting the Miss America Pageant dumped copies of *Cosmopolitan*, *Playboy*, and *Vogue*, along with dishcloths, bras, false eyelashes, and high-heeled shoes into a larger container symbolically marked the "Freedom Trash Can."

The Pill

The development and diffusion of oral contraceptives also marked the sexual revolution. The Pill, as it came to be known, was approved by the Food and Drug Administration in 1960 as a contraceptive. The drug was largely the brainchild of physiologist Gregory Pincus, who in 1951 was asked by Margaret Sanger to undertake the invention of a foolproof birth control that would help stem population growth in underdeveloped parts of the world. Sanger worried that available female methods were too complicated for uneducated populations, whose procreation advocates of population control most wanted to check. In the late 1950s, clinical trials of the Pill were conducted on hundreds of impoverished Puerto Rican and Haitian women (some of whom received a placebo instead of the standard 10 mg of progestin), partly to see if poor, uneducated women could "comply" with a once-a-day contraceptive regimen (Tone, 1999).

Ironically, when the drug was released in the United States, it was initially priced beyond the reach of the poorest Americans. But this did not stop it from becoming the favored birth control of the middle class. By mid-1964 oral contraceptives, available only by prescription,

had become the most popular contraception in the country. An estimated 3.5 million women were taking them, constituting one-fourth of all couples practicing contraception in the United States. Women flocked to doctors' offices for prescriptions because they believed they would personally benefit from a contraceptive that was more effective and simpler to use than previous methods. Unlike the diaphragm, the Pill promised almost 100% efficacy. Small, simple, and discreet, it did not require direct male cooperation. And because it could be swallowed any time of the day, independent of the act of intercourse, it uncoupled sex from conception more directly than had any previous contraceptive.

The popularity of the Pill launched a national debate on women's health and sexual morality. As Pill-related problems from migraine headaches to nausea to strokes made the national news, many feminists portrayed Pill users as unwitting "medical guinea pigs," pawns of a pharmaceutical industry profiting from women's desperate search for effective birth control. Why, they asked, must women unilaterally shoulder the personal and physiological costs of pregnancy prevention? Why weren't there more contraceptives for men? At the same time, several African-American leaders denounced the Pill as a technology of racial genocide and warned that, like sterilization, oral contraceptives were being pushed on women of color to thwart the expansion of the black community. The Catholic Church proclaimed the Pill to be contrary to church teachings, and moralists warned that oral contraceptives had spawned a generation of promiscuous single women who, following the dictates of Helen Gurley Brown, regarded "sex without worry" as a laudable practice.

LEGAL LIBERALIZATION

Griswold v. Connecticut

The debate had scarcely been launched when in 1965 the Supreme Court handed down its landmark decision in *Griswold v. Connecticut*, a decisive victory for champions of sexual liberty and birth control. The case challenged the constitutionality of Connecticut's 1879 mini-Comstock law which proscribed the use of any "drug, medicinal article or instrument for the purpose of preventing conception." Purposefully violating the statute, Estelle Griswold, executive director of the Planned Parenthood League of Connecticut, and D. Led Buxton, chair of the Department of Obstetrics at the Yale University School of Medicine, opened a birth control clinic for married women in New Haven on November 1. On June 7, 1965, the Supreme Court invalidated the Connecticut law, declaring that a constitutional right to privacy for married couples fell within the "penumbra" of the Bill of Rights, understood in this context to be the right to matrimonial privacy in the bedroom. "Would we allow the police to search the sacred precincts of marital bedrooms for telltale signs of the uses of contraceptives?" Mr. Justice Douglas, writing for the majority, asked. "The very idea is repulsive to the notions of privacy surrounding the marriage relationship." In 1972, the Supreme Court's decision in *Eisenstadt v. Baird* did for contracepting singles what *Griswold v. Connecticut* had done for married couples. After activist Bill Baird offered containers of free contraceptive foam at a public lecture at Boston University in violation of Massachusetts's "crimes against chastity law," the Supreme Court ruled that "if the right of privacy means anything, it is the right of the individual, married or single, to be free from unwarranted governmental intrusion into matters so fundamentally affecting a person as the decision whether to bear or beget a child." With this ruling, a woman's right to use birth control became the law of the land (Tone, 1997).

Roe v. Wade

The last legal restrictions on abortion fell a year later with the Supreme Court's ruling in *Roe v. Wade*. In 1972, an estimated 2500 American women were having abortions daily, many traveling to New York and California, states that had recently legalized abortion. Others unable to afford to travel were forced to have illegal "back-alley" abortions. Poor women and women of color were most vulnerable to the accompanying medical hazards; in 1969, they constituted 75% of those who died from botched procedures and unhygienic conditions.

Texas was one of many states that permitted a woman to have an abortion only if it was necessary to save her life. In 1969, Norma McCorvey (using the alias "Jane Roe" to protect her anonymity), a single, pregnant woman, agreed to serve as plaintiff in a case to test the legality of the Texas statute. McCorvey's lawyers, Linda Coffee and Sarah Weddington, recent graduates of the University of Texas Law School, argued that the law violated the Constitution's implied right to privacy as articulated in *Griswold v. Connecticut* and *Eistenstadt v. Baird*. This right, they insisted, protected a woman from being forced by the state to continue an unwanted pregnancy. Coffee and Weddington argued that the safety concerns that had propelled the passage of abortion legislation in the nineteenth century were no longer relevant; advances in medical technology had made abortion significantly less dangerous than carrying a pregnancy to term. The Court agreed with their logic, declaring that the right to privacy included the right of a woman, in consultation with her physician, to terminate a pregnancy without state interference in her first trimester (Tone, 1997). Ironically, Norma McCorvey delivered her baby long before the Court handed down its decision.

Roe v. Wade overturned existing state proscriptions on abortion, but it did not guarantee all women equal access to the procedure. In the aftermath of *Roe*, the pro-life movement gained momentum and support. By September 1973, eighteen bills sponsoring constitutional amendments against abortion had been introduced in Congress. Although the constitutional campaign ultimately failed, pro-lifers succeeded in 1977 in passing the Hyde Amendment. Introduced by Representative Henry Hyde (R-IL), as an amendment to the Department of Health,

Education, and Welfare's appropriations bill, the measure banned federal funding for abortions in all cases except where rape or incest had been promptly reported to police or where the mother's life was in danger. Although the 20,000-member National Abortion Rights Action League immediately denounced the restrictive measure as "inhumane and quite possible unconstitutional," the Supreme Court upheld the law's constitutionality in 1981 in *Harris v. McRae*. The Hyde Amendment created a two-tier system of abortion care in the United States. From this point forward, only women with adequate financial resources could afford to exercise their legal "right to choose" (Tone, 1997).

CONCLUSIONS

Since the 1970s, advancements in women's sexual and reproductive health have been mixed. Access to safe, medical abortions has been compromised by escalating clinic violence and doctor and patient intimidation. While *Roe v. Wade* continues to govern abortion policy, new state laws mandating 24-hour waiting periods and parental notification have circumscribed its reach. In addition, the health insurance industry continues to ignore or downplay women's reproductive health needs. While a growing number of insurers cover the expensive male impotence drug Viagra, most still refuse to cover women's infertility treatments and reversible contraceptives. Both areas of reproductive health have undergone a technological revolution in the last two decades, offering women choices that include *in vitro* fertilization, the injectable contraceptive Depo-Provera, and the chemical implant Norplant. The unwillingness of most health insurance plans to cover these options have forced women to pay for them out-of-pocket, exacerbating the class and gender gap in access to reproductive medicine. Insurance trends have also encouraged poorer women to select nonreversible methods such as tubal ligations, which most plans, including Medicaid, cover. (Insurance companies have deemed

it cheaper to pay for women to be sterilized than to risk having to pay the higher costs associated with pregnancy and childbirth.) Since the late 1970s, despite the availability of new contraceptive technologies, voluntary sterilization has become the most frequently used form of birth control in the nation.

Moreover, in the aftermath of class-action suits against the manufacturers of the Dalkon Shield, an intrauterine device whose design flaws and inadequate testing left many American women in the early 1970s pregnant, sick, or infertile, the pace of contraceptive research in the United States has slowed. Manufacturers concerned with profits have to worry about both consumer litigation and health insurance coverage before committing to the manufacture of breakthrough devices and drugs. Still, new research, much of it funded by public sector entities, has yielded promising results. In the next decade, we may see a barrage of new choices on the contraceptive market: mechanical and chemical barriers that are both spermicidal and microbicidal (thereby protecting women against pregnancy and sexually transmitted diseases), immunocontraception, improved oral contraceptives, and even hormonal birth control—pills or injections—for men (Harrison and Rosenfield, 1996).

REFERENCES

Brodie, J. F. (1994). *Contraception and abortion in nineteenth-century America*. Ithaca, NY: Cornell University Press.
Coontz, S. (1992). *The way we never were: American families and the nostalgia trap*. New York: Basic Books.
D'Emilio, J., Freedman, E. B. (1989). *Intimate matters: A history of sexuality in America*. New York: Harper and Row.
Friedman, L. (1993). *Crime and punishment in American history*. New York: Basic Books.
Gilfoyle, T. (1992). *City of eros: New York City, prostitution, and the commercialization of sex, 1790–1920*. New York: W. W. Norton.
Gordon, L. (1977). *Woman's body, woman's right: A social history of birth control in America*. New York: Penguin Books.
Harrison, P. F., & Rosenfield. A. (1996). *Contraceptive research and development: Looking to the future*. Washington: National Academy Press.

McCann, C. R. (1994). *Birth control politics in the United States, 1916–1945*. Ithaca, NY: Cornell University Press.

Mohr, J. C. (1978). *Abortion in America: The origins and evolution of national policy, 1800–1900*. New York: Oxford University Press.

Odem, M. (1995). *Delinquent daughters: Protecting and policing adolescent female sexuality in the United States, 1885–1920*. Chapel Hill: University of North Carolina Press.

Reagan, L. J. (1991). "About to meet her maker": The state's investigation of abortion in Chicago, 1867–1940. *Journal of American History*, 77(March 1991): 1240–1264.

Roberts, D. (1997). *Killing the black body: Race, reproduction, and the meaning of liberty*. New York: Vintage.

Solinger, R. (1992). *Wake up little Susie: Single pregnancy and race before Roe v. Wade*. New York: Routledge.

Tone, A. (1997). *Controlling reproduction: An American history*. Wilmington, DE: Scholarly Resources.

Tone, A. (1999). Violence by design: Contraceptive technology and the invasion of the female body. In M. Bellesiles (Ed.), *Lethal imagination: Violence and brutality in American history* (pp. 372–391). New York: New York University Press.

Tone, A. (2001). *Devices and desires: Women, men, and the commercialization of contraception*. New York: Hill & Wang.

3

Adolescent Girls' Sexual Development

JULIA A. GRABER and JEANNE BROOKS-GUNN

ADOLESCENT GIRLS' SEXUAL DEVELOPMENT

Adolescence is a period of development when the body has the most rapid change in physical growth second only to infancy. Along with dramatic physical changes at the entry into adolescence, the adolescent decade is defined by the restructuring of social roles, expectations, and relationships within the family, peer group, and school environment (e.g., Adams, Montemayor, & Gullotta, 1989–2000; Feldman & Elliott, 1990; Graber, Brooks-Gunn, & Petersen, 1996). Notably, the pubertal transition, which has often been used to define the beginning of adolescence, has also been viewed as the impetus for other behavioral and social changes with which puberty co-occurs and precedes (Brooks-Gunn & Petersen, 1983; Petersen & Taylor, 1980). Changes within an individual's social environment are in some part attributable to the re-

sponse of family, friends, and teachers to a more adultlike appearance. Clearly, an adultlike appearance is an indication of reproductive capacity as well as signs that new behaviors relating to sexual feelings and interest are emerging. Internal rather than external pubertal processes have also been considered an impetus for behavioral change; for example, emotional lability and arousal have been associated with hormonal changes (Brooks-Gunn, Graber, & Paikoff, 1994; Buchanan, Eccles, & Becker, 1992; Susman, Dorn, & Chrousos, 1991). Given the range and possibilities for interaction among the biological, social, and psychological substrates of development, it is clear that how pubertal development is traversed may be a potent determinant of subsequent behaviors, feelings, and experiences of adolescents.

An important aspect of the developmental experiences of adolescents is the formation of a sexual identity and sense of self as a sexual being (Graber, Brooks-Gunn, & Galen, 1998; Katchadourian, 1990). Whether or not they have had any sexual experience, sex has great meaning in the lives of youth (Graber et al., 1998). Although sexuality, in terms of both desires and identity, is a part of earlier phases of life, these issues become particularly salient in the adolescent years for several reasons: pubertal development results in reproductive capability; iden-

JULIA A. GRABER • Department of Psychology, University of Florida, Gainesville, Florida 32611. **JEANNE BROOKS-GUNN** • Institute for Child Psychology, Child Development, and Education, Teachers College, Columbia University, New York, New York 10027.

Handbook of Women's Sexual and Reproductive Health, edited by Wingood and DiClemente. Kluwer Academic / Plenum Publishers, New York, 2002.

tity development in adolescence includes the formation of a sexual identity; sexual exploration (be it kissing, intercourse, or just dreaming) usually occurs during the adolescent years; and the negotiation of autonomy and intimacy will take place within sexual situations (Brooks-Gunn & Paikoff, 1993, 1997; Graber *et al.*, 1998).

Parents of adolescents in general feel tension over sexual behavior, and girls, in particular, seem to experience greater constraints and pressures around the regulation of sexuality, at least within the United States. In many ways, reproductive (and therefore sexual) transitions are central to women across the life span from menarche, to childbearing, to menopause (Graber & Brooks-Gunn, 1996). For girls, outward signs of impending sexual transitions begin during mid- to late childhood with the appearance of breast buds. Thus, the identification of girls as sexual beings occurs early in the life course. In addition, girls often bear the pressure to regulate sexual behavior due to the risk of pregnancy and the problems that may result from pregnancy during the adolescent years. Thus, adolescent girls frequently face unique challenges in integrating sexuality into their developing identities and behaviors.

The present chapter examines how the pubertal transition is linked to girls' emerging sexuality with attention to the risks and challenges that may occur for some girls. First, we describe the nature of adolescent development and puberty for girls. Then we examine how pubertal development connects with emerging sexuality and how sexual development is interconnected with multiple aspects of adolescent development. Drawing upon this background for girls' sexuality, we discuss program approaches that have sought to promote healthy development in girls. Finally, we consider the longer-term outcomes of different developmental trajectories of girls' sexual development along with policy implications of understanding girls' sexual behavior as part of a developmental trajectory for healthy or unhealthy behaviors and outcomes.

EPIDEMIOLOGY

Adolescence is one of the most fascinating and complex transitions in the life span: a time of accelerated growth and change second only to infancy; a time of expanding horizons, self-discovery, and emerging independence; a time of metamorphosis from childhood to adulthood.... The events of this crucially formative phase can shape an individual's life course and thus the future of the whole society (Carnegie Foundation, 1996, p. 7).

As demonstrated by this quote from the Carnegie Council on Adolescent Development, adolescence has frequently been viewed as a critical period of development on the road to successful adult outcomes. Clearly entry into adolescence is defined by the physical changes of puberty. However, it is notable that for some time across several cultures and contexts the transition to adult reproductive capacity has not resulted in the automatic conference of adult status on individuals (Schlegel & Barry, 1991). Rather, the period of adolescence, although changing in length and to a lesser extent purpose over history, has been an intermediary period between childhood and adulthood in which youth are expected to master the skills they will need to enter the world of work, financial independence, partnership, and parenthood (Modell & Goodman, 1990). Of course, some individuals will make these transitions earlier or later than their peers, having either truncated or extended periods of adolescence.

The entire period of adolescence is usually referred to as the second decade of life, but usually adolescence is divided into three phases: entry into/early adolescence, mid-adolescence, and late adolescence. There are no definitive demarcations for different phases of adolescence; ages are included as guidelines. The entry into adolescence is most commonly associated with pubertal development, changes in school environment, and commensurate relationship and role changes with parents and peers. Typically, entry into adolescence or early adolescence is from ages 11–14. Mid-adolescence (ages 15–17 or 18) most often encompasses the high school years in the United States and is typified by greater independence with lower conflict with parents. Youth in this period of adolescence often initiate part-time employment, engage in extracurricular activities out of school, and become licensed drivers. Late adolescence (ages 18–20) is frequently defined by the transition to adulthood, which itself may be a lengthy period of multiple transitions as individuals first make decisions about continuing their education past high school, entering the world of work, and living independently. By the early twenties, most youth are clearly in transition to adulthood and are either attaining adult roles, making decisions as to which roles they want to attain, and/or engaging in behaviors that constrain or enhance the attainment of some adult roles. Because of the variation among individuals during late adolescence and young adulthood (e.g., completing or not completing high school, entering work or the military or college, etc.), the entire period from 18–25 has been considered an extended transitional period of life (Arnett, 2000).

Notably, for each of these developmental periods, development of sexuality and a sexual sense of self is inherently, if not specifically, a part of each. By the end of early adolescence, most individuals have usually begun sexual exploration with a partner such as kissing and touching of breasts, or having breasts touched (Coles & Stokes, 1995; Feldman, Turner, & Araujo, 1999; Westney, Jenkins, & Benjamin, 1983). These activities are likely to occur in mixed-gender situations where young adolescents have gone out in groups or are at a party (Spreadbury, 1982). Only a subset of young adolescents will progress to intercourse during early adolescence; based on data compiled by the Alan Guttmacher Institute (AGI, 1994), about one in five 14-year-olds has had intercourse. Although there have been recent declines in the number of youth who have had intercourse, girls in this age group have caught up with rates reported by boys (Terry & Manlove, 1999).

By mid-adolescence, most individuals will have begun to go out with other youth in social and sexual situations with less adult supervision. Being able to drive and potentially having a disposable income via after-school jobs afford youth in mid-adolescence greater autonomy in their social activities. Kissing and petting behaviors progress during this period of development to vaginal and penile touching (Feldman et al., 1999; Katchadourian, 1990). A number of adolescents will progress to intercourse during mid-adolescence with percentages increasing with age; for example, for girls and boys, respectively, 25% and 27% of 15-year-olds, 39% and 45% of 16-year-olds, and 52% and 59% of 17-year-olds have had intercourse (AGI, 1994; Terry & Manlove, 1999).

By late adolescence, the majority of youth will have engaged in sexual intercourse, as well as other sexual behaviors. Specifically, by age 18, 68% of boys and 66% of girls will have had intercourse; by age 19, the rates are up to 85% for boys and 77% for girls (Terry & Manlove, 1999). Thus, the transition of first intercourse occurs for many youth prior to the completion of high school or shortly thereafter. By this point in development, expression of sexual desires is one aspect of more complex intimate relationships (Furman & Simon, 1999). Across adolescence, cognitive development progresses with increasing abilities to understand future outcomes, planning and decision making, and abstract thinking. These developmental advances interconnect with changes in feelings and behaviors as youth develop their identities and intimate relationships.

As youth become adults, there is the expectation of forming committed relationships and eventually of becoming a parent. The median age of first marriage is 26.7 for men and 25.0 for women as of 1998 Census Bureau estimates (Lugaila, 1998). For individuals who are between the ages of 18 and 24, about 22% of young women and 12% of young men are married. Whereas most youth and young adults expect to postpone childbearing for one to two years after marriage (Graber, Britto, & Brooks-Gunn, 1999), young adults ages 20–24 have the highest rates of out-of-wedlock childbearing (Darroch & Singh, 1999; Terry & Manlove, 1999). Hence, typical patterns of young adult transitions may not hold for all individuals, with some making transitions earlier or later than others. Of course not all individuals become parents or form stable, committed relationships as adults (Graber et al., 1999).

The percentage of youth who engage in sexual intercourse is a narrow view of the emergence and development of sexual behaviors and feelings (Graber et al., 1998). Certainly, the focus on intercourse is heterocentric, although it should be noted that most gay men report having had vaginal intercourse during adolescence (Savin-Williams, 1995); less is known about the sexual histories of lesbians. In addition, there are variations among adolescents for engaging in intercourse or other sexual behaviors. For example, there has, historically, been a gender difference in the age of first intercourse, with boys on average engaging in intercourse at an earlier age than girls. However, gender disparities have progressively decreased over the past few decades (AGI, 1994; Oliver & Hyde, 1993; Terry & Manlove, 1999).

Variations in timing of intercourse have also been reported by race and ethnicity. In this case, African-American youth have earlier ages of first intercourse than other youth; however, controlling for socioeconomic differences among study samples often greatly reduces these differences. Some studies have also reported different sequencing of sexual behaviors by racial and/or ethnic group. Smith and Udry (1985) found that White adolescents progressed through a sequence of kissing and fondling, oral sex, then intercourse, whereas Black adolescents were less likely to engage in noncoital activities prior to intercourse. In contrast, Feldman and colleagues (1999) reported that the sequencing of sexual behaviors during adolescence was quite similar for African-American, Asian, White, and Latino youth. Interestingly, rather than the order of the activities, it was the age of onset of initial sexual behaviors and the rate of progression through these activities that demonstrated larger race/ethnicity differences. After controlling for sociodemographic factors, African-

American youth did, as expected, engage in each behavior at the youngest ages but these ages were usually not significantly different from the ages reported by White or Latino youth. However, significant differences in age of initiation of a behavior were almost always between Asian-Americans and the other youth. That is, Asian-American youth initiated each sexual activity at a significantly older age than their counterparts. Notably, African-American youth had the most rapid progression of sexual activities, initiating kissing a little before 14 years of age and intercourse by 15.5 years of age; in contrast other youth took about 2–2.5 years for this progression.

Regardless of race, ethnicity, gender, or socioeconomic differences among adolescents, emerging sexuality is perhaps the most challenging aspect of adolescent development for parents and adults living and working with youth. Based on the previous description of the initiation of sexual behaviors across adolescence, it seems that sexual behaviors and feelings are a normative part of development. Of course, whereas an interest in sexual activities may be normative for adolescents, parents also have a normative interest in regulating these behaviors. Adolescents frequently engage in unprotected intercourse or other sexual activities (AGI, 1994). In addition, experimentation with drugs and alcohol in social situations impairs judgment about sexually healthy behavior. These types of health-compromising behaviors are one factor that make the regulation of adolescent sexual behavior a concern not only to parents but to society in general.

PUBERTAL DEVELOPMENT

Sexual behaviors and feelings are present during puberty. Puberty involves physiological and structural changes in nearly all systems of the body, including changes in height and weight, the central nervous system, the cardiovascular system, and the reproductive organs (Marshall & Tanner, 1986). Coupled with these changes are myriad psychological and social changes that also happen either concurrently with, or as a result of, puberty. In order to understand the ways in which puberty may influence the course of adolescent development and development of sexual behaviors, identities, and feelings, a description of pubertal development is provided.

Hormonal Changes at Puberty

Puberty encompasses a number of interrelated physiological processes that serve to restructure the body from that of a child to that of a reproductively capable adult. Maturation and adult reproductive functioning are controlled by the reproductive endocrine system via the hypothalamus–pituitary–adrenal (HPA) axis and the hypothalamus–pituitary–gonadal (HPG) axis. Activation of the reproductive endocrine system involves increases in sex-steroid hormone secretion (e.g., estrogen and testosterone) through two independent processes: (a) adrenarche and (b) gonadarche (Reiter & Grumbach, 1982). Adrenarche involves increases in production of adrenal androgens, via the maturation of the adrenal cortex, beginning by 7–8 years of age in girls and boys (Grumbach & Styne, 1998). Approximately two years later, gonadarche occurs with increased secretion of gonadal steroids.

During the prenatal period, the hypothalamus and pituitary glands in the brain develop specialized areas that function to regulate reproductive development at puberty. These systems are also involved in the initial development of the external genitalia and reproductive systems that are in place at birth. Maturation of the reproductive system results in the production of gonadotropin-releasing hormone (GnRH) by the hypothalamus. GnRH acts as a chemical signal to the pituitary, which responds by releasing pulsatile bursts of gonadotropins, LH and FSH. LH and FSH are secreted at low levels by the pituitary during childhood, but episodic nocturnal bursts of LH of low amplitude are characteristic of the early stages of puberty. At this time, the gonads also become more responsive to the gonadotropins, resulting in in-

creased secretion of the gonadal hormones. In girls, the primary gonadal hormone is estradiol. Testosterone production also begins to rise in girls, but most of the testosterone produced in girls comes from conversion of hormones secreted by the adrenal glands (i.e., androstenedione; see Grumbach and Styne, 1998, for a comprehensive review of hormonal and metabolic changes at puberty). The adultlike pattern of hormonal regulation of reproduction in girls (and boys) involves the monitoring of levels of circulating sex steroids (e.g., estradiol) by the hypothalamus, which then responds via alterations in release of the gonadotropins, which in turn, act on the gonads to stimulate increases in sex steroids.

Pubertal Status

As a result of the development of the reproductive hormonal system at puberty, external signs of puberty (i.e., secondary sexual characteristics) become apparent to girls and those around them. Exactly when and how quickly individuals will experience puberty varies greatly among individuals (Marshall & Tanner, 1969). For girls, the first external sign of puberty is usually breast budding followed a few months later by the first growth of pubic hair. Some girls will experience pubic hair growth prior to breast budding; such variations are not considered atypical. Although puberty has usually been viewed as an indicator of the transition into adolescence, for girls pubertal development most often begins in the late childhood years.

On average, White girls in the United States begin breast development at 9.96 years of age and pubic hair growth at 10.51 years of age (Herman-Giddens et al., 1997; Kaplowitz et al., 1999). In contrast, African-American girls in the United States begin development about one year earlier than their White counterparts, with breast development beginning at 8.87 years of age and pubic hair growth at 8.78 years of age, on average (Herman-Giddens et al., 1997; Kaplowitz et al., 1999).

Despite the fact that nearly everyone will

go through puberty, normative data have been sporadic and not comprehensive. That is, only a few studies have documented the average age for initiation of different secondary sexual characteristics, and many of these have been relatively small studies of specific populations of children (e.g., white, middle-class, or institutionalized youth in England). Most recently, two larger, representative studies in the United States have found that initiation of pubertal development in girls is earlier than previously reported and that a consistent racial difference in timing of onset existed at this time (Herman-Giddens et al., 1997; The National Heart, Lung, & Blood and Health Study Research Group, 1992). Thus, the ages of onset reported here reflect information from these most recent studies.

Most individuals will take four to five years to traverse from the initiation of external signs of development to completed development (Marshall & Tanner, 1969; Grumbach & Styne, 1998). Even though pubertal growth is a continuous process or multiple processes, Tanner developed a rating scale for categorizing girls' (and boys') pubertal development into stages for specific characteristics. For girls, both pubic hair growth and breast development are typically classified into stages ranging from stage 1, indicating that development on this characteristic has not begun, to stage 5, indicating that the mature status has been reached (Tanner, 1962). Typically, girls will experience the growth spurt or peak height velocity in the earlier stages of puberty (between stages 2 and 3 of breast and pubic hair development). The growth spurt for boys is about two years later than that for girls.

Girls will also experience a "spurt" in weight with gains in both body fat and lean muscle mass (Grumbach & Styne, 1998). However, in comparison to boys, girls gain more fat and less muscle. In addition, fat is distributed to the hips changing the body shape to form a more curved figure. On average, girls will gain 24 pounds during the fat spurt (Warren, 1983); this rapid change in weight and body shape has often been cited as a precursor to increased dieting in adolescent girls (Tyrka, Graber, & Brooks-Gunn, 2000).

Just after the peak in height velocity and around stage 4 of pubic hair and breast development, girls have their first menstruation, or menarche (Grumbach & Styne, 1998). Thus, menarche occurs near the end of pubertal development. The same recent studies that have reported racial differences and younger ages than previously thought for girls in age of onset of pubic hair growth and breast development have also found racial differences in age at menarche. The average age at menarche is about 12.2 for African-American girls and 12.7–12.8 for White girls in the United States (Herman-Giddens et al., 1997; National Center for Health Statistics, 1997). Menarche does not inherently translate to reproductive capacity in that many girls will not ovulate regularly with each menstrual cycle during the first two years after menarche (Grumbach & Styne, 1998). Of course, girls themselves are not aware of whether or not their cycles are fertile.

Timing of Onset of Puberty

As indicated, there is enormous variation among girls in the timing of onset and rate of progression through each of these aspects of puberty. The ages of key events are provided to indicate average ages for these events, but girls must be substantially earlier or later than these ages of development for puberty to be considered abnormal or requiring treatment for medical reasons. The ordering of events, again, is typical, but variations occur among girls. Perhaps some of the most perplexing issues in the study of pubertal development are associated with recent reports of earlier development for girls and the racial difference among girls both of which have only been reported in the past decade. For the racial difference, it is feasible that there was insufficient examination of girls from different racial and ethnic backgrounds in prior studies. Thus, differences may have existed, but only recently have studies been undertaken that would identify these differences.

One issue in studies of race/ethnicity differences is that such differences may be accounted for by differences in SES. It is difficult to determine the source of racial differences given that race and ethnicity are frequently confounded with income, such that African-American girls and women are disproportionately represented in the lower end of the income distribution, and White girls and women are disproportionately represented in the upper end of income. As yet, there are only a few studies that have examined both SES and race/ethnicity and findings have not been consistent among these studies. In a study of girls that sampled by race/ethnicity and high, low, and middle SES, controlling for SES reduced differences in age at menarche between Latina and White girls (Obeidallah, Brennan, Brooks-Gunn, Kindlon, & Earls, 2000). However, this study did not find an initial race difference in age at menarche for White and African-American girls. In contrast, a study of a large, nationally representative sample of girls recruited as part of an investigation of cardiovascular risk found a race difference in onset of pubertal development, consistent with that found by Herman-Giddens and her colleagues (1997; National Heart, Lung, & Blood and Health Study Research Group, 1992); the race difference was not accounted for by SES. However, while this study had a nationally representative sample, indices of economic factors were not assessed in as much depth as was done for the study by Obeidallah and her colleagues (2000). As such, further examination of race/ethnicity and SES factors need to be considered in understanding pubertal timing differences among girls.

Interestingly, in examining the ages of menarche reported by women who participated in the 1995 National Survey of Family Growth, there is no race or ethnic difference among the oldest group of women (ages 40–44; National Center for Health Statistics, 1997). Specifically, women in this age group had average ages of menarche of 12.7 for white, non-Hispanic women, 12.5 for Hispanic women, and 12.6 for non-Hispanic black women. The youngest group (ages 15–19) in this study had much younger ages as well as ethnic differences in menarche, with 12.4 for white, non-Hispanic women, 12.1 for Hispanic women, and 12.0 for non-Hispanic black women. These data support the notion that puberty has been getting earlier for girls

over the past few decades and suggest that the racial/ethnic difference has also been developing over this time period. Notably, there is only sparse evidence that the onset of pubertal development is changing for boys either over the last few decades or by race/ethnicity (Kaplowitz et al., 1999). Data on this issue are limited as only two larger studies of boys' puberty in racially diverse samples have been conducted in the past few years (Biro, Lucky, Huster, & Morrison, 1995; Herman-Giddens, Wang, & Koch, 2001).

There are many hypotheses to explain earlier onset of puberty in girls. First, the onset of puberty does have some associations across generations that are assumed to be at least in part due to genetic factors. That is, mothers' and daughters' ages of menarche usually have a moderate correlation (e.g., Brooks-Gunn & Warren, 1988; Zacharias & Wurtman, 1969). However, genetic factors are less likely to explain why the time of onset is changing. Second, there are data that suggest that exposure to environmental toxins may stimulate pubertal development in girls by mimicking estrogens in the body (e.g., Gladen, Ragan, & Rogan, 2000). Third, perinatal factors have also been found to play a role in subsequent pubertal development (e.g., Persson et al., 1999). In this case, girls who were smaller at birth but had a rapid "catch-up" period of growth between birth and age 6 were earlier maturers. Although the exact mechanisms through which this works are not known, given that sex hormones are active prenatally in organizing the brain for subsequent pubertal development and reproductive functioning, it seems likely that the prenatal environment will influence subsequent timing of onset of development. In addition, the effect of rapid growth in childhood found in the Persson et al. study (1999) may have also been partially due to the influence of body fat on pubertal timing. That is, as a fourth hypothesis, it has been suggested that higher body fat is associated with earlier maturation potentially via the hormone leptin (Clayton & Trueman, 2000). Leptin, which is associated with weight gain and influences gonadotropin activity in the brain, increases dramatically in girls as normative weight gain occurs during puberty (Horlick *et al.*, 2000). With increasing rates of obesity in childhood, it has been suggested that more girls would be expected to mature at earlier ages due to elevated leptin levels. Of course, not all heavier girls will mature early. Also, it may be more likely that changes in leptin levels are not the trigger for pubertal onset but rather a product of pubertal onset (Clayton & Trueman, 2000). That is, leptin increases are a normative part of pubertal development and leptin undergoes changes when other pubertal systems are turned on.

While there are probably numerous other hypotheses, the final one that we will discuss is that of psychosocial or environmental stress. In several studies, social stressors, in particular, stressful family situations, have been linked to earlier onset of puberty (Graber, Brooks-Gunn, & Warren, 1995; Moffitt, Caspi, Belsky, & Silva, 1992; Surbey, 1990). Father absence in the childhood years as well as lower quality of family relations result in earlier maturation for girls. Some of this work has been retrospective (Surbey, 1990) or did not control for the possibility that puberty may have already begun when the studies were initiated (Moffitt *et al.*, 1992). In our own work, we have found that lower warmth in parent–child relationships resulted in earlier age at menarche after controlling for the effect of maternal age at menarche and level of breast development (Graber *et al.*, 1995). Again, mechanisms have not been defined. It is likely that for each of these explanations influences on estrogens may be the likely conduit of environmental toxin or stress on puberty as there is an increasing body of evidence demonstrating effects of stress on estrogen systems in adults (e.g., McEwen, 1994).

PSYCHOSOCIAL CORRELATES OF PUBERTY

Perhaps the most pervasive belief about adolescence is that pubertal development results in "raging hormones" that are thought to cause any and all difficulties that youth, parents, and/or teachers may experience. Whereas

this belief may be prevalent, evidence supporting it has not been nearly as pervasive. Rather, behavioral and affective changes at puberty may in part be the result of hormonal changes but are also the result of physical development occurring within a social context (e.g., Brooks-Gunn, Petersen, & Eichorn, 1985; Jones & Mussen, 1958). How girls adapt to puberty or navigate early adolescence is in part associated with the values that friends, family, and society place upon different types and tempos of pubertal development. Just as we have identified three aspects of pubertal development—hormonal changes, status, and timing of puberty—we also examine how each aspect of puberty is associated with adjustment and behavioral changes during early and mid-adolescence. Whereas some of the hormonal studies have included sexual feelings, masturbation, and a range of behaviors, much of this work looks at initiation of intercourse. In fact, the study of sexual behavior in adolescence has focused extensively on intercourse and "problems of sexuality" with little attention to issues such as desire or interest.

Hormonal Effects on Behavior

Models delineating the influence of pubertal development on sexual behavior (and adjustment) outline several potential paths (Brooks-Gunn *et al.*, 1994; Buchanan *et al.*, 1992). The first hypothesis linking puberty to behaviors, emotions, and sexual interest proposes direct effects such that hormonal changes at puberty are thought to result in increased moodiness and potentially poorer mental health as well as interest and engagement in sexual behaviors.

As only a limited number of research groups have actually examined hormone-behavior links, supporting evidence for hormone effects on desire and sexual behavior is not extensive but does exist. Much of this work has considered direct associations of hormones to behavior. However, an underlying assumption is that the effects of hormones on behavior that have been observed were not really direct effects but rather were the result of indirect pathways. For example, hormonal changes at puberty may result in changes in sexual or emotional arousal (Brooks-Gunn *et al.*, 1994; Brooks-Gunn & Warren, 1989; Buchanan *et al.*, 1992; Udry, 1988; Udry, Billy, Morris, Groff, & Raj, 1985); it may be that it is the arousal that subsequently leads to behavioral or affective outcomes. Other research has examined interactive models that incorporate arousal with social controls and consider potential biologically based influences on sexual behavior that may or may not be via hormonal effects on sexual arousal (Udry & Campbell, 1994).

Initial investigations of the hormonal stimulation of sexuality were based on the adult literature, suggesting that testosterone was directly associated with sexual interest or drive in men; that is, men with very low sexual interest increased their sexual activity upon receiving testosterone supplements (Kwan, Greenleaf, Mann, Crapo, & Davidson, 1983). (See Udry and Campbell, 1994, for a review of this literature.) Udry and colleagues (1985) conceptualized adolescents as being in a low testosterone state and expected them to respond to the normatively occurring increase in testosterone with increased sexual activity (across a range of behaviors) until reaching adult hormonal levels.

Initial examinations of this model appeared to find support for direct hormonal effects on sexual behavior at least for boys (Udry *et al.*, 1985). In their cross-sectional study of young adolescent boys, testosterone was positively correlated with engaging in more advanced sexual behaviors (i.e., coital behaviors). However, it was immediately apparent that the same direct link between hormones and behavior was not present for girls (Udry, Talbert, & Morris, 1986). In order to explain the sexual activity of comparably aged girls, the addition of social factors needed to be included in the models. Androgen effects were found on noncoital behaviors such as kissing, but engagement in coital behaviors was better explained by variables tapping social controls. In this case, Udry and colleagues (1986) asserted that girls received greater pressure by parents, friends, and the culture at large to inhibit sexual activity with greater constraints on opportunity for intercourse.

However, subsequent examination of social controls in boys and longitudinal examination of hormone and behavior links suggested that the direct-effect model did not, in fact, apply to boys very well either (Udry & Campbell, 1994). Specifically, Halpern and her colleagues (Halpern, Udry, Campbell, Suchindran, & Mason, 1994) found that the effect of initial testosterone level was moderated by level of attendance at religious services much the way that religious service attendance (Halpern, Udry, & Suchindran, 1997) or social/family controls (Udry *et al.*, 1986) mediated girls' sexual behaviors. Notably, girls in the more recent study by Halpern and her colleagues (1997) were in the advanced stages of puberty when they began the study.

Thus, hormone effects have been mixed and are clearly not direct effects; rather sexual behaviors are best explained via moderated and mediated models. Moreover, desire or sexual arousal in girls has yet to be predicted by hormones at all in these studies. Few studies of hormones and behavior have been conducted with adolescents; furthermore, much of this work, especially with girls, has studied individuals in the advanced or postpubertal years.

Pubertal Status Effects on Behavior

The second way in which puberty may influence behavior during early adolescence is via the changes in status or secondary sexual characteristics. The observable physical changes of puberty may serve as a social stimulus to the adolescent and her peers that the individual is more adultlike. Based on what adolescents view as normative behavior, including sexual behavior, they may engage in behaviors that fit these expectations. It may also be that external signs of puberty are a signal to others of the adolescent's desirability; the more advanced her development, the more interest other youth will have in this individual.

Certainly, pubertal hormones are responsible for the changes in secondary sexual characteristics that are visibly observable to the adolescent and those around her, and it is likely that the experience of development in this social context is linked to behavior (Brooks-Gunn & Reiter, 1990). Menarche is the most commonly investigated pubertal experience even though it is not an event that others notice unless they are told. In general, most girls will have an initial emotional reaction to menarche that may range from excitement, pride, sadness, apprehension, or happiness (Petersen, 1983; Brooks-Gunn & Ruble, 1982). For most girls, initial emotional experiences subside rather quickly. In particular, girls who received adequate information via programs at school and/ or discussions with their mothers seem to have few difficulties with menarche itself. Girls who did not have this type of preparation either because they reached menarche before programs were conducted or before mothers spoke to them about menstruation reported more discomfort with menstruation in general and more negative emotions around menarche (Brooks-Gunn & Ruble, 1982; Rierdan & Koff, 1985).

Other studies of how girls' changes in secondary sexual characteristics are experienced have focused on breast development, although the literature is sparser in this area than for menarche. Also, in contrast with the experience of menarche, breast development is clearly noticeable to those around girls. As such, about half of all girls in the mid-to-later stages of breast development report that they have been teased about this aspect of puberty by peers or family members (Brooks-Gunn, 1984). Little is known about the consequences of the teasing or whether some girls experience more severe forms of teasing than others. Observations made by Peggy Orenstein (1994) in two middle schools in California indicate that some teasing about breast development progresses to sexual harassment with physical aggression (e.g., grabbing a girl's breast in gym class). To date, formal investigation of the frequency and effect of teasing has not been made.

Studies have found that pubertal status was associated with intercourse for both girls and boys, although effects appear to be weaker for boys than for girls (e.g., Flannery, Rowe, & Gulley, 1993). The gender difference is not surprising in that breast development is a highly noticeable pubertal change for girls, whereas the most noticeable change for boys is a growth spurt. In their most recent study of young adolescent girls (beginning at age 13), Udry and Campbell (1994) found that level of pubertal development was associated with sexual activity via what they term an "attractiveness" effect. More advanced sexual behaviors (i.e., coital) did not occur until girls had reached more advanced levels of development, suggesting that physical signs of maturity attract attention from boys and perhaps signal that sexual behavior is more appropriate for someone of this level of development. However, this study examined pubertal status in a sample of girls in the advanced stages of puberty and had very few girls at the beginning of puberty.

Pubertal Timing Effects on Behavior

Previously we discussed cohort and subgroup changes in the timing of the onset of puberty. However, within an age cohort of girls, variations in the timing of pubertal development also exist. In addition, it has been suggested that the timing of puberty may be particularly salient for differentiating who will have difficulties navigating adolescence, and who will initiate or advance in sexual behaviors. In this case, timing of pubertal development refers to going through puberty earlier, at about the same time, or later than one's peers. How individuals cope with and are influenced by puberty depends upon their emotional and cognitive skills when the transition occurs (Brooks-Gunn *et al.*, 1985; Petersen & Taylor, 1980). When looking at adjustment outcomes for girls, several studies have found that early-maturing girls in comparison to on-time and late-maturing girls (and boys) are experiencing difficulties during adolescence (Caspi & Moffitt, 1991; Graber, Brooks-Gunn, Paikoff, & Warren, 1994; Petersen, Sarigiani, & Kennedy, 1991; Simmons & Blyth, 1987; Stattin & Magnusson, 1990). In addition, such reports have demonstrated that the effects are particularly strong at the more severe end of the adjustment spectrum. Specifically, early-maturing girls have higher lifetime prevalence of major depressive disorder, conduct disorder, eating disorders, and suicide attempts in comparison to on-time and late-maturing girls by the time they are in high school (Graber, Lewinsohn, Seeley, & Brooks-Gunn, 1997), as well as concurrent depressive disorders in middle school (Hayward et al., 1997).

In the case of sexual behaviors and feelings, again, the literature has focused almost exclusively on age of first intercourse. Several studies have, in fact, found early maturation effects for both boys and girls such that earlier puberty was associated with earlier initiation of intercourse. In this case, early maturation may result in increased desire and initiation of sexual behaviors, while at the same time early maturers may be poorly prepared to manage these feelings and situations. The result may be poor choices in sexual situations. In particular, early-maturing girls are most at risk for having poor coping strategies and early initiation of sexual behaviors as they mature earlier than any other group of adolescents (Stattin & Magnusson, 1990). In contrast, it has been suggested that late-maturing girls may experience delays in initiation of heterosocial behaviors such as dating (e.g., Simmons & Blyth, 1987). These girls also seem to spend more time on schoolwork (Dubas, Graber, & Petersen, 1991b; Graber et al., 1997), perhaps because they are not going out with boys or mixed-gender groups of adolescents as often as other girls.

It is important to remember when looking at timing effects on sexuality that such effects are also subject to social constraints as described in studies of hormone effects on behavior. That is, early maturation does not necessarily lead to earlier initiation of sexual behaviors. Although some studies have found this association (Zabin & Hayward, 1993), in our own work with upper-middle-class girls, there was no association between age at menarche and age at first intercourse (Graber & Brooks-Gunn, 1996). This is not to say our sample was problem free

or low risk; rather these girls had fairly high rates of subclinical eating problems and co-occurring eating and depressive problems both of which were associated with earlier pubertal maturation (Graber & Brooks-Gunn, 2001; Graber et al., 1994). Thus, in order to understand why pubertal timing is associated with adverse outcomes, experiences of subgroups of girls and of girls in different contexts must be considered.

Processes or mechanisms through which pubertal timing influences girls have begun to amass. Stattin and Magnusson (1990) have found that it was early-maturing girls who associated with older peers (especially older boys) who were more likely to engage in problem behaviors at earlier ages than their peers. Others have found that going through puberty just before making a school change was predictive of having a depressive episode or problems in late adolescence (Petersen et al., 1991; Simmons & Blyth, 1987). Because of the timing of the middle school transition in many districts, this school transition is most likely to overlap with the peak of pubertal development for early-maturing girls. Brooks-Gunn (1991) has also found that girls frequently demonstrated increases in the experience of stressful life events during the pubertal years (ages 12–14); in this study, such co-occurring events—puberty and stressful life events—predicted increases in depressive affect over time. Other contextual factors have also been identified as correlates or moderators of the effects of pubertal timing. For example, Brooks-Gunn and her colleagues have found that links between dating and pubertal timing were not as strong for adolescent girls who were ballet dancers as for other girls (Gargiulo, Attie, Brooks-Gunn, & Warren, 1987). In this case, the salience of another area of life, that is, dancing, was protective against earlier engagement in dating. In addition to the immediate context or environment in which puberty occurs, Caspi and Moffitt (1991) demonstrated that prior behavioral problems may be accentuated by early maturation. In their study, early-maturing girls who did not have prior behavioral problems in middle childhood did not go on to have serious behavioral problems during adolescence. Instead, the girls with the most behavioral problems as adolescents were early-maturing girls who had prior behavioral problems.

These models are a few of the possible explanations for why early maturation may be a risk to healthy development for adolescent girls. As indicated in the study by Caspi and Moffitt (1991), adjustment, coping skills, and biological predispositions existing in middle childhood combine with different types of pubertal transitions and may influence longer-term developmental outcomes. The models described have mostly been used to explain poor mental health or behavior problems. We know very little about how puberty, in general, or pubertal timing, more specifically, influences multiple aspects of sexual behavior and feelings. Rather we have some idea of how puberty influences age of first intercourse and to a much lesser extent initial sexual feelings and explorations. It is still necessary to begin to understand how girls are interpreting physiological arousal and translating it into desires and behaviors (Graber, Brooks-Gunn, & Warren, in press).

PSYCHOLOGICAL SEQUALAE

As noted, aspects of the pubertal transition may have important influences on the mental health and behaviors of adolescent girls during the adolescent decade. In particular, we noted that off-time developers, especially early-maturing girls were experiencing significant psychopathology and may be at risk for early initiation of sexual behaviors. However, despite an increased interest in the lives of adolescents over the past 20–30 years, there is still a dearth of studies that have followed the same children through puberty and adolescence into adulthood. Thus, there are many studies of adolescent girls and many studies of young adult women but little continuity between the two. Unfortunately, some of the studies that followed girls from adolescence into young adulthood did not include pubertal development in the adolescent assessments (e.g., Allen & Hauser, 1996).

Given the severity of problems that may plague early-maturing girls, it is likely that these experiences may have long-term consequences. In our own work, early-maturing girls were likely to have the most persistent or recurrent eating problems although levels tapered off by age 22–23 (Graber et al., 1994). Recent studies have found associations between experiencing a depressive episode in adolescence and the likelihood of having a recurrent episode in young adulthood (Lewinsohn, Rohde, Seeley, Klein, & Gotlib, 2000). As yet, it is not known whether pubertal timing is a factor in this pattern, although early- and late-maturing girls in this sample had higher rates of concurrent depression than on-time maturers when they were in high school; early maturers had higher rates of psychopathology across several domains in this study (Graber et al., 1997).

Stattin and Magnusson (1990) have conducted one of the few studies that followed girls in Sweden from early adolescence into adulthood as far as age 30. Interestingly, this group found moderating effects of peer influence and pubertal timing on alcohol use and sexual behaviors. That is, early maturers who associated with older peers were the most likely to engage in these behaviors at earlier ages. By late adolescence, timing did not differentiate girls on these types of behaviors as it was more normative for all girls to do these things. In adulthood, Stattin and Magnusson (1990) examined the education and career outcomes for this sample. At age 30, women who had been early maturers in puberty had less education and lower level careers than other women. Furthermore, during adolescence, these girls had not differed from one another on school achievement or other indicators of educational ability, yet the early-maturing women had lowered outcomes in adulthood. There were some indications that these women married at earlier ages and this may have been a factor that curtailed their education and subsequent career trajectories.

It may be that girls in this country may enter onto similar trajectories based on findings that link early maturation with early initiation of intercourse. Early initiation has been associated with engagement in sexual risk behaviors. Adult outcomes of adolescent sexual risk behaviors are a bit unclear with the exception of teen pregnancy. Certainly, adolescent girls who have children are at risk for school dropout and hence lowered educational attainment followed by potentially lifelong struggles with poverty and unemployment (Brooks-Gunn & Chase-Lansdale, 1995; Hofferth & Hayes, 1987). Much of this hypothetical pathway has yet to be determined from the existing data. Rather, it seems to be a possible trajectory from early maturation to adult outcomes. It is important to remember that not all studies find links between early pubertal maturation and sexual behavior (e.g., Graber & Brooks-Gunn, 1996). Thus, the social or contextual constraints that protect early-maturing girls from entering this pathway deserve further investigation.

When asking individuals to think about the nature of their pubertal development or their adolescence, it seems that some early adolescents have difficulty making sense of the process. For example, when asking adolescents whether they were early, on-time, or late maturers, reports seem to fluctuate during early adolescence but are more accurate by late adolescence, in comparison to an objective measure of development that is not based on adolescent report (Dubas, Graber, & Petersen, 1991a). Some studies have also found that girls may not divulge that they have reached menarche when asked close to the event but will accurately report after more time has passed (e.g., Petersen, 1983). Thus, in order to illustrate what a few women felt about their development, we have asked an older adolescent/young adult and an adult woman to describe their puberty and how it connected with their adolescent experience. The distance from events is likely to alter how women construct or reconstruct their stories about their adolescence; however, the following brief stories by two women illustrate some of the findings that have been reported in this chapter.

The first report is from a young woman, age 18, who is white and a freshman in college. Based on her age at menarche, she is considered an on-time maturer.

The second report is from an adult woman who is also white and college educated. Based on her age at menarche, she was an early maturer.

Again, while these are only two stories, they seem to illustrate many of the findings seen in the literature. The fact that both individuals are white and middle-class during their childhood and adolescence is in many ways typical of the literature as fewer studies that connect puberty to adjustment or sexuality have been able to look at diversity. More recently, more studies that will be able to address diversity in race/ethnicity and income are under way. In these stories, there are clear differences between the on-time and early maturer in terms of severity of risk behaviors and problems that are identified. However, even the young woman who is on time reports feelings of awkwardness and teasing that seem to be the typical experience of puberty. It is also interesting to hear this woman speak of "raging hormones," highlighting the pervasiveness in the belief in their existence even if data have been less conclusive. While the early maturer may have had a tumultuous adolescence, longer-term outcomes are not apparent from her statements. As she points out, other factors such as intelligence may have been protective for her.

Overall, the field seems to be on the brink of being able to identify more of the underlying processes that place girls at risk during adolescence as well as the long-term outcomes of their adolescent experiences. This is not to say that we do not already know quite a bit. At this point, there is and has been sufficient information to advise parents, teachers, and policymakers on programming that would help adolescent girls navigate this decade of life.

PREVENTION

As the prior section suggests, the entry into adolescence and the pubertal transition

I was 12 when I first got my period and in the middle of seventh grade. I knew exactly what it was when it happened and I remember crying because I knew that it meant I was getting older. My mother assured me that it was a good thing. Of course it became a big topic of conversation with my girl friends, both those who had it already and those who didn't. I was happy that I wasn't the first or the last of my friends to get my period because I would have felt left out either way. We considered it an extremely big deal when someone got it for the first time. I don't really know when it was exactly that I started developing pubic hair or breasts, but I have a feeling it was around fifth and sixth grade. I definitely felt awkward during this stage of my life. Probably this was mostly attributed to my feelings of nonexistence to boys. Looking back on that now, it seems very sad that they had any control over my self-image. Around seventh grade I began to have boyfriends and be friends with boys. This made me feel better about my ever-changing body. I was lucky because I didn't develop too quickly or too slowly. Girls whose breasts were large were constantly made fun of and the same with girls whose breasts were very small. The teasing was mostly generated by the boys who were obviously insecure also. Girls are very catty and fickle around that age because of the raging hormones, and I think that I was probably affected in this way also. I really enjoyed junior high, but there was a lot of pettiness involved in friendships with other girls. I definitely tended to be much more emotional than I am now and my parents received the brunt of that emotion. It was harder to look at the big picture during my adolescent years, and little problems or issues that I had consumed my world. Things that I would now get over extremely quickly would affect me for days. I do think of my adolescence as a very fun period of my life however, despite the internal roller coasters.

may be difficult for some girls. Most girls will have no major difficulties as they navigate this period of development. These girls, however, may have minor bumps along the way as seen in reports of teasing, dips in self-esteem or body image, and/or simply feeling more self-conscious as their bodies change. Whereas these girls would undoubtedly benefit from a range of prevention programming that would help them build skills to address the challenges of adolescence, this group of girls, actually the majority, are not on the pathway to significant health problems.

In contrast, the experiences of two other groups of girls are of more concern. As indicated, some girls are having emotional or behavioral difficulties prior to adolescence. These girls frequently continue on a poor trajectory during adolescence and for some, additional challenges at puberty such as early development

accentuates these difficulties (e.g., Caspi & Moffitt, 1991). Because studies of the psychosocial impact of puberty on development have generally been conducted with adolescents already in middle or junior high school, little is known about how many girls enter puberty on this trajectory. We are presently investigating girls' entry into puberty by following a group of girls from third through sixth grades in order to examine the causes, correlates, and outcomes of this pathway in more depth.

The other group that is of concern, especially from a prevention perspective, consists of those girls who are doing relatively well prior to puberty but find the transition to adolescence very difficult. These girls move from a healthy to an unhealthy trajectory. Unfortunately, it may not be simple to differentiate these girls from the majority of girls who have minor difficulties. That is, if some self-consciousness,

It's funny how well I remember when I got my first period even though I have a hard time remembering the age. It was the Fourth of July weekend the summer between fourth and fifth grades—I guess I was 10. My best friend and I both got our periods that same weekend. I suppose I was really unusual because it was my father who had told me about menstruation about a year before that; I think my mother was relieved that she didn't have to explain much but could just give me "products." I can't say that I thought a lot about my physical development, per se, but I do remember that by sixth and seventh grades I had this intense desire to hang out with older kids, usually older boys. I wanted to DO something and life seemed really boring. My older sister had an older boyfriend and sometimes I could hang out with them. I tried pot for the first time when I was 12. I could usually convince people I was 15 when I was in seventh grade and I started hanging out with other girls who looked older. We would hang out at the beach in the summer and look for boys. I think back on it now and realize how lucky I was that something really bad didn't happen. Sometimes we would go off with older boys and drive around. Often we were drinking or smoking pot. And sometimes I would end up making out with one of these boys. I just wanted a boyfriend, to have some fun, and to be cool. That sounds so ridiculous now but it would be dishonest to deny it. By high school, I sort of wised up. I still smoked pot and drank but I started having steady boyfriends (and sex) but I kept a low profile so my parents assumed I was doing OK. Overall, I was pretty unhappy during the teen years; at times, I guess depressed. I had a hard time fitting in at school even though I got good grades; I was always searching for a group where I belonged. It wasn't until college that I really found my niche. It was around that time that I started to pull it together emotionally. As a child I had a lot of insecurities, and when I think about it now, being so physically mature when I was in junior high school probably combined with the insecurities and that's what caused some of my problems. On the other hand, I think the fact that I was always pretty smart helped me keep my behaviors under control.

moodiness, or poor body image is normative, at what point do minor disturbances become problems? Furthermore, is it possible to identify these girls prior to the development of more serious problems? From the research to date, early pubertal timing appears to be one factor that separates girls who are more likely to develop more serious problems during the entry into adolescence from girls who will experience normative bumps along the road. Of course, other factors need to be identified.

Hypothetically, some girls may have difficulties prior to adolescence and then have improvements during this period. These girls may experience fewer challenges during adolescence, have more supports, or may receive interven-tion that helps them move from an unhealthy to a healthy trajectory. This group, however, is almost never studied and we have little idea how many girls fit this pattern or what factors are associated with this pattern.

Prevention Programming for Girls

One question has been how to move girls from unhealthy developmental trajectories to healthy trajectories or how to keep girls on a healthy track. First, it is often difficult to differentiate girls who will maintain a healthy trajectory from those who will not. Prevention, when a universal approach is used, includes both groups. The following are some examples of programs that have focused on girls during their entry into adolescence. One of these focuses on eating disorders and symptoms, another on exercise, healthy eating, and body image, and others on personal growth and achievement.

As unhealthy eating practices escalate with the entry into adolescence, this has been a target outcome for some projects seeking to improve health for girls. For example, Killen and his colleagues (1993) conducted a large, school-based prevention program with girls in middle school (sixth and seventh grades). Overall, the program did not demonstrate effects; however, it did reduce symptoms in girls who had elevated symptom levels at the pretest assessment. Thus, the targeted approach seemed to work for the subgroup of girls who had already entered an unhealthy pathway for eating problems. In contrast, in a pilot project, we were able to reduce increases in dieting practices in a somewhat younger sample of girls who engaged in informational sessions on puberty and developmental challenge, along with curricula typical for programs targeting eating problems (Schuman, Contento, Graber, & Brooks-Gunn, 1994).

In our own work, we have tried to promote healthy lifestyles by targeting exercise/ activity patterns, healthy eating, and most recently cigarette smoking prevention. Through this work, our goal has been to develop healthy behaviors again while helping girls understand the challenges of adolescence. In a collaborative project with a fitness center, African-American and Latina girls from an urban, public school received an hour of physical activity (e.g., swimming, dance, aerobics) followed by health promotion programming. Girls in seventh and eighth grades received sessions on elements of physical fitness, healthy eating, puberty, body image, and goal setting. Older girls (ninth and tenth grades) received sessions on stress reduction and alternatives to drug, alcohol, and tobacco use. In general, girls responded positively to the sessions, especially those on puberty and body image (Archibald, Harris, Graber, & Brooks-Gunn, 1998). Based on curricula development and preliminary analysis of this project, we have

conducted a pilot study of the appropriateness of "girl" focused curricula in tobacco prevention in a community setting. Process data suggest that girls were particularly engaged in sessions on mood management and stress reduction (Archibald, Cole, Graber, Brooks-Gunn, & Schinke, 2000).

In addition, organizations like Girl Scouts of America, Girls Inc., and others have developed a breadth of programming targeting personal growth and school achievement, and in some cases information sessions on puberty (see *http://www.girlsinc.org* for information on Girls Inc. and *http://www.gsusa.org* for Girl Scouts of America). Unfortunately, these programs more often enroll elementary school girls rather than adolescent girls. Recently, the Ms. Foundation launched an initiative to evaluate programs that specifically targeted adolescent girls mainly focusing on personal growth and development.

There are several issues that are raised by this sampling of programming for girls. One consideration is what age is best for prevention programs. Certainly, early prevention may be desirable especially given the ages at which girls begin puberty. However, programs may be more effective once girls begin to face the other challenges of adolescence such as change to a middle school environment. There is also often a loss of continuity from elementary school to middle school as girls entering middle school are less likely to continue to participate in out of school programs (e.g., Girl Scouts). Furthermore, prevention initiatives have often targeted specific behaviors rather than broader development issues. Although these types of initiatives may prove to be effective for reducing eating problems, alcohol use, or use of tobacco, girls who have difficulties in early adolescence may be at risk for a variety of different problems. The specific pathway that some girls are on may not be addressed by a single initiative.

The programs we described also varied on another dimension: some were school based, whereas others were community based. Younger adolescents are still likely to be enrolled in school, which allows for inclusion of nearly all youth via school-based approaches. In contrast, community-based approaches may be better able to target the needs of specific subgroups of girls or provide programming that schools can not (Roth, Brooks-Gunn, Murray, & Foster, 1998). It should also be noted that while there has been a groundswell in the establishment of community-based or youth development programs, high-quality evaluation research demonstrating if and how programs are effective has been lacking (Roth *et al.*, 1998; Kirby & Coyle, 1997b). Programs working in poorer communities with minimal funding have not had the resources to conduct extensive evaluations. Several private foundations (e.g., Annie E. Casey Foundation, W. T. Grant Foundation, Robert Wood Johnson Foundation and others) have devoted funding to evaluation efforts. Finally, prevention curricula frequently lack a strong connection to developmental theory in content and delivery of programs (Roth & Brooks-Gunn, 2000).

Prevention of Sexual Risk in Girls

In considering how parents, schools, and society are preparing girls for the challenges of puberty, sexuality, and adolescence, more generally, there is a mix of approaches and programs. It should be noted that nearly every school system offers a basic 1–2 hour informational session on puberty and reproduction (e.g., "the film"). In addition, nearly every state in the United States either recommends or requires sexuality education and all 50 states require or recommend HIV/AIDS education programming in schools (Kirby & Coyle, 1997a). Given concerns around teen pregnancy and unhealthy sexual behaviors, there seems to be widespread acceptance of prevention programming. Rather, it is the content of programming that seems to cause the most debates among adults. Thus, district by district, adolescent girls receive very different types of programming to help them manage adolescent transitions effectively.

In the case of sexuality focused programs, two interrelated approaches have been common. One approach targets adolescent sexuality (with a focus on intercourse) as a problem behavior often in isolation from other behaviors and developmental influences. At the same time, models of adolescent risk behavior have considered sexual behavior and its timing as part of a constellation or cluster of behaviors (Irwin & Millstein, 1986; Jessor, 1992). From this perspective, a sexual behavior such as intercourse may not have a specific poor outcome when it is examined out of the context of other behaviors and experiences. Instead, for many adolescents multiple problems seem to group together. Thus, in order to structure prevention programs or health promotion effectively, it is important to understand how behaviors are associated, what leads to these clusters, when these behaviors begin within an adolescent's life (again, the issue of timing of a transition being important), and what are the protective factors that keep adolescents from entering into a lifestyle of unhealthy behaviors that is likely to have serious long-term effects on health (Jessor, 1992).

However, there has been debate about the nature of the co-occurrence of sexual and problem behaviors (e.g., Ensminger, 1990; Stanton *et al.*, 1993). Specifically, sexual behaviors may not cluster with other problem behaviors for subgroups of adolescents, in particular, African-American girls (Stanton *et al.*, 1993). Ensminger (1990) also found that African-American girls whose only "risk" behavior was early intercourse were better off on other dimensions than girls who engaged in early sex and other behaviors.

Despite increased school-based programming for adolescents about sexual and HIV risks, it is often unclear which strategies might best reach those adolescents who have not been responsive to present approaches and for whom programs are most effective (Brooks-Gunn & Paikoff, 1993). In particular, initial work in this area has focused on the prevention of specific outcomes (e.g., pregnancy) rather than on health promotion as a comprehensive endeavor. We have argued that models for understanding health-compromising behaviors may be applicable across several types of behavior (Graber *et al.*, 1998); however, this hypothesis has not been thoroughly tested. Moreover, there are likely to be multiple pathways to sexual risk behaviors.

In a recent review of school-based programs targeting sexual risk behaviors, Kirby and Coyle (1997a) point out that most programs have been fairly focused on the outcomes targeted—promoting abstinence, delaying initiation of intercourse, or increasing contraception use. While focused programs have demonstrated effectiveness at reaching the specific goal, programs that have included broader developmental issues such as puberty, dating, or family relationship changes have not been evaluated to the same extent. Notably, increasing both abstinence and healthy sexual behaviors have been associated with decreasing teen pregnancy (Darroch & Singh, 1999). Kirby and Coyle (1997a) also note that effective programs typically use theoretical or conceptual models that have been employed effectively with other behavioral outcomes. In this case, commonalities included a focus on skill building to meet the challenges of sexual situations and changing group norms for behavior (e.g., Botvin, 1995).

Overall, programming for adolescent girls has either not been specific for girls or not well evaluated. In addition, most school-based health programs are designed for boys and girls rather than one or the other. As such, unique experiences for either group are often not emphasized although other challenges of adolescent development may be included. Thus, it is difficult to determine which approaches work for which outcomes. We have advocated for health promotion programming with girls that includes information on puberty and normative developmental challenges within programs that also build skills that may translate across behavioral outcomes. Of course, programs casting a wider net of outcomes would still need to help girls (and boys) learn information and skills appropriate to specific situations. For example, refusal skills are important in alcohol, tobacco, and drug use prevention as well as delaying intercourse. However, adolescents are likely to need the opportunity to practice skills specific to each context. For example, it is not the same negotiation task for a girl to tell a friend she doesn't want a cigarette (when the friend may not have an investment in whether the girl smokes or not) versus telling her boyfriend she isn't ready to have intercourse. Unfortunately, schools usually set aside curricula time for mandated programs such as drug prevention or sexual risk reduction, but comprehensive programming that is continuous, building skills over time and introducing new topics while rehearsing prior topics are nearly nonexistent. If these programs do exist, they are often established by individual schools with little or no evaluation.

School and community programs are not the only mechanisms through which adolescent girls find supports and build skills for healthy development. Nearly two thirds of youth indicate that they have discussed sex with their parents. For girls, discussions with mothers are most common. In addition, it has been suggested that parent–child communication is one effective method of increasing healthier sexual behaviors, or at least reducing teen pregnancy (Terry & Manlove, 1999). The combination of parental guidance and support with alternative sources of information and developmentally appropriate curricula is likely to be the most effective method for keeping girls on healthy trajectories or moving them onto these pathways.

CONCLUSION

The focus of this chapter has been on the experiences of girls at puberty and the connection of these experiences to health trajectories. In the course of considering prevention, we have highlighted programs for girls. Adolescence is a challenging period for all youth. Certainly, boys face many challenges when they enter adolescence and as they navigate this decade of life; some challenges are the same as those for girls and others are unique. The emphasis on developmental issues for girls and incorporating these concepts into health promotion for girls does not negate the need for similar attention to the developmental experiences of boys and how these factors may set boys on the course for healthy and unhealthy trajectories. While it is important to examine unique experiences, it is equally important not to engage in a girl-versus-boy debate.

In this chapter we have focused on only a few areas of adolescent development. In understanding sexuality, clearly other factors such as same and mixed-gender peer relationships are of great importance. Ultimately, a major challenge for most adolescents will be to find effective ways to regulate their sexual desires, interests, and behaviors, while also finding satisfaction and enjoyment in the interpersonal relationships in which sexuality is expressed. Given that many adults have difficulty with this challenge, the task facing adolescents is daunting. On the other hand, most youth will manage adolescence effectively without experiencing serious health problems. However, the assessment of whether an individual "manages" usually does not include how well they are able to negotiate sexuality but rather whether they negotiated it well enough to avoid pregnancy or sexually transmitted diseases. Perhaps it is time for a more elaborated concept of successful adolescent development and a focus on the breadth of skills that will make this possible for more, if not all, youth.

ACKNOWLEDGMENTS. The authors were supported by grants from the National Institute of Mental Health (MH56557) and the National Institute of Child Health and Human Development (HD32376).

REFERENCES

Adams, G. R., Montemayor, R., & Gullotta T. (Eds.) (1989–2000) *Advances in adolescent development*: Vols. 1–7. Newbury Park, CA: Sage.

Alan Guttmacher Institute (1994). *Sex and America's teenagers*. New York: Author.

Allen, J. P., & Hauser, S. T. (1996). Autonomy and relatedness in adolescent-family interactions as predictors of young adults' states of mind regarding attachment. *Development & Psychopathology, 8,* 793–809.

Arnett, J. J. (2000). Emerging adulthood: A theory of development from the late teens through the twenties. *American Psychologist, 55,* 469–480.

Archibald, A. B., Cole, K., Graber, J. A., Brooks-Gunn, J., & Schinke, S. (2000). *Girls and smoking: Curriculum manual.* New York: School of Social Work, Columbia University.

Archibald, A. B., Harris, J., Graber, J. A., & Brooks-Gunn, J. (1998). *Building better bodies: Curriculum manual.* New York: Asphalt Green.

Biro, F. M., Lucky, A. W., Huster, G. A., & Morrison, J. A. (1995). Pubertal staging in boys. *Journal of Pediatrics, 127,* 100–102.

Botvin, G. J. (1995). School-based health promotion: Substance abuse and sexual behavior. *Applied and Preventive Psychology, 4*(3), 167–184.

Brooks-Gunn, J. (1984). The psychological significance of different pubertal events to young girls. *Journal of Early Adolescence, 4,* 315–327.

Brooks-Gunn, J. (1991). How stressful is the transition to adolescence for girls? In M. E. Colten & S. Gore (Eds.), *Adolescent stress: Causes and consequences* (pp. 131–149). Hawthorne, NY: Aldine de Gruyter.

Brooks-Gunn, J., & Chase-Lansdale, P. L. (1995). Adolescent parenthood. In M. H. Bornstein (Ed.), *Handbook of parenting: Vol. 3. Status and social conditions of parenting* (pp. 113–149). Mahwah, NJ: Erlbaum.

Brooks-Gunn, J., Graber, J. A., & Paikoff, R. L. (1994). Studying links between hormones and negative affect: Models and measures. *Journal of Research on Adolescence, 4*(4), 469–486.

Brooks-Gunn, J., & Paikoff, R. L. (1997). Sexuality and developmental transitions during adolescence. In J. Schulenberg, J. Maggs, & K. Hurrelmann (Eds.), *Health risks and developmental transitions during adolescence* (pp. 190–219). New York: Cambridge University Press.

Brooks-Gunn, J., & Paikoff, R. L. (1993). "Sex is a gamble, kissing is a game": Adolescent sexuality and health promotion. In S. G. Millstein, A. C. Petersen, & E. O. Nightingale (Eds.), *Promoting the health of adolescents: New directions for the twenty-first century* (pp. 180–208). New York: Oxford University Press.

Brooks-Gunn, J., & Petersen, A. C. (Eds.) (1983). *Girls at puberty: Biological and psychosocial perspectives.* New York: Plenum Press.

Brooks-Gunn, J., Petersen, A. C., & Eichorn, D. (1985). The study of maturational timing effects in adolescence. *Journal of Youth and Adolescence, 14*(3), 149–161.

Brooks-Gunn, J., & Reiter, E. O. (1990). The role of pubertal processes. In S. Feldman & G. Elliott (Eds.), *At the threshold: The developing adolescent* (pp. 16–53). Cambridge, MA: Harvard University Press.

Brooks-Gunn, J., & Ruble, D. N. (1982). Developmental processes in the experience of menarche. In A. Baum & J. E. Singer (Eds.), *Handbook of psychology and health* (Vol. 2, pp. 117–147). Hillsdale, NJ: Erlbaum.

Brooks-Gunn, J., & Warren, M. P. (1988). Mother-daughter differences in menarcheal age in adolescent girls attending national dance company schools and nondancers. *Annals of Human Biology, 15*(1), 35–43.

Brooks-Gunn, J., & Warren, M. P. (1989). Biological contributions to affective expression in young adolescent girls. *Child Development, 60*, 372–385.

Buchanan, C. M., Eccles, J. S., & Becker, J. B. (1992). Are adolescents the victims of raging hormones? Evidence for activational effects of hormones on moods and behavior at adolescence. *Psychological Bulletin, 111*, 62–107.

Carnegie Council on Adolescent Development. (1996). *Great transitions: Preparing adolescents for a new century.* New York: Carnegie Corporation.

Caspi, A., & Moffitt, T. E. (1991). Individual differences are accentuated during periods of social change: The sample case of girls at puberty. *Journal of Personality and Social Psychology, 61*, 157–168.

Clayton, P. E., & Trueman, J. A. (2000). Leptin and puberty. *Archives of Disease in Childhood, 83*, 1–4.

Coles, R., & Stokes, G. (1995). *Sex and the American teenager.* New York: Harper & Rowe.

Darroch, J. E., & Singh, S. (1999). Why is teenage pregnancy declining? The roles of abstinence, sexual activity, and contraceptive use. *Occasional report, No. 1.* New York: The Alan Guttmacher Institute.

Dubas, J. S., Graber, J. A., & Petersen, A. C. (1991a). A longitudinal investigation of adolescents' changing perceptions of pubertal timing. *Developmental Psychology, 27*, 580–586.

Dubas, J. S., Graber, J. A., & Petersen, A. C. (1991b). The effects of pubertal development on achievement during adolescence. *American Journal of Education, 99*, 444–460.

Ensminger, M. E. (1990). Sexual activity and problem behaviors among Black, urban adolescents. *Child Development, 61*(6), 2032–2046.

Feldman, S., & Elliott, G. (Eds.) (1990). *At the threshold: The developing adolescent.* Cambridge, MA: Harvard University Press.

Feldman, S. S., Turner, R. A., & Araujo, K. (1999). Interpersonal context as an influence on sexual timetables of youths: Gender and ethnic effects. *Journal of Research on Adolescence, 9*, 25–52.

Flannery, D. J., Rowe, D. C., & Gulley, B. L. (1993). Impact of pubertal status, timing, and age on adolescent sexual experience and delinquency. *Journal of Adolescent Research, 8*, 21–40.

Furman, W., & Simon, V. A. (1999). Cognitive representations of adolescent romantic relationships. In W. Furman, B. B. Brown, & C. Feiring (Eds.), *Contemporary perspectives on adolescent relationships* (pp. 75–98). New York: Cambridge University Press.

Gargiulo, J., Attie, I., Brooks-Gunn, J., & Warren, M. P. (1987). Girls' dating behavior as a function of social context and maturation. *Developmental Psychology, 23*, 730–737.

Gladen, B. C., Ragan, N. B., & Rogan, W. J. (2000). Pubertal growth and development and prenatal and lactational exposure to polychlorinated biphenyls and dichlorodiphenyl dichloroethene. *Journal of Pediatrics, 136*, 490–496.

Graber, J. A., Britto, P. R., & Brooks-Gunn, J. (1999). What's love got to do with it? Adolescents' and young adults' beliefs about sexual and romantic relationships. In W. Furman, B. B. Brown, & C. Feiring (Eds.), *Contemporary perspectives on adolescent relationships* (pp. 364–395). New York: Cambridge University Press.

Graber, J. A., & Brooks-Gunn, J. (1996). Reproductive transitions: The experience of mothers and daughters. In C. D. Ryff & M. M. Seltzer (Eds.), *The parental experience in midlife* (pp. 255–299). Chicago: University of Chicago Press.

Graber, J. A., & Brooks-Gunn, J. (2001). Co-occurring eating and depressive problems: An 8-year study of adolescent girls. *International Journal of Eating Disorders, 30*, 37–47.

Graber, J. A., Brooks-Gunn, J., & Galen, B. R. (1998). Betwixt and between: Sexuality in the context of adolescent transitions. In R. Jessor (Ed.), *New perspectives on adolescent risk behavior* (pp. 270–316). New York: Cambridge University Press.

Graber, J. A., Brooks-Gunn, J., & Petersen, A. C. (Eds.) (1996). *Transitions through adolescence: Interpersonal domains and context.* Mahwah, NJ: Erlbaum.

Graber, J. A., Brooks-Gunn, J., Paikoff, R. L., & Warren, M. P. (1994). Prediction of eating problems: An eight year study of adolescent girls. *Developmental Psychology, 30*, 823–834.

Graber, J. A., Brooks-Gunn, J, & Warren, M. P. (1995). The antecedents of menarcheal age: Heredity, family environment, and stressful life events. *Child Development, 66*, 346–359.

Graber, J. A., Brooks-Gunn, J., & Warren, M. P. (in press). Pubertal effects on adjustment in girls: Moving from demonstrating effects to identifying pathways. *Journal of Youth & Adolescence.*

Graber, J. A., Lewinsohn, P. M., Seeley, J. R., & Brooks-Gunn, J. (1997). Is psychopathology associated with the timing of pubertal development? *Journal of the American Academy of Child and Adolescent Psychiatry, 36*, 1768–1776.

Grumbach, M. M., & Styne, D. M. (1998). Puberty: Ontogeny, neuroendocrinology, physiology, and disorders. In J. D. Wilson, D. W. Fostor, & H. M. Kronenberg (Eds.), *Williams textbook of endocrinology* (pp. 1509–1625). Philadelphia: W. B. Saunders.

Halpern, C. T., Udry, J. R., Campbell, B., Suchindran, C., & Mason, G. A. (1994). Testosterone and religiosity as predictors of sexual attitudes and activity among adolescent males: A biosocial model. *Journal of Biosocial Science, 26*, 217–234.

Halpern, C. T., Udry, J. R., & Suchindran, C. (1997). Testosterone predicts initiation of coitus in adolescent females. *Psychosomatic Medicine, 59*, 161–171.

Hayward, C., Killen, J. D., Wilson, D. M., Hammer, L. D., Litt, I. F., Kraemer, H. C., Haydel, F., Varady, A., Taylor, C. B. (1997). Psychiatric risk associated with early puberty in adolescent girls. *Journal of the Ameri-*

can Academy of Child & Adolescent Psychiatry, 36, 255–262.

Herman-Giddens, M. E., Slora, E. J., Wasserman, R. C., Bourdony, C. J., Bhapkar, M. V., Koch, G. G., & Hasemeier, C. M. (1997). Secondary sexual characteristics and menses in young girls seen in office practice: A study of pediatric research in office settings network. Pediatrics, 99, 505–512.

Hofferth, S. L., & Hayes, C. D. (Eds.) (1987). Risking the future: Adolescent sexuality, pregnancy and childbearing, Vol. 2. Washington, DC: National Academy Press.

Horlick, M. B., Rosenbaum, M., Nicolson, M., Levine, L. S., Fedun, B., Wang, J., Pierson, R. N., Jr., & Leibel, R. L. (2000). Effect of puberty on the relationship between circulating leptin and body composition. Journal of Clinical Endocrinology & Metabolism, 85, 2509–2518.

Irwin, C. E., & Millstein, S. G. (1986). Biopsychosocial correlates of risk-taking behaviors during adolescence: Can the physician intervene? Journal of Adolescent Health Care, 7 (6, supplement), 82–96.

Jessor, R. (1992). Risk behavior in adolescence: A psychosocial framework for understanding and action. In D. E. Rogers & E. Ginzberg (Eds.), Adolescents at risk: Medical and social perspectives (pp. 19–34). Boulder, CO: Westview.

Jones, M. C., & Mussen, P. H. (1958). Self-conceptions, motivations, and interpersonal attitudes of early- and late-maturing girls. Child Development, 29, 491–501.

Katchadourian, H. (1990). Sexuality. In S. Feldman & G. Elliott (Eds.), At the threshold: The developing adolescent (pp. 330–351). Cambridge, MA: Harvard University Press.

Kaplowitz, P. B., Oberfield, S. E., & The Drug and Therapeutics and Executive Committees of the Lawson Wilkins Pediatric Endocrine Society. (1999). Reexamination of the age limit for defining when puberty is precocious in girls in the United States: Implications for evaluation and treatment. Pediatrics, 104, 936–941.

Killen, J. D., Taylor, C. B., Hammer, L. D., Litt, I., Wilson, D. M., Rich, T., Hayward, C., Simmonds, B., Kraemer, H., & Varady, A. (1993). An attempt to modify unhealthful eating attitudes and weight regulation practices of young adolescent girls. International Journal of Eating Disorders, 13, 369–384.

Kirby, D., & Coyle, K. (1997a). School-based programs to reduce sexual risk-taking behavior. Children & Youth Services Review, 19, 415–436.

Kirby, D., & Coyle, K. (1997b). Youth development programs. Children & Youth Services Review, 19, 437–454.

Kwan, M., Greenleaf, W. J., Mann, J., Crapo, L., & Davidson, J. M. (1983). The nature of androgen action on male sexuality: A combined laboratory and self-report study in hypogonadal men. Journal of Clinical Endocrinology and Metabolism, 57, 557–562.

Lewinsohn, P. M., Rohde, P., Seeley, J. R., Klein, D. N., & Gotlib, I. H. (2000). Natural course of adolescent Major Depressive Disorder in a community sample: Predictors of recurrence in young adults. American Journal of Psychiatry, 157, 1584–1591.

Lugaila, T. A. (1998). Marital status and living arrangements: March 1998 (Update). Current Population Reports. (U.S. Bureau of the Census Publication No. P20-514.) Washington, DC: U.S. Department of Commerce.

Marshall, W. A., & Tanner, J. M. (1969). Variations in the pattern of pubertal changes in girls. Archives of Disease in Childhood, 44, 291–303.

Marshall, W. A., & Tanner, J. M. (1986). Puberty. In F. Falkner & J. M. Tanner (Eds.), Human growth: Vol. 2, Postnatal growth neurobiology (pp. 171–209). New York: Plenum.

McEwen, B. S. (1994). How do sex and stress hormones affect nerve cells? Annals of the New York Academy of Sciences, 743, 1–18.

Modell, J., & Goodman, M. (1990). Historical perspectives. In S. Feldman & G. Elliott (Eds.), At the threshold: The developing adolescent (pp. 93–122). Cambridge, MA: Harvard University Press.

Moffitt, T. E., Caspi, A., Belsky, J., & Silva, P. A. (1992). Childhood experience and the onset of menarche: A test of a sociobiological model. Child Development, 63, 47–58.

National Center for Health Statistics (1997). Fertility, family planning and women's health: New data from the 1995 National Survey of Family Growth (DHHS Publication No. (PHS) 97-1995.) Hyattsville, MD: U.S. Department of Health and Human Services.

The National Heart, Lung, and Blood Institute Growth and Health Study Research Group. (1992). Obesity and cardiovascular disease risk factors in black and white girls: The NHLBI growth and health study. American Journal of Public Health, 82, 1613–1620.

Obeidallah, D. A., Brennan, R., Brooks-Gunn, J., Kindlon, D., & Earls, F. E. (2000). Socioeconomic status, race, and girls' pubertal maturation: Results from the Project on Human Development in Chicago Neighborhoods. Journal of Research on Adolescence, 10, 443–464.

Oliver, M. B., & Hyde, J. S. (1993). Gender differences in sexuality: A meta-analysis. Psychological Bulletin, 114 (1), 29–51.

Orenstein, P. (1994). School Girls: Young women, self-esteem, and the confidence gap. New York: Doubleday.

Persson, I., Ahlsson, F., Ewald, U., Tuvemo, T., Qingyuan, M., von Rosen, D., & Proos, L. (1999). Influence of perinatal factors on the onset of puberty in boys and girls: Implications for interpretation of link with risk of long term diseases. American Journal of Epidemiology, 150, 747–755.

Petersen, A. C. (1983). Menarche: Meaning of measures and measuring meaning. In S. Golub (Ed.), Menarche: The transition from girl to woman (pp. 63–76). Lexington, MA: Lexington Books.

Petersen, A. C., Sarigiani, P. A., & Kennedy, R. E. (1991). Adolescent depression: Why more girls? Journal of Youth and Adolescence, 20, 247–271.

Petersen, A. C., & Taylor, B. (1980). The biological approach to adolescence: Biological change and psychological adaptation. In J. Adelson (Ed.), *Handbook of adolescent psychology* (pp. 117–155). New York: Wiley.

Reiter, E. O., & Grumbach, M. M. (1982). Neuroendocrine control mechanisms and the onset of puberty. *Annual Review of Physiology*, *44*, 595–613.

Rierdan, J., & Koff, E. (1985). Timing of menarche and initial menstrual experience. *Journal of Youth and Adolescence*, *14*, 237–244.

Roth, J., & Brooks-Gunn, J. (2000). What do adolescents need for healthy development?: Implications for youth policy. *Social Policy Report*, *14*(1). Ann Arbor, MI: Society for Research in Child Development.

Roth, J., Brooks-Gunn, J., Murray, L., & Foster, W. (1998). Promoting healthy adolescents: Synthesis of youth development program evaluations. *Journal of Research on Adolescence*, *8*(4), 423–459.

Savin-Williams, R. C. (1995). An exploratory study of pubertal maturation timing and self-esteem among gay and bisexual male youths. *Developmental Psychology*, *31*(1), 56–64.

Schlegel, A., & Barry, H. III. (1991). *Adolescence: An anthropological inquiry*. New York: Free Press.

Schuman, M., Contento, I., Graber, J. A., & Brooks-Gunn, J. (1994). *Eating disorder prevention in adolescent girls*. Paper presented at the annual meeting of the Society for Nutrition Education.

Simmons, R. G., & Blyth, D. A. (1987). *Moving into adolescence: The impact of pubertal change and school context*. New York: Aldine.

Smith, E. A., & Udry, J. R. (1985). Coital and non-coital sexual behaviors of white and black adolescents. *American Journal of Public Health*, *75*, 1200–1203.

Spreadbury, C. L. (1982). First date. *Journal of Early Adolescence*, *2*(1), 83–89.

Stanton, B., Romer, D., Ricardo, I., Black, M., Feigelman, S., & Galbraith, J. (1993). Early initiation of sex and its lack of association with risk behaviors among adolescent African-Americans. *Pediatrics*, *92*(1), 13–19.

Stattin, H., & Magnusson, D. (1990). *Paths through life: Vol. 2. Pubertal maturation in female development*. Hillsdale, NJ: Erlbaum.

Surbey, M. K. (1990). Family composition, stress, and the timing of human menarche. In T. E. Ziegler & F. B. Bercovitch (Eds.), *Socioendocrinology of primate reproduction* (pp. 11–32). New York: Wiley.

Susman, E. J., Dorn, L. D., & Chrousos, G. P. (1991). Negative affect and hormone levels in young adolescents: Concurrent and predictive perspectives. *Journal of Youth and Adolescence*, *20*, 167–190.

Tanner, J. M. (1962). *Growth at adolescence*. New York: Lippincott.

Terry, E., & Manlove, J. (1999). Trends in sexual activity and contraceptive use among teens. *Child trends research briefs*. Washington, DC: Child Trends. Retrieved November 9, 2000, from the World Wide Web: http://www.childtrends.org/PDF/teentrends.pdf

Tyrka, A. R., Graber, J. A., & Brooks-Gunn, J. (2000). The development of disordered eating: Correlates and predictors of eating problems in the context of adolescence. In A. J. Sameroff, M. Lewis, & S. M. Miller (Eds.), *Handbook of developmental psychopathology*, 2nd ed. (pp. 607–624). New York: Plenum.

Udry, J. R. (1988). Biological predispositions and social control in adolescent sexual behavior. *American Sociological Review*, *53*, 709–722.

Udry, J. R., Billy, J. O. G., Morris, N. M., Groff, T. R., & Raj, M. H. (1985). Serum androgenic hormones motivate sexual behavior in boys. *Fertility and Sterility*, *43*, 90–94.

Udry, J. R., & Campbell, B. C. (1994). Getting started on sexual behavior. In A. S. Rossi (Ed.), *Sexuality across the life course. The John D. and Catherine T. MacArthur Foundation series on mental health and development: Studies on successful midlife development* (pp. 187–207). Chicago: University of Chicago Press.

Udry, J. R., Talbert, L., & Morris, N. M. (1986). Biosocial foundations of adolescent female sexuality. Paper presented at the annual meeting of the American Sociological Association, Washington, D.C.

Warren, M. P. (1983). Physical and biological aspects of puberty. In J. Brooks-Gunn & A. C. Petersen (Eds.), *Girls at puberty: Biological and psychosocial perspectives* (pp. 3–28). New York: Plenum.

Westney, O. E., Jenkins, R. R., & Benjamin, C. A. (1983). Sociosexual development of preadolescents. In J. Brooks-Gunn & A. C. Petersen (Eds.), *Girls at puberty: Biological and psychosocial perspectives* (pp. 273–300). New York: Plenum.

Zabin, L. S., & Hayward, S. C. (1993). *Adolescent sexual behavior and childbearing*. Newbury Park, CA: Sage.

Zacharias, L., & Wurtman, R. J. (1969). Age at menarche: Genetic and environmental influences. *New England Journal of Medicine*, *280*, 868–875.

4

The Social Organization of Women's Sexuality

EDWARD O. LAUMANN and JENNA MAHAY

INTRODUCTION

Women's sexual behavior, while typically thought of as a matter of personal and individual choice, is fundamentally organized by social factors. This chapter examines how selected social factors, including religious preference, racial or ethnic group membership, and educational attainment, as well as age and marital status, shape women's sexual desires, sexual partnerships, sexual acts, and subjective understanding of these facets of sexual experiences. While fully acknowledging the significance of biological factors in sexuality, we shall stress in this chapter the role social groups and contexts play in shaping women's sexual conduct through their impact on the production and enforcement of socially constructed and shared conceptions of appropriate sexual behavior.

Some of the questions we want to explore include the following: How do education and racial/ethnic group membership shape women's sexual practices? How do single women's sexual

experiences differ from those of women in long-term, committed marital relationships? What are the trends in women's sexual practices and experiences over time, and has women's sexual behavior changed in response to the HIV/AIDS epidemic? In light of women's greater involvement in religious matters (in comparison to men), what impact does religious affiliation have on women's attitudes toward sexuality, actual sexual practices, and even sexual preferences? Furthermore, in general, we shall demonstrate how the gender categories themselves exert perhaps the most powerful influence on women's sexual behavior.

Because public attention and efforts at social control have always been more focused on women's sexuality than on men's (Nathanson, 1991), gender centrally organizes almost all aspects of sexual behavior and crosscuts all the other social categories. Not only do women and men engage in different sexual behaviors, they also experience sexual practices differently and understand their actions often from contrasting normative positions. Distinctive gendered perspectives may in part be rooted in biological differences between women and men, but they in large measure also arise from particular cultural assumptions about the meaning of being female or being male that guide sexual conduct in everyday settings. Gender is thus both an outcome and a determinant of sexual experi-

EDWARD O. LAUMANN and JENNA MAHAY • Department of Sociology, University of Chicago, Chicago, Illinois 60637.

Handbook of Women's Sexual and Reproductive Health, edited by Wingood and DiClemente. Kluwer Academic / Plenum Publishers, New York, 2002.

ence. Although the focus of this chapter is on how women's sexuality is socially organized in the United States, most of the tables include men for comparative purposes since women's sexual practices and experiences often take on meaning only in relation to men's, and vice versa.

This chapter first examines women's sexual desire, as reflected in their sexual preferences and objects of erotic attraction. We then analyze women's actual sexual behavior, from the formative experiences of first sex to current adult practices, including masturbation, number of partners, frequency and duration of sex, oral and anal sex, and orgasm. Finally, we examine women's normative orientations toward sexuality. In the past, most of the studies of women's sexuality have drawn their data from rich descriptions of female patients in clinics or other laboratories (cf. Goldman & Milman, 1969; Kaplan, 1995; Masters & Johnson, 1966). Other studies have collected information using in-depth interviews or discussion groups with volunteers and have a limited number of respondents (cf. Blumstein & Schwartz, 1985; Fisher, 1973; Maltz & Boss, 1997; Rubin, 1982; Sterk-Elifson, 1994; Wyatt, 1982, 1993). These types of studies, while they reveal a great deal about particular women, draw their data from a sample that is highly selective and biased and thus not representative of the general population of women. Even many of the larger surveys that have been conducted did not use probability sampling, but instead recruited respondents in selective ways (Hite, 1979; Kinsey *et al.*, 1953). For example, the famous Hite Report on female sexuality distributed questionnaires through certain magazines and had only a 3% response rate (Hite, 1979). In such studies, the lack of probability sampling in such studies means that they cannot generalize from their sample to the rest of the population. These studies can tell us little about the sexual behavior of women in the general population.

It was in large part with the objective of providing some baseline knowledge about sexual attitudes, behaviors, and experiences of the population at large that the National Health and Social Life Survey (NHSLS) was conducted. The NHSLS is a nationally representative sample of 1749 women and 1410 men aged 18 to 59 living in noninstitutional households throughout the United States in 1992, and included an oversample of racial and ethnic minorities to allow for comparison. The sample completion rate was greater than 78%, with no notable sampling biases. The interviews were conducted in person, each lasting about 90 minutes, and included a self-administered section for especially sensitive topics such as forced sex, same-gender sex, and extramarital affairs.* This chapter examines the social organization of women's sexuality both through new analyses of the NHSLS and using the findings regarding women's sexuality from *The Social Organization of Sexuality* (Laumann, Gagnon, Michael, & Michaels, 1994), which first reported the results of this survey.

WOMEN'S SEXUAL DESIRE

Sexual desire, often considered one of the most basic biological "drives," is fundamentally shaped by social context. We all must learn what to regard or understand as being sexual or nonsexual. What some people see as sexually appealing or erotic, others find repulsive or a "turnoff." Cultural factors not only influence one's sexual fantasies but also prescribe the sequence of acts, postures, objects, and gestures that elicit and sustain sexual arousal (Simon & Gagnon, 1987). Cultural conceptions of gender exert such powerful influences on sexual desire that women in the United States are usually regarded as having a lower "sex drive" than men, and this expectation may frame women's own desire in reference to men.

Gender also organizes attraction to and choice of sexual partners so that the majority of women are attracted to and choose partners of the "opposite" sex. Those who do not conform to this heterosexual standard are subject to ex-

*For more detail on the survey design and methodology, see Laumann, Gagnon, Michael, & Michaels (1994).

pressions of social disapproval. This section will examine women's sexual preferences and fantasies first, and then examine women's sexual attraction to others, their choice of partners, and their sexual identity.

Sexual Preferences

The NHSLS included a number of questions about sexual preferences, which fall into three general categories. First, we consider preferences for particular sexual techniques, such as vaginal, oral, and anal sex, as well as manual stimulation of the anus and the use of vibrators. Second, we inquire into preferences for certain types of visual stimulation, including watching a partner undress or seeing other people engage in sexual acts. Finally, we examine the appeal of different types of sexual partners or sexual relationships: same-gender sex, sex with a stranger, or group sex. Respondents were asked whether they found the above sexual practices "very," "somewhat," "not," or "not at all" appealing. Overall, women report finding only an average of 1.64 of these practices very appealing, compared with an average of 2.57 practices for men. One possible reason for this may be that women have more interest in acts such as hugging, kissing, and body stroking that were not included in this survey.* In addition, "very appealing" may set too high a threshold of "appeal" for women, given the cultural conception of women having lower sex drives than men, which may, in turn, influence the way that women think about or represent their own sexuality. Thus, Table 1 reports the percentage of

women who found each sexual practice either "very" or "somewhat" appealing.

In terms of sexual acts, vaginal intercourse was the most commonly appealing for women, with about 95% finding it at least somewhat appealing (although only 77% of women found it "very" appealing). This percentage drops slightly, however, for women between the ages of 55 and 59, of whom about 90% find vaginal intercourse at least somewhat appealing, and only 67% find it very appealing. This may be a result of either declining interest or a reflection of the desexualization of older women in our culture, which affects not only how others view older women but also how older women view their own sexuality. It must be kept in mind that preferences for sexual acts may also be affected by whether the respondent is in a long-term, satisfying relationship. For example, married and cohabiting women were the most likely to find vaginal intercourse appealing (98% and 96%, respectively), while never-married, noncohabiting women were the least likely to find vaginal intercourse appealing (88%).

The other sexual acts that substantial percentages of women found appealing were watching their partner undress and oral sex. Approximately 77% of women found watching their partner undress appealing, 61% found cunnilingus appealing, and 50% found fellatio appealing. Thus, on average, women were less likely to find giving oral sex appealing as receiving it. It is also important to note in terms of the negotiation of sexual practices between women and men that women were much less likely than men to find either giving or receiving oral sex appealing.

Women's interest in oral sex and watching their partner undress increased from their early twenties to their late twenties and then gradually declined with age. Interest in oral sex is especially low among women in their fifties. This may be due to both a cohort and a period effect. Older women may not find these sexual practices appealing either because they have lost interest or because they came of sexual age before the so-called Sexual Revolution of the

*Pilot interviews with several hundred subjects that were conducted in developing the interview schedule for the NHSLS revealed that "hugging" and "kissing" were so universally appealing to both men and women (with 85% or more reporting these activities appealing) that it was decided not to include them in the list of sexual practices because variation in appeal was likely to be so limited that it would not provide useful discriminating information across different statuses. It is certainly true, however, that there is still the possibility of gender bias in the list of practices because, among other things, auditory contexts involving music and singing were excluded and these might elicit differential gender responses.

TABLE 1. The Social Organization of Sexual Preferences (Percentage Who Found Selected Practices "Very" or "Somewhat" Appealing)

Social characteristics	Vaginal intercourse		Watching partner undress		Receiving oral sex		Giving oral sex		Anus stimulated by partner's finger		Watching other people do sexual things	
	Women	Men	Women	Men	Women	Men	Women	Men	Women	Men	Women	Men
Total population	94.9	95.2	77.2	91.6	60.7	77.4	49.9	71.0	18.0	20.6	17.7	37.5
Age												
18–24	94.6	93.8	79.4	93.3	66.4	82.7	50.7	70.7	15.3	17.0	16.3	35.6
25–29	96.1	94.6	83.3	93.3	73.4	84.7	64.7	81.0	18.1	19.4	20.5	41.7
30–34	95.5	92.8	82.2	89.3	71.1	81.6	60.6	76.7	17.4	19.8	18.6	38.9
35–39	96.2	98.0	80.2	94.6	67.7	84.0	56.5	76.5	21.5	23.3	22.7	40.4
40–44	95.6	97.3	78.2	94.0	59.4	79.7	51.1	75.3	17.5	31.9	18.8	44.6
45–49	94.0	94.2	76.1	90.7	54.5	71.0	43.7	64.5	21.0	18.7	18.0	30.0
50–54	94.3	96.3	58.9	82.6	36.7	54.6	27.3	51.4	18.7	13.8	13.5	33.9
55–59	89.9	95.6	64.7	89.0	27.0	52.8	16.8	45.1	13.9	16.5	6.5	22.8
Marital status												
Never married, not cohabiting	87.5	89.8	74.9	90.1	58.7	79.2	45.3	69.2	13.7	19.5	19.4	39.4
Never married, cohabiting	95.8	93.3	82.2	93.3	75.3	90.0	61.6	86.7	13.7	26.7	16.4	50.8
Married	98.1	98.0	78.2	91.5	60.5	75.1	50.9	70.9	17.7	20.3	17.6	36.5
Divorced/separated/widowed, not cohabiting	92.9	97.0	76.6	94.5	60.7	75.6	48.4	68.3	22.1	21.3	15.2	30.9
Divorced/separated/widowed, cohabiting	96.4	94.7	76.8	94.7	58.9	86.5	53.6	75.7	26.8	21.1	23.2	44.7

Education												
Less than high school	89.3	88.8	66.4	82.5	37.9	55.9	26.3	48.4	14.8	13.9	9.0	28.0
High school graduate or equivalent	94.5	95.3	74.7	90.6	57.1	73.0	44.1	67.8	18.5	19.4	14.1	32.0
Some college/vocational school	96.1	96.0	79.3	93.7	67.4	83.8	56.9	76.1	18.8	24.0	20.6	37.4
Finished college	97.8	97.5	86.0	94.5	69.7	87.7	61.4	81.8	15.9	18.6	21.4	51.1
Master's/advanced degree	96.3	97.5	78.7	95.0	69.8	81.5	62.3	77.3	23.6	26.9	28.4	45.8
Religion												
None	95.4	92.3	80.1	88.7	76.8	83.5	68.2	76.8	22.3	25.3	29.1	47.9
Type I Protestant[a]	95.7	96.3	81.6	94.1	63.0	81.3	53.6	75.4	18.0	22.3	17.5	39.3
Type II Protestant	94.5	96.1	74.4	91.1	52.0	67.0	38.7	58.9	17.9	17.5	13.7	30.8
Catholic	94.9	95.4	76.9	91.2	64.1	81.9	54.0	77.0	16.7	18.8	19.0	37.9
Jewish	*	*	*	*	*	*	*	*	*	*	*	*
Other	86.1	90.0	70.3	92.5	61.1	75.0	50.0	75.0	19.4	30.0	16.2	36.6
Race/ethnicity												
White	95.9	95.8	79.1	93.2	64.9	82.2	55.4	76.9	18.9	21.5	19.4	39.1
Black	92.9	93.0	70.3	84.6	40.1	55.1	24.4	39.7	14.5	16.0	13.6	29.9
Hispanic	92.5	93.1	75.2	88.2	62.1	68.3	48.5	59.0	17.4	17.8	11.3	34.0
Asian	86.7	94.1	58.6	82.4	43.3	70.6	43.3	73.5	*	26.5	20.0	35.3
Native American	*	*	*	*	*	*	*	*	*	*	*	*
N	1730	1396	1733	1398	1728	1391	1727	1391	1726	1393	1742	1404

(continued)

TABLE 1. (*Continued*)

Social characteristics	Using a dildo or vibrator		Stimulate partner's anus		Sex with a stranger		Group sex		Same-gender partner		Anal sex (passive)	
	Women	Men	Women	Men	Women	Men	Women	Men	Women	Men	Women	Men
Total population	16.1	22.4	13.8	24.6	8.4	31.2	7.8	42.1	5.6	4.5	4.3	9.8
Age												
18–24	9.1	14.4	10.6	17.9	9.1	32.9	8.0	48.9	4.4	6.2	2.6	7.8
25–29	12.5	22.1	13.8	22.5	6.8	36.0	9.9	51.1	5.1	4.9	7.8	10.0
30–34	18.2	24.7	12.5	26.1	10.3	34.5	6.2	48.7	6.2	8.4	5.6	13.7
35–39	18.8	27.0	15.4	27.4	10.3	30.5	11.0	39.9	7.6	2.0	3.9	10.0
40–44	19.4	30.1	14.9	39.0	11.8	32.1	9.2	44.0	7.0	3.8	2.6	12.9
45–49	24.6	25.4	16.2	25.2	7.8	30.7	7.8	39.3	7.8	3.6	5.4	8.8
50–54	16.1	11.9	16.6	13.8	2.1	21.1	3.6	21.1	2.8	1.8	2.9	3.7
55–59	11.0	19.8	13.1	18.7	3.6	20.7	2.9	17.6	2.2	1.1	2.9	5.6
Marital status												
Never married, not cohabiting	14.0	19.4	10.1	22.9	8.3	37.0	7.2	49.0	6.8	9.2	4.0	11.7
Never married, cohabiting	6.9	33.9	12.3	33.9	12.3	44.3	9.6	60.7	8.2	16.4	2.8	17.2
Married	16.4	21.2	13.4	24.3	8.3	26.7	7.3	37.5	4.3	1.7	3.7	8.2
Divorced/separated/widowed, not cohabiting	17.9	26.4	18.2	25.0	7.1	29.7	7.1	37.8	5.2	1.8	5.2	8.1
Divorced/separated/widowed, cohabiting	21.4	31.6	21.4	26.3	12.5	36.8	14.3	42.1	14.3	0.0	12.5	8.1

Education												
Less than high school	8.2	16.9	13.2	18.2	4.5	26.5	5.8	30.2	2.1	2.7	4.2	8.1
High school graduate or equivalent	12.9	19.0	13.8	23.3	7.5	28.5	6.7	39.8	4.1	2.2	3.9	6.8
Some college/vocational school	17.9	27.2	13.8	25.6	9.2	32.7	8.7	44.2	5.6	6.7	4.3	12.0
Finished college	19.1	23.3	14.1	26.7	9.6	35.2	7.8	52.7	8.5	4.6	5.1	11.3
Master's/advanced degree	30.2	23.5	15.1	30.3	13.8	34.5	11.9	40.0	11.0	5.8	3.8	11.1
Religion												
None	21.5	28.4	15.3	29.9	18.0	39.2	15.9	51.0	12.6	8.3	6.7	15.2
Type I Protestant[a]	18.4	27.2	13.2	28.4	8.1	31.0	6.0	43.0	2.8	4.6	4.6	8.2
Type II Protestant	13.7	17.0	14.7	20.5	5.1	25.2	5.9	33.4	5.1	3.6	2.6	6.1
Catholic	13.8	20.9	12.5	21.7	8.0	33.6	7.8	47.2	5.9	2.4	5.5	9.6
Jewish	*	*	*	*	*	*	*	*	*	*	*	*
Other	22.2	15.4	11.1	32.5	18.9	30.0	10.8	41.5	13.5	12.2	2.9	30.0
Race ethnicity												
White	18.7	24.5	14.4	25.6	8.8	31.4	8.0	56.8	5.6	4.7	4.5	9.9
Black	7.4	13.0	13.3	21.2	6.6	30.6	8.7	58.6	6.2	4.5	3.7	6.6
Hispanic	8.4	18.8	12.9	21.8	9.0	29.1	5.3	65.1	6.0	3.9	5.3	11.0
Asian	*	18.2	*	26.5	6.7	29.4	6.7	64.7	0.0	2.9	*	20.6
Native American	*	*	*	*	*	*	*	*	*	*	*	*
N	1723	1387	1727	1391	1742	1403	1739	1403	1743	1404	1724	1370

Note. * indicates that base N is under 30 cases. This table includes all respondents, regardless of sexual orientation.

[a] Type I Protestants are those belonging to most mainline denominations, such as Methodists, Lutherans, Presbyterians, Episcopalians, and United Church of Christ; Type II Protestants consist of more fundamentalist denominations, such as Baptists, Pentacostals, Churches of Christ, Assemblies of God, those belonging to nondenominational churches, and those who have been "born again." (See Laumann *et al.* 1994 for detailed coding.)

late 1960s and therefore did not incorporate these acts into their sexual scripts.

As with vaginal intercourse, women currently in cohabiting or marital relationships are also the most likely to find watching their partner undress and oral sex appealing. In addition, highly educated women and women with no religious affiliation were much more likely to find these acts appealing. There was also a strong association between race and the appeal of oral sex; African-American women were noticeably less likely to find either giving or receiving oral sex appealing. The racial/ethnic difference in the percentage who found cunnilingus and fellatio appealing remains even after we control for other characteristics, such as age, education, marital status, and religion (Mahay, Laumann, & Michaels, 2001).

Fewer women found the other sexual practices appealing. Between 10% and 20% of women found manual stimulation of the anus, watching other people do sexual things, or using a dildo or vibrator appealing. Sex with a stranger, group sex, sex with another woman, and anal sex were the least popular, with less than 10% of women finding them appealing. In sum, women who are 25 to 29 years of age, white, and well educated found the most sexual practices appealing. African-American women were the least likely to find many of these sexual acts appealing, a sharp contradiction to the cultural stereotypes about African-American women's sexuality (see Wyatt, 1982, for a discussion of the cultural myths of African-American women's sexuality).

Sexual Fantasy

Like sexual preferences, sexual fantasies are not isolated from the cultural context in which one lives; fantasies depend on social sources for their form, from the learned cultural scenarios that specify certain types of people, acts, and contexts as "sexual" (Simon & Gagnon, 1987). The majority of women (67%) report that they think about sex between a few times a month to a few times a week. And almost 20% of women think about sex once a day or more. Women who are under 35 years old are the most likely to think about sex this frequently, as are women who have never married but are cohabiting. Women who are divorced and not cohabiting and women who have less than a high school education, on the other hand, are the most likely to rarely or never think about sex.

There has been much theorizing about gender differences in the content of women's and men's sexual fantasies. We found that women were somewhat more likely than men to report that their sexual fantasies involved stories, 21% of women compared to 14% of men. However, both women and men were much more likely to report that their fantasies involved images or pictures (49% of women and 56% of men). In addition, a substantial proportion of both women and men reported that their fantasies involved both stories and images/pictures (15% and 19%, respectively).

Sexual Attraction

The question of sexual attraction is a difficult one to answer because feelings of attraction, identity, and behavior are so variable over time and context. The NHSLS asked two quite different questions about sexual attraction to same- and opposite-gender partners. The first question asked about the appeal of sex with someone of the same gender, the second about the gender of the people to whom the respondent is sexually attracted. As shown in Table 1, 5.6% of women report finding the idea of sex with another woman appealing. For the question on sexual attraction, 4.4% of women reported being sexually attracted to other women. In all, 7.5% of women report one or the other form of same-gender sexual attraction or interest.

The rates of reporting some degree of same-gender desire are higher, however, for women than their rates of reporting same-gender partners. Only 1.3% of the sexually active women reported having a female partner in the last year, 2.2% report a same-gender partner in the last five years, and 4.1% of women reported having any female partners since turning 18. The rates of same-gender desire are also considerably higher than the proportions of women who explicitly self-identify with same-gender sexuality; only 1.4% of women reported identifying as a homosexual, lesbian, bisexual or other identity denoting at least some same-gender sexuality.

Figure 1 illustrates the interrelation between these components of attraction, behavior, and identity. The three circles each represent a dimension or component of same-gender sexuality. The total of 150 women (8.6% of the total sample) who report any same-gender desire, behavior, or identity are distributed across all the possible mutually exclusive combinations of the three categories. Desire with no corresponding adult behavior is the largest category for women, with about 59% of the women in this cell. About 13% of these women report a same-gender partner since turning 18, but no current desire or identity. However, 0% reported having only a homosexual identity. Finally, about 15% of these women are found in the intersection of all three circles. This analysis raises provocative questions about both how homosexuality is organized as a set of behaviors

and how it is experienced subjectively among women. While there is a core group of 1.3% of women in the survey who define themselves as homosexual or bisexual, have same-gender partners, and express homosexual desires, there are also sizable groups of women who do not consider themselves either homosexual or bisexual but have had adult homosexual experiences or express some degree of same-gender desire.

WOMEN'S SEXUAL EXPERIENCES

Formative Sexual Experiences

The sexual experiences of women and men begin to diverge early in the life course. For women, first sex has traditionally been a landmark event surrounded by a complex set of moral strictures and normative concerns about the meaning of virginity, the loss of innocence or purity, the transition to womanhood, and the assumption of responsibility for procreation and the next generation. Men's first sexual experiences, in contrast, are assumed to be relatively straightforward and expected upon achieving sexual maturity in response to the pressing needs for sexual outlets in adolescence and the provision of needed experience in learning the mature procreative roles required of adults. Cultural taboos about discussing sexuality, however, have limited what we actually know about young women's (as well as men's) first sexual experiences. While other national surveys (e.g., Hofferth, 1990; Hofferth & Hayes, 1987) have asked a few questions about first sex, usually sufficient to determine age of first intercourse and not much else, the NHSLS went into much greater detail with both female and male respondents so that we can form a more nuanced picture of this key life transition and how it may have changed over the past 40 years.

Age at First Sex

The age at which women first have sex is important and has been found to relate to a

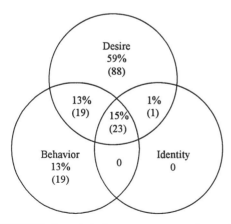

FIGURE 1. Interrelation between components of women's homosexuality. For 150 women (8.6% of the total 1749) who report any adult same-gender sexuality. From Laumann, Gagnon, Michael, & Michaels (1994, p. 299). Copyright 1994 by Edward O. Laumann, Robert T. Michael, CSG Enterprises, Inc., and Stuart Michaels. Reprinted with permission.

number of adult outcomes (Joyner & Laumann, 2001). There is a trend toward earlier experiences of first intercourse for women since the 1950s. For women who came of age in the 1950s and 1960s, 19% had intercourse by the age of 16 and 55% by the age of 19. The modal age of first sex for women in this age cohort was about 18. For women who came of age in the 1970s and 1980s, however, 37% of women had intercourse by the age of 16, and 83% by the age of 19. For this age cohort, the modal age of first intercourse for women is about 17. Although the mean age at first intercourse has traditionally been higher for women than for men, this difference has decreased over time for all racial/ethnic groups. And, African-American women have traditionally had a lower mean age at first intercourse than white women, although this difference is also decreasing.

Context of First Sex

While the age at first intercourse is important, it is necessary to understand the context in which this first intercourse occurred. The NHSLS asked whether first intercourse was something that the respondent wanted to happen at the time, something that she did not want but went along with, or something that she was forced to do against her will. At the same time that the age at first intercourse has declined, greater proportions of women report not wanting their first sexual experiences. As shown in Table 2, almost one quarter, 24.5%, of women reported that their first sexual intercourse was something they did not want but went along with. Another 4.2% of women reported that their first intercourse was forced. Further, a much larger percentage of African-American women report not wanting their first sexual intercourse to happen when it did than women of other racial and ethnic groups, 41% compared to an average of 29%. And these are all much higher percentages than for men.

The reasons that women gave for having had their first intercourse were also much different from those given by men. Table 3 breaks down the reasons given for first intercourse by

TABLE 2. First Intercourse Wanted, Not Wanted, or Forced (Percentages)

First intercourse	Women	Men
Wanted	71.3	92.1
Not wanted but not forced	24.5	7.6
Forced	4.2	0.3
N	1337	1689

Note. From Lauman, Gagnon, Michael, & Michaels (1994; p. 329). Copyright 1994 by Edward O. Laumann, Robert T. Michael, CSG Enterprises, Inc., and Stuart Michaels. Reprinted with permission.

gender and whether they wanted it or not. For those who wanted their first intercourse, the vast majority of women said they had their first sex because of affection for their partner or because it was their wedding night (68.6%), while only 31.8% of men gave these reasons. Interestingly, only about 3% of the women said that physical pleasure was their main reason for having first intercourse, compared to four times as many men who said this (12%). Among those whose first intercourse was not wanted, but something they went along with, most women listed affection for partner (39%), peer pressure (25%), and curiosity/readiness for sex (25%) as the reasons they went along with it. The data on first sexual intercourse demonstrate, at a minimum, that young women come to sex with quite different expectations and desires than do young men, which may lead to conflict or exploitation in the sexual encounter.

In discussing first sexual experiences, we must also recognize that some women's first sexual experience occurred as a child in the form of "adult–child sexual contact." About 12% of women in the NHSLS reported experiencing adult–child sexual contact, defined as sexual contact before puberty with someone at least four years older than themselves (Browning & Laumann, 1997). These sexual experiences have long-term consequences for women's sexual health; women who have experienced some form of adult–child sexual contact are more sexually active in both adolescence and adulthood, are more likely to experience STDs, and

TABLE 3. Reasons for Having First Intercourse,
by Gender and Desire Status

Attributed reasons	Wanted first intercourse		Not wanted but not forced	
	Women	Men	Women	Men
Affection for partner	47.5	24.9	38.5	9.9
Peer pressure	3.3	4.2	24.6	28.6
Curiosity/readiness for sex	24.3	50.6	24.9	50.5
Pregancy	0.6	0.5	0	0
Physical pleasure	2.8	12.2	2.1	6.6
Under the influence of alcohol/drugs	0.3	0.7	7.2	3.3
Wedding night	21.1	6.9	2.7	1.1
N	1147	1199	374	91

Note. From Lauman, Gagnon, Michael, & Michaels (1994; p. 329). Copyright 1994 by Edward O. Laumann, Robert T. Michael, CSG Enterprises, Inc., and Stuart Michaels. Reprinted with permission.

more likely to experience forced sex later on (for a detailed analysis of the life course effects of adult–child sexual contact, see Browning & Laumann, 1997; Browning, 1997).

Forced Sex

A substantial proportion of women have also experienced sex they did not want in adulthood. Like first sexual experiences, these later experiences have been shown to have an impact on subsequent sexual behavior, and thus we consider them formative as well. The NHSLS asked respondents whether they had ever been forced to do something sexual that they did not want to do. As shown in Table 4, about 22% of women, or more than 1 in 5, have experienced what they consider to be an incident in which they were forced to do something sexual that they did not want to do. Rates of forced sex for women vary only modestly by other demographic variables. By age, there is a hint of lower rates at older ages, suggesting an upward trend in sexual assault, since the period of greatest risk of sexual assault on women is thought to be in the late teens and early twenties. However, Hispanic and Asian women report notably lower rates than white women, with African-American women reporting rates between those extremes. Catholic women also report a rate for forced sex

that is only half that of women who have no current religious affiliation.

The most intriguing pattern may be the relatively low rate of forced sex reported by women living in central cities compared to the much higher rate for women living in smaller urban areas. This pattern is not consistent with the perception that women living in the largest cities are at the greatest risk of sexual assault. A vast majority of the reported forced sex occurs with someone the respondent knows rather than with a stranger, which is the more typical circumstance thought to occur in large cities. Only 4% of the women forced to do something sexual were forced by a stranger; the majority (55%) report that the person who forced them was either someone with whom they were in love or their spouse. These findings are consistent with those reported in other studies of sexual assault (Bureau of Justice Statistics, 1984; Koss, 1988; Koss, Dinero, Seibel, & Cox, 1988; Russell, 1984).

Adult Sexual Behavior

Masturbation

Popular orientations toward masturbation assume that masturbation is an indication of an inherent and insistent sex drive that needs to be

TABLE 4. Distribution of Women Ever Forced Sexually by a Man, by Master Status

	Respondent ever forced to do something sexual by a man		
	Yes	No	N
All women	22	77	1749
Age			
18–24	25	75	276
25–29	22	78	234
30–34	24	75	291
35–39	26	74	266
40–44	22	78	229
45–49	18	81	168
50–54	17	81	143
55–59	18	81	140
Education			
Less than high school	26	74	246
High school graduate or equivalent	17	83	512
Some college/vocational school	26	74	588
Finished college	22	77	281
Master's/advanced degree	23	77	109
Religion			
None	31	68	152
Type I Protestant[a]	21	79	422
Type II Protestant	25	74	592
Catholic	17	83	476
Race/ethnicity			
White	23	76	1338
Black	19	80	342
Hispanic	14	86	184
Asian	17	83	30
Size of place			
Central city/12 largest SMSAs	16	82	154
Central city/100 largest SMSAs	29	71	244
Suburb/12 largest SMSAs	19	80	211
Suburb/100 largest SMSAs	29	81	307
Other urban	25	74	642
Rural	18	81	191

Note. From Lauman, Gagnon, Michael, & Michaels (1994; p. 329). Copyright 1994 by Edward O. Laumann, Robert T. Michael, CSG Enterprises, Inc., and Stuart Michaels. Reprinted with permission.

Percentages do not add to 100 because of missing data and because women who were ever forced by a woman are excluded.

[a]Type I Protestants are those belonging to most mainline denominations, such as Methodists, Lutherans, Presbyterians, Episcopalians, and United Church of Christ; Type II Protestants consist of more fundamentalist denominations, such as Baptists, Pentecostals, Churches of Christ, Assemblies of God, those belonging to nondenominational churches, and those who have been "born again." (See Laumann *et al.*, 1994, for detailed coding).

expressed one way or another. In our view, however, masturbation is driven primarily by a variety of social factors both in adolescence and adulthood; it is practiced in a complex environment of condemnation and elicitation, and varies significantly with age, marital status, education, race/ethnicity, and religion.

For example, in Table 5 we see that while about 60% of women with no religious affiliation had masturbated in the last year, only about half as many women (33%) who had a conservative Protestant affiliation had done so. The effect of education is also dramatic. Almost 60% of women with graduate degrees have masturbated in the last year, a proportion that declines to 25% among those who have not finished high school. Moreover, while 44% of white women masturbated in the last year, only 32% of African-American women and 34% of Hispanic women did so. Thus, masturbation is most frequent among white, more educated, and nonreligious women. These findings demonstrate quite clearly that the incidence and frequency of masturbation are functions of variations in social location. It is also interesting to note that while women's sexual "coming of age" in terms of partnered sexual activity typically occurs in adolescence, it is women in their thirties and early forties who are the most likely to have masturbated in the last year.

The two most frequent reasons that women gave for masturbating were to relieve sexual tension (63%) and for physical pleasure (42%).* Despite secular trends in the amount and frequency of masturbation among younger cohorts, about half the women who masturbate report feeling guilty about it. Age, in fact, is not related to guilt; that is, older women are no more likely to report feeling guilty about masturbation than young women. This may be because those who feel very guilty are those who are most likely to stop masturbating, leaving only those who do not feel as guilty. Another factor may be that feelings of guilt decline as masturbation becomes a more routine part of adult lifestyles.

*Respondents were allowed to choose more than one reason, and the percentages therefore add up to more than 100.

Number of Sexual Partners

The number of sexual partners is an important aspect of sexual behavior that reflects the breadth of sexual experience and the nature of a person's sexual relationships. It also has important implications for the risk of sexually transmitted infections (STIs). Overall, the median number of sexual partners since age 18 for adult women is two, compared to a median of six partners for men. A single number, however, cannot effectively capture the complex history of individual maturation and change; in particular, it cannot reflect the highly variable process by which one selects sex partners at different stages in the life course. By placing sexual behavior in its social, demographic, and economic context and by determining whether these partnerships occurred concurrently or sequentially, we can be far better informed about the reasons for, and the likely consequences of, that behavior.

Table 5 presents the number of sexual partners for women of different ages, marital statuses, educational levels, religious affiliations, and racial/ethnic groups. In a given year, almost 14% of women aged 18 to 59 have no sex partner, and 75% have only one; just about 2% have five or more partners. This table demonstrates the tremendous influence of age and marital status on the number of partners women have in the past year and five years. Women who are 18 to 24 years old have the highest number of sexual partners; roughly 43% of women in this age group had two to four partners in the last five years, and another 23% had five or more partners in the last five years. These proportions drop dramatically among women in their late twenties and continue to drop for older women. There is also a higher rate of acquiring many sexual partners in the lifetime for women in the more recent birth cohorts, suggesting a period effect. While only 1% of women in the 1933–1942 birth cohort had five or more partners by age 20 (and 3% by age 30), 12% of women in the 1953–1962 cohort had acquired five or more partners by age 20 (and 22% by age 30).

As would be expected, married women are

TABLE 5. Distribution of Women's Sexual Practices by Selected Social Characteristics

| Social characteristics | Frequency of masturbation | | Felt guilty after masturbation | No. of partners past 12 months | | | | No. of partners past 5 years | | | | Frequency of sex in the past year | | | Duration of last event | |
	Not at all	Once a week	%	0	1	2–4	5+	0	1	2–4	5+	A few times per year/not at all	A few times per month	Two or more times a week	Fifteen minutes or less	One hour or more
All women[a]	58.3	7.6	46.8	13.6	74.7	10.0	1.7	8.7	59.4	24.3	7.7	29.7	37.2	33.0	14.7	14.8
Age																
18–24	64.4	9.4	56.4	9.4	62.3	21.7	6.5	11.6	22.9	43.1	22.5	27.3	31.5	41.2	7.3	22.6
25–29	58.3	9.9	52.7	3.4	84.6	10.7	1.3	4.5	50.2	34.5	10.8	14.8	38.1	47.1	10.2	19.0
30–34	51.1	8.6	38.4	7.9	78.4	12.4	1.4	3.5	60.8	29.0	6.7	24.7	34.6	40.7	13.1	15.4
35–39	52.3	6.6	48.8	10.9	80.0	7.6	1.5	6.9	68.2	20.0	4.9	26.5	37.8	35.7	16.7	10.1
40–44	49.8	8.7	45.7	14.4	79.0	6.6	0.0	7.7	73.8	15.4	3.2	30.1	46.1	23.7	12.2	15.3
45–49	55.6	8.6	35.4	17.3	75.6	6.6	0.6	10.4	71.2	15.3	3.1	32.2	41.0	26.7	17.9	10.5
50–54	71.8	2.3	53.3	21.0	74.8	4.2	0.0	12.5	75.7	11.8	0.0	40.0	40.0	20.0	25.9	9.3
55–59	77.6	2.4	50.0	41.4	57.1	1.4	0.0	18.6	75.2	5.4	0.8	63.2	29.6	7.2	35.9	2.6
Marital status																
Never married, not cohabiting	51.8	12.3	48.1	29.6	42.6	22.8	5.0	22.1	21.1	36.0	20.8	53.7	26.0	20.3	6.6	32.8
Never married, cohabiting	54.9	12.7	51.4	1.4	83.6	12.3	2.7	1.4	40.9	45.1	12.7	8.3	31.9	59.8	17.7	11.8
Married	62.9	4.7	49.2	2.7	94.8	2.1	0.3	2.5	82.0	13.1	2.4	14.9	46.5	38.5	16.1	7.8
Divorced/separated/widowed, not cohabiting	52.7	9.6	41.3	34.8	45.2	18.4	1.6	15.3	39.5	37.8	7.5	57.5	21.9	20.5	16.5	25.8
Divorced/separated/widowed, cohabiting	50.9	12.7	35.5	1.8	76.8	19.6	1.8	5.5	36.4	45.5	12.7	9.4	39.6	50.9	13.7	13.7

Education																
Less than high school	75.1	7.6	44.2	17.1	69.5	11.4	2.0	12.5	58.8	20.2	8.6	33.2	36.2	30.7	25.9	14.2
High school graduate or equivalent	68.4	5.6	46.1	11.3	79.1	7.8	1.8	8.5	62.1	24.5	5.0	26.7	37.7	35.6	16.7	14.0
Some college/ vocational school	51.3	6.9	49.8	13.0	74.1	10.7	2.2	7.2	57.5	24.7	10.5	29.4	37.7	32.9	12.3	16.1
Finished college	47.7	10.2	49.0	13.5	74.4	11.7	0.4	6.8	58.7	28.0	6.4	30.8	33.5	35.8	9.0	14.1
Master's/advanced degree	41.2	13.7	34.9	18.4	70.6	9.2	1.8	13.3	60.0	20.0	6.7	33.6	44.6	21.8	8.4	13.3
Religion																
None	41.4	13.8	51.1	9.9	71.1	13.8	5.3	3.5	50.0	29.9	16.7	29.0	36.5	34.5	13.2	20.2
Type I Protestant[b]	55.1	7.4	43.9	12.8	76.3	9.2	1.7	9.1	60.6	22.7	7.6	30.3	39.8	29.8	14.2	12.0
Type II Protestant	67.3	5.8	46.8	14.3	73.2	11.0	1.6	8.9	61.4	23.0	6.7	29.1	36.0	34.9	16.9	14.4
Catholic	57.3	6.6	50.7	15.1	76.3	7.8	0.8	9.6	59.2	24.9	6.3	30.0	37.0	32.9	13.7	15.8
Jewish	*	*	*	*	*	*	*	*	*	*	*	*	*	*	*	*
Other	52.9	17.6	*	16.2	73.0	10.8	0.0	16.7	61.1	16.7	5.6	*	*	*	*	*
Race/ethnicity[c]																
White	55.7	7.3	47.7	13.2	76.1	9.2	1.5	8.1	61.8	23.1	7.0	29.1	38.1	32.9	14.1	13.5
Black	67.8	10.7	35.6	16.1	64.0	17.5	2.3	11.1	49.4	28.1	11.4	36.1	33.1	30.9	17.5	21.5
Hispanic	65.5	4.7	51.4	10.9	76.1	10.9	2.2	10.4	60.7	20.8	8.1	23.0	34.1	42.9	18.2	15.6
Asian	*	*	*	16.7	83.3	0.0	0.0	*	*	*	*	*	*	*	*	*
Native American	*	*	*	*	*	*	*	*	*	*	*	*	*	*	*	*
N	1649		760				1748		1669			1664				1461

Note. Columns 1–3 and 12–16 from Laumann, Gagnon, Michael, & Michaels (1994; pp. 82, 88–89, and 94). Copyright 1994 by Edward O. Laumann, Robert T. Michael, CSG Enterprises, Inc., and Stuart Michaels. Reprinted with permission.

[a]Cross section $N = 1749$.

[b]Type I Protestants are those belonging to most mainline denominations, such as Methodists, Lutherans, Presbyterians, Episcopalians, and United Church of Christ; Type II Protestants consist of more fundamentalist denominations, such as Baptists, Pentecostals, Churches of Christ, Assemblies of God, those belonging to nondenominational churches, and those who have been "born again." (See Laumann *et al.*, 1994, for detailed coding).

[c]With oversample, $N = 1921$. * indicates that the base N for the cell was under 30 cases.

the most likely to have had only one partner in the last 12 months and the last 5 years, while single women are more likely to have either no partners or two or more partners in these time periods. African-American women are somewhat more likely than women of other races to have had two or more partners in the last 12 months and 5 years, probably due to the lower rate of marriage among African-American women.

About 15% of women reported having had an extramarital affair, compared with 25% of men.* Somewhat surprisingly, in light of the alleged effects of the Sexual Revolution on women's liberation, the percentage of women who reported having had extramarital sex does not change dramatically across the four age cohorts, being 12.4% among those 50 to 59 years of age, 19.9% among those 40 to 49 years old, 14.5% among those 30 to 39 years old, and 11.7% among those 18 to 29 years old. That is, rates of marital defection are fairly low and stable across the cohorts. Recall, however, that the question asks whether the respondent ever had extramarital sex during the marriage and older women are likely to be reviewing their behavior in marriages that are of much longer durations than younger women's marriages. Another way to consider the matter of marital infidelity is to note that the percentage of the currently married women who report two or more partners in the current year at each year of age is roughly a constant rate of about 2.4% per year.

Frequency of Partnered Sex

Closely related to number of sexual partners is the frequency of sex. Table 5 reports the frequency of sex in the past year by age, race, religion, and marital status. Women fall roughly into three levels of activity in partnered sex. About 33% have sex with their partner at least two or more times a week, 37% have sex a few times per month, and the remaining 30% have sex only a few times per year or not at all. Con-

trary to the historically popular stereotypes of group differences in rates of sexual conduct, we found only minor variations in the frequency of partnered sex across race and ethnicity, religious affiliation, and level of education.

Social characteristics that were related strongly to women's reported frequencies of partnered sexual activity were age and marital status. Age is curvilinearly related to having had no sex in the last year. While 11% of women 18 to 24 years old had no partnered sex in the last year, rates of sexual activity rise for women 24 to 29 years of age, of whom only 5% had no sexual activity in the last year. Rates of sexual activity then begin to decline for women starting in their early thirties, with an especially dramatic drop in sexual activity for women in their late fifties, of whom 41% had no sexual activity in the last year. This is very different than for men, whose rates of sexual inactivity remain relatively low, and rise to only about 16% in their late fifties. While the sexual activity among older women may certainly be influenced by the biological processes of aging, an understanding of the normative effects of aging for women provides a more complete explanation of the different experiences of older women compared to older men. Researchers need to examine how the cultural conceptions of older women's sexuality affect their likelihood of having sex. How can older women overcome the deeply ingrained cultural bias against their participation in the sexual marketplace?

In addition, the patterns we see revealed by age may also represent an underlying relationship with another crucial factor in explaining the frequency of sex—marital status. We find that married and cohabiting women are the most sexually active women in the sample. This may be both because of proscriptions against sexual intercourse for women outside of marriage or a marriage-like relationship among some segments of the population, and because living with a partner ensures that the option of sex, at least, may be available on a fairly regular basis. Over time, however, sex in marriage may become increasingly competitive with childcare responsibilities and increasing work and financial responsibilities as the family grows

---

*These percentages are based on responses to the question, "Have you ever had sex with someone other than your husband or wife while you were married?"

(Goldscheider & Waite, 1991), leading to a decline in the frequency of sex among older married women. The decline in sexual activity for older women may also partially be due to the fact that this age group encompasses a higher number of divorced or widowed women. Divorce or the death of a spouse, combined with social proscriptions against sexual assertiveness, leaves a significant proportion of middle-aged women without access to a sex partner.

Duration of Partnered Sex

The number of partners and the frequency of sex do not tell us the amount of time invested in partnered sexual events, however. Sexual events that respondents reported as lasting 15 minutes or less are defined as shorter sexual events, while those lasting an hour or more are defined as extended sexual events.*

Age is strongly associated with the duration of sexual events; the proportion of women reporting extended sexual events (an hour or more) drops from 23% of 18- to 24-year-old women to only 3% of 55- to 59-year-old women. There are at least three general interpretations of these data. First, age may be seen to influence one's energy, interest, or physical stamina for sexual activity. However, differences in women's reported duration of sexual events may be more effectively explained through reference to variation in the social circumstances and cultural constructions of sexual interaction. For instance, as we discuss later in this chapter, older women are less likely to engage in such practices as oral sex. To the extent that the practice of oral sex is associated with other forms of foreplay or non-genitally-oriented sexual techniques, older women will tend to have considerably shorter sexual encounters.

Third, younger women are more likely to be involved in short-term or relatively new relationships in which the perceived length of sexual events may include kissing and petting, disrobing, and extended foreplay, activities that are less likely to form a major component of sexual events with a familiar partner. Indeed, significant discrepancies are found when considering the relation between length of last sexual event and marital status. Thirty-three percent of never-married, noncohabiting women reported extended sexual events, compared to only 12% of cohabiting women and 8% of married women. These fairly dramatic declines in the reported length of sexual events indicate that the third explanation discussed may be of particular import in understanding the organization and perception of time spent on sexual activity.

Partnered Sexual Techniques

So far we have examined only the number of partners, the frequency, and the duration of partnered sex, but not the actual substance of sexual behavior. The NHSLS elicited information on the occurrence and incidence of four basic techniques utilized in sex between women and men: vaginal intercourse, fellatio, cunnilingus, and anal intercourse.† These are sexual practices that occur at the level of the partnership or dyad, and should therefore be seen as a result of an explicit or tacit negotiation between two (or more) people who embody specific social locations and cultural understandings. Table 6 presents the lifetime percentages of these sexual practices by the master status

---

*People's reports of the length of time that their last sexual event took are unlikely to be especially precise with respect to the number of minutes elapsed. People are focused on other things than keeping track of time, and there are inherent and unresolved ambiguities in defining the beginning and the end of a sexual event. We do believe, however, that people can provide reasonable indications of the relative amounts of time spent involved in sexual activity, and we have therefore focused on people's sense of the event being very brief (less than 15 minutes) or quite long (over an hour).

†Since the NHSLS was designed, in part, to fill significant gaps in our knowledge of sexual behavior associated with the AIDS virus, the questions were slanted toward those sexual practices that could be demonstrably related to the transmission of the infection. This disease-centered emphasis led to the omission of significant nongenital sexual practices that are often independent sources of physical and emotional pleasure and satisfaction, such as hugging, kissing, and body stroking. We view this as a serious limitation of our study and will incorporate a more inclusive list of sexually relevant techniques in our future work.

TABLE 6. Distribution of Sexual Techniques by Selected Social Characteristics (Women Only)[a]

Social characteristics	Occurrence of active oral sex (%)		Occurrence of receptive oral sex (%)		Occurrence of anal sex (%)[b]			Occurrence of orgasm with primary partner (%)			
	Life	Last event	Life	Last event	Life	Last year	Last event	Always	Usually	Sometimes	Rarely or never
All women[c]	67.7	18.8	73.1	19.9	20.4	8.6	1.2	28.8	41.9	20.9	8.4
Age											
18–24	69.1	19.1	74.7	24.2	16.2	10.1	0.9	21.9	39.3	25.9	13.0
25–29	76.2	23.8	79.8	24.3	20.3	11.9	2.4	31.7	39.9	20.6	7.8
30–34	76.6	19.1	83.1	22.3	21.2	8.1	1.2	28.9	40.8	20.0	10.4
35–39	71.3	21.0	73.7	23.3	27.5	9.5	0.0	28.8	40.6	24.0	6.6
40–44	72.7	16.9	76.8	12.6	23.2	8.3	0.5	33.0	43.3	17.0	6.7
45–49	65.2	21.6	72.7	18.3	26.1	9.5	3.2	34.6	44.9	15.4	5.2
50–54	48.5	11.7	59.4	12.6	14.4	1.9	0.0	26.6	48.6	20.2	4.6
55–59	38.9	5.5	44.3	6.9	9.2	2.5	1.4	25.6	44.9	19.2	10.2
Marital status											
Never married, not cohabiting	59.4	21.0	67.7	26.8	19.1	11.8	2.0	26.0	31.1	26.0	17.0
Never married, cohabiting	72.2	21.5	76.4	22.7	18.1	7.4	3.0	23.6	43.1	30.6	2.8
Married	70.7	16.9	73.9	16.9	21.3	7.3	1.0	28.9	46.5	18.3	6.4
Divorced/separated/widowed, not cohabiting	64.1	25.4	73.1	24.2	20.0	10.2	0.6	34.4	33.9	21.9	10.0
Divorced/separated/widowed, cohabiting	79.6	16.3	85.2	20.4	22.2	13.5	0.0	23.6	45.5	23.6	7.2

Education											
Less than high school	41.1	10.1	49.6	13.2	12.7	8.5	0.5	30.8	34.9	26.7	7.7
High school graduate or equivalent	59.6	16.4	67.1	18.5	16.6	7.4	1.7	34.5	38.6	17.9	8.9
Some college/vocational school	78.2	20.7	81.6	22.2	24.6	10.2	1.1	25.3	43.4	21.7	9.6
Finished college	78.9	22.9	83.1	20.7	21.8	7.2	0.9	24.4	46.2	22.7	6.7
Master's/advanced degree	79.0	28.8	81.9	27.0	28.6	8.3	1.3	29.1	52.3	12.8	5.8
Religion											
None	77.9	29.2	83.3	30.6	36.1	16.7	2.5	21.8	48.1	21.8	8.3
Type I Protestant[d]	74.5	19.6	77.4	18.7	20.4	7.7	0.6	27.3	44.1	19.7	9.0
Type II Protestant	55.6	12.9	64.8	16.1	16.8	5.9	1.2	32.8	37.3	22.3	7.6
Catholic	73.6	21.5	76.6	21.8	19.8	9.8	1.1	27.0	43.3	20.0	9.8
Jewish	*	*	*	*	*	*	*	*	*	*	*
Other	65.7	*	65.7	*	25.7	*	*	*	*	*	*
Race/ethnicity[e]											
White	75.3	21.0	78.9	21.2	23.2	8.4	1.2	26.4	44.5	20.4	8.7
Black	34.4	9.3	48.9	13.1	9.6	6.0	1.5	38.9	33.8	21.1	6.2
Hispanic	59.7	18.7	63.7	22.0	17.0	12.5	0.7	34.4	34.4	22.1	9.1
Asian	*	*	*	*	*	*	*	*	*	*	*
Native American	*	*	*	*	*	*	*	*	*	*	*
N	1661	1380	1660	1384	1658	1477	1383				1471

Note. Columns 1–7 from Laumann, Gagnon, Michael, & Michaels, (1994, 98–99). Copyright 1994 by Edward O. Laumann, Robert T. Michael, CSG Enterprises, Inc., and Stuart Michaels. Reprinted with permission.

* indicates that the base N for the cell was under 30 cases.

[a]Percentages are calculated on the basis of three time periods: over the life course, over the past year, and during the last sexual event. The relevant sample varies over the different time periods. Lifetime inquiries are based on the entire cross-section; the last event and the last year include only those respondents who engaged in opposite-gender partnered sex in the last year.

[b]Questions concerning the occurrence of anal sex in the last year are partner-specific—we ask only whether anal sex occurred within the "primary" or "secondary" partnership last year. To the extent that respondents experienced anal sex in partnerships other than primary or secondary, the percentages reported may slightly underestimate the true sample proportion of respondents who experienced anal sex in the last year.

[c]Cross section N = 1749.

[d]Type I Protestants are those belonging to most mainline denominations, such as Methodists, Lutherans, Presbyterians, Episcopalians, and United Church of Christ; Type II Protestants consist of more fundamentalist denominations, such as Baptists, Pentecostals, Churches of Christ, Assemblies of God, those belonging to nondenominational churches, and those who have been "born again." (See Laumann et al., 1994, for detailed coding.)

[e]With oversample, N = 1921.

variables alongside the proportion reporting the occurrence of the specified technique in the last event.* This juxtaposition provides some indication of the extent to which the practice in question constitutes a regular, episodic, or an isolated occurrence in the sex life of the respondent.

Vaginal Intercourse

Vaginal intercourse was excluded from Table 6 owing to the lack of notable variation in its distribution across the master status variables. Ninety-seven percent of women reported a lifetime incidence of vaginal intercourse, with only marginally fewer women reporting its occurrence in the last sexual event. These findings highlight the near universality of vaginal intercourse as a defining sexual technique of heterosexuality. Of women who had a sexual partner in the last year, only a few groups report an incidence of vaginal sex in the last event lower than 95%. These include women who have never been married and are not living with a partner (13% of whom report a sexual event that did not include vaginal intercourse), and the most educated women (11% of whom report a sexual event that did not include vaginal intercourse). The view in popular sexual practice and belief that vaginal intercourse is sex tends to be confirmed by these data, although a significant minority of some groups of women had sexual events that did not involve vaginal intercourse.

Oral Sex

While the ultimate goal in sexual events appears to remain vaginal intercourse, there has been a dramatic increase in the incidence and frequency of oral sex. The emergence of oral sex as a widespread technique practiced by opposite-gender sex partners probably began in the 1920s, and over the past 70 years it has become

*These two analyses are based on different populations: the former on all respondents regardless of current partnership status, the latter on those respondents with an opposite-gender last-event sex partner.

more common among most social groups. The trends in oral sex can be seen when we control for age. We can think of the effect of age as an indication of when the respondent became sexually active. Table 6 displays the percentages of women who have experienced cunnilingus and fellatio in their lifetime by birth cohort. The overall trend reveals a rapid change in sexual techniques, if not a revolution. For example, the proportion of women receiving oral sex in their lifetime increases from 44% of those born between 1933 and 1937 to 77% of those born between 1948 and 1952. The significant increase in lifetime experience occurs for women coming of sexual age (18 to 24) just prior to 1968. Indeed, no substantial increase in lifetime experience occurs for respondents born after 1948–52. The timing of changes in sexual techniques appears to have been responsive to cultural changes in the late 1950s through the 1970s, when they approached saturation level in the population. The lower rate among the youngest group in our survey are not necessarily evidence of a decline in oral sex; it may just be that these women have not yet engaged in sexual relationships in which oral sex has become likely.

The growth in rates of lifetime occurrence of oral sex has by no means been uniform across all social categories, however. Both the youth-oriented urban cultures of the early 1960s (cf. Lofland, 1970) and their more politically oriented counterparts of the late 1960s were confined largely to white middle- and upper-class populations. Less-educated women and women of other racial groups are significantly less likely to have experienced oral sex in their lifetime. The proportion of women with less than a high school degree who have performed fellatio on a partner is only 41%, compared to almost twice as many, 79%, of women with at least a college education. Analysis of the effect of race on lifetime experience of both receiving and performing oral sex also reveals significant differences. White women have rates of lifetime experience of oral sex that are at least 30 percentage points higher than those of African-

American women. While these differences are due in part to the significant discrepancies in educational level between the two races, multivariate analyses confirm the independent effect of race on the lifetime incidence of oral sex. Finally, religion is also associated with lifetime incidence of oral sex, suggesting that normative constraints on oral sex continue to have an effect.

Although most people have experienced oral sex at some point in their lifetime, the status of oral sex as a regular practice remains somewhat ambiguous. While the proportion of women reporting any lifetime incidence of cunnilingus and fellatio was roughly 70%, the proportion of women for whom oral sex is a current activity (as measured by its occurrence in the last sexual event) is roughly 50 percentage points lower, at around 20%. Oral sex, then, is a technique with which most people have at least some familiarity, but it has in no sense become a defining feature of sex between women and men (as vaginal intercourse or, perhaps, kissing, is). The uncertainty surrounding oral sex, the ongoing potential problem of reciprocity, and the differential symbolic meanings of oral sex have immediate implications for relations between women and men. However, Table 6 shows that in the last sexual event about the same percentage of women reported receiving oral sex as reported performing it, although both proportions are about 8 percentage points lower than the figures reported by men.

Anal Sex

Unlike oral sex, anal sex has not entered into the repertoire of regular sexual practices for most women in the United States. Anal sex is not only far less frequently experienced over the life course but also far less likely to become a common or even an occasional sexual practice once it has been experienced. Table 6 reports the incidence of heterosexual anal intercourse over the life course in the past year and in the last sexual event. In contrast to oral sex, only about 20% of women have experienced anal sex in their lifetime, and far fewer have had anal

sex in the last year (9%), or in the last sexual event (1%).

Controlling for cohort membership reveals a fairly steady increase in the proportion of women ever experiencing anal sex for those born in the 1933–37 cohort (women aged 55 to 59) through the 1953–57 cohort (women 35 to 39)—from 9% to 28%. However, the proportion declines for the younger cohorts rather than remaining stable (as was the pattern for oral sex). While these lower rates of anal sex among more youthful cohorts may be a result of the role of anal sex in HIV transmission, it could as likely be that experience with anal sex requires a longer engagement in partnered sex and a larger number of sex partners among whom an interested partner might be found. This latter hypothesis is supported by the fact that the decline in lifetime experience with anal sex occurs for cohorts that were sexually active in the 1970s and early 1980s, before the onset of the HIV/AIDS epidemic.

The practice of anal intercourse, then, is a highly socially structured phenomenon. As we can see from Table 6, women with higher levels of education, white women, women with no religious affiliation, and women in their thirties and forties are most likely to have had an experience in their lifetime with anal sex. These characteristics, however, do not appear to structure the incorporation of anal sex into the regular sexual repertoires of women, indicating that lifetime experience with anal sex may for most women be an isolated experimental incident facilitated by the more open sexual climate of the 1960s.

Sexual Satisfaction

Orgasm

Orgasm is a response to a complex set of socially contextualized stimuli. For any individual, there will be a variety of sources of both physical and mental stimulation. While this is true for both women and men, orgasm among women is a form of experience that is poorly taught and has limited bases of social support. With the changing sexual and gender roles since the 1960s, however, women's orgasm became a highly politicized issue involving feminists, researchers, and clinicians. In this section we simply try to establish some parameters for this aspect of sexual pleasure, and examine its occurrence for women of various social groups and different types of sexual relationships.

Data on the frequency of orgasm with a specific partner in the last year are presented in Table 6.* Only 29% of women report that they always have orgasm during sex with their primary sex partner, compared with 75% of men. With female orgasm now often considered both a right for women and a responsibility for men, this discrepancy may generate considerable intergender, interpersonal tension.† However, although only 29% of women "always" have an orgasm, another 42% of women report "usually" having an orgasm with their partner, and only 8% report rarely or never having an orgasm. The percentages of rarely or never having an orgasm with their partner are highest among the younger and single women, perhaps reflecting relative inexperience with partnered sex in general or with their specific partner. Women in their fifties also report slightly reduced rates of consistent orgasm. This decline may reflect either a cohort, an age, or a partner's age effect. Similarly, while there are other differences in the experience of orgasm on the part of women, none of these are easily interpreted. For instance, there is variability among women of different educational levels but no systematic and direct effect of education. Indeed, women who might be expected to have more frequent orgasm because of their more elaborated sexual

techniques—the better educated and white—have slightly lower rates.

Religion may also have an independent effect on rates of female orgasm in sexual relationships. Women without religious affiliation were the least likely to report always having an orgasm with their primary partner—only 1 in 5. On the other hand, the proportion of conservative Protestant (Type II) women who reported always having an orgasm was the highest, at nearly one third. However, the highly discrepant educational (and ethnic) backgrounds of the different religious groupings must be kept in mind when interpreting rates of orgasm by religious background.

Orgasm, however, is only one aspect of sexual satisfaction. The experience of orgasm may be of highly variable significance in the overall level of physical or emotional satisfaction felt in a particular sexual partnership. Overall, about 40% of women report being "extremely" physically satisfied with their sexual partner, and about the same proportion of women reported being "extremely" emotionally satisfied. These proportions are comparable to those of men who report being "extremely" physically and emotionally satisfied. While frequency of orgasm is indeed correlated with physical satisfaction, characteristics of the relationship, such as the level of emotional investment, sexual exclusivity, stability of the relationship, and union status, also play a significant role in predicting overall physical and emotional satisfaction (Waite & Joyner, 2001).

On the opposite side of sexual satisfaction is sexual dysfunction, which is also quite common among women. About 43% of women have experienced sexual dysfunction for several months or more in the last 12 months, including lacking desire for sex, difficulty becoming aroused (i.e., lubricated), physical pain during intercourse, not finding sex pleasurable, and anxiety (Laumann, Paik, & Rosen, 1999). Like sexual satisfaction, sexual dysfunction is highly correlated with relationship status; women who have never married are significantly more likely to have sexual problems than married women (Laumann, Paik, & Rosen, 1999).

---

*These specific partners may be marital partners, cohabitational partners, partners selected as "primary" by those who had two or more partners and no marital or cohabitational partner, or the partner of those with only one partner who is not a marital or cohabitational partner. Each individual respondent is represented by only one partnership. For the sake of brevity, we refer to this as the primary partnership.

†This is not, however, to suggest that orgasm is necessarily always the primary "goal" of sexual interaction.

WOMEN'S SEXUAL ATTITUDES

Normative Orientations toward Sexuality

Like sexual behaviors and desire, women's sexual attitudes may be both part of what defines them as feminine, as well as a result of their membership in the social category of women. Laumann *et al.* (1994) conducted a cluster analysis of respondents' attitudes toward nine issues related to sexuality: premarital sex, teenage sex, extramarital sex, same-gender sex, pornography, sex without love, the influence of religious beliefs on sexual behavior, abortion in the case of rape, and abortion for any reason. This analysis found that people's sexual attitudes cannot be characterized by a unidimensional scale of permissiveness. Instead, as shown in Table 7, people typically fell into three major normative orientations toward sexuality: traditional, relational, and recreational (cf. DeLamater, 1987).

Each normative orientation is based on a fundamental assumption about the purpose of sexual activity. Those with a traditional normative orientation regard reproduction as the sole purpose of sex, which should take place only within marriage. Prohibitions are placed on those behaviors that do not lead (or are not intended to lead) to conception, such as masturbation, oral sex, homosexuality, sex outside of marriage, and the use of birth control. This orientation has traditionally been rooted in the Roman Catholic and more conservative Protestant churches, but may now also be justified simply by an appeal to traditional moral values. Second, a relational orientation toward sexuality is based on the idea that sexual activity is a natural component of a loving, intimate relationship. Unlike the traditional orientation, a relational orientation allows for premarital sex within the context of a loving relationship; it is inconsistent, however, with extramarital sex and with activities such as group sex and casual sex without love. Third, a recreational orientation is based on the premise that pleasure is the primary purpose of sexual activity. Although it may be accompanied by a proscription against forcing others to comply, this orientation essentially allows for any type of sexual activity among consenting adults.

The Traditional Orientation

In the cluster analysis, those in the traditional clusters have high proportions believing that premarital sex, teenage sex, extramarital sex, and same-gender sex are always wrong, that religious beliefs guide their sexual behavior, and that there should be laws against pornography. Among those with this traditional orientation, there was a major distinction with regard to beliefs about abortion, however. The first cluster, referred to as the conservative cluster, had conservative attitudes toward abortion. About 17% of all women belonged to this particular cluster. The other cluster, referred to as pro-choice, is still generally conservative with regard to most of the attitude measures, but differs in that all the women in this cluster reported that women should be able to obtain legal abortions in all cases, and they were less likely to say that premarital sex is always wrong. This profile accounted for another 16% of women. With these two clusters combined, about one third of all women have a traditional orientation, with about half of those being conservative when it comes to abortion, and the other half being pro-choice. The proportion of women with traditional orientations is much higher than for men, of whom only about one quarter are traditional. These first-order gender differences are consistent with previous research demonstrating greater religious involvement among women and greater permissiveness toward both premarital and extramarital sexuality among men.

Among women, African-Americans are more likely than whites or Hispanics to have a traditional orientation, with almost 45% of African-American women with this orientation. This finding gives a very different impression from previous research claiming that African-American women are more sexually permissive than white women (e.g., Klassen, Williams, & Levitt, 1989; Smith, 1994). This

TABLE 7. Women's Attitude Cluster Membership, by Selected Social Characteristics (Percent Distribution)

Social characteristics	Traditional			Relational		Recreational		N
	Conservative	Pro-choice	Religious	Conventional	Contemporary religious	Pro-life	Libertarian	
All women	17.3	16.4	21.7	15.5	10.4	4.5	14.2	1564
Age								
18–29	12.8	12.2	20.2	23.2	9.7	5.5	16.4	475
30–44	16.1	17.7	21.3	14.4	11.7	4.8	14.0	694
45–59	24.6	19.0	24.4	8.4	8.9	2.8	11.9	394
Marital status								
Never married	11.4	15.4	15.8	23.2	10.4	5.0	18.8	298
Cohabiting[a]	1.5	19.7	22.7	19.7	7.6	0.0	28.8	66
Married	20.4	15.8	24.5	13.9	9.7	4.5	11.3	849
Divorced/separated/widowed	17.0	18.8	20.3	12.4	12.4	4.5	14.5	330
Education								
Less than high school	23.3	13.2	29.5	14.1	4.0	8.4	7.5	227
High school graduate or equivalent	20.0	18.3	21.6	17.4	7.0	5.7	10.0	459
Some college/vocational school	14.4	18.3	21.6	15.9	10.8	3.4	15.7	529
Finished college	14.5	14.9	14.9	14.0	18.2	1.7	21.9	242
Master's/advanced degree	12.5	8.3	21.9	12.5	20.8	3.1	20.8	96
Religion								
None	3.0	7.4	8.9	25.9	9.6	5.2	40.0	135
Type I Protestant[b]	11.7	19.2	20.0	16.1	15.3	2.9	14.8	385
Type II Protestant	31.8	18.6	22.5	11.2	4.7	5.0	6.1	537
Catholic	9.1	13.1	28.6	16.7	12.6	5.5	14.3	419
Race/ethnicity								
White	16.7	13.8	22.0	15.1	11.1	4.6	16.6	1184
Black	18.0	26.6	21.0	16.4	8.4	3.3	5.6	214
Hispanic	20.3	20.3	16.9	16.9	9.3	5.9	10.2	118

Note. Adapted from Laumann, Gagnon, Michael, & Michaels (1994, pp. 520–521). Copyright 1994 by Edward O. Laumann, Robert T. Michael, CSG Enterprises, Inc., and Stuart Michaels. Adapted with permission.

[a]Includes only those who have never been married. Those who have been married but are now divorced, widowed, or separated are included in the last row.

[b]Type I Protestants are those belonging to most mainline denominations, such as Methodists, Lutherans, Presbyterians, Episcopalians, and United Church of Christ; Type II Protestants consist of more fundamentalist denominations, such as Baptists, Pentecostals, Churches of Christ, Assemblies of God, those belonging to nondenominational churches, and those who have been "born again." (See Laumann *et al.*, 1994, for detailed coding.)

difference is due largely to the fact that other studies have focused primarily on the partial effects of race after other variables have been controlled. Indeed, our own multivariate analyses (not shown) indicate that African-Americans have somewhat lower odds of being in the conservative cluster after taking into account the effects of gender, age, marital status, and religion. However, great care must be taken in interpreting such multivariate models when they are applied to survey data. Our data shows that as a group, African-American women still have more traditional orientations toward sexuality than white women.

The likelihood of being in either traditional cluster also increases with increasing age. As we have already discussed, this likely reflects both a cohort effect and the fact that increasing age is accompanied by a higher probability of being married and having children, events that tend to be associated with a higher degree of sexual conservatism. Those with higher education, however, are less likely to be in the conservative cluster.

The Relational Orientation

The most common orientation among women is the relational orientation, encompassing almost half of all women. The primary distinction between the traditional clusters and those that we have labeled relational is that respondents in the latter almost uniformly believe that there are certain situations in which premarital sex is not wrong (most believe that it is wrong only sometimes or not at all). However, with respect to other items, there is considerable variation among the relational clusters. For example, the first relational cluster is labeled religious because the majority of its members reported that religious beliefs shape their sexual behavior and because their attitudes against such activities as same-gender sex and abortion are consistent with the formal positions of many religious groups. About 22% of women fall into this cluster. In contrast, those in the following cluster are more tolerant than those in the religious cluster with regard

to teenage sex, homosexuality, pornography, and abortion, and are much less likely to report that religious beliefs influence their sexual conduct. We refer to this cluster as conventional since most still report that both extramarital and same-gender sex—behaviors that many would view as unconventional—are always wrong. About 16% of women fall into this cluster.

The remaining relational cluster is much more tolerant of homosexuality. Surprisingly, however, all women in this cluster report that religious beliefs shape and guide their sexual behavior, more than in any other cluster. We therefore refer to this cluster as contemporary religious since its opinions regarding premarital sex, teenage sex, extramarital sex, same-gender sex, pornography, and abortion reflect not traditional religious doctrine but rather the newly adopted positions of more liberal denominations (Roof, 1993). About 10% of women fall into this cluster.

Women are more likely than men to subscribe to the religious or contemporary religious orientations, while there is little difference with respect to the conventional orientation. In terms of age, much of the increase in the traditional orientation comes from the sharp decrease in the conventional cluster. In fact, from the youngest to the oldest age category, the conventional cluster is reduced to between half and one third of its original size. It may be that, for some, the conventional orientation represents a modern, nonreligious alternative to the traditional orientation. Regardless, the fact that this cluster contains almost one quarter of the women under age 30 suggests that it deserves special attention.

The percentages of those in the contemporary religious cluster increase steadily with increasing education. This result largely reflects the positive association between education and approval of homosexuality since one of the major differences between this cluster and the other two relational clusters is that those in the former are considerably more tolerant of same-gender sex. However, it is also significant that this is the only cluster to combine religious influence on sexual behavior with a relatively tolerant position on several items. Together with the educational composition of this cluster, we interpret this as reflecting either membership in a liberal parish or a willingness to rethink and perhaps reject particular elements of church doctrine.

The Recreational Orientation

Finally, about 19% of women have what can be called a recreational orientation. Just as the primary distinction between the traditional and the relational clusters is disapproval of premarital sex, the primary distinction between the relational clusters and those that we have labeled recreational is that most of those in the latter do not consider love to be a necessary prerequisite for engaging in sex. The first of the clusters within this orientation is interesting since it combines relatively liberal positions on extramarital sex and pornography with relatively conservative positions on homosexuality and abortion. For this reason, we call this cluster pro-life. Only about 5% of women fall into this cluster. In contrast, the second recreational cluster reflects consistently liberal views on each of the nine items. We therefore refer to it as libertarian. Fourteen percent of women fall into this cluster.

Women are much less likely than men to report either of these recreational orientations. Among women, white women are the most likely to have a libertarian orientation, while African-Americans are the least likely. Being married, while increasing one's chances of being in the conservative cluster, decreases one's chances of being in the libertarian cluster. Cohabitation has the opposite effect, consistent with the interpretation of the decision to cohabit as reflecting a more liberal orientation toward sexuality.

The libertarian orientation is most common among women with no religious affiliation, where the percentage is more than double that for the other groups. The percentage of women in the libertarian cluster also generally increases with education. This is consistent

with prior work demonstrating positive associations between education and approval of premarital sexuality, extramarital sexuality, and same-gender sex.

Overall, the fact that the clusters are quite homogeneous indicates that much of the variation in these data can be described in terms of a few discrete sets of individuals who share a particular profile of responses. This reflects in part the relatively high association among many of the attitudes. In addition, it shows that women's sexual attitudes have more than one dimension, which reflects the different ways in which women understand certain sexual behaviors.

In general, women have more traditional normative orientations toward sexuality than men, and this gender difference crosscuts other social categories, such as racial/ethnic groups, educational groups, and religious groups, although the gender difference does vary within these groups. Women's more traditional attitudes may reflect the sexual double standard that places more restrictions on women's sexuality than on men's. The fact that women and men are entering into sexual relationships with different understandings of sexuality is important to keep in mind in any analysis of sexual relationships.

DISCUSSION

Women's sexuality is heavily conditioned by the social groups to which they belong. Gender is one of the most important social categories that shape sexual behavior; cultural definitions of femininity include conceptions of how women are supposed to act sexually. The NHSLS indeed found substantial differences between women and men in their sexual preferences, experiences, and understandings about sexuality. Women tended to find fewer of the sexual practices included in the survey appealing, had fewer sexual partners, were more likely to experience unwanted sex, and had more traditional attitudes about sex than men.

However, this chapter has also shown the

tremendous variations in sexual expression among women of different ages, marital statuses, educational levels, religions, and races/ethnicities. In general, women who are younger, white, well educated, and have no religious affiliation have the most elaborated sexual practices, being the most likely to have experienced cunnilingus, fellatio, and anal sex, and to find these acts appealing. Despite their more elaborated sexual scripts, these groups of women were not, however, the most likely to experience frequent orgasms with their partners.

Perhaps one of the most interesting findings from this analysis is how women's sexuality has changed since before the sexual revolution of the 1960s through the outbreak of HIV/AIDS. Since the 1950s, women have been experiencing sexual intercourse at younger ages, having a greater number of partners, and are more likely to have experienced oral and anal sex. Unfortunately, however, women in the more recent cohorts are also more likely to experience their first sex as unwanted, and slightly more likely to have experienced forced sex. These trends can have long-term consequences for women's later sexual behavior, physical and emotional satisfaction, and sexual health.

Finally, our discussion of sexual satisfaction and dysfunction leads to the question of what is normal sexual functioning for women. Analyses of both sexual satisfaction and dysfunction show that women's sexuality cannot be understood in isolation; women's sexual experiences are in large part a function of the particular sexual relationship in which she is embedded. Both partners' sexual attitudes, exclusivity, emotional investment, as well as characteristics of the relationship as a whole, such as marital or cohabitational status, are important elements in women's sexual satisfaction and functioning.

REFERENCES

Blumstein, P., & Schwartz, P. (1985). *American couples: Money, work, sex*. New York: Pocket Books.

Browning, C. R. (1997). *Trauma in transition: A life course perspective on the long-term effects of early sexual experiences*. Unpublished doctoral dissertation, University of Chicago.

Browning, C. R., & Laumann, E. O. (1997). Sexual contact between children and adults: A life course perspective. *American Sociological Review*, 62(4), 540–560.

Bureau of Justice Statistics (1984). *Criminal victimization in the United States, 1982*. Washington, DC: U.S. Department of Justice.

DeLamater, J. (1987). A sociological approach. In J. H. Geer & W. T. O'Donohue (Eds.), *Theories of human sexuality*. New York: Plenum Press.

Fisher, Seymour (1973). *The female orgasm: Psychology, physiology, fantasy*. New York: Basic Books.

Goldman, G. D., & Milman, D. S. (Eds.) (1969). *Modern woman: Her psychology and sexuality*. Springfield, IL: Charles C. Thomas.

Goldscheider, F. K., & Waite, L. (1991). *New families, no families? The transformation of the American home*. Berkeley and Los Angeles: University of California Press.

Hite, S. 1979. *The Hite report on female sexuality*. New York: Knopf.

Hofferth, S. (1990). Trends in adolescent sexual activity, contraception, and pregnancy in the U.S. In J. Bancroft & J. M. Reinisch (Eds.), *Adolescence and puberty*. Oxford: Oxford University Press.

Hofferth, S. L., & Hayes, C. D. (Eds.) (1987). *Risking the future: Adolescent sexuality, pregnancy, and childbearing*. Washington, DC: National Academy Press.

Joyner, K., & Laumann, E. O. (2001). Teenage sex and the sexual revolution. In E. O. Laumann & R. T. Michael (Eds.), *Sex, love, and health: Private choices and public policies* (pp. 41–71). Chicago: University of Chicago Press.

Kaplan, H. S. (1995). *The sexual desire disorders: Dysfunctional regulation of sexual motivation*. New York: Brunner/Mazel.

Kinsey, A. C., Pomeroy, W. B., Martin, C. E., & Gebhard, P. H. (1953) *Sexual behavior in the human female*. Philadelphia: Saunders.

Klassen, A. D., Williams, C. J., & Levitt, E. E. (1989). *Sex and morality in the U.S.: An empirical enquiry under the auspices of the Kinsey Institute* (H. J. O'Gorman, Ed.). Middletown, CT: Wesleyan University Press.

Koss, M. P. (1988). Hidden rape: Sexual aggression and victimization in a national sample of students in higher education. In A. W. Burgess (Ed.), *Rape and sexual assault II*. New York: Garland.

Koss, M. P., Dinero, T., Seibel, C., and Cox, S. (1988). Stranger and acquaintance rape: Are there differences in the victim's experience? *Psychology of Women Quarterly*, *12*, 1–24.

Laumann, E. O., Gagnon, J. H., Michael, R. T., & Michaels, S. (1994). *The social organization of sexuality: Sexual practices in the United States*. Chicago: University of Chicago Press.

Laumann, E. O., Paik, A., & Rosen, R. (1999). Sexual dysfunction in the United States: Prevalence and predictors. *Journal of the American Medical Association*, *281*, 537–544.

Lofland, J. (1970). The youth ghetto. In E. O. Laumann, P. M. Siegel, & R. W. Hodge (Eds.), *The logic of social hierarchies* (pp. 756–778). Chicago: Markham.

Mahay, J. W., Laumann, E. O., & Michaels, S. (2001). Race, gender, and class in sexual scripts. In E. O. Laumann & R. T. Michael (Eds.), *Sex, love, and health: Private choices and public policies* (pp. 197–238). Chicago: University of Chicago Press.

Maltz, W., & Boss, S. (1997). *In the garden of desire: The intimate world of women's sexual fantasies*. New York: Broadway Books.

Masters, W. H., & Johnson, V. E. (1966). *Human sexual response*. Boston: Little, Brown.

Nathanson, C. A. (1991). *Dangerous passage: The social control of sexuality in women's adolescence*. Philadelphia: Temple University Press.

Roof, W. C. (1993). *A generation of seekers: The spiritual journeys of the baby boom generation*. San Francisco: Harper-Collins.

Rubin, L. B. (1982). Sex and sexuality: women at midlife. In M. Kirkpatrick (Ed.), *Women's sexual experience: Explorations of the dark continent*. New York and London: Plenum Press.

Russell, D. (1984). *Sexual exploitation: rape, child sexual abuse and workplace harassment*. Newbury Park, CA: Sage.

Simon, W., & Gagnon, J. H. (1987). Sexual scripts: Permanence and change. *Archives of Sexual Behavior*, *15*(2), 97–120.

Sterk-Elifson, C. (1994). Sexuality among African-American women. In A. S. Rossi (Ed.), *Sexuality across the life course*. Chicago: University of Chicago Press.

Smith, T. W. (1994). Attitudes toward sexual permissiveness: Trends, correlates, and behavioral connections. In A. S. Rossi (Ed.), *Sexuality across the life course*. Chicago: University of Chicago Press.

Waite, L. J., & Joyner, K. (2001). Emotional and physical satisfaction with sex in married, cohabitating, and dating sexual unions: Do men and women differ? In E. O. Laumann & R. T. Michael (Eds.), *Sex, love, and health: Private choices and public policies* (pp. 239–269). Chicago: University of Chicago Press.

Wyatt, G. E. (1982). The sexual experience of Afro-American women. In M. Kirkpatrick (Ed.), *Women's sexual experience: Explorations of the dark continent*. New York and London: Plenum Press.

Wyatt, G. E. (1993). *Sexual abuse and consensual sex: Women's developmental patterns and outcomes*. Newbury Park, CA: Sage.

5

Cultural Influences on Women's Sexual Health

HORTENSIA AMARO, AMANDA M. NAVARRO,
KERITH JANE CONRON, and ANITA RAJ

CULTURAL INFLUENCES ON WOMEN'S SEXUAL HEALTH

The goal of this chapter is to provide the reader with an analysis of the role of culture on women's sexuality and sexual health in the United States. Due to the growing diversity of the U.S. population (U.S. Bureau of the Census, 1999) and the epidemiology of sexual health problems, there is a great need for information that can assist public health practitioners in understanding cultural factors that play a role in women's sexual health.

Our review of the published literature revealed that research on women's sexuality across the lifespan is limited, and studies of women's sexuality across cultural groups in the United States are almost nonexistent. Thus, with this imperfect body of work, it is not possible to represent a complete and thorough analysis of cultural influences on sexuality. Instead, we

identify and discuss culture, gender, race and class and their role in defining women's sexuality and therefore their sexual health. We also present a summary of existing research in four developmental periods: childhood, adolescence, adulthood, and the mature years. The final section provides a synthesis of the themes presented in the literature and discusses implications for research and public health practice.

CULTURE, GENDER, AND SEXUALITY

The Oxford American Dictionary (1980) defines culture as "the customs and civilization of a particular people or group (p.155)." Anthropologists describe culture as a "set of guidelines (both explicit and implicit) which individuals inherit as members of a particular society (or group), and which tells them how to view the world, how to experience it emotionally, and how to behave in it...." (Helman, 1994, p. 2). When sociologists discuss culture, they generally include norms, values, beliefs, and expressive symbols (Peterson, 1979). The following definition of culture by Bernad Ostry (1978) conveys how all encompassing the impact of culture is:

HORTENSIA AMARO, AMANDA M. NAVARRO, KERITH JANE CONRON, and ANITA RAJ • Department of Social and Behavioral Sciences, Boston University School of Public Health, Boston, Massachusetts 02118.

Handbook of Women's Sexual and Reproductive Health, edited by Wingood and DiClemente. Kluwer Academic / Plenum Publishers, New York, 2002.

Culture, however we define it, is central to everything we do and think. It is what we do and the
reasons why we do it, what we wish and why we
imagine it, what we perceive and how we express it,
how we live and in what manner we approach
death. It is our environment and the pattern of our
adaptation to it. It is the world we have created and
are still creating; it is the way we see that world and
the motives that urge us to change it. It is the way
we know each other and ourselves; it is our web of
personal relationships, it is the images and abstrac-
tions that allow us to live together in communities
and nations. It is the element in which we live. (p.1)

These definitions of culture acknowledge
that individuals often belong to more than one
cultural group and that culture can be based on
any unifying social phenomenon such as race/
ethnicity, gender, class, religion, sexual orientation, region, national origin, and age. Margaret
Mead described two types of social groups: abstract social groups, and concrete social classes
or subgroups, which are actually functioning
social units in terms of which of their individual members are directly related to one another
(Griswold, 1994). Subcultures emerge when relations between individuals in a social unit are
strong enough to counteract some of the influences of the societal generalized other. Subcultures operate with their own powerful set of
symbols, meanings, and behavioral norms—
often the opposite of those in the larger culture
(Griswold, 1994).

Thus, within any society there are numerous cultures and subcultures, and any given
individual can be affiliated with multiple cultures and subcultures. American cultures, for
example, include those of a variety of racial and
ethnic groups, immigrant culture, women's
culture, adolescent culture, lesbian culture, college culture, just to name a few. And an individual living in the United States may be a
Latina female, who is also an immigrant, an
adolescent, a lesbian and in college; therefore
her cultural makeup as an individual may be
comprised of all of these cultures as well as U.S.
American culture.

While culture can mean many things, in
the United States it is often defined as race/
ethnicity due to the diversity of racial/ethnic

groups as well as the history and continued
existence of racial hierarchy in the country.
Consequently, racial/ethnic groups are the primarily defined cultures of people in the United
States, and racial/ethnic identity is one of the
most common ways individuals define themselves. Further, ethnic identity development
and subsequent exploration, knowledge and acceptance of one's cultural group has been linked
to healthier psychological development of individuals of marginalized racial/ethnic groups
(Atkinson, Morten, & Sue, 1983; Cross, 1978;
Helms, 1985; Phinney, 1989, 1993).

While recognizing biological influences
on sexuality, scholars generally agree that sexuality is a social phenomenon based on prescribed arrangements and sexual scripts that
provide guidelines for gender appropriate behavior. These guidelines vary historically and
across cultures (Schneider & Gould, 1987). Socially approved sexual scripts provide individuals with clear guidelines for behavior, Gagnon
(1973) noted: "Sexual scripts are the plans that
people may have in their heads for what they are
doing and what they are going to do, as well as
being the devices for remembering what they
have done in the past."

Schneider and Gould (1987) point out that
"scripts vary by gender, from culture to culture,
and by subgroup within the culture" (pp. 6–9),
and individuals adherence to scripts may vary
from cultural prescriptions and across situations. They note that scripts whether sexual or
otherwise have the following five components:
(1) Who does a woman have sex with; that is,
what are the limits and constrains of appropriate partners? (2) What acts does a woman engage in sexually from the whole range of possible sexual acts? (3) When is sex done; that is,
at what times of the day, month, or year and in
one's life cycle? (4) Where, in setting or circumstance, does sex occur? (5) Why do people have
sex; that is, what are the culturally approved
accounts for doing sexual things that people
provide for themselves and others? (Gagnon,
1973).

As a social phenomenon, women's sexuality is embedded in and reflects women's as-

cribed lower social status. Schneider & Gould (1987) note that "gender domination suggests that women's sexual meanings and sexual language flow from male experience and male definitions of desire" (p.130). They identify the following four major assumptions as the basis of the current understanding of sexuality: (1) maleness and masculinity provide the normative baseline for understanding human sexuality; (2) heterosexuality is viewed as the only normal expression of sexual intimacy; (3) confusing sexuality with reproduction blurs the intricate meanings of both phenomena, especially for women; and (4) it is empirically unsound and conceptually unwise to detach sexuality from economic and political relations (Schneider & Gould, 1987).

RACE, CLASS, GENDER, AND SEXUALITY

As mentioned above, social arrangements that favor one group over another based on race, ethnicity, class and gender have an overwhelming impact on the health, including the sexual health, of populations in the United States (Williams, Lavizzo-Mourey, & Warren, 1994; Krieger & Fee, 1994). Race and class are powerful social categories clearly recognized as playing a primary role in shaping not only health but also many aspects of an individual's life experience. Turner and Kramer (1995) remind us of the importance of not only the individual acting out of prejudices, but also of the even more powerful effects of systemic domination of one group over another based on race:

> The word prejudice has come to mean negative attitudes toward a specific group without sufficient warrant, whereas the work discrimination refers to the acting out of prejudices to the detriment of a specific group and its members. The most comprehensive meaning of racism however must also include the concepts of power, stratification, and oppression. That is, inordinate power is held by one racial group; society is stratified according to race; and the dominant racial group uses its power to maintain this system and to oppress those who have been subordinated against their will. (p. 5)

The dynamics of racial and class oppression and their resulting impact on beliefs, attitudes and behaviors among so called "racial and ethnic minority groups" are often confused with the influence of culture. Through time it can become difficult to disentangle the threads of what we observe in a group as "cultural" and what beliefs, attitudes and behaviors result from survival strategies, adaptation to life conditions, or internalization of negative attributes ascribed to one's cultural group. For example, researchers have documented social conditions from slavery to modern times which shaped values related to motherhood and marriage, all of which led to higher acceptance of adolescent pregnancy among African-Americans in the United States (Anderson, 1990; Frazier, 1996; Hardy & Zabin, 1991; Ladner, 1971; Williams, 1991).

Specific manifestations of racism in reproductive health have been documented and include the critical and scientifically supported role of the eugenics movement and its role in reproductive control of nondesirable groups, including poor immigrants and other racial/ethnic minority groups (Bulhan, 1985; Galton, 1952; Hasian, 1996; Paul, 1995). These efforts include U.S. government–led sterilization targeted to women of color (Aptheker, 1974; Health Research Group, 1973; Herold, Warren, Smith, Rochat, Martinez, & Vera, 1986; Lopez, 1985; Schenshul, Borrero, Barrera, Backstrand, & Guarnaccia, 1982; Rodriguez-Trias, 1984; U.S. General Accounting Office, 1976; Warren, Westoff, Herold, Rochat, & Smith, 1986), the recent CRACK project that provides payment for sterilization to poor African-American and Latina mothers addicted to crack, and the infamous Tuskegee Study that prevented African-Americans in Alabama from receiving syphilis treatment (Gamble, 1993).

Racism has played an important role in the social control of sexuality among racial and ethnic minority groups. A common dynamic of oppression is the dominant groups' ascription of negative attributes to the subservient group (Amaro & Raj, 2000). Included in these negative ascriptions are characteristics related to the sexuality and or sexual behavior of racial and ethnic minority groups such as promiscuity, sexual properness, size of sexual organs and libido, uncleanness, and lack of sexual impulse control (Bulhan, 1985). Similarly, sexism has played an important role in the social control of women's sexuality. Research on stereotypes of women has demonstrated that regardless of race, in comparison to men, women are rated as less ambitious, competent, intelligent, self-confident, and hostile (Landrine, 1985, 1999). Further, there is also evidence that people hold different stereotypes of women based on their perception of women's race and class background. A study by Landrine (1999) showed that the stereotypes of lower-class women and black women were consistently more unfavorable than those held about middle-class and white women. These stereotypes are also reflected in the well-documented gender bias (Baker Miller, 1986), racism (Bulhan, 1985), and class bias (Freire, 1970) evident in the scientific and practice-based disciplines in the social sciences, medicine, and public health (Broverman, Broverman, Clarkson, Rosenkrantz, & Vogel, 1970; Reid, 1993; Reiker & Jankowski, 1995; Townsend, 1995; Turner & Kramer, 1995).

Consequently, one cannot discuss women's sexuality without acknowledging the influences of culture, societal oppression (i.e., racism, ethnocentrism, classism, and sexism), and institutional oppression such as biases in public health research and practice. Thus, a cultural analysis of women's sexual health recognizes these influences across the life span.

SEXUAL HEALTH THROUGHOUT THE LIFE SPAN

Childhood

While it is generally accepted that the foundation for healthy sexual development starts early in life, the empirical literature on children's development is rich in nearly every aspect of development with the exception of sexual development. Although, traditional the-oretical formulations in psychology (e.g., psychoanalytic theory) have given attention to the importance of very early healthy sexual development, these are not generally grounded in scientific inquiry or systematic study. In this section, we first discuss gender identity and gender role socialization, through which children learn culturally ascribed gender roles, expectations, sexual scripts, and behaviors. Next we discuss research on early childhood sexuality, and end the section with the impact of sexual abuse on children's sexual development. Where research identifies differences across cultural groups, we present and discuss these findings.

Gender Identity and Gender Role Socialization

Gender identity "is the individual's private experience of his or her socially defined gender: the concept of the self as male or female" (Lips, 1997, p. 145). Existing evidence indicates that gender identity forms out of the early experience of being assigned and consistently treated as male or female (Collaer & Hines, 1995; Money & Ehrhardt, 1996) rather than by hormonal or biological factors. Thus, through gender role socialization, boys and girls gain an understanding of how the society in which they live view women and men, what attributes they are ascribed, and what roles they are expected to play. This early assumption of gender identity sets the stage and the scripts for sexual behavior in childhood, adolescence, and adulthood.

Gender role socialization, the process of learning what are considered appropriate or inappropriate attitudes, behaviors, and values based on one's biological sex, starts early in life. At birth, parents as well as others view and treat infants differently based on their biological sex (O'Brien & Huston, 1985; Pomerleau, Bolduc, Malcuit, & Cossette, 1990; Rubin, Provenzano, & Luria, 1974; White & Brinkerhoff, 1981). This socialization defines girl babies as fragile, passive and desiring affection, where male children are ascribed as stronger, aggressive, and requiring less affection. This socialization may differ between mothers and fathers. Bronstein

(1999) found fathers but not mothers differed significantly in their interactions with girls and boys. Fathers paid more attention to the boys and showed more achievement/cognitive orientation with them than with the girls. Girls were treated gently, were not given full attention, and had opinions and values imposed on them. Thus, as mentioned previously, girls are relegated to the subordinate position in society.

Other powerful social sources that influence children's gender socialization are media influences, i.e., children's books and children television programs. Earlier studies show that female characters were virtually invisible in children's books (St. Peter, 1979; Stockard & Johnson, 1980; Weitzman, Eifler, Hokada, & Ross, 1972). Some research indicated that more children's stories are boy-centered rather than girl-centered, and males are portrayed as adventurous, brave, and competent, while girls are shown as incompetent, fearful, and dependent (Davis, 1984; Peterson & Lach, 1990). Although recent studies have shown more egalitarian depictions (Crabb & Bielawski, 1994; Davis, 1984; Dougherty & Engel, 1987; Kortenhaus & Demarest, 1993; Oskamp, Kaufman, & Wolterbeek, 1996), the majority of children's books continue to reflect traditional gender roles (Crabb & Bielawski, 1994; Davis, 1984; Dougherty & Engel, 1987; Kortenhaus & Demarest, 1993). Studies of children's television programs have also shown that females are less commonly depicted than males, that when females are depicted it is while they interact with males, and that both females and males depicted usually portray traditional gender stereotypes (Durkin, 1985; Lott, 1989).

As a consequence of socialization by parents and media, children are generally able to distinguish between the two sexes by the end of the first year. By ages 3 to 4, most are also able to use gender labels to classify themselves and others (Maccoby, 1998; Money & Ehrhardt, 1996). At this same age children begin to seek out and play with playmates of their own sex and avoid children of the opposite sex (Maccoby, 1998). The tendency to prefer same-sex playmates becomes progressively stronger throughout the preschool years and until grade school (Maccoby, 1998). These segregated interactions reinforce traditional sex roles and affect early male–female interactions, which have an impact on later male–female relationships (Maccoby, 1990, 1998).

There is some evidence that gender socialization patterns are not consistent among different socioeconomic and racial/ethnic groups in the United States. For example, gender stereotyping tends to be stronger and restrictions greater for females in working class families than in middle class families (McBroom, 1981). There is also some evidence showing a less rigid pattern of gender role socialization with African-American women due to the possible presence of extended kinship bonds. More women in African-American families may be involved in the socialization of children who are not their biological children, providing the children with several alternative role models (Greene, 1994b). In addition, unlike traditional gender expectations held by the dominant White culture, African-American girls are socialized to have more economic responsibility and a commitment to employment than White girls (Greene, 1994b; Myers, 1989; Smith, 1982). Conflicting findings have been seen among gender role studies with Latinos and Whites. One study found that Latinos are socialized differently than Whites, for example Mexican families in the United States seem to promote more pronounced traditional sex roles than White Americans (Uribe, Medardo, LeVine, & LeVine, 1994). In contrast, Bronstein (1999) found similar patterns of parental interaction for Mexican and American families. However, both studies indicated a stronger influence of gender role socialization from the father.

Overall, research on gender role socialization indicates that girls are socialized by dominant society to be passive and subordinate, resulting in increased invisibility and reduced autonomy. Furthermore, findings indicate that messages from racial/ethnic minority groups can sometimes deviate from those provided by dominant society. These conflicting messages combined with the pervasive racism of society can further contribute to the sexist messages received by girls, such that girls are forced to develop in a climate that represses their individual control of self and limits their identity formation.

Early Sexuality

Ernest Borneman (1990) suggests that the first phase of sexual development is the cutaneous phase in which an infant's skin is considered a "single erogenous zone." Between six months to one year, infants begin to touch their genitals, sometimes producing sexual excitement and orgasm. From ages 3 to 6 they can be flirtatious and like to play-act love affairs with their playmates, and during the middle years of childhood they are likely to attempt intromission (Money & Ehrhardt, 1996). Parents' reactions to these different behaviors directly influence subsequent sexual attitudes and behavior (Money & Ehrhardt, 1996).

Typically, gender role stereotypes make it more acceptable for male children rather than female children to engage in these types of early sexual behaviors. Research shows that compared to boys, girls interested in romance and sex during childhood create more anxiety and alarm in adults (Borneman, 1990; Goldman & Goldman, 1982). Such feelings in girls are often seen as unnaturally precocious and inappropriate. Research also shows that, although masturbation is common among young children (Galenson & Roiphe, 1976; Kleeman, 1975) and parents are aware that children masturbate (Gagnon, 1985), few parents report that their own children masturbate, especially their female children (Gagnon, 1985). Clearly, societal repression of female sexuality starts early in girls' lives, creating a climate for females in which their sexual autonomy cannot easily develop.

Sexual Abuse

Sexual abuse during childhood is a pervasive phenomenon among girls and this has a direct and serious impact on their sexual development and sexual health. Recent studies with adolescents demonstrated that girls are approximately three times more likely than boys to report having been sexually abused, with approximately 30% of the girls reporting having been victimized (Thomas, Nelson, & Summers, 1994; Raj, Silverman, & Amaro, 2000). Retrospective studies of adult women have indicated rates of childhood sexual abuse ranging from 6% (Siegel, Sorenson, Golding, Burnham, & Stein, 1987) to 62% (Wyatt, 1985). In addition, numerous studies also indicate that childhood sexual abuse is also associated with a variety of high risk sexual behavior and sexual health concerns during adolescence and adulthood (Cunningham, Stiffman, Dore, & Earls, 1994; Golding, 1996; Irwin *et al.*, 1995; Plichta & Abraham, 1996; Raj *et al.*, 2000; Zierler, Feingold, Laufer, & Velentgas, 1991). High-risk behaviors include not using condoms or contraceptives, earlier first coitus, and having a greater number of sex partners. Sexual health concerns include unwanted pregnancy, STDs, HIV, and cervical cancer.

Minimal research has been conducted on race/ethnicity and sexual abuse and that which has been conducted focuses on epidemiological differences. Research findings showing that incidence of sexual abuse varies according to racial/ethnic group is conflicting. For example, similar rates were found among Latina, African–American, or White women (Arroyo, Simpson, & Aragon, 1997; Romero, Wyatt, Loeb, Carmona, & Solis, 1999; Russell, 1986; Wyatt, 1985). However, Seigel *et al.* (1987) reported that non-Hispanic White women were more than twice as likely than Hispanics to report childhood victimization. In contrast, Kercher and McShane (1984) reported a significantly higher rate of sexual abuse among Latino residents of Texas than among their White counterparts. In Lindholm and Willey's (1986) study, African-American girls were less likely to be reported for sexual abuse than Anglo or Latina girls, while Tzeng and Schwarzin (1990) found African-American children to be more vulnerable to being reported. Russell (1983) found that Asian women reported a lower rate of childhood victimization than did White women.

In addition, specifics of the abuse have also led to contradictory findings. One study found that African-American girls were younger than White or Latina girls when their abuse began (DeJong, Hervada, & Emmett, 1982). African-American children reported for sexual abuse were younger, had their abuse reported sooner, and were more likely to deny the abuse than White children (Pierce & Pierce, 1984). In contrast, Wyatt (1985) found that White women were abused at a younger age than African-American counterparts. Also, while some studies (Rao, DiClemente, & Ponton, 1992) have found that having a male relative as an abuser was most likely for Asians and least likely for Whites and Hispanics; others (Russell, 1986; Tzeng & Schwarzin, 1990) report that African-American girls were less likely to be abused by a biological father than White girls. Mennen (Mennen, 1994; Mennen & Meadow, 1995) found that race/ethnicity does have a relationship with the duration of abuse, with White girls tending to be abused longer than their Latina or African-American peers.

Some differences in levels of trauma by race/ethnic group have been noted in retrospective studies with women. For example, Wyatt (1990) reported few differences in African-American and White women in the initial effects of sexual abuse. However, Russell (1986) found a significant relationship between race/ethnicity and degree of trauma. Latinas had the highest percentage of subjects reporting considerable trauma, followed in order by African-American, Asians, and Whites. In addition, one study found higher rates of rape associated with a prior history of child sexual abuse among White, African-American, and Latina women, but not for Asian-American women (Urquiza & Goodlin-Jones, 1994).

Conflicting findings across studies of racial and ethnic minority women may be attributed to methodological flaws or difference. Use of different types of samples, different tools, and different data acquisition techniques yields different findings for this type of sensitive topic. In addition, socioeconomic status may not have been taken into account and, thus,

may have confounded findings. Further, different racial and ethnic groups may have different comfort levels in reporting victimization. However, certain findings appear to be common across all groups: Girls reporting a history of sexual abuse tend to have been victimized by an older male familiar, experience long-term trauma as a consequence, and report higher-risk sexual behavior and greater sexual health concerns. Again, this appears to be a direct consequence as well as a reinforcement of women's lower status in society, and this appears to cut across racial and ethnic groups.

Adolescence

Adolescence, typically described as ages 13 to 18, is more commonly recognized as a time of sexual exploration for youth. Consequently, more sexuality research has been conducted with adolescents. However, due to the stigmatization of sexuality, this research has primarily focused on adolescent sexual development and exploration as negative, with many of the studies marking racial and ethnic minority females as "problematic". The following section will focus on the epidemiology of adolescent sexual behavior, how self-esteem, body image, and attitudes toward menstruation influence racial and ethnically diverse adolescent girls' sexual development, and sexual preference identity development in adolescent girls.

Adolescent Sexual Behavior

Recent Massachusetts Youth Risk Behavior Survey (YRBS) data indicate that 42.4% of adolescent girls and 46.8% of adolescent boys have engaged in sexual intercourse (Raj et al., 2000). Rickert, Jay, & Gottlieb (1990) found that 20% of adolescent girls and 33% of adolescent boys have had sexual intercourse by age 15. Although rates vary for racial and ethnic groups, higher rates of sexual activity for males are consistent across racial and ethnic groups. Black and Hispanic males were more likely than Black and Hispanic females to have had sexual intercourse and had multiple sex partners. However, Black female students were more likely than Hispanic and White female students to have had sexual intercourse, had first coitus at an earlier age, and had multiple sex partners. The few studies with Asian-American youth indicate greater sexual conservatism for this population. Asian youth initiate sexual activity later, are less likely to be sexually active (Cochran, Mays, & Leung, 1991; Moore & Erikson, 1985; Yap, 1986), and report lower HIV knowledge than other youth (DiClemente, Zorn, & Temoshok, 1987). Within racial or ethnic group differences have not been well explored (e.g., within Asian, Latino, or Black groups) and may vary based on cultural and other influences in these groups.

Increased sexual behavior and number of sex partners among males as compared with females may be a consequence of increased acceptance of these behaviors for males. Female sexual development is shaped by socialization such that they repress or fail to report their natural sexual behavior. Differences in rates for racial and ethnic minority groups may also be a consequence of societal expectations and stereotypes.

Self-Esteem

Much research has been conducted on the role of girls' self esteem on their development including their sexual development. This research, conducted on mostly White middle class girls in the United States, has shown that girls pay close attention to the dominant culture's messages of being timid and fragile (Brown & Gilligan, 1992; Rogers, 1993). Feingold (1994) reports that in childhood girls have higher self-esteem than boys, but during adolescence this trend reverses. For the most part, girls are pressured by the dominant White culture to be compliant and silent (Baker Miller, 1986). During adolescence, girls tend to show a loss of self-confidence, loss of "voice" and courage to "speak one's mind" (Baker Miller, 1986; Gilligan, 1982; Gilligan, Lyons, & Hammer, 1990; Gilligan, Rogers, & Tolman, 1991). During this time, girls also begin experiencing more

depression than males (Nolen-Hoeksema, 1987; Seigel *et al.*, 1998), with girls from lower socioeconomic backgrounds experiencing greater depression due to more stressful life events (Garrison, Schuchter, Schoenbach, & Kaplan, 1989; Gore, Aseltine, & Colton, 1992; Seigel *et al.*, 1998). Brown and Gilligan (1992) suggest that this reduced self-esteem and increased depression are a consequence of the gender role socialization labeling them as less than males. As a result, many girls desire male attention as proof of their increased value.

However, several studies have shown that gender differences in self-esteem do not follow the same patterns across all racial and ethnic groups. Dukes and Martinez (1994) examined the impact of "ethgender"—the combination of ethnicity, race, and gender—on junior high and high school students and found that ethnicity, race and gender interact to produce different levels of core and public self-esteem. Black and Hispanic males had the highest levels of global self-esteem, and Asian and Native American females had the lowest. Asian and Native American females also had the lowest public self-esteem, while White and Black males had the highest levels. All females, except Black females, had lower levels of both global and public self-esteem than did males. Brown *et al.* (1998) examined the changes in self-esteem in White and Black girls, ages 9 to 14, and also found that self-esteem does not follow the same developmental pattern in Black as in White girls. Black girls had higher and more stable self-worth and greater satisfaction with their physical appearance in comparison to White girls. The AAUW survey (1995) revealed similar findings. This study showed that as girls went from elementary to high school, Whites and Hispanics reported lower self-esteem, where Black girls reported minimal change.

Way's (1995) findings with a group of urban poor and working-class girls show similar trends to those reported by Dukes & Martinez (1994), Brown *et al.* (1998) and AAUW (1995). However, her qualitative analysis revealed that this reaction too was based on the threat to girls' self-esteem. Further, some girls reporting that although they considered themselves "outspoken" could not speak their minds with boys for fear of losing relationships or of being betrayed. Unlike White girls, maintaining a "voice" is crucial for girls that are not only marginalized by their gender but also by their race, ethnicity, or class. Way (1995) argues that African-American and Puerto Rican parents teach their daughters to be outspoken and strong because if they are passive they may be pushed further into the margins of society. However, Way (1995) found that in the context of relationships with boyfriends, African-American girls also silenced themselves for fear of causing conflict and losing relationships with boys.

Body Image

Poor body image is a significant factor influencing girls' self-esteem and self-confidence. Negative body image among females is very common and often said to be a state of "normative discontent" (Cash & Pruzinsky, 1990; Rodin, Silberstein, & Streigel-Moore, 1985). During puberty, the change that girls experience such as an increase in body mass, particularly around the hips and thighs, contradicts the dominant White culture's standard of beauty, which may lead to body dissatisfaction and distress (Attie, Brooks-Gunn, & Petersen, 1990; Blythe, Simmons, & Zakin, 1985; Rosenblum & Lewis, 1999; Wardle & Marsland, 1990).

Much research indicates that poor body image is more a part of White culture than the cultures of other racial and ethnic groups in the United States. Researchers found in the comparison of body perceptions between White and African-American girls that more White girls perceived themselves as overweight and were more likely to engage in unhealthy dieting practices (Neff, Sargent, McKeown, Jackson, & Valois, 1997). While African-American females expressed their desire to gain weight, White females wanted to lose weight. Studies have also shown that African American and Caribbean men and women value a larger size

body and normal-weight females are less likely to consider themselves overweight (Coogan, Bhalla, Sefa-Dedah, & Rothblum, 1996; Furnham & Baguma, 1994; Rucker & Cash, 1992; Smith & Cogswell, 1994; Thompson, Sargent, & Kemper, 1996). However, among more highly acculturated and higher socioeconomic status African-American and Hispanic girls and women (i.e., those more closely tied with White culture), poor body image and subsequent eating disorders are more common (Bowen, Tomoyasu, & Cauce, 1991). Further, additional research indicates that within Latino and Asian groups, many females share some of the preference for thinness exhibited by the dominant culture (Cash & Henry, 1995; Joiner & Kashubeck, 1996; Wardle, Bindra, Fairclough, & Westcombe, 1993), and are at greater risk of developing eating disorders (Robinson *et al.*, 1996).

Overall, research on body image indicates that while not as much a factor for racial and ethnic minority girls as it may be for White girls, it is still an issue, especially for more acculturated girls of color. Further, this research is limiting by defining body image solely by weight. Factors such as skin color/shade or hair texture play a larger role in attractiveness within non-White cultures than in the dominant White culture (Bond & Cash, 1992; Sahay & Piran, 1997); hence they may be more accurate measures of body image for some cultures. Regardless, body image is based on unrealistic expectations of one's body. Again, it is a socialization that reduces girls' perceptions of control over their own bodies, where only unnatural interventions (i.e., eating disorders, hair chemicals, skin bleaches) can help. And it further reduces girls' self-esteem by defining beauty by what they are naturally not, based on gender as well as race and ethnicity.

Menstruation

Menstruation is a natural event that signifies girls' healthy adolescent development. It is a marker of puberty and a girl's ability to conceive a child. By the time that girls experience menarche, they are conscious of the rules and taboos of menstruation (Stoltzman, 1986). Such rules include shame and discomfort, requiring that the girl feel she has something to hide (Brooks-Gunn & Ruble, 1980). Numerous religions disallow women and girls from attending services when they are menstruating due to the "impurity" of it. However, most researchers and health professionals agree that a girl's first period is an important turning point in her life, changing her feelings about her body, her sexuality, and her identity as a woman (Golub, 1983; Rierdan & Koff, 1980; Taylor & Woods, 1991). Thus, the social rules of menstruation reinforce the messages that for girls sex is shameful, impure, and something she must hide.

Sexual Preference Identity Development

Research on adolescent sexual behavior primarily focuses on behavior between males and females. Outside of the HIV literature, research on gay, lesbian, and bisexual adolescent sexuality has been virtually nonexistent (see Rosario, Meyer-Bahlburg, Hunter, Exner, Gwadz, & Keller, 1996). The little research that has been conducted has been on biased samples of teens willing to report being gay or bisexual. These teens are the minority, as indicated by a 1985 survey in which only 1 in over 1000 checked the "homosexual identity" box (Coles & Stokes, 1985).

Although relatively few adolescents who report same-sex attractions, fantasies, or activities acknowledge that they are gay, lesbian, or bisexual, those who do report higher self-esteem (Savin-Williams, 1990). Unfortunately, representative youth data indicate that those who identify as lesbian or bisexual females also report increased sexual risk behavior (Rosario, Meyer-Bahlburg, Hunter, &, Gwadz, 1999). Some researchers argue that sexual development is particularly difficult for gay, lesbian, and bisexual adolescents of color, as they must integrate their ethnic, cultural, and racial background with their sexual orientation and identity (Savin-Williams & Rodriguez, 1993). How-

ever, others report no racial/ethnic differences in gay-related stree in youth (Rosario, Rotherman-Borus, & Reid, 1996; Rosario, Meyer-Bahlburg, *et al.*, 1996).

ADULTHOOD

Adulthood is the socially sanctioned time in life for women's sexual activity. Thus there is much research on the sexual behavior of racial and ethnic minority women. The research perspective tends to focus on these women's sexual activities as negative, emphasizing the outcomes of disease and welfare children. However, as with the adolescent research, this is also primarily focused on health practices and concerns rather than on women's sexual satisfaction. The following section will focus on contraception and STD/HIV prevention, gender roles, and lesbians.

Contraception and Condom Use

As mentioned above, racial and ethnic minority women are commonly identified as problem contraceptors; consequently, more effective methods of contraception such as injections and sterilization are urged for these groups (Forrest, 1994; Henshaw, 1998). A recent study by Piccinino and Mosher (1998) revealed that overall contraceptive use, including sterilization (male and female combined), did not vary substantially by race/ethnicity among adult women. Nonetheless, this same study also found that Blacks were most likely to use implants (Norplant) and injectables (Depo-Provera), whereas Whites were most likely to use the pill. Further, although overall sterilization did not differ across groups, female sterilization rates were considerably higher among Hispanic and Black women as compared with White women, regardless of socio-economic status (Piccinino & Mosher, 1998).

Although the use of methods that provide longer-term contraceptive protection is more common among Black and Hispanic women, unintended pregnancies and abortion are more common among these groups as well (Henshaw, 1998). This may be a consequence of cultural differences in the acceptability of unintended pregnancy, consistent contraceptive use, and in some cases being pressured to practice long-term contraception. Amaro (1988) and Kuss (1997) found in their studies with Latinas and Asians that, despite holding pronatal values, women felt compelled to use contraception and limit family size due to financial limitations.

Condom use, more often used by Black women than White or Hispanic women (Anderson, Wilson, Doll, Jones, & Barker, 1999; Piccinino & Mosher, 1998), are more commonly associated with STD/HIV protection rather than contraceptive use. Researchers found that among Hispanics, condom use was more likely to be successful if used for contraceptive reasons, rather than for disease prevention (Fleisher, Senie, Minkoff, & Jaccard, 1994). Nonetheless, condom use remains stigmatized by most cultures, including among Blacks and Hispanics, as a marker of casual relationships (Catania et al., 1994; Carovano, 1991; Fullilove, Fullilove, Haynes, & Gross, 1990; Marin, Tschann, Gomez, & Gregorich, 1998; Sobo, 1995). Further, studies with Hispanic women indicate that they report unprotected sex with their partners even when they knew their partners were infected with HIV because unprotected sex represents love and intimacy (Yeakley & Gant, 1997; Yep, 1992).

Gender Role Stereotypes

Gender role stereotypes starting early in life define the female role as the "sexual gatekeeper" while males are to be the sexual aggressor (Erickson, 1998–1999). Only "bad" women are allowed to enjoy sex, but these women do not warrant respect or consideration by men. Good women are to be dominated by males sexually, placing them at risk for sexual violence. The dichotomy of women's sexual roles as Madonna/Whore places all women at greater sexual risk by reducing her sexual control. Researchers have documented the presence of a Madonna/Whore belief system among both

African-American women and Latinas (Fullilove, Fullilove, Haynes, & Gross, 1990; Lown, Winkler, Fullilove, & Fullilove, 1993; Erickson, 1998–1999).

Fullilove et al.'s (1990) study with African-American women and girls found that "Madonnas" were women in steady relationships in which condoms were not used. These women were monogamous, though their partners might not be. "Whores" were substance users who engaged in sex with multiple partners. These women were more likely to use condoms, although consistent condom use and lower-risk partners were unlikely. In contrast, some studies of Latino groups suggest that culture impacts the acceptability of woman initiated communication about sexual activity and pleasure. "Proper" women are expected to be ignorant about sex and serve as "gatekeepers" to sexual activity (Erickson, 1998–1999). A Hispanic woman who carries condoms may be viewed as "prepared for sex" and thus believed to be promiscuous and undesirable (Mays & Cochran, 1988; Weeks, Schensul, Williams, Singer, & Grier, 1995). However, research on gender roles and their impact on condom use across cultural groups is in its infancy and delineating many of the culturally specific predictors of gender role influences and their impact on condom use require further research.

While culture may limit women's comfort in protecting themselves from HIV, gender role norms require that women take primary responsibility for sex, including contraceptive use. Recent surveys with men reveal that Black men, in particular, believe that women are more responsible for decisions about contraception (16% compared to 6% of White men and 4% of Hispanic men) (Grady, Tanfer, Billy, & Lincoln-Hanson, 1996). However, at the same time, researchers have documented the presence of a negative attitude by Hispanic and Black men toward woman initiated condom use (Catania et al. 1991; Gilmore, DeLamater, & Wagstaff, 1996; Weeks et al., 1995; Whitehead, 1997). Studies also show that male attitudes toward the use of protection are related to the likelihood of using protection (Amaro, Lopez-Gomez,

Conron & Cabral, 1998; Fleisher *et al.*, 1994). Thus, a "proper" woman is expected to take responsibility for sex, but at the same time she is not permitted control over the sexual situation with men. Therefore, women are at increased risk for sexual violence as well as sexual/reproductive health concerns including STD/HIV as a direct consequence of gender role stereotypes and sexism.

Lesbians

Gender roles impact not only women's sexual health, but also the ease with which women may form sexual relationships with other women. Gender roles vary across ethnic cultures to affect the acceptability of same-sex relationships. Heterogeneity of religious beliefs and acculturation within ethnic groupings may also affect the acceptability of same-sex relationship (Greene, 1994a; Solarz, 1999). For example, according to Liu and Chan (1996), sexual desires are obstacles to salvation under a Buddhist belief system. Same-sex behavior is believed to reflect the impurity of pursuing sexual desire, but homosexuality itself is not a sin. However, from a Taoist perspective, a balance of yin and yang is necessary to maintain harmony. This balance is reflected in the natural marriage of men and women; hence same-sex relationships are unbalanced and unnatural. Savin-Williams (1996) suggest that for African-Americans, strong family allegiance and strong religious beliefs may make it more difficult to come out as a lesbian, yet family bonds may decrease the likelihood that a lesbian will be rejected by her family or church. For Latinas, lesbianism may be perceived as a threat to the Latina gender role which values women who embrace motherhood and the nurturing of others (Morales, 1996); thus, lesbianism, viewed as antichildbearing, may be considered a threat to the highly valued family unit. Furthermore, Espin (1984) observes that claiming a lesbian identity requires acknowledgment of women's sexuality, which is often denied in Latino culture. According to Greene (1994a), Native American cultures are fairly accepting of varied gender roles, including a lesbian sexual orientation. However, contemporary attitudes, which are more influenced by the larger multicultural American culture, may be less accepting (Greene, 1994a).

MATURE WOMEN

The sexuality of women age 50 and older is largely unacknowledged by society. However, population-based data indicate frequent sexual activity for older married participants (Binson, Pollack, & Catania, 1997; Marsiglio & Donnelly, 1991), with no differences across racial and ethnic groups (Marsiglio & Donnelly, 1991). In fact, older women reported dysfunction comparable to that of younger women on a large national survey of sexual functioning (Laumann, Paik, & Rosen, 1999). Nonetheless, research on the sexuality of mature women has primarily focused on menopause and sexual dysfunction; thus, these will be the topics presetned in this section.

Menopause

Despite the finding by researchers that many women define menopause as a neutral or positive life event, a biomedical model of disease and decline pervades studies on this topic (Berg & Taylor, 1999; Kaufert, Boggs, Ettinger, Woods, & Utian, 1998). Further, biases in the research are primarily a result of menopausal research being dominated by those who stand to profit from medicalizing a natural process. Hence, the major themes appearing in the study of menopause are age of onset, estrogen-related symptoms (sweats and vaginal dryness), sexual interest and function, and treatment, particularly estrogen-replacement therapy (Pariser & Niedermier, 1998). In general, women are presented as a homogenous group in the literature (Kaufert *et al.*, 1998) and information is scant on women of minority ethnic groups in the United States (McKinlay, 1996). Culture is minimally considered as a lens that shapes interpretation of menopausal symptoms and attitudes toward symptom treatment.

Berg and Taylor's (1999) menopausal study of Filipinas, Thai women, and White women revealed the importance of cultural attitudes on menopausal symptomatology. Filipina Americans were least likely to report distressing symptoms of the three groups. Filipino culture also views "perimenopausal symptoms as a part of a normal life stage that does not warrant concern." However, Im and Lipson (1997) suggest that as Asian cultural attitudes change with acculturation, views of menopause change. In Korean culture, for instance, menopause is welcomed as a sign of age because as women grow older, they gain greater respect and power within the family and community. However, as Korean-American society becomes more acculturated and elders are less respected, the authors suggest that women may be prone to depression related to role devaluation. Unfortunately, these studies do not indicate how cultural attitudes toward menopause influence the sexual pleasure and functioning of mature women.

DISCUSSION

This chapter sought to provide a selective summary of what is known about women's sexual health within a life-span developmental framework. Available research reveals that much of the existing work related to women's sexual health is focused on "risk" behaviors and "problem" populations. In other words, sexual health research, practice and policy focuses on sexuality primarily from a disease perspective and approaches the sexuality of racial/ethnic groups from the perspective of "fixing" a problem. This research is generally void of a contextual understanding of women's sexuality and women's experiences and relies primarily on limited methods largely defined by political agendas that have impeded real progress in this field of scientific inquiry and public health application (di Mauro, 1995). With these limitations in mind, a number of major themes

emerge in the literature. In this section we discuss some of the overarching themes and areas for future research.

First, the review of the existing literature on the cultural variations in sexuality and health proved extremely disappointing. Since the comprehensive review conducted in 1996 by Wiederman, Maynard, & Fretz (1996), which found that only 25% of published sexuality research articles between 1971 and 1995 reported the ethnic composition of the sample, we found little progress in the field. Even fewer studies (7.3%) considered ethnicity a relevant variable (Wiederman et al., 1996). We found that while some studies included the most basic information (i.e., race and/or ethnicity) in the description of the study sample, very few had sufficiently large samples to conduct systematic comparisons or had focused study questions on the cultural aspects of sexuality and sexual health (di Mauro, 1996; Tiefer, 1994). Existing research has revealed little about cultural differences in sexual norms, socialization of children around sexuality and sexual behaviors. While some of this body of research provides data on racial and sometimes ethnic differences in sexual behaviors, it tells us little about how culture within and across various groups shapes sexual norms, expectations, and behaviors. Instead racial or ethnic differences are reported without consideration of their cultural meanings. Further, socioeconomic differences across groups are not considered, and these are interpreted as reflecting underlying cultural factors that determine the sexual behaviors reported. Despite an adequate empirical base, we found many examples of undocumented claims of cultural differences in sexual behavior and sexual norms—many of which were aligned with common stereotypes of women of color (e.g., discussions of gender role restrictions were more often explored in discussions of sexuality among Latinas).

The research found also had a number of notable methodological limitations, further restricting our understanding of culture and sexuality. We have already mentioned the problems of sampling with survey research. Much current data on sexual behavior and sexual health has been collected as part of larger disease specific studies whose primary focus is not sexuality or overall sexual health (di Mauro, 1995). Thus they have provided very circumscribed information that is often decontextualized from cultural and social factors that would help us to understand the underlying processes that shape them. Further, sample selection that relies on volunteers, response bias in self-administered questionnaires, and sample bias in studies using face-to face interviews present methodological challenges and biases in human sexuality research (Strassberg & Lowe, 1995). There is also a need for methods development to improve the reliability and validity of measures. For example, much of the research on children uses parent and child self-reporting and interviewing, but some recent studies have shown through observational data that the information given by parents and children is quite different from what is directly observed (Broderick, 1966; Hunt, 1974; Kinsey *et al.*, 1948, 1953). Although most parents state that they would not treat their child any differently because of gender, observational data presents a very different picture. Finally, assumptions underlying the biomedical model and health models of sexuality, which often ignore the contextual, cultural and social aspects of sexual behavior, the methods used in sexuality and sexual health research have resulted in a general absence of women's voices (Ehrhardt, 1996; Irvine, 1994; Krieger & Fee, 1994; McCormick, 1996; Schneider & Gould, 1987; Tiefer, 1991, 1994; Weis, 1998).

Second, existing research on sexuality is almost exclusively limited to "sexual bookkeeping" (Schneider & Gould, 1987), which was evident in the research initiated by Kinsey *et al.* (1948, 1953) and later continued in survey research. This research has focused almost exclusively on documenting the initiation and frequency of heterosexual intercourse, contraceptive use, and condom use to the near exclusion of almost all other aspects of sexuality. For example, in contrast to studies that document sexually related public health problem and risk be-

haviors, there is a striking dearth of studies of sexual attitudes, beliefs, and values, and the cultural and socialization processes and contexts that shape them (di Mauro, 1995; Parker & Gagnon, 1995; Irvine, 1994; Schneider & Gould, 1987; Tiefer, 1994). Further, even the "sexual bookkeeping" studies have been limited by the lack of generalizability of nonrepresentative samples, lack of attention to sexual behavior across the life cycle, and inadequate inclusion of varied populations based on race, ethnicity, sexual preference and other characteristics (di Mauro, 1995; Irvine, 1994; Peplau, Cochran, & Mays, 1997; Schneider & Gould, 1987; Strunin, 1994; Wyatt, 1994).

Third, there are major gaps in knowledge with respect to sexual behaviors and sexual health in the context of society and culture (di Mauro, 1995; Strunin, 1994; Tiefer, 1994). The Social Science Research Council Report *Sexuality Research in the United States: An Assessment of the Social and Behavioral Sciences* (di Mauro, 1995) concluded that research on sexual behavior should be both based on a framework of society and culture and be developmental in nature. The lack of such a framework has resulted in little information on various critical issues throughout the life cycle. For example, during childhood and adolescence little is known about what and how family and other institutions teach and influence sexual attitudes, norms, values and behaviors among children and adolescents of varying ethnic and cultural groups. In adolescence and adulthood, there has been very limited research beyond that on reproduction, contraception, disease control, and sexual dysfunction. Furthermore, in the older years, most research on women has centered on physiological changes related to menopause, almost completely ignoring these women as sexual beings.

Fourth, there is a lack of acknowledgment of and attention to issues of power and control in women's sexual realities; thus, there is potential danger for misdirected research to further contribute to this end. Perhaps the repeated attempts and strategies to control the sexuality and reproductive potential of groups that are not in power are understood best when one considers the implications of growth of a subordinate group. Lal (1995) notes that:

> Race prejudice is aroused when members of a dominant group perceive a real or an imaginary threat to an existing set of institutional arrangements and to a style of life as a result of claims by member of a subordinate and/or oppressed group for a greater share of material resources such as jobs, housing, and education and/or unfettered participation and greater inclusion in economic and political life.

From this perspective, the analyses of population growth and reproductive health problems must consider the interests of different social groups in identifying certain behaviors as public health problems. Griswold (1994) argues that adolescent pregnancy is an example of a social problem that is culturally constructed. She notes that labeling of "teenage pregnancy" as a social problem in the United States is not shared internationally where the social problem may be defined as not being married by age 20 (Nigeria) and having a female child (China). Kristen Luker's (1991) analysis of teen pregnancy in the United States concludes that concern about babies having babies have more to do with public disapproval of the welfare system, racial prejudices, and concerns about teen sexuality than with actual demographic changes of rising teen pregnancy. Luker (1991) challenges the view that teen pregnancy causes school dropout and poverty for young mothers and argues that it is the other way around. Griswold (1994) reminds us that when issues are defined as social problems, it is critical to question who creates the definition of the problem, who receives and interprets it, what meaning does it contain, and what is the social world in which it is meaningful (p. 95). She notes that social problems are identified or named based on American ideas and institutions, the same event or happening may get labeled differently as a problem or not in various settings and or even the analyses of the fault for the event may be different (p. 96). The conditions that get defined as a social problem, those that get selected are or can be made dramatic; resonate with deep mythic themes in the culture; and

they are politically viable, often because they are linked with powerful interest groups.

Finally, an often unquestioned assumption in most sexual health research is the designation of sexuality as a matter of health (Tiefer, 1994). It is clear that viewing sexuality within the context of public health and medicine has provided opportunities for research that otherwise might not have been supported. However, some feminist scholars have voiced great concern with the disadvantages that such models for framing issues of sexuality (Rothman, 1987; Tiefer, 1994; Schneider & Gould, 1987). Tiefer (1994) argues that assumptions of the biomedical model critiqued by Mishler (1981): norms and deviance, universality, individualism, and biological reductionism, render the study of women's sexuality at risk for great misuse and disservice. More than ever the rising rates of sexually transmitted disease, HIV infection, and continued public concern with adolescent pregnancy, have contributed to women's sexual health being assumed by the fields of public health and medicine and biomedical models of disease. The slow progress in advancing a culturally contextualized understanding of women's health was discussed in a comprehensive, but now 14-year-old, critique of the study of female sexuality by Schneider and Gould (1987). Unfortunately, their critique is still largely applicable today and the research and theoretical agenda that they set forth is still a valuable guide for the future of women's sexual health research. Some of the critiques of sexuality research made at that time continue to be noted in more recent reviews (Ehrhardt, 1996; Money & Ehrhardt, 1996).

Despite the limitations of much of the current sexuality and sexual health research, there is an emerging body of work that has sought to decipher the complex interplay between class, race, and sexuality and others who have sought to understand factors that help us to understand within-group differences in sexuality. Essed's research (1991) documents ways in which "racism and sexism interact to create specific ways in which women and men of various racial and ethnic groups create ideological constructions of racially specific femininity and sexuality, representing the opposite models of White middle class womanhood" (Essed, 1991, pp. 31–33). Her research documented "everyday racism" (p. 2) as a "process routinely created and reinforced through everyday practices," which include sexual violence involving verbal and nonverbal threats, sexual harassment, and the myth of sexual pathology of Blacks (p. 250). Other more recent contributions in the field of sexuality and sexual health research have also attended to contextual social and cultural issues in more nuanced and specific ways (Espin, 1999; Greene, 1997; Irvine, 1994; Wyatt, 1989; 1994).

While some attention on the influence of culture is evident in these more recent theoretical and scientific works on sexuality and sexual health, less attention has been given to the meanings of and daily realities and life conditions relevant to sexual health among culturally different groups. A critical reading of the reproductive health and sexuality literature demands that we understand the social and political context of sexuality. Advances in the understanding of cultural influences on sexual health and sexuality require that we develop more advanced scientific methods and integrative theoretical frameworks that help us to understand culture, oppression, and sexuality and their impact on sexual health. Thus, future work on culture and sexuality must include recognition of the following:

1. *Sexuality is a social and cultural construct* defined largely by each cultural group and their expectations and norms regarding what it means to be male and female.
2. *Dynamics of oppression based on class and race/ethnicity also shape sexuality for groups ascribed socially subservient positions.* The meaning of being female or male is shaped not only by specific cultural meanings but also by meanings imposed on subservient groups by the dominant group based on color, ethnicity, and class.
3. *Discerning the cultural vs. oppression influences on sexual behavior* requires the parallel development in knowledge regarding sexuality, and the processes of adaptation, survival, and

resistance by racial and culturally oppressed groups who are ascribed sexual and other characteristics by the more powerful social group. Through internalization of ascribed characteristics, influences of oppression on sexuality and sexual health can be erroneously interpreted as culturally based.

REFERENCES

American Association of University Women (AAUW) (1995). *How schools shortchange girls: The AAUW report.* Marlowe & Company.

Amaro, H. (1988). Women in the Mexican-American community: religion, culture, and reproductive attitudes and experiences. *Journal of Community Psychology, 16,* 6–20.

Amaro, H., Lopez-Gomez, A., Conron, K., & Cabral, H. (1998). Study of clients presenting for HIV counseling and testing in MDPH funded agencies. Unpublished report. Boston: Massachusetts Department of Public Health.

Amaro, H. & Raj, A. (2000). On the margin: Power and women's HIV risk reduction strategies. *Sex Roles, 42,* 723–749.

Anderson, E. (1990). *Streetwise: Race, class, and change in an urban community.* Chicago: University of Chicago Press.

Anderson, J. E., Wilson, R., Doll, L., Jones, S., & Barker, P. (1999). Condom use and HIV risk behaviors among U.S. adults: Data from a national survey. *Family Planning Perspectives, 31,* 24–28.

Aptheker, H. (1974). Sterilization, experimentation and imperialism. *Political Affairs, 53,* 37–48.

Arroyo, J. A., Simpson, T. L., & Aragon, A. S. (1997). Childhood sexual abuse among Hispanic and non-Hispanic white college women. *Hispanic Journal of Behavioral Sciences, 19,* 57–68.

Atkinson, D., Morten, G., & Sue, D. W. (1983). *Counseling American minorities.* Dubuque, IA: Wm. C. Brown.

Attie, I., Brooks-Gunn, J., & Petersen, A. (1990). A developmental perspective on eating disorders and eating problems. In M. Lewis & S. M. Miller (Eds.), *The handbook of developmental psychopathology.* New York: Plenum Press.

Baker Miller, J. (1986). *Toward a new psychology of women.* Boston: Beacon Press.

Berg, J. A., & Taylor, D. L. (1999). Symptom experience of Filipino American midlife women. *Menopause: The Journal of the American Menopause Society, 6,* 105–114.

Binson, J., Pollack, L., & Catania, J. A. (1997). AIDS-related risk behaviors and safer sex practices of women in midlife and older in the United States: 1990 to 1992. *Health Care for Women International, 18,* 343–354.

Blythe, D. A., Simmons, R. G., & Zakin, D. F. (1985). Satisfaction with body image for early adolescent females: The impact of pubertal timing within different school environments. *Journal of Youth and Adolescence, 4*, 207–225.

Bond, S. & Cash, T. F. (1992). Black beauty: Skin color and body images among African American college women. *Journal of Applied Social Psychology, 22*, 874–888.

Borneman, E. (1990). Progress in empirical research on children's sexuality In M. E. Perry (Ed.), *Childhood and adolescent sexology: Handbook of sexology. Vol. 7*. Amsterdam: Elsevier.

Bowen, D. J., Tomoyasu, N., & Cauce, A. M. (1991). The triple threat: A discussion of gender, class, and race differences in weight. *Women and Health, 17*(4), 123–143.

Broderick, C. B. (1966). Sexual behavior among pre-adolescents. *Journal of Social Issues, 22*(2), 6–21.

Bronstein, P. (1999). Differences in mothers' and fathers' behaviors toward children: A cross cultural comparison. In L. A. Peplau, S. C. DeBro, R. C. Veniegas, & P. L. Taylor (Eds.), *Gender, culture, and ethnicity: Current research about women and men*. Mountain View, CA: Mayfield.

Brooks-Gunn, J., & Ruble, D. N. (1980). The menstrual attitude questionnaire. *Psychosomatic Medicine, 42*(5), 503–512.

Broverman, I. K., Broverman, D. M., Clarkson, F. E., Rosenkranz, P. S., & Vogel, S. R. (1970). Sex-role stereotypes and clinical judgements of mental health. *Journal of Consulting and Clinical Psychology, 34*, 1–7.

Brown, L. M., & Gilligan, C. (1992). *Meeting at the crossroads: Women's psychology and girls' development*. Cambridge, MA: Harvard University Press.

Brown, K. M., McMahon, R. P., Biro, F. M., Crawford, P., Schreiber, G. B., Similo, S. L., Waclawiw, M., & Striegel-Moore, R. (1998). Changes in self-esteem in black and white girls between the ages of 9 and 14 years. *Journal of Adolescent Health, 23*, 7–19.

Bulhan, H. A. (1985). *Franz Fanon and the psychology of oppression*. New York: Plenum Press.

Carovano, K. (1991). More than mothers and whores: Redefining the AIDS prevention needs of women. *International Journal of Health Services, 21*, 131–142.

Cash, T. F., & Pruzinsky, T. (1990). *Body images: Development, deviance and change*. New York: Guilford Press.

Cash, T. F., & Henry, P. E. (1995). Women's body images: The results of a national survey in the USA. *Sex Roles, 33*, 19–28.

Catania, J. A., Coates, T. J., Golden, E., Dolcini, M., Peterson, J., Kegeles, S., Siegel, D., & Fullilove, M. T. (1994). Correlates of condom use among black, Hispanic, and white heterosexuals in San Francisco: The AMEN longitudinal survey. *AIDS Education and Prevention, 6*, 12–26.

Catania, J. A., Coates, T. J., Kegeles, S., Fullilove, M. T., Peterson, J., Marin, B., Siegel, D., & Hulley, S. (1991). Condoms use in multi-ethnic neighborhoods of San Francisco: The population-based AMEN (AIDS in multi-ethnic neighborhoods) study. *American Journal of Public Health, 81*, 284–287.

Cochran, S. D., Mays, V. M., & Leung, L. (1991). Sexual practices of heterosexual Asian American young adults. *Archives of Sexual Behavior, 20*, 381–391.

Coles, R., & Stokes, G. (1985). *Sex and the American teenager*. New York: Harper & Row.

Collaer, M. L., & Hines, M. (1995). Human behavioral sex differences: A role for gonadal hormones during early development? *Psychological Bulletin, 118*, 55–107.

Coogan, J. C., Bhalla, S. K., Sefa-Dedah, A., & Rothblum, E. D. (1996). A comparison study of United States and African students on perceptions of obesity and thinness. *Journal of Cross-Cultural Psychology, 27*, 98–113.

Crabb, P. B., & Bielawski, D. (1994). The social representation of material culture and gender in children's books. *Sex Roles, 30*, 69–79.

Cross, W. E., Jr. (1978). The Thomas and Cross models of physical nigrescence: A literature review. *Journal of Black Psychology, 4*, 13–31.

Cunningham, R. M., Stiffman, A. R., Dore, P., & Earls, F. (1994). The association of physical and sexual abuse with HIV risk behaviors in adolescence and young adulthood: Implications for public health. *Child Abuse and Neglect, 18*, 233–245.

Davis, A. J. (1984). Sex-differentiated behaviors in nonsexist picture books. *Sex Roles, 11*, 1–16.

DeJong, A. R., Emmet, G., & Hervada, A. R. (1982). Sexual abuse of children: Sex-, race-, and age-dependent variations. *American Journal of Disabled Children, 136*, 129–134.

DiClemente, R. J., Zorn, J., & Temoshok. L. (1987). The association of gender, ethnicity, and length of residence in the Bay Area to adolescents' knowledge and attitudes about acquired immune deficiency syndrome. *Journal of Applied Social Psychology, 17*, 216–230.

di Mauro, D. (1995). *Sexuality research in the United States: An assessment of the social and behavioral sciences*. The Sexuality Research Assessment Project. New York: The Social Science Research Council.

DiMauro, D. (1996). Executive summary of sexuality research in the United States: An assessment of the social and behavioral sciences. *Sexuality and Disability, 14*, 117–118.

Dougherty, W. H., & Engel, R. E. (1987). An 80s look for sex equality in Caldecott winners and honor books. *Reading Teacher, 40*, 394–398.

Dukes, R. L., & Martinez, R. (1994). The impact of ethgender on self-esteem among adolescents. *Adolescence, 29*, 105–115.

Durkin, K. (1985). Television and sex-role acquisition: I. Content. *British Journal of Social Psychology, 24*, 101–113.

Ehrhardt, A. A. (1996). Our view of adolescent sexuality: A focus on risk behavior without the developmental context. *American Journal of Public Health, 86*, 1523–1525.

Erickson, P. (1998–1999). Cultural factors affecting the negotiation of first sexual intercourse among Latina adolescent mothers. *International Quarterly of Community Health Education, 18,* 121–137.

Espin, O. (1984). Cultural and historical influences on sexuality in Hispanic/Latina women: Implications for psychotherapy. In C. Vance (Ed.), *Pleasure and danger: Exploring female sexuality* (pp. 149–163). London: Routledge & Kegan Paul. In B. Greene (1994). *Ethnic minority lesbians and gay men: Mental health and treatment issues.* In B. Greene (Ed.) (1997). *Ethnic and cultural diversity among lesbians and gay men. Psychological perspectives on lesbian and gay issues, Vol. 3.* Thousand Oaks, CA: Sage.

Espin, O. (1999). *Women crossing boundaries: A psychology of immigration and transformations of sexuality.* New York: Routledge.

Essed, P. (1991). *Understanding everyday racism: An interdisciplinary theory.* London: Sage.

Feingold, A. (1994). Gender differences in personality: A meta-analysis. *Psychological Bulletin, 116,* 429–456.

Fleisher, J. M., Senie, R. T., Minkoff, H., & Jaccard, J. (1994). Condom use relative to knowledge of sexually transmitted disease prevention, method of birth control, and past or present infection. *Journal of Community Health, 19*(6), 395–407.

Forrest, J. D. (1994). Preventing unintended pregnancy: The role of hormonal contraceptives. Epidemiology of unintended pregnancy and contraceptive use. *American Journal of Obstetrical Gynecology, 170,* 1485–1489.

Frazier, E. F. (1966). *The Negro family in the United States.* Chicago: University of Chicago Press.

Freire, P. (1970). *Pedagogy of the oppressed.* New York: Seabury Press.

Fullilove, M. T., Fullilove R. E., Haynes, K., & Gross, S. (1990). Black women and AIDS prevention: A view towards understanding the gender rules. *The Journal of Sex Research, 27,* 46–64.

Furnham, A., & Baguma, P. (1994). Cross-cultural differences in the evaluation of male and female body shapes. *International Journal of Eating Disorders, 15,* 81–89.

Gagnon, J. H. (1973). Scripts and the coordination of sexual conduct. *Nebraska Symposium on Motivation, 21,* 27–59.

Gagnon, J. H. (1985). Attitudes and responses of parents to pre-adolescent masturbation. *Archives of Sexual Behaviour, 14,* 451–466.

Galenson, E., & Roiphe, H. (1976). Some suggested revisions concerning early female development. *Journal of American Psychoanalysis Association (suppl), 24,* 29–57.

Galton, F. (1952 {1892}). The comparative worth of different races. In *Hereditary genius: An inquiry into its laws and consequences* (pp. 325–337). New York: Horizon Press.

Gamble, V. N. (1993). A legacy of distrust: African Americans and medical research. *American Journal of Preventive Medicine, 9, 6 Suppl,* 35–38.

Garrison, C. Z., Schuchter, M., Schoenbach, V. J., & Kap-

lan, B. K. (1989). Epidemiology of depressive symptoms in young adolescents. *Journal of American Academy of Child Adolescent Psychology, 28,* 343–351.

Gilligan, C. (1982). *In a different voice: Psychological theory and women's development.* Cambridge, MA: Harvard University Press.

Gilligan, C., Lyons, N. P., & Hanmer, T. J. (1990). *Making connections: The relational worlds of adolescent girls at Emma Willard School.* Cambridge, MA: Harvard University Press.

Gilligan, C., Rogers, A. G., & Tolman, D. L. (1991). *Women, girls, and psychotherapy: Reframing resistance.* New York: Haworth Press.

Gilmore, S., DeLamater, J., & Wagstaff, D. (1996). Sexual decision-making by inner city Black adolescent males: A focus groups study. *Journal of Sex Research, 33*(4), 363–371.

Golding, J. M. (1996). Sexual assault history and women's reproductive and sexual health. *Psychology of Women Quarterly, 20,* 101–121.

Goldman, R. J., & Goldman, J. D. (1982). How children perceive the origin of babies and the roles of mothers and fathers in procreation: A cross-national study. *Child Development, 53,* 491–504.

Golub, S. (1983). Menarche: The beginning of menstrual life. *Women and Health, 8,* 17–36.

Gore, S., Aseltine, R. H., Jr., & Colton, M. E. (1992). Social structure, life stress, and depressive symptoms in a high school-aged population. *Journal of Health Social Behavior, 33,* 97–113.

Grady, W. R., Tanfer, K., Billy, J. O. G., & Lincoln-Hanson, J. (1996). Men's perceptions of their roles and responsibilities regarding sex, contraception, and child-rearing. *Family Planning Perspectives, 28,* 221–226.

Greene, B. (1994a). Ethnic minority lesbians and gay men: Mental health and treatment issues. In B. Greene (Ed.), *Ethnic and cultural diversity among lesbians and gay men. Psychological perspectives on lesbian and gay issues, Vol. 3* (pp. 216–239). Thousand Oaks, CA: Sage.

Greene, B. (1994b). African-American women. In L. Comas-Diaz & B. Greene (Eds.), *Women of color: Integrating ethnic and gender identities in psychotherapy.* New York: Guilford Press.

Greene, B. (Ed.) (1997). *Ethnic and cultural diversity among lesbians and gay men. Psychological perspectives on lesbian and gay issues, Vol. 3.* Thousand Oaks, CA: Sage.

Griswold, W. (1994). *Cultures and societies in a changing world.* London: Pine Forge Press.

Hardy, J. B., & Zabin, L. S. (1991). *Adolescent pregnancy in an urban environment.* Washington, DC: Urban Institute Press and Baltimore–Munich: Urban and Schwarzenberg.

Hasian, M. A. (1996). Race and African-American interpretation of eugenics. In *The rhetoric of eugenics in Anglo American thought* (pp. 51–88). Athens: University of Georgia Press.

Health Research Group (1973). *A Health Research Group*

study of surgical sterilization: Present abuses and proposed regulations. Washington, DC: Health Research Group.

Helman, C. G. (1994). *Culture, health and illness: An introduction for health professionals* (3rd ed.). Oxford: Butterworth Heinemann.

Helms, J. (1985). *Black and White racial identity: Theory, research, and practice.* Westport, CT: Praeger.

Henshaw, S. K. (1998). Unintended pregnancy in the United States. *Family Planning Perspectives, 30*, 24–29.

Hunt, M. (1974). *Sexual behavior in the 1970's.* Chicago: Playboy Press.

Im, E., & Lipson, J. G. (1997). Menopausal transition of Korean immigrant women: A literature review. *Health Care for Women International, 18*, 507–520.

Irvine, J. M. (1994). Cultural differences and adolescent sexualities. In J. M. Irvine. *Sexual cultures and the construction of adolescent identities* (pp. 3–28). Philadelphia: Temple University Press.

Irwin, K. L., Edlin, B. R., Wong, L., Faruque, S., McCoy, H V., Word, C., Schilling, R., McCoy, C. B., Evans, P. E., & Holmberg, S. D. (1995). Urban rape survivors: Characteristics and prevalence of human immunodeficiency virus and other sexually transmitted infections. *Obstetrics and Gynecology, 85*, 330–336.

Joiner, G. W., & Kashubeck, S. (1996). Acculturation, body image, self-esteem and eating disorder symptomalogy in adolescent Mexican-American women. *Psychology of Women Quarterly, 20*, 419–435.

Kaufert P., Boggs, P., Ettinger B., Woods N. F., & Utian, W. H. (1998). Women and menopause: Beliefs, attitudes, and behaviors. The North American menopause society 1997 menopause survey. *Menopause: The Journal of the North American Menopause Society, 5*, 197–202.

Kercher, G. A., & McShane, M. (1984). The prevalence of child sexual abuse victimization in an adult sample of Texas residents. *Child Abuse and Neglect, 17*, 7–24.

Kinsey, A., Pomeroy, W. B., & Martin, C. E. (1948) *Sexual behavior in the human male.* Philadelphia: W. B. Saunders.

Kinsey, A., Pomeroy, W. B., Martin, C. E., & Gebhard, P. (1953) *Sexual behavior in the human female.* Philadelphia: W. B. Saunders.

Kleeman, J. (1975). Genital self-stimulation in infant toddler girls. In I. Marcus & F. Francis (Eds.). *Masturbation: From infancy to senescence.* New York: International University Press.

Kortenhaus, C. M., & Demarest, J. (1993). Gender role stereotyping in children's literature: An update. *Sex Roles, 28*, 219–232.

Krieger, N., & Fee, E. (1994). Man-made medicine and women's health: The biopolitics of sex/gender and race/ethnicity. In E. Fee & N. Krieger (Eds.), *Women's health politics and power: Essays on sex/gender, medicine, and public health* (pp. 11–30). New York: Baywood.

Kuss, T. (1997). Family planning experiences of Vietnamese women. *Journal of Community Health Nursing, 14*, 155–168.

Ladner, J. A. (1971). Tomorrow's tomorrow: The black woman. Garden City, NY: Doubleday.

Lal, B. B. (1995). Symbolic interaction theories. *American Behavioral Scientist, 38*, 421–441.

Landrine, H. (1985). Race/class stereotypes of women. *Sex Roles, 13*, 65–75.

Landrine, H. (1999). Race/class stereotypes of women. In L. A. Peplau, S. C. DeBro, R. C. Veniegas, & P. L. Taylor (Eds.), *Gender, culture, and ethnicity. Current research about women and men* (pp. 38–61). Mountain View, CA: Mayfield.

Laumann, E. O., Paik, A., & Rosen, R. C. (1999). Sexual dysfunction in the United States: Prevalence and predictors. *Journal of the American Medical Association, 281*, 537–544.

Lindholm, K. J., & Willey, R. (1986). Ethnic differences in child abuse and sexual abuse. *Hispanic Journal of Behavioral Sciences, 8*, 111–125.

Lips, H. M. (1997). *Sex & gender: An introduction* (3rd ed.). Mountain View, CA: Mayfield.

Liu, P., & Chan, C. S. (1996). Lesbian, gay, and bisexual Asian Americans and their families. In J. Laird & R. J. Green (Eds.), *Lesbians and gays in couples and families: A handbook for therapists* (pp. 137–152). San Francisco: Jossey-Bass. In A. L. Solarz (Ed.) (1999). *Lesbian health: current assessments and directions for the future.* Institute of Medicine. Washington, DC: National Academy Press.

Lopez, I. (1985). Sterilization among Puerto Rico women: A case study in New York city. (Doctoral dissertation, Columbia University, 1985). *Dissertation Abstracts International, 47*, 960A.

Lott, B. (1989). Sexist discrimination as distancing behavior: II. Primetime television *Psychology of Women Quarterly, 13*, 341–355.

Lown, E. A., Winkler, K., Fullilove, R. E., & Fullilove, M. T. (1993). Tossin' and tweakin': Women's consciousness in the crack culture. In C. Squire (Ed.), *Women and AIDS: Psychological perspectives* (pp. 90–105). London: Sage.

Luker, K. (1991). Dubious conceptions: The controversy over teen pregnancy. *The American Prospect, 5*, 73–83.

Maccoby, E. E. (1990). Gender and relationships: A developmental account. *American Psychologist, 45*, 513–520.

Maccoby, E. E. (1998). *The two sexes: Growing apart, coming together.* Cambridge, MA: Harvard University Press.

Marin, B. V., Tschann, J. M., Gomez, C. A., & Gregorich, S. (1998). Self-efficacy to use condoms in unmarried Latino adults. *American Journal of Community Psychology, 26*, 53–71.

Marsiglio, W., & Donnelly, D. (1991). Sexual relations in later life: A national study of married persons. *Journal of Gerontology, 46*, S338–344.

Mays, V., & Cochran, S. D. (1988). Issues in the perception of AIDS risk and risk reduction activities by Black and Hispanic/Latina women. *American Psychologist, 43*, 949–957.

McBroom, W. H. (1981). Parental relationships, socioeconomic status, and sex role expectations. *Sex Roles, 7,* 1027–1033.

McCormick, N. B. (1996). Our feminist future: women affirming sexuality research in the late twentieth century. *Journal of Sex Research, 33,* 99–102.

McKinlay, S. M. (1996). The normal menopause transition. *Maturitas, 23,* 137–145.

Mennen, F. E. (1994). Sexual abuse in Latina girls. *Hispanic Journal of Behavioral Sciences, 16,* 475–486.

Mennen, F. E., & Meadow, D. (1995). The relationship of abuse characteristics to symptoms in sexually abused girls. *Journal of Interpersonal Violence, 10,* 259–274.

Mishler, E. (1981). Viewpoint: Critical perspectives on the biomedical model. In E. G. Misher, L. R. Amara Singham, S. T. Hauser, R. Liem, S. D., Osherson, & N. E. Waxler), *Social context of health, illness, and patient care* (pp. 1–23). Cambridge: Cambridge University Press.

Money, J., & Ehrhardt, A. A. (1996). *Man & woman, boy & girl: Gender identity from conception to maturity.* Northvale, NJ: Jason Aronson.

Moore, D. S., & Erickson, P. I. (1985). Age, gender, and ethnic differences in sexual and contraceptive knowledge, attitudes, and behaviors. *Family and Community Health, 8,* 38–51.

Morales, E. (1996). Gender roles among Latino gay and bisexual men: Implications for family and couples relationships. In J. Laird & R. J. Green (Eds.), *Lesbians and gays in couples and families: A handbook for therapists* (pp. 272–297). San Francisco: Jossey-Bass.

Myers, L. W. (1989). Early gender role socialization among black women: Affective or consequential? *The Western Journal of Black Studies, 13,* 173–178.

Neff, L. J., Sargent, R. G., McKeown, R. E., Jackson, K. L., & Valois, R. F. (1997). Black–white differences in body size perceptions and weight management practices among adolescent females. *Journal of Adolescent Health, 20,* 459–465.

Nolen-Hoeksema, S. (1987). Sex differences in unipolar depression: Evidence and theory. *Psychological Bulletin, 101,* 259–282.

O'Brien, M., & Huston, A. C. (1985). Development of sex-typed play behavior in toddlers. *Developmental Psychology, 21,* 866–871.

Oskamp, S., Kaufman, K., & Wolterbeek, L. A. (1996). In R. Crandall (Ed.), *Handbook of gender research. Journal of Behavior and Personality, 11,* 27–39.

Ostry, B. (1978). *The cultural connection.* Toronto: McClelland and Stewart.

Pariser, S. F., & Niedermier, J. A. (1998). Sex and the mature woman. *Journal of Women's Health, 7,* 849–859.

Parker, R. G., & Gagnon, J. H. (1994). *Conceiving sexuality: Approaches to sex research in a postmodern world.* Florence, KY: Taylor & Francis/Routledge.

Paul, D. B. (1992). Eugenic anxieties, social realities, and political choices. *Social Research, 59,* 663–683.

Paul, D. B. (1995). Whose country is this? Eugenics and race. In M. Jacob & S. Weart (Eds.), *Controlling human heredity: 1865–the present* (pp. 97–114). Jersey City, NJ: Humanities Press.

Peplau, L. A., Cochran, S. D., Mays, V. M. (1997). A natural survey of the intimate relations of African American lesbians and gay men. A look at commitment, satisfaction, sexual behavior and HIV disease. In B. Greene (Ed.), *Ethnic and cultural diversity among lesbians and gay men. Psychological perspectives on lesbian and gay issues.* Vol. 3 (pp. 11–38). Thousand Oaks, CA: Sage.

Peterson, R. (1979). Revitalizing the culture concept. *Annual Review of Sociology, 5,* 137–166.

Peterson, S. B., & Lach, M. A. (1990). Gender stereotypes in children's books: Their prevalence and influence on cognitive and affective development. *Gender and Education, 2,* 185–197.

Phinney, J. S. (1989). Stages if ethnic identify in minority group adolescents. *Journal of Early Adolescence, 9,* 34–49.

Phinney, J. S. (1993). A three-stage model of ethnic identity development in adolescence. In M. B. Bernal and G. P. Knight (Eds.), *Ethnic identity: Formation and transmission among Hispanics and other minorities* (pp. 61–79). New York: State University of New York.

Piccinino, L. J., & Mosher, W. D. (1998). Trends in contraceptive use in the United States: 1982–1995. *Family Planning Perspectives, 30,* 4–10, 46.

Pierce, L. H., & Pierce, R. L. (1984). Race as a factor in the sexual abuse of children. *Social Work Research Abstracts, 20,* 9–14.

Plichta, S. B., & Abraham, C. (1996). Violence and gynecological health in women <50 years old. *American Journal of Obstetrics and Gynecology, 174,* 903–907.

Pomerleau, A., Bolduc, D., Malcuit, G., & Cossette, L. (1990). Pink or blue: Environmental gender stereotypes in the first two years of life. *Sex Roles, 22,* 359–367.

Raj, A., Silverman, J., & Amaro, H. (2000). The relationship between sexual abuse and sexual risk among high school students: Findings from the 1997 Massachusetts Youth Behavior Survey. *Maternal and Child Health Journal, 4,* 125–134.

Rao, K., DiClemente, R. J., & Ponton, L. E. (1992). Child sexual abuse of Asians compared with other populations. *Journal of American Academy of Child & Adolescent Psychiatry, 31*(5), 880–886.

Reid, P. (1993). Poor women in psychological research: Shut up and shut out. *Psychology of Women Quarterly, 17,* 133–150.

Reiker, P. P., & Jankowski, M. K. (1995). Sexism and women's psychological status. In C. V. Willie, P. P. Reiker, B. M. Kramer, & B. S. Brown (Eds.), *Mental health, racism and sexism* (pp. 27–50). Pittsburgh: University of Pittsburgh Press.

Rickert, V. I., Jay, M. S., & Gottlieb, A. A. (1990). Adolescent wellness: Facilitating compliance in social morbidities. *Adolescent Medicine, 74,* 1135–1148.

Rierdan, J., & Koff, E. (1980). The psychological impact of menarche: Integrative versus disruptive changes. *Journal of Youth and Adolescence, 9,* 49–58.

Robinson, T. N., Killen, J. D., Litt, I. F., Hammer, L. D., Wilson, D. M., Haydel, K. F., Hayward, C., & Barr Taylor, C. (1996). Ethnicity and body dissatisfaction: Are Hispanic and Asian girls at increased risk for eating disorders? *Journal of Adolescent Health, 19,* 384–393.

Rodriguez-Trias, H. (1984). The women's health movement: Women take power. In V. Sidel & R. Sidel (Eds.), *Reforming medicine: Lessons of the last quarter century* (pp. 107–126). New York: Pantheon.

Rodin, J., Silberstein, L. R., & Streigel-Moore, R. (1985). Women and weight: A normative discontent. In T. B. Sonderegger (Ed), *Nebraska Symposium on Motivation: Vol. 32. Psychology and Gender.* Lincoln: University of Nebraska Press.

Rogers, A. G. (1993). Voice, play, and a practice of ordinary courage in girls' and women's lives. *Harvard Educational Review, 63*(3), 265–295.

Romero, G. J., Wyatt, G. E., Loeb, T. B., Carmona, J. V., & Solis, B. M. (1999). Prevalence and circumstances of child sexual abuse among Latina women. *Hispanic Journal of Behavioral Sciences, 21,* 351–365.

Rosario, M., Meyer-Bahlburg, H. F. L., Hunter, J., Exner, T. M., Gwadz, M., & Keller, A. M. (1996). The psychosexual development of urban lesbian, gay, and bisexual youths. *The Journal of Sex Research, 33*(2), 113–126.

Rosario, M., Meyer-Bahlburg, H. F. L., Hunter, J., & Gwadz, M. (1999). Sexual risk behaviors of gay, lesbian, and bisexual youths in New York City: Prevalence and correlates. *AIDS Education and Prevention, 11*(6), 476–496.

Rosario, M., Rotherman-Borus, M. J., & Reid, H. (1996). Gay-related stress and its correlates among gay and bisexual male adolescents of predominantly Black and Hispanic background. *Journal of Community Psychology, 24,* 136–159.

Rosenblum, G. D., & Lewis, M. (1999). The relations among body image, physical attractiveness, and body mass in adolescence. *Child Development, 70,* 50–64.

Rothman, B. K. (1987). Reproduction. In B. B. Hess & M. M. Ferree. *Analyzing gender: A handbook of social science research* (pp. 154–170). Thousand Oaks, CA: Sage.

Rubin, J., Provenzano, F., & Luria, Z. (1974). The eye of the beholder: Parents' views on sex of newborns. *American Journal of Orthopsychiatry, 44,* 512–519.

Rucker, C. E., & Cash, T. F. (1992). Body images, body-size perceptions and eating behaviors among African-American and White college women. *International Journal of Eating Disorders, 12,* 291–299.

Russell, D. E. H. (1983). The incidence and prevalence of intrafamilial and extrafamilial sexual abuse of female children. *Child Abuse and Neglect, 7,* 133–146.

Russell, D. E. H. (1986). *The secret trauma: Incest in the lives of girls and women.* New York: Basic Books.

Sahay, S., & Piran, N. (1997). Skin-color preferences and body satisfaction among South Asian–Canadian and European–Canadian female university students. *Journal of Social Psychology, 137,* 161–172.

Savin-Williams, R. C. (1990). *Gay and lesbian youth: Expressions of identity.* Washington, DC: Hemisphere.

Savin-Williams, R. C. (1996). Ethnic and sexual minority youth. In R. C. Savin-Williams & K. M. Cohen (Eds.), *The lives of lesbians, gays, and bisexuals: Children to adults* (pp. 152–165). Forth Worth, TX: Hartcourt Brace. In A. L. Solarz (Ed.). (1999). *Lesbian health: Current assessments and directions for the future.* Institute of Medicine. Washington, DC: National Academy Press.

Savin-Williams, R. C., & Rodriguez, R. G. (1993). A developmental, clinical perspective on lesbian, gay male, and bisexual youths. In T. P. Gullotta, G. R. Adams, & R. Montemayor (Eds.), *Adolescent sexuality: Advances in adolescent development. Vol. 5.* Newbury Park, CA: Sage.

Schenshul, S., Borrero, M., Barrera, V., Backstrand, J. & Guarnaccia, P. (1982). A model of fertility control in a Puerto Rican community. *Urban Anthropology, 11,* 81–100.

Schneider, B. E., & Gould, M. (1987). Female sexuality: Looking back into the future. In B. B. Hess & M. M. Ferree (Eds.), *Analyzing gender: A handbook of social science research* (pp. 120–153). Newbury Park, CA: Sage.

Seigel, J. M., Sorenson, S. B., Golding, J. M., Burnham, M. A., & Stein, J. A. (1987). The prevalence of childhood sexual assault. *American Journal of Epidemiology, 126,* 1141–1153.

Seigel, J. M., Aneshensel, C. S., Taub, B., Cantwell, D. P., & Driscoll, A. K. (1998). Adolescent depressed mood in a multiethnic sample. *Journal of Youth and Adolescence, 27,* 413–427.

Smith, E. J. (1982). The black female adolescent: A review of the educational, career, and psychological literature. *Psychology of Women Quarterly, 6,* 261–288.

Smith, D. E., & Cogswell, C. (1994). A cross-cultural perspective on adolescent girls' body perception. *Perceptual and Motor Skills, 78,* 744–746.

Sobo, E. J. (1995). *Choosing unsafe sex: AIDS-risk denial among disadvantaged women.* Philadelphia: University of Pennsylvania Press.

Solarz, A. L. (Ed.). (1999). *Lesbian health: Current assessments and directions for the future.* Institute of Medicine. Washington, DC: National Academy Press.

St. Peter, S. (1979). Jack went up the hill ... but where was Jill? *Psychology of Women Quarterly, 4,* 256–260.

Stockard, J., & Johnson, M. M. (1980). *Sex role: Sex inequality and sex role development.* Englewood Cliffs, NJ: Prentice Hall.

Stoltzman, S. M. (1986). Menstrual attitudes, beliefs, and symptom experiences of adolescent females, their peers, and their mothers. In V. L. Olesen & N. F. Woods (Eds.), *Culture, society and menstruation: Health care for women international publication.* Washington, DC: Hemisphere.

Strassberg, D. S., & Lowe, K. (1995). Volunteer bias in

sexuality research. *Archives of Sexual Behavior, 24,* 369–382.

Strunin, L. (1994). Culture, context, and HIV infection: Research on risk taking among adolescents. In J. M. Irvine (Ed.), *Sexual cultures and the construction of adolescent identities* (pp. 3–28). Philadelphia: Temple University Press.

Taylor, D. L., & Woods, N. F. (1991). *Menstruation, health and illness.* Washington, DC: Hemisphere.

Thomas, M. C., Nelson, C. S., & Sumners, C. M. (1994). From victims to victors: Group process as the path to recovery for males molested as children. *Journal for Specialists in Group Work, 19*(2), 102–111.

Thompson, S. H., Sargent, R. G., & Kemper, K. A. (1996). Black and white adolescent males' perceptions of ideal body size. *Sex Roles, 34,* 391–406.

Tiefer, L. (1991). Commentary on the status of sex research: Feminism, sexuality, and sexology. *Journal of Psychology and Human Sexuality, 4,* 5–42.

Tiefer, L. (1994). Women's sexuality: Not a matter of health. In A. Dan (Ed.), *Reframing women's health* (pp. 151–162). London: Sage.

Townsend, J. (1995). Racial, ethnic, and mental illness stereotypes: Cognitive process and behavioral effects. In C. V. Willie, P. P. Reiker, B. M. Kramer, & B. S. Brown (Eds.), *Mental health, racism and sexism* (pp. 51–118). Pittsburgh, PA: University of Pittsburgh Press.

Turner, C. B., & Kramer, B. M. (1995). Connections between racism and mental health. In C. V. Willie, P. P. Reiker, B. M. Kramer, & B. S. Brown (Eds.), *Mental health, racism and sexism* (pp. 3–26). Pittsburgh, PA: University of Pittsburgh Press.

Tzeng, O., & Schwarzin, H. (1990). Gender and race differences in child sexual abuse correlates. *International Journal of Intercultural Relations, 14,* 135–161.

Uribe, F., Medardo, T., LeVine, R. A., & LeVine, S. E. (1994). Maternal behavior in Mexican community: The changing environments of children. In P. M. Greensfield & R. R. Cocking (Eds.), *Cross-cultural roots of minority child development.* Hillsdale, NJ: Erlbaum.

Urquiza, A. J., & Goodlin-Jones, B. L. (1994). Child sexual abuse and adult revictimization with women of color. *Violence and Victims, 9,* 223–232.

U.S. General Accounting Office (1976). *Report to Honorable James G. Abourezk,* B164031 {5}, November.

Wardle, J., & Marsland, L. (1990). Adolescent concerns about weight and eating: A social developmental perspective. *Journal of Psychosomatic Research, 34,* 377–391.

Wardle, J., Bindra, R., Fairclough, B., & Westcombe, A. (1993). Culture & body image: Body perception and weight concerns in young Asian and Caucasian women. *Journal of Community and Applied Social Psychology, 3,* 173–181.

Warren, C. W., Westoff, C. F., Herold, J. M., Rochat, R. W., & Smith, J. C. (1986). Contraceptive sterilization in Puerto Rico. *Demography, 23,* 351–356.

Way, N. (1995). "Can't you see the courage, the strength I have?": Listening to urban adolescent girls speak about their relationships. *Psychology of Women Quarterly, 19,* 107–128.

Weeks, M. R., Schenshul, J. J., Williams, S. S., Singer, M., & Grier, M. (1995). AIDS prevention for African-American and Latina women: Building culturally and gender-appropriate interventions. *AIDS Education and Prevention, 7,* 251–263.

Weiss, D. L. (1998). The use of theory in sexuality research. *Journal of Sex Research, 35,* 109.

Weitzman, L. J., Eifler, D., Hokada, E., & Ross, C. (1972). Sex-role socialization in picture books for preschool children. *American Journal of Sociology, 77,* 1125–1150.

White, L., & Brinkerhoff, D. (1981). The sexual division of labor: Evidence from childhood. *Social Forces, 60,* 170–181.

Whitehead, T. (1997). Urban low-income African-American men, HIV/AIDS, and gender identity. *Medical Anthropology Quarterly, 11,* 411–447.

Wiederman, M. W., Maynard, C., & Fretz, A. (1996). Ethnicity in 25 years of published sexuality research: 1971–1995. *Journal of Sex Research, 33,* 339–343.

Williams, C. W. (1991). *Black teenage mothers: Pregnancy and child rearing from their perspective.* Lexington, MA: D. C. Heath.

Williams, D. R., Lavizzo-Mourey, R., & Warren, R. C. (1994). The concept of race and health status in America. *Public Health Reports, 109,* 26–41.

Wyatt, G. E. (1985). The sexual abuse of Afro-American and White-American women in childhood. *Child Abuse Neglect, 9,* 507–519.

Wyatt, G. E. (1989). Reexamining factors predicting Afro-American and White American women's age at first coitus. *Archives of Sexual Behavior, 18*(4), 271–298.

Wyatt, G. E. (1990). The aftermath of child sexual abuse of African-American and White American women: The victim's experience. *Journal of Family Violence, 5,* 61–81.

Wyatt, G. E. (1994). The sociocultural relevance of sex research: Challenges for the 1990's and beyond. *American Psychologist, 49*(8), 748–754.

Yap, J. G. (1986). Philippine ethnoculture and human sexuality. *Journal of Social Work and Human Sexuality, 4*(3), 121–134.

Yeakley, A., & Gant, L. (1997). Cultural factors and program implications: HIV/AIDS interventions and condom use among Latinos. *Journal of Multicultural Social Work, 6*(3–4), 47–71.

Yep, G. (1992). Communicating the HIV/AIDS risk to Hispanic populations: A review and integration. *Hispanic Journal of Behavioral Sciences, 14,* 403–420.

Zierler, S., Feingold, L., Laufer, D., & Velentgas, P. *et al.* (1991). Adult survivors of childhood sexual abuse and subsequent risk of HIV infection. *American Journal of Public Health, 81,* 572–575.

6

Mass Media and Adolescent Female Sexuality

JANE D. BROWN and SUSANNAH R. STERN

INTRODUCTION

Jessica, 16, wakes up to the music on her clock radio. This morning Britney Spears sings "Baby hit me one more time" and then Brandy asks "What do I gotta do to get you in my arms, baby?" as Jessica stumbles out of bed to the shower. Later, as she gobbles a Poptart for breakfast, the TV on the kitchen counter flashes images of the scene of a rape and murder the night before. On the drive to school, Jessica glances at a billboard that in big red letters declares: "Virgin: Teach your kids it's not a four-letter word." During homeroom, Jessica and her friends laugh about the awkward kiss on the new WB program *Jack & Jill* they all watched on TV the night before, and they ponder if Joey will lose her virginity on *Dawson's Creek* this season. At lunch, they pore over the latest issue of *Glamour* magazine, wishing they were as thin as the perfect models and celebrities and giggling at the tips for how to "get the guy." In health class a video about the benefits of waiting to have sex until marriage makes them all snicker. After school, Jessica goes online to do some research for a class project, but ends up in a chat site talking about the virtues of boys who know how to be romantic. Jessica's boyfriend comes over later with a video and they snuggle up on the couch in the family room to watch *American Pie*.

The extent to which a variety of media and sexual images saturate the life of an adolescent like Jessica is not unusual. In fact, most teen girls in the United States are in contact with some kind of media during most of their waking hours. Much of the media content they come in contact with contains messages, images, and ideas about sex and sexuality.

In this chapter we look at what research tells us about the sexual content in the media adolescent girls attend to, and we consider how this content may affect adolescent girls' sexual knowledge, attitudes, and behaviors.

SEXUALITY AND FEMALE ADOLESCENTS' HEALTH

We define sex and sexuality broadly to include not only sexual intercourse and the consequences of sexual intercourse, but also the norms and values, such as sexual orientation,

---

JANE D. BROWN • School of Journalism and Mass Communication, University of North Carolina at Chapel Hill, Chapel Hill, North Carolina 27599-3365.   SUSANNAH R. STERN • Communications Department, Boston College, Chestnut Hill, Massachusetts 02467.

Handbook of Women's Sexual and Reproductive Health, edited by Wingood and DiClemente. Kluwer Academic / Plenum Publishers, New York, 2002.

attractiveness, romantic scripts, dating rituals, and sexual violence that inform and influence sexual experiences. Given this broad definition of sexuality, most adolescent girls in the United States are leading sexual lives—with real-life consequences. Consider the following statistics:

- Half of adolescent girls have dieted, most because they want to look better rather than because lower weight will enhance their health (Commonwealth Fund, 1999).
- Thirteen percent of early adolescent girls and 18% of middle and late adolescent girls report having binged and purged (Commonwealth Fund, 1999).
- The average age of first intercourse is 17 for females and 16 for males (Alan Guttmacher Institute, 1994).
- Only about one third of girls use contraceptives every time they have intercourse, and not all of these use condoms. One in five *never* use contraceptives (Kaiser Family Foundation, 1998a).
- For both biological and social reasons, girls are more likely than boys to contract a Sexually Transmitted Disease (STD) from an infected partner, are less likely to notice symptoms, and more likely to suffer long-term health consequences, including infertility, tubal pregnancies, and cervical cancer (Kaiser Family Foundation, 1998b).
- A teenaged girl who has unprotected sex with an infected partner just one time has a 1% chance of contracting HIV, a 30% chance of contracting genital herpes, and a 50% chance of contracting gonorrhea (Alan Guttmacher Institute, 1994).
- Although teen pregnancy rates are declining in the United States, the country continues to have one of the highest rates of teen pregnancy of any Westernized country in the world (Piot & Islam, 1994).
- Native American girls have the highest birth rates, and Asian-American girls the lowest. Although the birth rate for unmarried Black girls has been declining, the birth rate for Black and Hispanic teenage girls is twice that for White girls (Commonwealth Fund, 1999).
- In a national survey, 8% of high school girls and 5% of boys said they had been forced by a date to have sex against their will; 12% of the girls and 5% of the boys said they had been sexually abused at some point in their lives (Commonwealth Fund, 1999).
- Girls who have unwanted sexual experiences are more likely than those who don't to have many sexual partners and greater vulnerability to STDs and early pregnancy (Abma, Driscoll, & Morre, 1997).

The Media as Sex Educators

Does the media play a role in the pattern of adolescent sexual behavior conveyed by these statistics? In a country where the mass media discuss and depict sex around the clock, it seems inevitable that adolescent girls will find at least some of what they see as applicable to their own sexual lives. Mass media channels are numerous and expanding rapidly, thanks to cable, satellite, the Internet, laser and CD-ROM technologies. The sexual media menu is varied and accessible.

Research suggests that adolescents do learn about sexuality from the media, and some deliberately turn to the media for information that is difficult to obtain elsewhere. In a national sample of high school students, more than half said they had learned about birth control, contraception, or preventing pregnancy from magazines and/or television (Sutton, Brown, Wilson, & Klein, 2001). School health classes, parents, and friends were the only other sources that were cited more frequently. But parents often broach sexual topics awkwardly, if at all, and schools tend to address sexuality in clinical terms rather than in the context of relationships, emotions, and desire. Television, movies, music and music videos, magazines, and web sites, in contrast, capitalize on topics considered taboo in other social situations, thus often making sexual media fare especially attractive for younger consumers.

ADOLESCENTS' MEDIA USE

Although we often tend to discuss "adolescents" or "teenagers" as a homogenous cluster of like-minded people, we know that they actually are a diverse group of individuals whose media use differs dramatically. Steele & Brown (1995) and Steel (1999) developed a model to help explain how teens choose and use sexual media content (see Figure 1).

The model has three features that distinguish it from more traditional approaches to studies of mass media effects. First, the model is circular because it assumes that most media use is active in a number of ways: first through *selection* of which medium and genre to attend to, second through *interacting* and making sense of what is seen and/or heard, and third, by *applying* or rejecting some or all of what is attended to. The circle also represents the idea of the reciprocal nature of media effects; that is, rather than a linear process of only the mass media affecting the passive receiver, it is assumed that the adolescent receiver is both affected by and affects the media she uses.

Second, the model assumes that an adolescent's current and emerging sense of self or *identity* is a compelling component as decisions are made about what media will be selected and interacted with. Typically, studies of the effects of the mass media assume similarity in selection, exposure and interpretation of media content. The Media Practice approach, however, assumes that adolescents choose media and interact with media based on who they are or who they want to be at the moment and these motivations will affect what is learned and applied.

Finally, media practice is seen as occurring within the context of a range of other factors that influence and are embodied in the individual who is engaged in media use. We call these factors "lived experience." Lived experience accounts for the complex ways in which race, class, gender, developmental stage, and many other factors differentiate one person's experience of day-to-day occurrences from another person's. Here we move through each phase of the model and discuss the potential for media to have an impact on adolescent girls' sexual health.

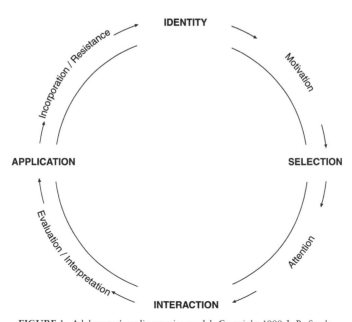

FIGURE 1. Adolescents' media practice model. Copyright 1999 J. R. Steele.

Teens' Access to and Selection of Sexual Media Content

At the beginning of the new millennium, youth have increased access to many more media channels than ever before. The videocassette recorder (VCR), the remote control and portable compact disc players also have given teens much more control over when and where the media will be used. Almost all teens have their own source of music, many subscribe to at least one magazine, and more than half have their own television, frequently hooked up to cable and a VCR, usually in their bedroom (Kaiser Family Foundation, 1999) (see Table 1).

Teens spend up to half the time they are awake with some form of media and some even sleep with their radios on. Many use more than one medium simultaneously, e.g., a girl will flip through *YM* while listening to the radio Top 40 countdown. It is important to note that although television is viewed on average 2 to 3 hours a day, television use tends to decline in early adolescence in favor of more portable and more teen-oriented media, especially music, movies, and magazines. Advertising also is an important part of most media content, and teens say they "read" advertisements to learn

about the latest trends (Zollo, 1995). The Internet is also becoming an important way for teens to communicate with one another and find information on diverse subjects, including sex.

Teens' Media Diets

Given the vast array of media material available today, teens must make choices about which media and content they will pay attention to. In Figure 2 we use the familiar USDA food group pyramid to illustrate some possible dimensions of what we call adolescents' *media diets*. At the bottom of the triangle is what Paul Willis (1990) refers to as "the common culture"—the images, styles, ideas that most youth will attend to in the media.

When television first became a family staple, the "bread and grains" category was a larger part of a teen's media diet than it is today. In the mid-1950s, teen girls had no choice but the three TV networks and *Seventeen* magazine, while today's teen girls can choose from 30 to 300 television channels and at least 10 magazines that are designed to appeal especially to young women. Recorded music has been highly specialized for some time, so that many large markets have a number of stations program-

TABLE 1. Availability, Frequency of Use, and Attractive Attributes of Mass Media Used by Adolescent Females (14–18 Years Old)

Medium	Availability and average use[a]	Attractive attributes
Music[b]	Almost all (88–94%) have radio, tape player, and/or CD player in bedroom; 2–3 hrs/day; 20+ hrs/week	Highly specialized; portable; arousing
Television[c]	Two thirds (65%) have TV in bedroom; 3½ hrs/day, 20+ hrs/week	Favorite shows familiar, relaxing, funny
Movies	About one third (33–38%) have VCR and/or cable TV in bedroom; ½ hr/day[d]; 1/mo in theaters	Favorite media stars; relevant; arousing
Magazines	15 min/day; most reading teen girls' and women's magazines	Shows trends, sets standards; portable
Internet	44% have Internet at home; average use ½–1 hr/day	Information; chat groups; porn (?)
Advertising	In all media; estimated 20 ads/hr[e]	Signals trends, what's cool

[a]Source: Kaiser Fmaily Foundation (1999).
[b]Includes radio, CDs, and tapes.
[c]Includes broadcast and cable television, taped TV shows, and commercial videos.
[d]Includes commercial videos, movies on TV, and in theaters.
[e]Source: Potter (1998).

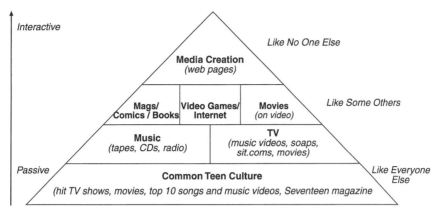

FIGURE 2. Adolescent females' media diet pyramid.

ming for different segments of the youth audience (e.g., Alternative Rock, Hot 100 (or Top 40), Rap, Country Western).

What we see today is a smorgasbord of media from which teens may choose idiosyncratic diets. In the middle of the media diet pyramid are the increasingly specialized media "food groups" from which teens may choose. The Media Practice Model predicts that these choices are governed primarily by the teen's developing sense of self or identity. The development of a firm sense of identity is a central task of adolescence. Exploring personal values and beliefs about sexuality and interpersonal relationships is a core piece of this identity work. Some adolescent development theorists have suggested that each teen is learning in what ways she is *like all other people, like some others,* and *like no others* (Gallatin, 1975). The media may be used as virtual tool kits of identity possibilities. At the common culture level, a teen is (or yearns to be) like all other people.

At the next level, though, the teen is like only some others, e.g., "popular girls" who read *Elle* and *Vogue* and watch *The Young and the Restless* soap opera. We know, for example, that teen girls' media diets differ dramatically by race. Blacks and Whites choose very different television diets, especially since the early 1990s when a number of cable channels began providing more shows with Black characters. In 1999, for example, the highest-rated show in Black households was *The Steve Harvey Show* on the WB network, but that situation comedy ranked 154th among White TV viewers ("Gap between," 1999). Black and Hispanic girls today also have a number of different magazines, such as *Black Hair* and *Latina* to choose from.

At the top of the pyramid is where youth can express their desires to *be like no one else.* Many teen girls have kept diaries in the past; now computer technology gives teens the opportunity to express their uniqueness in semi-public ways, such as on personally designed web pages and 'zines (privately produced, limited circulation magazines) that they can distribute to their friends or post on the Internet.

Interaction with Sexual Media Content

The second major step in media practice is Interaction: once content is selected, how is it understood? What aspects of the content are attended to, engaged with? A few studies of teens' interpretations of the frequent sexual content in the media, and a large body of work on the concept of selective perception, tells us that all members of an audience will not see or interpret the same message in the same way (Livingstone, 1989; Zillmann & Bryant, 1985).

One striking example was the differing interpretations of one of Madonna's early music videos, *Papa Don't Preach.* When first released, columnist Ellen Goodman called it "a commercial for teenage pregnancy," while the antiabortion groups said it was a stand against abortion. College students who saw the video differed in their "reading" of the video, too. Although most White females thought the video was about a teen girl deciding to keep her unborn child ("baby"), Black males were more likely to think the girl (Madonna) in the video was singing about wanting to keep her boyfriend "baby" (Brown & Schulze, 1990). Since the young men were identifying primarily with the dilemma of the boyfriend in the video, they were less likely than the female viewers to see or hear the cues that suggested pregnancy.

Other studies conclude that young males and females interpret media content differently. Monique Ward and her colleagues (2000) have shown college students portions of situation comedies such as *Roseanne* and *Martin*. They find that young women are more likely than young men to think the sexual scenes they see are realistic, and the women are more approving than the men of behaviors that are relationship maintaining (e.g., jealous husband protecting wife) and less approving of relationship threats (e.g., man contemplating cheating).

How girls will select and interpret sexual media content probably is related to their developmental level and real-world experience with sexual relationships. In an ethnographic study of 11- to 15-year-old middle class White girls, three patterns of interaction with sexual media content were identified (Brown, White, & Nikopoulou, 1993). The younger, less sexually experienced girls were the most likely to say that they thought kissing and nudity in the media were "gross" and "disgusting." Other girls who were slightly more physically mature and had participated in some preliminary erotic experience (e.g., hand holding and kissing) typically had plastered their bedroom walls with images similar to the ones the disinterested girls had eschewed (e.g., scantily clad models, women and men embracing). Another set of girls, however, typically the most physically mature and sexually experienced, was critical of the mainstream media's "romantic myth." These girls sought alternative media such as comic books with strong heroines and 'zines published by girls who had themselves grown weary of the limiting gender roles and relationships reflected in the more traditional media venues.

Application of Sexual Media Content

As teens attend to and interpret sexual media content, they also evaluate and sometimes incorporate what they are seeing into their own developing sense of sexuality. This is the step that we traditionally have referred to as media effects. We ask, does the sexual content in the media influence how adolescents behave sexually? Does the talk about and the images of love, sex and relationships promote irresponsible sexual behavior? Are the media responsible for teenagers having sex earlier, more frequently, without protection or commitment?

The answer to all of these questions is a qualified "yes." Qualified, because even though we know a fair amount about the ubiquity and explicitness of sexual content in the media, we still have only sparse research on the effects of sexual media content per se. According to classic social scientific methods, an ideal test of the effect of sexual media content would involve either randomized assignment to different media diets, or longitudinal surveys. Such studies would establish whether media exposure or behavior came first, and would allow for generalizations about what kinds of media content cause what kinds of behaviors.

Unfortunately, the perceived sensitivity of sex as a research topic and a focus on television to the exclusion of other media has restricted the kind of research that has been done. Most of the work has been analyses of content, and we can only speculate about what effects the content may have on audiences. But the few studies that go beyond content to address how audiences respond to and incorporate sexual content in their lives suggests that the media may, indeed play a role in the sexual lives of adolescent girls.

THEORIES OF MASS MEDIA EFFECTS

Traditional communication research and a growing body of interdisciplinary work by psychologists, anthropologists, sociologists, and cultural theorists emphasize three theoretical perspectives that explain how people can be affected by the media: (1) agenda setting/framing, (2) cultivation, and (3) cognitive social learning.

Agenda Setting

Agenda setting and framing theories propose that the media tell people both what is important in the world around them, and how to think about the events and people who inhabit that world (McCombs & Shaw, 1993; Kosicki, 1993). Singular events become bigger than life when shown on TV or blown up on the front page of a newspaper. People use such stories as reference points against which to compare what they already know, or think they know. The result often reinforces stereotypes and helps define what is considered appropriate and inappropriate behavior in the culture (Entman, 1994).

Although rarely thought of as sex educators, the news media at the least help keep sexual behavior salient. The American public and policy makers frequently are faced with news stories about abandoned babies, abortion clinic violence, and even presidential sexual affairs. The media are in a unique position to get people thinking and talking about specific issues while keeping other issues from the public eye.

Framing

As professional storytellers, the news media control not only which stories get told, but also how they get told. This "framing" helps shape understanding of events and may affect behavior (Iyengar, 1991; Neuman, Just, & Crigler, 1992). For instance, suppose a headline read "College Student Disposes of Newborn in Dumpster. Says Baby Would Interfere with Career Plans." Such a headline predisposes readers to think of the girl as a monster, an "antimother" who should be charged with murder (Tsing, 1990). A different reaction probably would result from this headline: "Fetus Found in Dumpster: Distraught Student Has No Recollection of Birth." Reading this, a reader might feel sympathy for the mother and think that psychological counseling rather than a jail sentence was in order (Brown & Steele, 1996).

The Cultivation Hypothesis

According to cultivation theory, television is the most powerful storyteller in the culture, one that continually repeats the myths and ideologies, the facts and patterns of relationships that define and legitimize the social order. TV tells its stories through news programs as well as in prime-time situation comedies and serials, daytime soap operas and talk shows, and the steady stream of commercials that fuel the entire industry. According to the cultivation hypothesis, a steady dose of television, over time, acts like the pull of gravity toward an imagined center. Called mainstreaming, this pull results in a shared set of conceptions and expectations about reality among otherwise diverse viewers. Tests of the hypothesis have found, for example, that frequent or "heavy" television viewers are more likely to believe the world is a mean and dangerous place, apparently because they are exposed to a high frequency of violence on TV (Gerbner, Gross, Morgan & Signorelli, 1994).

A few studies also have asked whether heavy exposure to television's version of sexual behavior cultivates a specific set of sexual beliefs. Researchers, for example, have found that college students who are soap opera fans are more likely than their nonviewing counterparts to overestimate the occurrence of divorce and illegitimate children. Soap fans also overestimated the number of abortions and the incidence of sexually transmitted disease in the real world (Buerkel-Rothfuss & Mayes, 1991; Buerkel-Rothfuss & Strouse, 1993). Studies of adolescents also have found that heavy television viewing is predictive of negative attitudes toward remaining a virgin (Courtright & Baran, 1980).

Cognitive Social Learning Theory

Cognitive social learning theory and its earlier variant, social learning theory, has been applied to the study of media effects for almost three decades. Basically, the theory predicts that people will imitate (model) behaviors of others when those models are rewarded or not punished for their behavior. Modeling will occur more readily when the model is perceived as attractive and similar and the modeled behavior is salient, simple, prevalent, has functional value and is possible (Bandura, 1994). Thus, the theory would predict that teens who attend to media content that includes depictions of attractive characters who enjoy having sexual intercourse with each other and rarely suffer any negative consequences will be likely to imitate the behavior. Others have suggested that the media provide cognitive "scripts" for sexual behavior they may not be able to see anywhere else (Gagnon & Simon, 1973). Teens may watch to fill in the gaps in their understanding about how a particular sexual scenario might work (e.g., kissing goodnight at the end of a date, having sex with a new partner).

SEXUAL CONTENT AND EFFECTS

Given these explanations of how the media may affect girls' sexual beliefs and behaviors, we turn to look more closely at what research has found. Here we review findings from the numerous content analyses of the media most often attended to by adolescent girls and the fewer studies that have examined how that content is interpreted and applied. See Table 2 for a summary.

Sex on Television

Television has received the bulk of attention from those interested in portrayals of sexuality and their effects. After all, television is on about seven hours per day in the average home, and teenagers, in particular, spend about 2 hours per day watching television (Wartella, 1994), even though they show a growing preference for music as they grow older (Arnett, 1992; Larson, Kubey, & Colletti, 1989). The number of hours teens watch television tells only a fraction of the story, however. The more important questions are: What do adolescent girls see on the screen? How do they interpret and apply what they see?

Prime Time

Content analyses of various television day parts and genres reveal that sexuality, broadly defined, is a frequent ingredient across the television dial. More than half of television programming contains sexual content (either talk or behavior); more than one third contains at least one scene with substantial emphasis on sex (Kunkel et al., 1999). The television shows teens watch most frequently during prime time (8 P.M. to 11 P.M. EST) are full of talk about and depictions of sexual activity. In 45 episodes of the top prime-time television shows that teens watched most frequently in 1996 (including *Friends*, *Seinfeld*, *Married with Children*), the primarily late teen and young adult characters talked about sex and engaged in sexual behavior in two thirds of the shows (Cope & Kunkle, 2001). However, most of the sexual content on television still is *talk*—characters discussing their own or others' current or future sexual activity. Women are more likely than men to be shown talking about romantic relationships (Children Now, 1997).

Sexual *behaviors* on primetime television, although frequent, are relatively modest, mostly flirting and kissing (Kunkle et al., 1999). Sexual intercourse rarely is depicted on these shows, but is sometimes implied (in the 45 episodes of top teen shows, sexual intercourse was depicted once and implied five times).

Talk Shows

Talk shows that frequently feature dysfunctional couples publicly disclosing their

TABLE 2. Sexual Media Content and Effects

	Sexual content	Effects
Television	1. Women most likely to be young[a] and thin[b]	1. Ideal body image programming and commercials affect girls' perceptions of their own bodies[f]
	2. Sexual talk is frequent; sexual behavior less frequent but common[c]	
	3. Negative consequences of sex are infrequently shown[d]	2. Gender role stereotypes are accepted by some viewers[g]
	4. Contraception and preplanning for sex are also rare[e]	3. Frequent soap viewers more likely to believe that single mothers have an easy life[h]
Magazines	1. One third of articles in teen girls' and women's magazines concern dating; one third focus on appearance[i]	1. Exposure to thin models in magazines can produce depression, stress, shame, and body dissatisfaction[l]
	2. 1 to 6 articles per issue focuses on sexual health[j]	2. Girls report that images in women's magazines make them feel bad about themselves[m]
	3. Women's magazines encourage females to put men's interests before their own[k]	
Music and music videos	1. Videos emphasize women musicians' appearance over musical ability[n]	1. Positive correlation between teen's exposure to MTV and permission attitudes about premarital sex[p]
	2. Frequent references to relationships and sexual behavior[o]	2. Exposure to stereotypical images of gender and sexuality in videos has been linked to greater acceptance of interpersonal violence[q]
	3. Less gender role stereotyping in videos, but females still more often affectionate, nurturing, and sexually pursued than males[o]	
Film	1. Romantic and sexual relations present in almost all top grossing movies[r]	
	2. Women more likely than men to talk about romantic relationships[s]	
	3. Older people rarely shown expressing tenderness or love for each other[r]	
Internet	1. Information about sex is abundant (i.e., pornography, sexual health)	

[a]Davis (1990). [b]Silverstein et al. (1986). [c]Kunkel et al. (1999). [d]Heintz-Knowles (1996); Kunkel et al. (1999). [e]Kunkel et al. (1999); [f]Myers & Biocca (1992). [g]Morgan (1982). [h]Larson (1996). [i]Children Now (1997). [j]Walsh-Childers et al. (2001). [k]Garner & Sterk (1998). [l]Shaw (1995); Stice & Shaw (1994). [m]Field et al. (1999). [n]Gow (1996). [o]Seidman (1999). [p]Greeson & Williams (1986). [q]Kalof (1999). [r]Pardun (2002). [s]Children Now (1997).

troubles and infidelities are another favorite television genre of teen audiences. These shows also talk about rather than explicitly depict sexual behavior, but the discussions often are detailed and racy. Recent studies have found that parent–child relations, marital relations and infidelity, other sexual relations, and sexual orientation are the most commonly talked about topics. Sexual themes are more frequent on the shows teens most prefer (e.g., *Geraldo Rivera*, *Jenny Jones*, *Rolonda Watts*, and *Jerry Springer*) rather than on others that attract older audiences (e.g., *Oprah Winfrey* and *Phil Donahue*). A number of the talk shows include professional therapists who are supposed to comment on how the problems might be solved, but these "experts" get less airtime than anyone

else on the set, including the audience (Greenberg & Smith, 2002).

Soap Operas

Soap operas, another popular teen girl genre, also have been targeted as programs with a prominent focus on sex. As with other television programming, soap operas depict more sexual talk than sexual behaviors, although sexual behaviors (ranging from kissing to sexual intercourse) are not altogether infrequent. Planning for sexual activity (such as visiting a health clinic, purchasing contraceptives) as well as negative consequences of sexual activity (such as the transmission of a STD or pregnancy) are rarely portrayed (Heintz-Knowles, 1996).

Types of Sexual Content Portrayed on Television

Unhealthy Sexuality

Despite their prolific portrayal of sexuality, most television programming neglects to realistically depict the risks that accompany sexual activity. Indeed, the American Academy of Pediatrics concluded that only 165 of the nearly 14,000 sexual references, innuendoes, and jokes the average teenager views on television per year dealt with topics such as birth control, self-control, abstinence, or STDs (cited in Sutton *et al.*, 2001).

Across the dial, most sexual intercourse depicted takes place between adults, but although more than half are in established relationships, a majority are not married to each other, and about 1 in 10 who are shown having sexual intercourse have only just met. In almost two thirds of programs in which characters have sex, no clear consequences are shown. When consequences are portrayed, they are almost four times as likely to be positive than negative. Only about one tenth of the programs include anything to do with sexual patience, sexual precaution, and/or depiction of risks and negative consequences of unprotected sex (Kunkle *et al.*, 1999).

Other patterns of sexual behavior on television also warrant concern. One study found that 40% of the sexual behaviors observed in prime-time comedies fit the legal definition of sexual harassment, often to the accompaniment of a laugh track. Although the sexual harassment rarely led to a successful sexual encounter, it did not lead to social sanctions either. Typically, the recipient (female or male) simply ignored or quietly rejected the unwelcome sexual advances (Skill, Robinson, & Kinsella, 1994).

Ward (1995) found that one in four of the speaking interactions between characters per episode of the top shows for children and adolescents (1992–1993 broadcast year) contained some sort of sexual message. The most frequently occurring types of messages equated masculinity with being sexual and/or commented on women's bodies as sexual objects. The picture of sexuality presented was one of sex as recreation, where competition and game playing are anticipated and the prize is physically attractive.

Standards of Beauty

Women on television, as in most other media, are unnaturally physically attractive and slim. The media-depicted ideal of female beauty has become thinner and thinner over the past 30 years, and the difference between the idealized body and the average young woman has increased: models used to weigh about 8% less than the "average" woman in the United States, yet now they weigh about 23% less (Seid, 1989; Silverstein, Perdue, Peterson, & Kelly, 1986). The current standard of attractiveness on TV and in magazines is slimmer for women than for men, and the standard is slimmer than it was in the past. One study found that more than one fourth of female models in television commercials had comments made about their looks compared to only 7% of males (*Media Report to Women*, 1999).

Sexual Aggression

Television females also frequently are depicted as victims and men as aggressors. In fact, television viewers are more than twice as likely to see a scene in which a male character predominates over a female rather than a female over a male. Men on television are also almost twice as likely as women to be shown using physical force. In the television world, women's power is their sexuality. Three times as many women as men are seen promising sex to men on TV (*Media Report to Women*, 1999; Children Now, 1997).

Effects of Exposure to Sex on Television

Such content studies can tell us only so much. We might speculate about the possible effects of this pattern of content on viewers, but the big question remains: How do viewers apply what they see about sex on television to their own sexual lives? Unfortunately, only a few studies have investigated the link between exposure to sexual media content and teens' sexual attitudes and behaviors. These few studies suggest that television depictions of sexuality do have an influence on beliefs that may influence behavior, but much more work remains to be done.

Body Dissatisfaction

Research has shown that the emphasis the media place on the thin ideal body image may be responsible for body size overestimations that women make, and indirectly cause increases in eating disorders such as anorexia nervosa and bulimia. In one study, just 30 minutes of exposure to ideal-body programming and commercials changed young women's moods and their perceptions of their own bodies. Unexpectedly, the young women who saw thin media models were *less* likely to overestimate the size of their own bodies and were *less* likely to be depressed than young women who had not seen the television ads. The researchers proposed that body-image disturbance may be at least a two-stage phenomenon in which viewers first absorb a representation of the ideal body which frequently is found in the media, but after an initial feeling of identification realize that their body does not measure up, and become dissatisfied, perhaps depressed, perhaps motivated to achieve the ideal through dieting or exercise (Myers & Biocca, 1992). In surveys of high school students, television viewing, magazine reading, and identification with thin models in the media have been related to body dissatisfaction, belief in ideal body stereotypes (e.g., slim for females, muscular for males), and dieting and exercising (Hofschire & Greenberg, 2001).

Ideas about Parenthood

Surveys also have found relationships between viewing daytime soap operas and beliefs about single parenthood. In one study, junior and senior high school students who frequently viewed daytime soap operas were more likely than those who watched less often to believe that single mothers have relatively easy lives, have good jobs, and do not live in poverty. The soap viewers also thought that the babies of single mothers would be as healthy as most babies, and will get love and attention from adult men who are friends of their mothers (Larson, 1996).

Marriage is not as pleasantly perceived as single motherhood by frequent television viewers. In another study, college students who watched more television were more likely than lighter viewers to be ambivalent about the possibility that marriage is a happy way of life (Signorielli, 1991).

Early Intercourse

Two correlational studies also suggest that heavier exposure to sexual content on television is related to earlier initiation of sexual intercourse (Brown & Newcomer, 1991; Peterson, Moore, & Furstenberg, 1991).

Sex in Teen Magazines

Magazines are an important part of most teen girls' daily media diets. *YM* has a circulation of 2.2 million and is exceeded in circulation only by *Seventeen*, whose readership climbed from 4.5 to 6.5 million in the 1990s (Schwartz, 1998). Analyses of teen girl magazines show that these magazines are designed primarily to tell girls that their most important function in life is to get sexually attractive enough to catch a desirable male (Peirce, 1995). The message (e.g., "What's your lovemaking profile?" "Perfect pickup lines: Never again let a guy get away because you can't think of anything to say") is repeated even more explicitly in the women's magazines, such as *Cosmopolitan*, *Glamour*, and *Mademoiselle* that many middle and older adolescent girls read.

One of the most comprehensive studies of teen girls' and women's magazines shows that these magazines are full of information about sexuality. Teen girl magazines, on average, include more than 80 column inches (one to six items) per issue on sexual topics. Women's magazines devote more than twice that amount (about 178 col. inches). Both teens' and women's magazines have increased their coverage of sexual topics since the mid-1980s (Walsh-Childers, Gotthoffer, & Ringer, 2001).

Surprisingly, teen girls' magazines may be doing a better job than the women's magazines of educating their readers about such sexual health topics as contraception, pregnancy, abortion, emergency contraception, and STDs. In women's magazines the average number of column inches devoted to sexual health content has decreased since the mid-1980s, while space for other sexual topics, such as how to improve sexual performance, has increased (Walsh-Childers et al., 2001).

These magazines are the standard bearers of unattainable beauty ideals. One in every three articles in leading teen girl magazines includes a focus on appearance, and half of the advertisements use and appeal to beauty to sell their products. One in three articles focus on dating compared to only 12% discussing either school or careers (Children Now, 1997). A close analysis of 175 articles and columns about health, sex and relationships appearing in *Glamour*, *Seventeen*, *Teen*, *Mademoiselle* and *YM* magazines in the 1970s, 1980s, and 1990s, concluded that the magazines were urging girls to be enthusiastic consumers in pursuit of perfection—perfect hair, perfect complexions, perfect wardrobes; were holding up thinner and thinner models as the ideal; and were serving as field guides for sexual indulgence (Garner, Sterk, & Adams, 1998).

Effects of Exposure to Sex in Magazines

The images in the magazines adolescent girls read tend to have a greater effect on them than on the adults who may be reading the same magazines (Shaw, 1995). In one study, female undergraduates were shown pictures from magazines containing either "ultra-thin" models, average-sized models, or no models. The young women who saw the thin models subsequently reported more depression, stress, guilt, shame, insecurity, and body dissatisfaction than the young women who saw other kinds or no models (Stice & Shaw, 1994). A survey of fifth through twelfth grade girls found that girls say magazines have a strong impact on their perceptions of their weight and shape. More than two thirds of the girls said that magazine pictures have influenced their idea of a perfect body shape, and almost half (47%) reported wanting to lose weight because of the pictures. The study found positive correlations between frequency of reading women's magazines and prevalence of having dieted or exercised to lose weight because of a magazine and/or magazine article (Field et al., 1999).

Sex in Teen Movies

Teens are one of the primary audiences for Hollywood movies in theaters and at-home movies on cable and videocassettes, and more than two thirds of the movies produced and rated each year in the United States are R rated, frequently because of the sexual content. Although only teens older than 16 technically are allowed to see R-rated movies unless accompanied by an adult, most children today have seen R-rated movies at least four years earlier (Greenberg et al., 1993).

An analysis of R-rated movies popular with teens in the early 1980s found an average of 17.5 sexual portrayals per movie (Greenberg et al., 1993). Pardun (2002) found that in the top grossing movies of 1995, romantic and sexual relationships are present even in action adventure movies such as *Apollo 13*. Although Greenberg's analysis suggested that teens' movies are more sexually explicit than their television shows, in the movies Pardun analyzed, there was more talk than action. Much of the talk was third-party discussion—two people, usually women, talking about the relationships of other people (Children Now, 1997). Underlying these discussions are some basic ideas that romantic relationships are mysterious, difficult to sort out, and primarily for the young.

Even in the movies, where we might expect more thorough character and story development than on television, sexual relations tend to occur with little reference to why the characters are attracted to each other or what they might expect from each other in the future. Older people in long-term relationships are rarely shown expressing tenderness or love for each other, and precautions against unwanted outcomes are as rare as they are on television.

Sex in Music and Music Videos

Even before the gyrating hips of Elvis were censored on *The Ed Sullivan Show*, popular music has been almost synonymous with sex. Especially appealing to youth, popular music and now music videos contain frequent references to relationships, romance, and sexual behavior.

Music videos may be especially influential sources of sexual information for adolescents because they combine visuals of adolescents' favorite musicians with music, and many of the visual elements are sexual (Hansen & Hansen, 1990). Although adolescent girls are as frequent viewers as their male peers, popular music videos of the early 1990s continued to underrepresent women, with men outnumbering women in lead roles by almost a 5 to 1 margin. When women do appear, their physical appearance rather than musical ability is emphasized (Gow, 1996). Music video women are more affectionate, nurturing, and sexually pursued than males, and most wear revealing clothing (Seidman, 1999).

Music lyrics have drawn criticism from groups such as the Parents Music Resource Center (Gore, 1987), leading to some voluntary labeling of recorded music. For some teens, however, such warnings may represent a stamp of approval rather than a deterrent to buy. Roe (1995) proposed a theory of "media delinquency" that suggests some teens may gravitate toward socially devalued or outlawed media content for the same reasons they resist other aspects of the mainstream culture.

Some variants of rap music (e.g., gangsta rap) are particularly explicit about both sex and violence. Perry (1995) argues that the explicit "sexual speak" of Black women rappers follows in the liberating tradition of the "blues," which gave voice to Black women's sexual and cultural politics during the years of Black migration to northern states. This striving for empowerment may explain why some rap musicians have responded to concerns about unsafe sex and sexually related behavior and have included alternative messages. Some rap music includes talk of "jimmy hats," or condoms. In a song called *Safe Sex*, rapper Erick Sermon chants, "Let's get high as a kite and have safe sex." An album by the female rap group Salt 'n' Peppa is about the pleasures and responsibilities of sex. A video by the group TLC called *Unpretty* shows a young woman considering breast implants because her boyfriend wants her to have them (at the beginning of the video he's shown looking at women in pornography). By the end of the video, she decides not to have the implants after all.

The premiere music video channel, MTV, has sponsored safer-sex public service campaigns on the channel and features the nightly call-in sex information and counseling show, *Loveline* with Dr. Drew Pinsky. Despite the sometimes raunchy and irreverent context, Dr. Pinsky consistently champions abstinence as the best choice for adolescents' emotional health.

Frank discussions about sex, ranging from Dr. Joy Brown's on-air psychological counseling to the sexual banter of disc jockeys such as Howard Stern who are hired to capture the teen/young adult audiences as they drive to school or work, are common on radio as well. Content analyses are rare, however, given the diversity of local radio programming and the speed with which radio personalities rise and fall in popularity.

Effects of Exposure to Sex in Music Videos

Only a few studies have investigated how exposure to the sexual content of music and music videos is related to adolescents' sexual beliefs and behaviors. One experimental study did find that adolescents who were exposed to only a few music videos were more likely than those who had not to have more permissive attitudes about premarital sex (Greeson & Williams, 1986). Another study found that exposure to the stereotypical images of gender and sexuality in music videos had an influence on college women's sexual beliefs, especially greater acceptance of interpersonal violence (Kalof, 1999).

Sex on the Internet

Despite protest from legislators and parents regarding the proliferation of sexual sites on the Internet, relatively little research has addressed the sexual content currently available online. Pornographic sites certainly are prevalent on the Internet, but it is not yet clear if adolescents, particularly female adolescents, are drawn to such sites. It seems more likely that girls are using the Internet to learn about sex and sexual health in anonymous forums. Sites such as *Go Ask Alice* (http://www.goaskalice. columbia.edu/) created by Columbia University's Health Education Program offer teens a forum in which they can ask questions regarding sex and sexual health and receive thoughtful and instructive answers from an adult.

Home pages also present a space in which teen girls can explore their emergent sexuality. Stern (2001), for example, found that adolescent girls frequently use their home pages to express and reflect on various aspects of their sexuality, such as homosexuality, sexual behaviors, body image, and relationship concerns.

Some have suggested that the Internet may fundamentally change courtship rituals since interactions between potential partners can transpire electronically through e-mail, rather than in person or over the phone. Teens who know one another from settings such as school may use the Internet as a means to establish a comfort zone without the awkwardness often associated with dating. Online courtship also seems to be growing as teens from diverse geographic regions meet in chat rooms. Some

new media critics have suggested that teens who engage in "cybersex" may learn more about their sexual selves in a safe-sex forum, while others object that cybersex is equally emotional (although perhaps physically less risky) than actual intercourse.

RESISTING MEDIA MESSAGES

Although much of the research cited here suggests that adolescent girls' sexual health can be influenced, often negatively, by the mass media, some authors argue the "popular media not only reflect and perpetuate young women's social subordination, but also offer them opportunities for pleasure and resistance" (Carpenter, 1998, p. 4). Teens incorporate and sometimes resist the sexual content they attend to in the media. Two qualitative studies of how girls use the Internet (Stern, 2001; Wray & Steele, 2001) show that girls also can be astute media critics and producers. These studies illustrate what is meant by "resistance" in the Media Practice Model—opposition to the dominant ideas of attractiveness and the female's role in the dominant model of heterosexual relationships. The 'zines and web sites produced by teen girls show that teens can be oppositional readers of mainstream media, and can be even more active audience members as producers themselves. For example, one young female web author posted a game she called, "Make Kate Fat." Spoofing the waifish figure of supermodel Kate Moss, the game allowed site visitors to select various foods Kate Moss might choose for lunch. As they clicked on fattening food items, the model's photographic image was enhanced to make it look like she was gaining weight. This game presented a clever way for the web author to express her dissatisfaction with the often unrealistic and unhealthy beauty standards promoted by mainstream media.

In short, adolescents are at once influencing and being influenced by the ubiquitous sexual content in the media. Some are choosing less nutritious sexual media diets than others. Some are able to resist the temptations of the mainstream culture that say that women should be thin and beautiful, men strong, and both should be engaged in sexual activity, regardless of the consequences. Others are seduced and model their developing sexual lives on the frequently unhealthy sexual media content they consume.

WORKING WITH THE MEDIA FOR HEALTHY SEXUALITY

Could the media be used to enhance rather than undermine the sexual lives of adolescent girls? Health advocates have developed four strategies for working with the media in the interest of healthier media consumers: (1) public health campaigns, (2) media advocacy, (3) entertainment–education (edutainment), and (4) media literacy. Each strategy has its strengths and weaknesses.

Public Information Campaigns

Public information campaigns are the most common form of intentional use of the mass media for noncommercial purposes. Effective campaigns typically are similar to campaigns for commercial products in that they use a number of media channels and are designed to generate specific effects in a relatively large number of people within a specified period of time (Rogers & Storey, 1987). One of the best known media campaigns designed to reduce teen pregnancy has run in the Baltimore, Maryland, area since the mid-1980s. The "Campaign for Our Children" has been credited with contributing to a significant decrease in teen pregnancies in the region. The campaign has included dramatic billboards in strategic locations on Interstates and roads near schools. The frequent television and radio spots include such messages as: "Virgin: Teach your kids it's not a four-letter word," and "You can go farther when you do not go all the way." A number of other states have launched or are about to launch similar campaigns (National Campaign to Prevent Teen Pregnancy, 1997).

Extensive evaluation of such campaigns for a variety of health-related issues have concluded that they will be most effective when the media campaign is complemented by other activities at the individual, community and policy levels, and when the campaign can be sustained over the long term. The messages provided in safer sex or pregnancy prevention media campaigns will get lost in the sea of competing messages that promote irresponsible and unhealthy sexual behavior unless they are repeated extensively and reinforced by service providers and public policy.

Media Advocacy

Some health activists have begun to use the media as tools for bringing health issues to the attention of the public and policymakers. Media advocacy calls for understanding how the media work and using that knowledge to get issues on the media agenda. Rather than waiting for the media to cover an issue or to run a public service announcement, health activists generate news that attracts the attention of the news media. The focus of this approach is on public policies that affect health rather than on individual health behaviors (Wallack, 1990). The underlying rationale is that individuals will not be able to change unhealthy behavior unless policy supports the desired behaviors. Thus, for example, public policies that affect access to and affordability of sexuality education, STD prevention, and contraception could be important topics of media advocacy. Policymakers also could help make research monies available for development of more effective contraceptives, and work with media to ensure more responsible information about sexuality.

Entertainment–Education

Another way to reach the public is to incorporate sexually responsible messages in popular entertainment programming on television, movies, and music. Such strategies have been effective in promoting family planning in a number of developing countries in Africa, and in other parts of the world (Gilluly & Moore, 1986; Lettenmaier, Krenn, Morgan, Kols, & Piotrow, 1993). In India, popular soap operas have included long-running plots about family planning that have increased visits to family planning clinics and the use of contraceptives (Singhal & Rogers, 1989).

Some groups also have worked with writers and producers as advocates for more responsible sexual portrayals in the media. For example, the Kaiser Family Foundation and Advocates for Youth funds the Media Project in Los Angeles that has assisted writers for the popular programs *Dawson's Creek* and *Felicity* in developing episodes dealing with teen sexuality. The long-running hit show *Beverly Hills 90210*, with editorial consultation from the Media Project, included a number of episodes in which the high school characters either agreed to wait to have sex or use contraceptives. Paul Stupin, executive producer of *Dawson's Creek*, said, "If there's a way to insert a subtle message after our characters have had sex, without banging our viewers over the head—maybe see a condom wrapper on the table next to the bed—we absolutely try to" (MacGregor, 1999, p. B1).

Although the impact of such messages has not been evaluated systematically in the United States, the results of similar efforts in other countries and with other topics suggest that entertainment-education can be an effective strategy. The Harvard School of Public Health's campaign against drunk driving, which generated more than 80 television episodes that included dialogue or depiction of designated drivers, was successful in increasing awareness and use of designated drivers (DeJong & Winsten, 1990). When *Felicity* aired a two-part episode on date rape, the Media Project encouraged the producers to put an 800-number for a rape hot line at the end of the show. They received more than 1000 calls. On *ER*, a girl was treated with the morning-after pill after being raped. The two scenes she was in were on the air for less than one minute, but knowledge of emergency contraception among the viewers polled before and after the episode increased 17% (MacGregor, 1999).

The insertion of socially responsible messages in entertainment media is a potentially powerful way of affecting sexual behavior because the "selling" of a particular behavior is not as obvious as it may be in a public service advertisement, and thus, audiences may not be as likely to resist the message. "Edutainment," as it is sometimes called, also is more likely to reach and attract the attention of target audiences. The longer formats also allow more time for developing more complex messages, such as how to negotiate condom use (Brown & Walsh-Childers, 1994.) The primary drawback to such a strategy in the United States, however, is that the media are unlikely to include portrayals they consider potentially controversial (Wallack, 1990). Homosexuality, abortion, and the use of contraceptives to prevent pregnancy still are topics the mainstream media do not like to discuss for fear of offending some portions of their audiences and/or their advertisers.

Media Literacy

Another promising strategy that is gaining momentum in the United States is called media literacy—"the ability to access, analyze, evaluate and communicate messages in a variety of forms" (Hobbs, 1997, p. 7). Across the country local groups are working in schools and community centers teaching youth and parents how to be more discerning media consumers by showing them that:

1. Media messages are constructed and can be "deconstructed" to uncover the symbolism that conveys meaning.
2. Messages are produced within economic, social, and political contexts.
3. They can create media themselves (Center for Media Literacy, 1998).

So far, although more research is needed, evaluation studies have shown that children who are taught such concepts are less susceptible to the negative effects of subsequent media use (e.g., Austin & Johnson, 1997). Other countries around the world, such as Canada and Australia, have incorporated extensive media literacy curricula in their schools, and some states in the United States now include media literacy in their statewide educational goals. The American Academy of Pediatricians (1995) has issued policy statements on media effects on sexuality and contraception, and has embraced media literacy as an important strategy to improve public health. Their "Media Matters" campaign includes a media use inventory that pediatricians are encouraged to have their young patients fill out and discuss with their parents. The expectation is that awareness of current media patterns may alert youth, parents, and physicians to problems that may result from excessive use of potentially harmful media content. Ultimately, we would hope that a media-literate populace would demand healthier media fare.

CONCLUSION

In short, it is clear from this review of the content and effects of the variety of media used by adolescent girls that the media are an important part of how girls learn about sexual norms and expectations in the culture. From music to magazines, to television and now the Internet, sex is a staple and often, unfortunately, an unhealthy ingredient of teen girls' media diets. Although we still know relatively little about how this ubiquitous sexual content is used by and affects adolescent girls, existing research suggests that such media content can have powerful effects, especially when other sources of information are difficult to access or are less compelling. Most of the media adolescents attend to provide alluring and relatively-risk-free opportunities to learn more about sex than their parents, teachers or even friends are willing to talk about. Unfortunately, these portrayals rarely include accurate depictions of the emotional and physical risks that may be involved in sexual activity. In the media world, women still are engaged primarily in attracting and seducing men, but the costs of achieving the ideal look and of engaging in sexual behavior regardless of love, commitment, or protection

against pregnancy or disease are rarely addressed.

At least four approaches may help provide adolescent girls with the information and skills they need to negotiate successfully in such a media world. Public information campaigns aimed at individuals and media advocacy targeting policymakers could offer alternative points of view about early sexual behavior and promote access to and use of condoms and contraceptives for adolescents. The entertainment media should be commended when they depict adolescent sexuality in a responsible way, and should be encouraged to look for opportunities to portray adolescent girls as interested in more than achieving the right look and "getting" the guy. Finally, parents, schools, religious institutions, and health providers should do all they can to help girls use the media more effectively and to provide the sexual information teen girls seek, so the media are not the only comfortable alternative.

REFERENCES

Abma, J., Driscoll, A., & Moore, K. (1997). *Differing degrees of control over first intercourse and young women's first partners: Data from cycle 5 of the National Survey of Family Growth.* Paper presented to the Annual Meeting of Population Association of America, Washington, DC.

Alan Guttmacher Institute (1994). *Sex and America's teenagers.* New York: Author.

American Academy of Pediatrics (1995). Sexuality, contraception and the media (RE9505). Policy Statement, 95(2), 298–300. [Online]. Available: http://www.aap.org

Arnett, J. (1992). The soundtrack of recklessness: Musical preferences and reckless behavior among adolescents. *Journal of Adolescent Research, 7,* 313–331.

Austin, E., & Johnson, K. (1997). Immediate and delayed effects of media literacy training on third graders' decision making for alcohol. *Health Communication, 94*(4), 323–349.

Bandura, A. (1994). Social cognitive theory of mass communication. In J. Bryant & D. Zillmann (Eds.), *Media effects: Advances in theory and research.* Hillsdale, NJ: Erlbaum.

Brown, J., & Newcomer, S. (1991). Television viewing and adolescents' sexual behavior. *Journal of Homosexuality, 21*(1/2), 77–91.

Brown, J. D., & Childers, K. W. (1994). Effects of media on personal and public health. In J. Bryant and D. Zillmann (Eds.), *Media effects: Advances in theory and research* (pp. 389–415). Hillsdale, NJ: Erlbaum.

Brown, J. D., & Schulze, L. (1990). The effects of race, gender, and fandom on audience interpretation of Madonna's music videos. In B. Greenberg, J. D. Brown, & N. Buerkel-Rothfuss (Eds.) *Media, sex, and the adolescent* (pp. 263–276). Cresskill, NJ: Hampton Press.

Brown, J. D., & Steele, J. (1996). Sex and the mass media. In M. Smith, D. Besharov, K. Gardiner, & T. Hoff (Eds.), *Sex and Hollywood: Should there be a government role?* (pp. 1–38). Menlo Park, CA: Kaiser Family Foundation.

Brown, J. D., White, A., & Nikopoulou, L. (1993). Disinterest, intrigue, resistance: Early adolescent girls' use of sexual media content. In B. Greenberg, J. D. Brown, & N. Buerkel-Rothfuss (Eds.), *Media, sex, and the adolescent* (pp. 177–195). Cresskill, NJ: Hampton Press.

Buerkel-Rothfoss, N. L., & Mayes, S. (1981). Soap opera viewing: The cultivation effect. *Journal of Communication, 31*(3), 108–115.

Buerkel-Rothfuss, N. L., & Strouse, J. S. (1993). Media exposure and perceptions of sexual behaviors: The cultivation hypothesis moves to the bedroom. In B. S. Greenberg, J. D. Brown, & N. Buerkel-Rothfuss (Eds.), *Media, sex, and the adolescent* (pp. 225–247). Cresskill, NJ: Hampton Press.

Carpenter, L. (1998). From girls into women: Scripts for sexuality and romance in *Seventeen* magazine, 1974–1994. *The Journal of Sex Research, 35*(2), 158(11).

Center for Media Literacy (1998). *What everyone should know about media.* [brochure]. Los Angeles: Author.

Children Now (1997). *Reflections of girls in the media.* Los Angeles: Children Now and the Henry J. Kaiser Family Foundation.

Commonwealth Fund (1999). *Improving the health of adolescent girls: Policy report of the Commonwealth Fund Commission on women's health.* New York: Author.

Cope, K., & Kunkel, D. (2001). *Sexual messages in teens' favorite prime-time TV programs.* In J. D. Brown, J. R. Steele, & K. Walsh-Childers (Eds.), *Sexual teens, sexual media.* Hillsdale, NJ: Erlbaum.

Courtwright, J., & Baran, S. (1980). The acquisition of sexual information by young people. *Journalism Quarterly, 57*(1), 107–114.

Davis, D. (1990). Portrayals of women in prime-time network television: Some demographic characteristics. *Sex Roles: A Journal of Research, 23*(5–6), 325–332.

DeJong, W., & Winsten, J. (1990). The use of mass media in substance abuse prevention. *Health Affairs, 9*(2), 30–46.

Entman, R. (1994). Representation and reality in the portrayal of blacks on network television news. *Journalism Quarterly, 71*(3), 509–520.

Field, A., Cheung, L., Herzog, D., Gortmaker, S., & Col-

ditz, G. (1999). Exposure to the mass media and weight concerns among girls. *Pediatrics, 103*(3), 361–365.

Gagnon, J., & Simon, W. (1973). *Sexual conduct: The social sources of human sexuality.* Chicago: Aldine.

Gallatin, J. E. (1975). *Adolescence and individuality.* New York: Harper and Row.

Gap between Black and White TV viewing habits narrows. (1999, May 17). *Jet,* p. 65.

Garner, A., Sterk, H., & Adams, S. (1998). Narrative analysis of sexual etiquette in teenage magazines. *Journal of Communication, 48*(4), 59–78.

Gerbner, G., Gross, L., Morgan, M., & Signorelli, N. (1994). Growing up with television: The cultivation perspective. In J. Bryant and D. Zillmann (Eds.), *Media effects: Advances in theory and research* (pp. 17–41). Hillsdale, NJ: Erlbaum.

Gilluly, R., & Moore, S. (1986). Radio—spreading the word on family planning. *Population Reports, Series J., No. 32.* Baltimore: Johns Hopkins University, Population Information Program.

Gore, T. (1987). *Raising PG kids in an X-rated society.* Nashville: Abingdon Press.

Gow, J. (1996). Reconsidering gender roles on MTV: Depictions in the most popular music videos of the early 1990s. *Communication Reports, 9*(2), 151–161.

Greenberg, B. S., & Smith, S. (2002). Talk shows: Up close and in your face. In J. D. Brown, J. R. Steele & K. Walsh-Childers (Eds.), *Sexual teens, sexual media.* Hillsdale, NJ: Erlbaum.

Greenberg, B., Siemicki, M., Dorfman, S., Heeter, C., Stanley, C., Soderman, A., & Lisangan, R. (1993). Sex content in R-rated films viewed by adolescents. In B. S. Greenberg, J. D. Brown, & N. L. Buerkel-Rothfuss (Eds.), *Media, sex and the adolescent* (pp. 29–44). Cresskill, NJ: Hampton Press.

Greeson, L. E., & Williams, R. A. (1986). Social implications of music videos for youth: An analysis of the content and effects of MTV. *Youth & Society, 18*(2), 177–189.

Hansen, C. H., & Hansen, R. D. (1990). The influence of sex and violence on the appeal of rock music videos. *Communication Research, 17*(2), 212–234.

Heintz-Knowles, K. (1996). *Sexual activity on daytime soap operas: A content analysis of five weeks of television programming.* Menlo Park, CA: Henry J. Kaiser Family Foundation.

Hobbs, R. (1997). Literacy for the information age. In J. Flood, S. B. Heath, & D. Lapp (Eds.), *Handbook of research on teaching media literacy through the communicative and visual arts* (pp. 7–14). New York: Simon & Schuster Macmillan.

Hofschire, L. J. & B. S. Greenberg (2001). Media's impact on adolescents' body dissatisfaction. In J. D. Brown, J. R. Steele, & K. Walsh-Childers (Eds.) *Sexual teens, sexual media.* Hillsdale, NJ: Erlbaum.

Iyengar, S. (1991). *Is anyone responsible? How television frames political issues.* Chicago: University of Chicago Press.

Kaiser Family Foundation (1998a). *Kaiser Family Foundation and YM Magazine National Survey of Teens: Teens talk about dating, intimacy, and their sexual experiences.* Menlo Park, CA: Henry J. Kaiser Family Foundation.

Kaiser Family Foundation (1998b). *Sexually transmitted diseases in America: How many cases and at what cost?* Menlo Park, CA: Henry J. Kaiser Family Foundation.

Kaiser Family Foundation (1999). *Kids & media @ the new millennium: A comprehensive analysis of children's media use.* Menlo Park, CA: Henry J. Kaiser Family Foundation.

Kalof, L. (1999). The effects of gender and music video imagery on sexual attitudes. *The Journal of Social Psychology*, *139*(3), 366–378.

Kosicki, G. (1993). Problems and opportunities in agenda-setting research. *Journal of Communication*, *43*(2), 100–127.

Kunkel, D., Cope, K., Farinola, W., Beily, E., Rollin, E., & Donnerstein, E. (1999). *Sex on TV. Biennial Report to the Kaiser Family Foundation.* Menlo Park, CA: Henry J. Kaiser Family Foundation.

Larson, M. (1996). Sex roles and soap operas: What adolescents learn about single motherhood. *Sex Roles: A Journal of Research*, *35*(1/2), 97–121.

Larson, R., Kubey, R., & Colletti, J. (1989). Changing channels: Early adolescent media choices and shifting investments in family and friends. *Journal of Youth and Adolescence*, *18*(5), 583–600.

Lettenmaier, C., Krenn, S., Morgan, W., Kols, A., & Piotrow, P. (1993). Africa: Using radio soap operas to promote family planning. *Hygie*, *12*(1), 5–10.

Livingstone, S. M. (1989). Interpretive viewers and structured programs. *Communication Research*, *16*(1), 25–57.

MacGregor, H. (1999, October 25). Media project teaches safe screen sex. *Los Angeles Times*, p. B1.

McCombs, M., & Shaw, D. (1993). The evolution of agenda-setting research: Twenty-five years later in the marketplace of ideas. *Journal of Communication*, *43*(2), 58–67.

Media Report to Women (1999, Winter). 27(1), 19. Silver Spring, MD: Communication Research Associates, Inc.

Morgan, M. (1982). Television and adolescents' sex-role stereotypes: A longitudinal study. *Journal of Personality and Social Psychology*, *43*(5), 947–955.

Myers, P., & Biocca, F. (1992) The elastic body image: The effect of television advertising and programming on body image distortions in young women. *Journal of Communication*, *42*(3), 108–133.

National Campaign to Prevent Teen Pregnancy. (1997). *Sending the message: State-based media campaigns for teen pregnancy prevention.* Washington, DC.

Neuman, W., Just, M., & Crigler, A. (1992). *Common knowledge: News and the construction of political meaning.* Chicago: University of Chicago Press.

Pardun, C. (2002). Romancing the script: Identifying the romantic agenda in top-grossing movies. In J. D. Brown, J. R. Steele, & K. Walsh-Childers (Eds.) *Sexual teens, sexual media*. Hillsdale, NJ: Erlbaum.

Peirce, K. (1995). Socialization messages in *Seventeen* and *Teen* magazines. In C. M. Lont (Ed.), *Women and media: Content, careers, and criticism* (pp. 79–85). Belmont, CA: Wadsworth.

Perry, I. (1995). It's my thang and i'll swing it the way i feel! In J. G. Dines & J. M. Humez (Eds.), *Gender, race and class in media* (pp. 524–530). Thousand Oaks, CA: Sage.

Peterson, J., Moore, K., & Furstenberg, F. (1991). Television viewing and early initiation of sexual intercourse. Is there a link? *Journal of Homosexuality*, *21*(1–2), 93–118.

Piot, P., & Islam, M. (1994). Sexually transmitted diseases in the 1990s: Global epidemiology and challenges for control. *Sexually Transmitted Diseases*, *21*(2), S7–13.

Potter, W. J. (1998). *Media literacy.* Thousand Oaks, CA: Sage.

Roe, K. (1995). Adolescents' use of socially disvalued media: Towards a theory of media delinquency. *Journal of Youth and Adolescence*, *24*(5), 617–632.

Rogers, E., & Storey, D. (1987). Communication campaigns. In C. Berger & S. Chaffee (Eds.), *Handbook of communication science* (pp. 817–846). Newbury Park, CA: Sage.

Schwartz, J. (1998, July 5). Teen 'zines too sexy, experts say. *Chicago Sun-Times*, p.35.

Seid, R. P. (1989). *Never too thin: Why women are at war with their bodies.* New York: Prentice-Hall.

Seidman, S. (1999). Revisiting sex-role stereotyping in MTV videos. *International Journal of Instructional Media*, *26*(1), 11–25.

Shaw, J. (1995). Effects of fashion magazines on body dissatisfaction and eating psychopathology in adolescent and adult females. *European Eating Disorders Review*, *3*(1), 15–23.

Signorielli, N. (1991). Adolescents and ambivalence toward marriage: A cultivation analysis. *Youth and Society*, *23*, 121–149.

Signorelli, N. (1997). *Reflections on girls in the media.* Menlo Park, CA: Henry J. Kaiser Family Foundation.

Silverstein, B., Perdue, L, Peterson, B., & Kelly, E. (1986). The role of the mass media in promoting a thin standard of bodily attractiveness for women. *Sex Roles*, *14*(9–10), 519–532.

Singhal, A., & Rogers, E. (1989). Educating through television. *Populi*, *16*(2), 38–47.

Skill, T., Robinson, J., & Kinsella, C. (1994, November). *Sexual harassment in network television situation comedies: An empirical content analysis of fictional programming one year prior to the Clarence Thomas senate confirmation hearings for the U.S. Supreme Court.* A paper presented at the annual meeting of the Speech Communication Association, New Orleans.

Steele, J. R. (1999). Teenage sexuality and media practice: Factoring in the influences of family, friends, and school. *Journal of Sex Research*, *36*(4), 331–341.

Steele, J., & Brown, J. (1995) Adolescent room culture: Studying media in the context of everyday life. *Journal of Youth and Adolescence*, *5*, 551–576.

Stern, S. R. (2001). Sexual selves on the WWW: Adolescent

girls' home pages as sites for sexual expression. In J. D. Brown, J. Steele, & K. Walsh-Childers (Eds.), *Sexual teens, sexual media*. Hillsdale, NJ: Erlbaum.

Stice, E., & Shaw, H. (1994). Adverse-effects of the media portrayed thin-ideal on women and linkages to bulimic symptomatology. *Journal of Social and Clinical Psychology, 13*(3), 288–308.

Strouse, J., Buerkel-Rothfuss, N., & Long, E. (1995). Gender and family as moderators of the relationship between music video exposure and adolescent sexual permissiveness. *Adolescence, 30*, 505–521.

Sutton, M., Brown, J. D., Wilson, K., & Klein, J. (2001). Shaking the tree of knowledge for forbidden fruit: Where adolescents learn about sexuality and contraception. In J. D. Brown, J. R. Steele, & K. Walsh-Childers (Eds.) *Sexual teens, sexual media*. Hillsdale, NJ: Erlbaum.

Tolman D., & Higgins, T. (1996). How being a good girl can be bad for girls. In N. Maglin & D. Perry (Eds.), *"Bad girls", "good girls": Women, sex and power in the nineties*. Hillsdale, NJ: Rutgers University Press.

Tsing, A. (1990). Monster stories: Women charged with perinatal endangerment. In F. Ginsburg & A. Tsing (Eds.), *Uncertain terms: Negotiating gender in American culture* (pp. 282–299). Boston: Beacon Press.

Wallack, L. (1990). Improving health promotion: A critical perspective. In R. E. Rice & C. K. Atkin (Eds.), *Public communication campaigns* (2nd ed., pp. 353–367). Newbury Park, CA: Sage.

Walsh-Childers, K., Gotthoffer, A., & Ringer, C. (2001). From "just the facts" to "downright salacious:" Teens' and women's magazines coverage of sex and sexual health. In J. D. Brown, J. R. Steel, & K. Walsh-Childers (Eds.), *Sexual teens, sexual media*. Hillsdale, NJ: Erlbaum.

Ward, L. M. (1995). Talking about sex: Common themes about sexuality in the prime-time television programs children and adolescents view most. *Journal of Youth and Adolescence, 24*, 595–615.

Ward, L. M., Gorvine, B., & Cutron, A. (2001). Would that really happen? Adolescents' perceptions of several relationships according to prime-time television. In J. D. Brown, J. R. Steele, & K. Walsh-Childers (Eds.), *Sexual teens, sexual media*. Hillsdale, NJ: Erlbaum.

Wartella, E. (1994). Electronic childhood. In E. E. Dennis and E. C. Pease (Eds.), *Media studies journal: Children and the media* (pp. 33–43). New York: The Freedom Forum.

Willis, P. (1990). *Common culture*. Boulder, CO: Westview Press.

Wray, J., & Steele, J. R. (2001). What it means to be a girl: Teen girl magazines. In J. D. Brown, J. R. Steele, & K. Walsh-Childers (Eds.), *Sexual teens, sexual media*. Hillsdale, NJ: Erlbaum.

Zillmann, D., & Bryant, J. (1985). *Selective exposure to communication*. Hillsdale, NJ: Erlbaum.

Zollo, P. (1995). *Wise up to teens: Insights into marketing and advertising to teenagers*. Ithaca, NY: New Strategist.

7

Family Influences on Adolescent Females' Sexual Health

RICHARD A. CROSBY and KIM S. MILLER

INTRODUCTION

Sexual behavior that puts adolescents, particularly female adolescents, at risk for adverse health outcomes is an overwhelming public health problem in the United States. Sexual risk behaviors, including early sexual initiation, unprotected intercourse, and sex with multiple partners, place female adolescents at risk for unintended pregnancy and sexually transmitted diseases (STDs), including infection with the human immunodeficiency virus (HIV). Approximately one million teenagers become pregnant each year (Alan Guttmacher Institute, 1993) and 3 million adolescents, about one of every eight teens or one in four sexually active teens, acquire an STD annually (Eng & Butler, 1997). About 20% of all new HIV infections occur in young people under age 25 (Office of National AIDS Policy, 1996). Incidence of HIV infection is increasing more rapidly among adolescent and young adult women than among men of the same age; thus young women comprise a population at exceptionally high risk for HIV infection (Denning & Fleming, 1998; Rosenberg & Biggar, 1998; Wortley & Fleming, 1997).

Although issues related to the sexual and reproductive health risks of adolescent females are complex and multifaceted, the prevention messages provided to adolescents have often been simplistically judgmental, ambiguous, and not specifically tailored to the unique needs of adolescent females. A common judgmental message has been that female adolescents should not engage in sexual intercourse, implying that those who have are "promiscuous." Ambiguous messages are also common, for example, indicating that adolescents should "wait to have sex," but not indicating when this waiting period should end. Although prevention experts have long understood the importance of tailoring health-related messages in light of specific characteristics of the target audience, such as age, gender, race/ethnicity, sexual orientation, developmental status and sexual experience (Calamidas, 1992; DiClemente & Houston-Hamilton, 1989; Miller *et al.*, 1997; Whitaker, Miller, & Clark, in press), the two key prevention messages provided to female adolescents have been simplistic: "don't have sex" or "use condoms or birth control every time you have sex."

Many sex education programs for female adolescents are poorly suited to the unique

RICHARD A. CROSBY • Department of Behavioral Sciences and Health Education, Rollins School of Public Health, Emory Unviersity, Atlanta, Georgia 30322. KIM S. MILLER • Division of HIV/AIDS Prevention, Centers for Disease Control and Prevention, Atlanta, Georgia 30333.

Handbook of Women's Sexual and Reproductive Health, edited by Wingood and DiClemente. Kluwer Academic / Plenum Publishers, New York, 2002.

needs of adolescents and consist of too little, too late. For example, programs for female adolescents are often, simply as a matter of convenience, delivered in schools, in a set number of sessions, in a specific grade, typically involving very little planned interaction. These programs differ widely, but most focus on the discussion of facts and risks, without the accompanying opportunities to acquire and practice risk-reduction skills (Eng & Butler, 1997).

Although schools offer the best opportunity to provide comprehensive primary prevention programs to the most female adolescents, underlying political and programmatic constraints frequently preclude such programs (Yarber, 1992, 1995). A strong vocal minority promotes programs that focus exclusively on abstinence from sexual intercourse, typically until marriage. In these programs contraception is not discussed or the emphasis is on the failure of contraception to provide complete protection against pregnancy and STDs. Given that 77% of females initiate sexual intercourse by their 19th birthday (Alan Guttmacher Institute, 1993) and given the strong scientific evidence that effective sexuality programs are theory based and comprehensive (Eng & Butler, 1997; Joint United Nations Programme on HIV/AIDS, 1997; National Institutes of Health, 1997; Sex Information and Education Council of the United States, 1997), these politically driven messages and programs may leave female adolescents at high risk for infection with HIV or STD, or for unintended pregnancy.

Adolescents may also receive sex education from agencies that serve youth and in clinical settings. Many such agencies provide assistance to adolescents for a broad range of problems, often targeting hard-to-reach, high-risk populations in homeless or runaway shelters, juvenile detention facilities, and housing projects. Unfortunately, sex education programs for these youth may be limited because of sparse resources. Youth, for the most part, are seen in clinical settings after problem outcomes such as pregnancy and STDs have occurred. Thus, like schools, primary prevention efforts in these settings may be less than ideal.

THE FAMILY AS AN IDEAL PROVIDER OF PRIMARY PREVENTION

Various individual and social factors influence the sexual behavior of adolescent females. Peers, for example, are an important social influence; however, in this chapter we focus on the potential of the family to serve as the main provider of primary prevention for STDs and HIV infection and pregnancy. As will be shown, the family may protect against negative peer and other social influences.

In this chapter we use parents to refer to all those who serve in a parental role for adolescent females, whether they are biological parents, legal guardians, or other influential adults. Parents, unlike peers, teachers, counselors, and medical professionals, generally have unlimited access to their children and therefore have a unique opportunity to intervene early, repeatedly, and at times that best match the child's rapidly changing social and developmental status. The family can help address the inadequacies of the current primary prevention approaches for female adolescents.

Parents are the most powerful socializing agents in the lives of young teens. Parents are in a powerful position for shaping young people's attitudes and behaviors, and for helping them to become healthy adults. They can do this, in part, by providing accurate information about risks, consequences, and responsibilities and by imparting skills to their children that enable them to make responsible decisions about their health behavior. However, the potency of parental influence on promoting healthy sexuality relative to other information sources may arise from their unique and continual opportunities for engaging their children in dialogues about development and decision making. These dialogues should take place early (when the child first asks questions), continually (i.e., not one-time events), sequentially (i.e., building one upon the other as the child's cognitive, emotional, physical, and social development and experiences change), and should be time-sensitive (i.e., information is immediately responsive to the child's questions and anticipated needs rather than programmed, such as in a school curriculum).

Research increasingly shows that adolescents want to hear from their parents (Kaiser Family Foundation, 1999). Parents are safe from political pressures about what to say or when they say it. In addition, parents can advocate programs that give children and adolescents the messages, skills, and tools for healthy sexuality. Parents can become a "vocal majority," sending messages about the importance of sexual health for adolescents to schools, churches, and policymakers. In summary, parents are potential key agents for changing society's view of how to incorporate issues concerning sexual health into the socialization of adolescents.

Defining the Family

A family is defined less by its structure than its purpose. Thus, a family need not have a set number of members. A family may have a single parent and only one child or may be comprised of two or more parent figures (e.g., grandparents, uncles, aunts) and a large number of children. Families may thus be better defined by purpose than by structure (Becvar & Becvar, 1993). One definition of a family might be "those who provide a caring and nurturing environment that supports the growth and well-being of the members." When a family includes children or adolescents, a primary goal of the family unit should be the fostering of healthy development for these young people.

Family Influences on Female Adolescents' Sexuality

The family is a primary part of adolescents' socialization to sexual values, sex roles, and expected sexual behaviors. Adolescents' sexual health depends to an extent on what is communicated and what is not communicated by parents. Evidence suggests that adolescent females' sexual health may be particularly influenced by their mothers (DiIorio, Kelley, & Hockenberry-Eaton, 1999; Dutra, Miller, &

Forehand, 1999; Miller, Kotchick, Dorsey, Forehand, & Ham, 1998a). For example, a recent study (see Table 1) indicated that mothers were more likely than fathers to communicate with their adolescents about sex-related topics (e.g., STD and AIDS, partner selection, sexual development) and that daughters were more likely than sons to report that they talked with their mother about these topics (Miller *et al.*, 1998a). Moreover, mothers may be a primary source of adolescents' information about sex, an influence rivaled only by that of friends (Reinisch & Beasley, 1990).

Family and maternal influences most likely compete with social influences, particularly peers, to shape adolescents' sexual behavior (Eng & Butler, 1997). Thus, the sexual risk behavior of adolescent females' may be viewed as being shaped by both family (particularly maternal) and social influences.

Social influences on female adolescents' sexuality may be particularly strong. For example, as adolescents mature and naturally pull

TABLE 1. Percentage of Adolescents Who Reported Discussing Sex-Related Topics with Their Mothers, by Gender

Topic	Discussions with mother	
	Daughters % (n = 519)	Sons % (n = 388)
When to start having sex	60	42*
Birth control	57	31*
Condoms	64	68
HIV/AIDS	81	76
Reproduction	71	51*
Physical/sexual development	51	25*
Masturbation	15	15
STDs	74	66*
Pressure to have sex	67	36*
Choosing sex partners	53	48

*Significantly ($p < .01$) more daughters than sons discussed the topic with their mothers.

Note. Miller, K. S., Kotchick, B.S., Dorsey, S., Forehand, R., & Ham, A. Y. (1998). Family communication about sex: What are parents saying and are their adolescents listening? *Family Planning Perspectives*, 30, 220.

away from the influence of their families, peer influences on sexual behavior become more prominent (Forehand & Wierson, 1993). Thus, it is important to optimize the facets of the mother–daughter relationship that may protect the daughter from risky sexual behaviors during her adolescence and as she becomes an adult.

Figure 1 illustrates four possible results of combining maternal and social influences. The crucial question raised by the scenarios presented in Figure 1 is: "What are the specific forms of healthy family and maternal influences on female adolescents' sexuality?" Investigation of this research question has resulted in the

delineation of five factors that may independently or interactively influence female adolescents' sexual behavior (Kirby, 1999; Miller, 1998):

- Parental monitoring
- Parent–adolescent communication
- Mother–daughter relationship satisfaction
- Parental modeling of sexual values
- Family structure

Empirical investigations focusing on each of these factors are described in more detail later in this chapter. Although many of these studies are based on samples of male and female adoles-

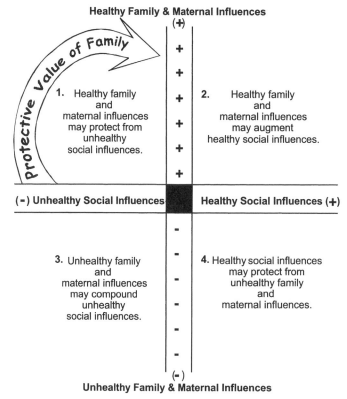

FIGURE 1. Four possible outcomes of interactions between family influences and social influences. Quadrant 1 illustrates the potential protective effect of healthy family and maternal influences from unhealthy peer and social influences. For example, recent research has indicated that healthy maternal influence protects adolescent females against unhealthy peer influences (Whitaker & Miller, 2000). This protective effect is not an issue when social influence is healthy (quadrant 2) and is nonexistent when family and maternal influence are unhealthy (quadrant 3). The figure also posits that healthy social influences may protect against unhealthy family and maternal influences (quadrant 4), but this possibility has not yet been addressed in published research.

cents, we summarize the findings as they relate to female adolescents.

Role of Ethnicity in Family Influences

Researchers have noted that studies have not investigated possible differences among ethnic groups in regard to female adolescents' sexual behavior (Dutra *et al.*, 1999; Kotchick, Dorsey, Miller, & Forehand, 1999). One exception is a study by Miller and colleagues (1998a) that found the number of female adolescents who discussed any one of nine sex-related topics (see Table 1 for a list of these topics) with their mothers did not differ among African-American and Hispanic adolescents. The only difference was in discussion about choosing sex partners: more of the Hispanic daughters reported that they had discussed this topic with their mother. Further research on differences in parenting style among parents of diverse ethnic backgrounds is needed (Forehand & Kotchick, 1996).

THE THEORETICAL BASIS

Studies have done little to increase our understanding of how factors from multiple systems of influence interact or combine with each other to shape the sexual behavior of female

adolescents. In this chapter, we examine the sexual behavior of female adolescents from a multisystem perspective. Such an approach is guided by Bronfenbrenner's (1979) ecological systems theory which emphasizes the reciprocal relations among multiple systems of influence on a person's behavior. According to this perspective, an accurate and comprehensive understanding of female adolescents' sexual and reproductive risk behavior must include some knowledge of the personal and environmental factors that may contribute to the decision to engage in sexual behaviors that put adolescents at greater or lesser risk for adverse health outcomes.

The ecological systems theory posits three systems of influence believed to be primary contributors to the sexual behavior of adolescents: the self, family, and extrafamilial systems (Bronfenbrenner, 1979). Figure 2 expands upon these three systems and illustrates the relative proximity of family influences on adolescent females' decision making about sex and, subsequently, their sexual risk behaviors.

Typically, sexual health interventions for female adolescents have been focused on individual attributes. However, examining the real world of female adolescents involves understanding the competing or perhaps complementary influences of dating partners, peer groups, family, and community. Emerging evi-

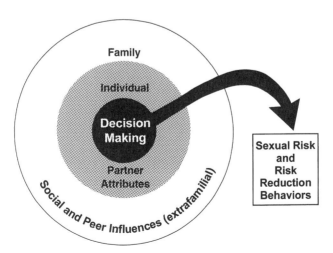

FIGURE 2. Proximity of family and other influences to the sexual risk behaviors of adolescent females.

dence suggests that family influence affects female adolescents' sexual behavior.

RESEARCH FINDINGS

Multiple research findings suggest that family influences are crucial determinants of the sexual behavior of female adolescents. Family influences are a multidimensional construct, comprising heterogeneous psychological and social factors. Factors such as parental monitoring, parent–adolescent communication, satisfaction with the mother–daughter relationship, parental modeling of sexual values, and family structure have been identified as influences on the sexual behavior of female adolescents.

Parental Monitoring

Female adolescents' perceptions of parental monitoring may be more important predictors of sexual risk behavior than parents' reports of parental monitoring. Although there is no uniform definition of parental monitoring, most studies measure at least two important aspects of parental monitoring: (a) adolescents' perceptions of their parents' knowledge of where they go and (b) adolescents' perceptions about parents' knowledge of whom they are with when the adolescent is not at home or in school. Parental monitoring is not the same as parental control of the adolescents' behavior at a psychological level. For example, Rodgers (1999) found that parental control was associated with increased sexual risk behavior of adolescent females, whereas parental monitoring was associated with decreased sexual risk behavior in the same sample.

Studies have documented that females' perceive higher levels of parental monitoring than adolescent males (Romer et al., 1994; Romer, Stanton, Galbraith, Feigelman, Black, & Li, 1999). Thus, the level of parental monitoring may be a particularly important influence on the sexual risk behaviors of female adolescents.

Romer and colleagues (1994) described an intriguing relationship between peer influences and parental monitoring in a sample of young adolescents (less than 15 years of age) in low-income neighborhoods. The number of females who had ever had sex increased with increasing age, particularly among adolescents who perceived that their peers were supportive of sexual activity and among those who perceived low parental monitoring.

In a later study of adolescent females in low-income neighborhoods, high levels of parental monitoring were related to lower odds of initiating sex before 11 years of age (Romer et al., 1999). In addition, continued parental monitoring was associated with a lower likelihood of sexual initiation as female adolescents grew older. This finding suggests that parental monitoring should continue throughout adolescence.

The relationship between parental monitoring and sexual initiation has also been investigated among female adolescents in junior and senior high schools (Small & Luster, 1994). A diverse collection of 13 factors were related to initiating sex (e.g., alcohol use, history of physical abuse, school attachment). Of these, the level of parental monitoring was one of the best discriminators of female adolescents who reported being sexually experienced and those who did not.

In addition to helping delay female adolescents' sexual initiation, parental monitoring has been shown to protect against other behaviors. In one study, parental monitoring was assessed by a questionnaire to female adolescents and their parents (Metzler, Noell, Biglan, Ary, & Smolkowski, 1994). Low parental monitoring was associated with a broad range of adverse sexual outcomes (e.g., STD infection) and risk-taking behaviors (e.g., multiple sex partners, sex with risky partners, and low frequency of condom and contraceptive use). Increased parental monitoring has been associated with fewer sex partners (Luster & Small, 1997) and less frequent intercourse (Benda & DiBlasio, 1994).

Parent–Adolescent Communication

Although at least one study has demonstrated that parent–adolescent communication can increase female adolescents' knowledge about a specific sex-related topic (e.g., AIDS), most studies related to adolescents' sexuality have investigated how such communication influences sexual risk behaviors. Collectively, studies assessing the relationship of parent–adolescent communication about sex and related issues to adolescents' sexual risk behavior have yielded mixed findings (Dittus, Jaccard, & Gordon, 1999; Kirby, 1999; Miller, 1998). However, this kind of communication has often been measured without the necessary attention to the specific content and nature of the communication process (Dittus et al., 1999). Improved measurement and study design have substantially added to the evidence that parent–adolescent communication about sex and sex-related topics has beneficial effects for the adolescent (Dutra et al., 1999).

A large number of studies have shown that the mothers serve as the primary parental agent of communication about sex with their adolescents; this finding seems to be particularly true for daughters (DiIorio et al., 1999; Dutra et al., 1999; Inazu & Fox, 1980; Miller et al., 1998a; Miller, Levin, Whitaker, & Xiaohe, 1998b; Nolin & Peterson, 1992; Noller & Callan, 1990; Whalen, Henker, Hollingshead, & Burgess, 1996; Whitaker, Miller, May, & Levin, 1999). For example, according to a survey of African-American adolescents, males and females preferred talking about sex-related topics with their mothers more than with their peers or with their fathers (DiIorio et al., 1999). Because some evidence has suggested that daughters may benefit more than sons from communication with their parents about sex and sex-related issues (Holtzman & Rubinson, 1995), recent research has focused on specific aspects of mother–daughter communication about sex and sexuality-related issues.

Overall, the evidence clearly suggests that mother–daughter communication can be an important determinant of female adolescents' sexual risk-taking behavior. Female adolescents who talk about sex-related topics with their mothers are (a) less likely to report being sexually experienced (DiIorio et al., 1999; Jaccard, Dittus, & Gordon, 1996; Leland & Barth, 1993), (b) likely to report less frequent penile-vaginal sex (Dutra et al., 1999; Holtzman &

Rubinson, 1995; Jaccard et al., 1996; Miller, Forehand, & Kotchick, in press), (c) more likely to report using condoms and other contraceptives (Dutra et al., 1999; Jaccard et al., 1996; Leland & Barth, 1993; Miller et al., 1998b), (d) less likely to become pregnant (Adolph, Ramos, Linton, & Grimes, 1995), and (e) likely to report fewer lifetime sex partners (Dutra et al., 1999; Holtzman & Rubinson, 1995).

Empirical investigations have suggested at least three reasons for these healthy outcomes. Mother–daughter communication may (a) improve communication between the daughter and her sex partner(s), (b) protect daughters from unhealthy peer influences on sexual behavior, (c) dissuade daughters from sexual initiation because of the mothers expressed disapproval.

Adolescents who talk with their mothers about sex-related topics are more likely to report talking with their dating partners about these topics. This communication increases the adolescents' odds of using a condom during first and later acts of intercourse (Dutra et al., 1999; Shoop & Davidson, 1994; Whitaker et al., 1999). Perceived self-efficacy in using condoms and other methods of preventing STDs and pregnancy has been positively associated with communication between sex partners about these methods (Lawrance, Levy, & Rubinson, 1990) and with implementation of these practices (Basen-Engquist & Parcel, 1992; Cobb, 1997; Rosenthal, Moore, & Flynn, 1991). However, these effects are probably mediated by the quality of the mother–adolescent relationship (Jaccard et al., 1996) and the degree of openness expressed during conversations (Dutra et al., 1999; Whitaker et al., 1999).

Mother–daughter communication may also protect adolescents from negative peer influences. A positive family-level influence may compensate for unhealthy peer influences. For example, in a study of students from schools in three geographically diverse, low-income, urban areas, Whitaker and Miller (2000) found that mother–daughter communication about sex reduced an otherwise strong relationship between self-reported sexual activity (e.g., age of sexual initiation and number of lifetime partners) and adolescents' perceptions of their peers' sexual activity. Thus, female adolescents who communicate with their mothers about sex and sex-related issues were less likely to be influenced by their perceptions that sexual activity is normative for adolescents. Similarly, mother–daughter communication about sex reduced an otherwise strong relationship between perceived norms against condom use and adolescents' reports of condom use.

The degree of a mother's disapproval of her adolescent daughter having sex is another influential aspect of mother–adolescent communication about sex and sex-related issues. For example, expressed maternal disapproval of premarital sex has been related to increased abstinence from sex and decreased frequency of sex among sexually active female adolescents (Jaccard et al., 1996). In an analysis of data from National Longitudinal Study of Adolescent Health (Add Health), female adolescents who reported that their mothers had not expressed disapproval of their having sex were significantly more likely (than those who reported that some degree of maternal disapproval had been expressed) to be infected by a sexually transmitted disease in the ensuing year (Crosby, Leichliter, & Brackbill, 2000).

Dittus and Jaccard (2000) who also analyzed the Add Health data, found that expressed maternal disapproval of the adolescent daughters' having sex decreased the odds that the daughters would have sex in the ensuing year (regardless of virginity status) and decreased the odds that the daughters would become pregnant in the ensuing year. Female adolescents were also more likely than male adolescents to accurately perceive maternal disapproval of the adolescent's having sex. Finally, satisfaction with the relationship with the mother had an equally important influence on the sexual risk behaviors of female adolescents.

Satisfaction with the Mother–Daughter Relationship

In another analysis of the Add Health data, the investigators used a variable they named

parent–family connectedness, defined as closeness to the parents, feeling loved by the family, and satisfaction with the parent–adolescent relationship (Resnick et al., 1997). Increased connectedness was associated with later age at first sexual intercourse. The last component of connectedness (satisfaction) has been used as a predictor variable by other researchers investigating the sexual behavior of female adolescents.

Dittus and Jaccard (2000) found that satisfaction with the mother–daughter relationship longitudinally predicted female adolescents use of contraception. In contrast, contraceptive use was not predicted by adolescents' perceptions of maternal disapproval of sex. Relationship satisfaction was also predictive of pregnancy and of whether the daughters had sex in the ensuing year. Similarly, Bull and Hogue (1998) found that poor mother–daughter relationships were associated with increased likelihood of repeat teen pregnancy in low-income families. These three studies suggest that female adolescents who like their mothers are less likely than their peers who do not like their mothers to report risky sexual behaviors or become pregnant.

Parental Modeling of Sexual Values

Another important factor influencing female adolescents sexual behavior is their perception of their parents' sexual values. The transmission of health-related behaviors from parents to adolescents has been documented in recent studies (Jessor, Turbin, & Costa, 1998; Wickrama, Conger, Wallace, & Elder, 1999). Unfortunately, few studies have investigated the influence of parental modeling of sexual values on adolescents' sexual behaviors (Kotchick et al., 1999). Nonetheless, evidence for the transmission of sexual behaviors—through adolescents' perceptions of maternal sexual values—has been documented in at least three recent studies.

Female adolescents perceptions of their parents' values about teen sex have been associated with whether the adolescents report being sexually experienced. As anticipated, perceiving that parents believe it is wrong for their daughter to have sex significantly predicted which adolescents were sexually inexperienced (Small & Luster, 1994). In a more detailed study in which Dittus and colleagues (1999) surveyed African-American adolescents and their mothers, the sexual values of the daughters tended to correspond to those of their mothers. The values included beliefs that pregnancy would lead to quitting school, sex would lead to a bad reputation and regrets because of not waiting, and having sex would lead a boyfriend to lose respect for the female partner. Maternal beliefs were associated with the daughters' motivations for sexual behaviors, independent of influences related to maternal communication about sex and sex-related issues. In turn, these motivations were associated with the daughters' sexual behaviors. These findings suggest that the sexual behavior of female adolescents is influenced by maternal beliefs and that this influence goes beyond the related influence of mother–daughter communication about sex.

In a related study, the mothers' sexual behaviors were associated with the sexual risk behaviors of their adolescent daughters (Kotchick et al., 1999). However, this association was not significant when the influence of mother–daughter communication about sex was included in the analysis. This finding illustrates the potential for interactive and complementary effects among the family factors that influence female adolescents.

Family Structure

The influence of single-parent versus dual-parent families on female adolescents' sexual risk behavior has been investigated in a limited number of studies, and the findings are conflicting. In a recent study, more of the female adolescents from dual-parent families, compared with those from single-parent families postponed the initiation of sexual intercourse (Lammers, Ireland, Resnick, & Blum, 1999). However, in another recent study, family structure (including parental income and education) was not associated with the sexual risk behavior of

female adolescents. In this same study, maternal monitoring and mother–daughter communication were associated with female adolescents' sexual risk behavior (Miller, Forehand, & Kotchick, 1999).

Other evidence also indicates that female adolescents from single-parent families may be no more likely than those from dual-parent families to engage in risky sexual behavior. Dutra and colleagues (1999) found that fathers were less likely than mothers to communicate with their daughters about sexual behavior. Thus, adolescents in single-parent families, headed by the mother, may experience levels of parent–adolescent communication about sex that are similar to the levels experienced by adolescents in dual-parent families. In a study of single mothers and their adolescent daughters, the levels of family protective influences were remarkably similar to those in other studies that included mother–daughter dyads in dual-parent families (Kotchick et al., 1999). If the single mother has time to spend with her adolescent daughter and if her levels of communication and monitoring are comparable to those of mothers in dual-parent families, no differences would be expected in the influence on daughters' sexual behavior.

LIMITATIONS OF EXISTING RESEARCH

A limitation of much of the research just described is that the data were collected at a single point in time. Thus, associations between family factors and the sexual behaviors of female adolescents are highly suggestive, but it cannot be said that causation has been demonstrated. Reliance on the validity of adolescents' self-reports of their sexual behaviors may lead to erroneous findings. For example, adolescents who perceive high levels of parental monitoring may be less likely to disclose that they have had sex, thus leading to a false relationship between high parental monitoring and later age at sexual initiation. In addition, little is known about the effect of family factors on aspects of female adolescents' sexuality other than sexual behavior. Finally, family influences have rarely been studied in the aggregate or with a great deal of attention to subtleties and nuance, so the full experience of the adolescent is rarely captured. The quality of research on the influences of the mother–daughter relationship on the daughters' sexuality can be improved by

- Using longitudinal study designs when feasible
- Using biological outcomes (e.g., pregnancy and STDs) as study endpoints when feasible
- Investigating the aggregate influence of the family factors—focusing on interactive effects of various sources of influence
- Assessing the effects of family factors on adolescent females' sexuality (e.g., sexual values, comfort levels with sexuality, comfort with a maturing body image) rather than investigating sexual behavior alone
- Increasing the resolution of predictor variables—focusing in greater detail on the family factors that may influence the sexual behavior of female adolescents

Communication Content and Process

Empirical inquiry into mother–daughter communication about sex and sex-related issues has begun to consider the role of communication content (what the communication is about) and process (how the communication occurs). Understanding the content of sex-related communication may be important in more precisely determining the specific influences of this communication on female adolescents' sexual behavior (Dutra et al., 1999). For example, discussing menarche and menstruation may diffuse embarrassment and confusion otherwise associated with early menstrual periods. Entirely different conversations may be required to promote the maturing adolescent's comfort with her sexuality, e.g., her changing body image, her sexual desires (including desires to masturbate), and her eventual decision to initiate sex with a partner.

Several process-related variables may affect the effectiveness of communication about sex. For example, the timing of the communication (Miller et al., 1998b), the breadth of the communication (Miller et al., 1999), parental responsiveness during the communication (Whitaker et al., 1999), and whether the messages are permissive or conservative (Jaccard et al., 1996) have each been related to the sexual behavior of female adolescents. Communication with adolescents may appropriately be viewed as a skill.

Indeed, maternal skill and comfort level in communicating about sex and sex-related issues with their daughters has been found to mediate the relationship between mother–adolescent communication and the adolescents' level of sexual communication with their sex partners (Whitaker et al., 1999). For example, Miller and colleagues (1998a) found that daughters' reports of discussing sex-related topics with their mothers corresponded more closely with the mothers' reports when the communicative process was open and receptive. Thus, the process of communicating is intertwined with the content of the discussion, implying that each plays a critical role in producing healthy outcomes.

Communication Skills

One way to improve communication skills relevant to sex is by first improving communication skills about general, perhaps less threatening, topics. For example, mother–daughter conversations about school or a recent movie may lay the groundwork for more in-depth discussions about love relationships and, perhaps eventually, about sex. In addition, recent evidence suggests that mother–daughter communication about general topics may positively influence adolescents' sexual behavior. Adolescents who engage in open communication with their mothers about general topics seem to have greater confidence in their ability to engage in communication about sex and sex-related issues with their mothers (Shoop & Davidson, 1994). Further, Miller and colleagues (in press) found that female adolescents who reported open communication with their mothers about general topics, compared with adolescents who did not, reported having sex less frequently.

Listening skills are another potentially important aspect of mother–daughter communication about sex that deserves investigation. Although listening is crucial in shared communication, empirical assessment of how careful attention to listening may improve mother–daughter communication about sex has not been conducted. Conceivably, thoughtful and responsive maternal listening may be an important influence on the sexual behavior of female adolescents. A key part of listening is understanding the emotions behind the words being expressed by the adolescent, a skill known as empathetic understanding (Rogers, 1986).

IMPLICATIONS FOR THE DESIGN OF PREVENTION PROGRAMS FOR ADOLESCENT FEMALES

A recent report from the Institute of Medicine recommended that attention to adolescents' sexual health should be a national priority (Eng & Butler, 1997). Thus, prevention programs should seek to promote sexual health rather than simply providing clinical and social services to address the aftermath of unsafe sexual behavior.

The sexual health of female adolescents can be promoted at several intervention points. Indeed, integrated, multiple-level interventions represent an ideal public health response to the high rates of unintended pregnancy and STD/HIV infection among adolescents (DiClemente & Wingood, 2000; Coates, DiClemente, Flay, Kirby, & Sittitrai, in press).

Psychological Intervention Points

Mothers have tremendous potential for influencing their daughters' sexual behavior. A primary guideline for producing a healthy influence on female adolescents' decision making about sex is to continually engage in the protective maternal behaviors (e.g., monitoring, open communication about sex), preferably beginning at a young age (i.e., at least before menarche). These maternal behaviors are amenable to improvement. For example, a brief intervention for parents (mothers and fathers) of low-income African-American adolescents has been shown to significantly improve the levels of parental monitoring (Stanton et al., 2000). Likewise, mothers can improve their communication skills and apply them to sex-related conversations with their daughters.

In addition, intervention programs designed to reduce female adolescents' risk for HIV/STD infection and teen pregnancy may benefit from including the mothers in the programs for their daughters. For example, clinic-based counseling for female adolescents who are receiving health care could include mothers. One goal of these programs, for example, might be to open the lines of communication about sex. Program success might then be indicated by long-term maintenance of this communication by the mother–daughter dyads.

A primary shortcoming of the psychological interventions that target the sexual risk behavior of female adolescents has been the failure to achieve long-term positive effects. Herein lies the strength of using the mother–daughter relationship as an intervention point. A high-quality mother–daughter relationship can become the basis for an ongoing and open dialogue about sex, continued maternal monitoring, and the teaching of maternal sexual values. Given the potential for a long-term, stable mother–daughter relationship, this form of prevention becomes the "intervention that never ends," thus moving beyond the shortcomings typical of other intervention points.

Social Intervention Points

Sociocultural taboos about discussing adolescent sexuality may be a common barrier for women who want to have a healthy influence on their daughters' sexuality. Transcending this barrier can be facilitated at the community level. For example, community and religious organizations can publicly advocate and encourage mothers to build positive relationships with their daughters and subsequently begin talking with them about sex and sex-related issues (e.g., AIDS, abortion, teen pregnancy). These same organizations can provide interventions and support for women who want to expand their own sexual comfort and skill levels in order to communicate more effectively with their daughters about sex. The media can also have a positive influence on women who have adolescent daughters. Media campaigns can motivate women to acquire skills for monitoring their daughters, communicating with them, developing positive relationships with them, and modeling healthy sexual values for them. These skills could be acquired in small-group interventions or workshops.

Public Policy Intervention Points

Community policies that involve parents in the sex education programs offered to children and adolescents in schools may be beneficial. For example, a youth development program that provided training to parents as well as their elementary school-aged children, decreased the odds of risky sexual behavior among these children as they progressed through adolescence (Hawkins, Catalano, Kosterman, Abbott, & Hill, 1999). Favorable outcomes included a lower likelihood of sexual experience, multiple sex partners, and pregnancy.

Policy changes at a much broader level may also be important. For example, women's disadvantages as wage earners may have a profound effect on the ability of single mothers to spend ample time with their adolescent daughters. Spending more time working to make ends meet typically translates into less time spent with the family. Thus, closing the salary gap between men and women may indirectly benefit the adolescent daughters of single mothers. Increased time at home allows the single mother to engage in an ongoing process of influencing her daughter's sexual behavior. Employers can also provide women who work with flexible

work schedules and, if applicable, the opportunity to telecommute. By educating the mothers of adolescent daughters we help move programs that address sexuality to a new level and create a new team of advocates who identify and help implement good programs for our daughters.

CONCLUSIONS

The sexual health of female adolescents can be significantly and positively influenced by their families, especially their mothers. This level of influence goes beyond the influence examined in most studies of adolescent sexual health which tend to focus on intrapersonal factors. Although several forms of positive familial influence have been investigated empirically, all of these forms point to the centrality of a high-quality mother–daughter relationship that nurtures ongoing and open dialogue about sex and that includes continued monitoring and the teaching of maternal sexual values. The positive influences of such a relationship seem to transcend the possible limitations of a single-parent family.

In the broad spectrum of public health, the family plays a pivotal role in protecting female adolescents from unintended pregnancy as well as from the epidemics of STD and HIV infection. Consequently, public health interventions that seek to optimize this pivotal role are more likely to be successful. This is particularly plausible because adolescents' exposure to the intervention (their family) is usually continuous and because the family is in an ideal position to teach values and skills to the female adolescent.

The Centers for Disease Control and Prevention (CDC) is currently developing and testing an intervention designed to promote effective parent–child communication about sexuality in order to promote sexual health among adolescents. Participants will be randomly assigned to participate in one of three interventions: a sexual health intervention, a brief sexual health intervention, and an intervention that focuses on general health promotion. Families will be followed longitudinally and the results from the study will help determine the immediate and long-term benefits of using the family as an intervention point to promote adolescent females' sexual health. The findings from these trials and from similar studies will become vital links in the present national effort to promote the sexual health of our nation's young women.

REFERENCES

Adolph, C., Ramos, D. E., Linton, K. L., & Grimes, D. A. (1995). Pregnancy among Hispanic teenagers: Is good parental communication a deterrent? *Contraception, 51,* 303–306.

Alan Guttmacher Institute. (1993). *Sex and America's teenagers.* New York: Author.

Basen-Engquist, K., & Parcel, G. (1992). Attitudes, norms and self-efficacy: A model of adolescents' HIV-related sexual risk behavior. *Health Education Quarterly, 19,* 263–277.

Becvar, D. S., & Becvar, R. J. (1993). *Family therapy: A systemic integration* (2nd ed.). Boston: Allyn and Bacon.

Benda, B. B., & DiBlasio, F. A. (1994). An integration of theory: Adolescent sexual contacts. *Journal of Youth and Adolescence, 23,* 403–420.

Bronfenbrenner, U. (1979). *The ecology of human development.* Cambridge, MA: Harvard University Press.

Bull, S., & Hogue, C. J. (1998). Exploratory analysis of factors associated with teens' repeated childbearing. *Journal of Health Care for the Poor and Underserved, 9*(1), 42–61.

Calamidas, E. (1992). Reaching youth about AIDS: Challenges confronting health educators. *Health Values, 15,* 55–60.

Coates, T. J., DiClemente, R. J., Flay, B., Kirby, D., & Sittirai, W. (in press). Prevention of sexually transmitted diseases among adolescents.

Cobb, B. K. (1997). Communication types and sexual protective practices of college women. *Public Health Nursing, 14,* 293–301.

Crosby, R. A., Leichliter, J. S., & Brackbill, R. (2000). Longitudinal prediction of STDs among sexually experienced adolescents: Results from a national survey. *American Journal of Preventive Medicine, 18,* 367–372.

Denning, P. F., & Fleming, P. L. (1998). Communities at risk—Estimating the impact of the HIV epidemic upon adolescents and young adults at the local level. Paper presented at the 126th annual meeting of the American Public Health Association.

DiClemente, R. J., & Wingood, G. M. (2000). Expanding the scope of HIV prevention for adolescents: Beyond individual-level interventions. *Journal of Adolescent Health, 26,* 377–378.

DiClemente, R. J., & Houston-Hamilton, A. (1989). Health promotion strategies for prevention of human immunodeficiency virus infection among minority adolescents. *Health Education, 20,* 39–43.

DiIorio, C., Kelley, M., & Hockenberry-Eaton, M. (1999). Communication about sexual issues: Mothers, fathers, and friends. *Journal of Adolescent Health, 24,* 181–189.

Dittus, P. J., & Jaccard, J. (2000). Adolescents' perceptions of maternal disapproval of sex: Relationship to sexual outcomes. *Journal of Adolescent Health, 26,* 268–278.

Dittus, P. J., Jaccard, J., & Gordon, V. V. (1999). Direct and nondirect communication of maternal beliefs to adolescents: Adolescent motivations for premarital sexual activity. *Journal of Applied Social Psychology, 29,* 1927–1963.

Dutra, R., Miller, K. S., & Forehand, R. (1999). The process and content of sexual communication with adolescents in two-parent families: Associations with sexual risk-taking behavior. *AIDS and Behavior, 3,* 59–66.

Eng, T. R., & Butler, W. T. (1997). *The hidden epidemic: Confronting sexually transmitted diseases.* Washington, DC: National Academy Press.

Forehand, R., & Kotchick, B. A. (1996). Cultural diversity: A wake-up call for parent training. *Behavior Therapy, 27,* 187–206.

Forehand, R., & Wierson, M. (1993). The role of developmental factors in planning behavioral interventions for children: Disruptive behavior as an example. *Behavior Therapy, 24,* 117–141.

Hawkins, J. D., Catalano, R. F., Kosterman, R., Abbott, R., & Hill, K. G. (1999). Preventing adolescent health-risk behaviors by strengthening protection during childhood. *Archives of Pediatrics & Adolescent Medicine, 153,* 226–234.

Holtzman, D., & Rubinson, R. (1995). Parent and peer communication effects on AIDS-related behavior among U.S. high school students. *Family Planning Perspectives, 27,* 235–240.

Inazu, J. K., & Fox, G. L. (1980). Maternal influence on sexual behavior of teen-age daughters: Direct and indirect sources. *Journal of Family Issues, 1*(1), 81–102.

Jaccard, J., Dittus, P. J., Gordon, V. V. (1996). Maternal correlates of adolescent sexual and contraceptive behavior. *Family Planning Perspectives, 28,* 159–165, 185.

Jessor, R., Turbin, M. S., & Costa, F. M. (1998). Protective factors in adolescent health behavior. *Journal of Personality and Social Psychology, 75,* 788–800.

Joint United Nations Programme on HIV/AIDS. (1997). Impact of HIV and sexual health education on the sexual behaviour of young people: A review update. Geneva, Switzerland.

Kaiser Family Foundation. (1999). Talking with kids about sex and relationships [on-line]. Available: http://www.talkingwithkids.org/sex.html.

Kirby, D. (1999). *Looking for reasons why: The antecedents of adolescent sexual risk-taking, pregnancy, and childbearing.* Washington, DC: The National Campaign to Prevent Teen Pregnancy.

Kotchick, B. A., Dorsey, S., Miller, K. S., & Forehand, R. (1999). Adolescent sexual risk-taking behavior in single-parent ethnic minority families. *Journal of Family Psychology, 13*, 93–102.

Lammers, C., Ireland, M., Resnick, M., & Blum, R. (1999). Influences on adolescents' decision to postpone onset of sexual intercourse: A survival analysis of virginity among youths aged 13 to 18 years. *Journal of Adolescent Health, 26*, 42–48.

Lawrance, L., Levy, S. R., & Rubinson, L. (1990). Self-efficacy and AIDS prevention for pregnant teens. *Journal of School Health, 60*, 19–24.

Leland, N. L., & Barth, R. P. (1993). Characteristics of adolescents who have attempted to avoid HIV and who have communicated with parents about sex. *Journal of Adolescent Research, 81*(1), 58–76.

Luster, T., & Small, S. A. (1997). Sexual abuse history and number of sex partners among female adolescents. *Family Planning Perspectives, 29*(5), 204–211.

Metzler, C. W., Noell, J., Biglan, A., Ary, D., & Smolkowski, K. (1994). The social context for risky sexual behavior among adolescents. *Journal of Behavioral Medicine, 17*, 419–431.

Miller, B. C. (1998). *Families matter: A research synthesis of family influences on adolescent pregnancy.* Washington, DC: The National Campaign to Prevent Teen Pregnancy.

Miller, K. S., Clark, L. F., Wendall, D. A., Levin, M. L., Gray-Ray, P., Velez, C. N., & Webber, M. P. (1997). Adolescent heterosexual experience: A new typology. *Journal of Adolescent Health, 20*, 179–186.

Miller, K. S., Kotchick, B. A., Dorsey, S., Forehand, R., Ham, A. Y. (1998a). Family communication about sex: What are parents saying and are their adolescents listening? *Family Planning Perspectives, 30*, 218–222, 235.

Miller, K. S., Levin, M. L., Whitaker, D. J., & Xiaohe, X. (1998b). Patterns of condom use among adolescents: The impact of mother–adolescent communication. *American Journal of Public Health, 88*, 1542–1544.

Miller, K. S., Forehand, R., Kotchick, B. A. (1999). Adolescent sexual behavior in two ethnic minority samples: The role of family variables. *Journal of Marriage and the Family, 61*, 85–98.

Miller, K. S., Forehand, R., & Kotchick, B. A. (in press). Adolescent sexual behavior in two ethnic minority samples: A multi-system perspective delineating targets for prevention. *Adolescence.*

National Institutes of Health. (1997). *NIH consensus development conference: Interventions to prevent HIV risk behaviors: Program and abstracts.* Bethesda, MD: Author.

Nolin, J. J., & Petersen, K. K. (1992). Gender differences in parent-child communication about sexuality: An exploratory study. *Journal of Adolescent Research, 7*, 59–79.

Noller, P., & Callan, V. J. (1990). Adolescents' perception of the nature of communication with parents. *Journal of Youth and Adolescents, 19*, 349–362.

Office of National AIDS Policy. (1996). *Youth and HIV/AIDS: An American agenda.* Washington, DC: Author.

Reinisch, J. M., & Beasley, R. (1990). *The Kinsey Institute new report on sex.* New York: St. Martin's Press.

Resnick, M. D., Bearman, P. S., Blum, R. W., Bauman, K. E., Harris, K. M., Jones, J., Tabor, J., Beuhring, T., Sieving, R. E., Shew, M., Ireland, M., Bearinger, L. H., & Udry, J. R. (1997). Protecting adolescents from harm: Findings from the National Longitudinal Study on Adolescent Health. *Journal of the American Medical Association, 278*, 823–832.

Rodgers, K. B. (1999). Parenting processes related to sexual risk-taking behaviors of adolescent males and females. *Journal of Marriage and the Family, 61*(1), 99–109.

Rogers, C. R. (1986). A theory of therapy, personality, and interpersonal relationships, as developed in the client-centered framework. In H. Kirschenbaum & V. L. Henderson (Eds.), *The Carl Rogers reader.* Boston: Houghton Mifflin.

Romer, D., Black, M., Ricardo, I., Feigelman, S., Kaljee, L., Galbraith, J., Nesbit, R., Hornick, R. C., & Stanton, B. (1994). Social influences on the sexual behavior of youth at risk for HIV exposure. *American Journal of Public Health, 84*, 977–985.

Romer, D., Stanton, B., Galbraith, J., Feigelman, S., Black, M. M., & Li, X. (1999). Parental influence on adolescent sexual behavior in high-poverty settings. *Archives of Pediatrics & Adolescent Medicine, 153*, 1055–1062.

Rosenberg, P. S., & Biggar, R. J. (1998). Trends in HIV incidence among young adults in the United States. *Journal of the American Medical Association, 279*, 1894–1899.

Rosenthal, D., Moore, S., & Flynn, I. (1991). Adolescent self-efficacy, self-esteem and sexual risk-taking. *Journal of Community & Applied Social Psychology, 1*, 77–88.

Sex Information and Education Council of the United States (1997). *SIECUS report.* New York: Author.

Shoop, D. M., & Davidson, P. M. (1994). AIDS and adolescents: The relation of parent and partner communication to adolescent condom use. *Journal of Adolescence, 17*, 137–148.

Small, S. A., & Luster, T. (1994). Adolescent sexual activity: An ecological, risk-factor approach. *Journal of Marriage and the Family, 56*, 181–192.

Stanton, B. F., Xiaoming, L. I., Galbraith, J., Cornick, G., Feigelman, S., Kaljee, L., & Zhou, Y. (2000). Parental underestimates of adolescent risk behavior: A randomized, controlled trial of a parental monitoring intervention. *Journal of Adolescent Health, 26*, 18–26.

Whalen, C. K., Henker, B., Hollingshead, J., & Burgess, S. (1996). Parent–adolescent dialogues about AIDS. *Journal of Family Psychology, 10*, 343–357.

Whitaker, D. J., & Miller, K. S. (2000). Parent–adolescent discussions about sex and condoms: Impact on peer influences of sexual risk behavior. *Journal of Adolescent Research, 15*, 251–273.

Whitaker, D. J., Miller, K. S., May, D. C., & Levin, M. L. (1999). Teenage partners' communication about sexual risk and condom use: Importance of parent-teenager discussions. *Family Planning Perspectives, 31*, 117–121.

Whitaker, D. J., Miller, K. S., & Clark, L. F. (in press). Reconceptualizing adolescent sexual behavior: Beyond did they or didn't they? *Family Planning Perspectives*.

Wickrama, K. A. S., Conger, R. D., Wallace, L. E., & Elder, G. H. (1999). The intergenerational transmission of health-risk behaviors: Adolescent lifestyles and gender moderating effects. *Journal of Health and Social Behavior, 40*, 258–272.

Wortley, P. M., & Fleming, P. L. (1997). AIDS in women in the United States: Recent trends. *Journal of the American Medical Association, 278*, 911–916.

Yarber, W. L. (1992). While we stood by ... the limiting of sexual information to our youth. *Journal of Health Education, 23*, 326–335.

Yarber, W. L. (1995). Principles for creating AIDS/sexuality education messages for youth. *Journal of Sex Research, 32*, 269–274.

8

Illicit Drug Use and Women's Sexual and Reproductive Health

KATHERINE P. THEALL, CLAIRE E. STERK,
and KIRK ELIFSON

INTRODUCTION

Historically, the use of drugs among women has been associated with prescription drugs, whereas drug use among men often is linked to the use of illegal substances such as cocaine, heroin, marijuana, and methamphetamine. Illicit drug use among women and the associated negative health consequences has only recently become a serious topic of investigation. Only since the 1960s have studies on the use of illicit drugs among women become common, a change that coincided with the second wave of the feminist movement in the western world. In most early 1960s/1970s studies, female drug users primarily were included as a comparison sample to male users. Consequently, the findings of these studies tended to emphasize differences between men and women, with female users typically being depicted as much more negative than their male counterparts. For example, women were described as weak, unable to con-

trol their drug use, and dependent on male users for the support of their drug habit (Sutter, 1966; Fiddle, 1976; File, 1976).

During the 1970s, much of the substance abuse research among women was based on the emancipation thesis, which assumes that as women become more "liberated," they also are more likely to become involved with criminal activities, including drug use (Adler, 1975). During this same decade, researchers in the drug field began emphasizing a link between drug use and crime (Goldstein, 1979). Whereas no studies confirmed a causal link between drug use and crime, the two phenomena were often presented as closely linked to each other. In addition, women who used drugs, independent of any involvement in other illegal activities, continued to be stigmatized far more than their male drug-using counterparts (Musto, 1973; Johnson *et al.*, 1985).

A criminal activity especially assumed to be connected to female drug use is prostitution (James, 1976; Goldstein, 1979). The drug use–prostitution connection has been used to create a double stigma for female users. They are accused of deviating from mainstream gender role expectations because of their use, as well as their involvement with prostitution.

Since the onset of the crack epidemic, the

KATHERINE P. THEALL, CLAIRE E. STERK, and KIRK ELIFSON • Department of Behavioral Sciences and Health Education, Rollins School of Public Health, Emory University, Atlanta, Georgia 30322.

Handbook of Women's Sexual and Reproductive Health, edited by Wingood and DiClemente. Kluwer Academic / Plenum Publishers, New York, 2002.

dynamics of the women's involvement in drug use and criminal activities further crystallized. This is partly due to the fact that women are more represented among crack cocaine users than among users of other drugs. It is also due to the financial drain caused by the need to support a crack cocaine habit. Compared to women who used other illicit drugs, female crack cocaine users are more likely to be involved in the drug business. The latter includes preparing, packaging, transporting, and, to a lesser extent, selling drugs (Inciardi, Pottieger, & Lockwood, 1993; Fagan, 1994; Sterk, 1999). Also, with the onset of the crack cocaine epidemic, a new form of prostitution emerged. Women began to exchange sex directly for crack cocaine (Inciardi, Pottieger, & Lockwood, 1993; Ratner, 1993; Sterk & Elifson, 1990; Sterk, 2000).

In many U.S. metropolitan areas, the emergence of the crack cocaine epidemic coincided with the beginning of the heterosexual spread of HIV. Prior to the onset of the AIDS epidemic, little attention was given to the health consequences of drug use. Previous concerns tended to be focused on the consequences for the users' families and society at large. Had the AIDS epidemic not occurred, the health consequences to drug users never may have received much attention. After all, observers appear to feel much more comfortable with female drug users as criminals than as patients.

The one health area that received particular attention, even prior to the AIDS epidemic, involved the reproductive health consequences of illicit drug use. The majority of the studies on reproductive health emphasized the negative impact of the women's drug use on the development of the fetus (Chasnoff, 1988; Chavkin, Allen, & Oberman, 1991; Garcia & Mur, 1991). For example, prenatal exposure to cocaine was associated with dysmorphia, growth retardation, and neurological damage (Chasnoff, 1988). Coles (1992) challenged these findings and stressed the potential negative impact of the sociocultural context, e.g., poor nutrition and disorganization in everyday life, on the development of the fetus and child. In much of this research, the focus appears to be on the regula-

tion of the reproductive behaviors of female drug users and on "fetal rights," which assume that a fetus is a person who has rights separate and independent from the pregnant woman carrying the fetus.

In addition to criminalizing women for drug use during pregnancy, they also are challenged in their role as mothers and many are declined the option to show they can be responsible mothers (Rosenbaum, 1981; Taylor, 1993; Kearney, Murphy, & Rosenbaum, 1994; Leib & Sterk-Elifson, 1993; Murphy & Rosenbaum, 1999; Sterk, 1999). Despite society's increasing concern for women drug users, their offspring, and their families, few resources are put aside to assist the women. For example, limited drug treatment options taking the unique needs of women into consideration are available.

In order to provide the reader with insight into some of the main issues surrounding illicit drug use among women, we will address a wide range of topics in this chapter. These include epidemiological, clinical, and ethnographic assessments of drug use, epidemiological profiles of female drug users, including age, race/ethnicity, sexual orientation, and pregnancy, research and theoretical perspectives of female drug use, health outcomes, and issues related to drug treatment. The chapter concludes with remarks and suggestions for future research.

ASSESSMENT AND EPIDEMIOLOGY OF FEMALE DRUG ABUSE

Assessment of Drug Abuse

Epidemiological Data

Drug use is a complex behavior, comprised of factors such as the frequency, quantity, and length of use by type of drug, the route of drug administration, the psychopharmacological effects of various classes of drugs, and the use of multiple drugs simultaneously or sequentially. Drug use patterns and experiences also vary depending on the company and the setting in which the drugs are taken. In addition, drug use is not a static phenomenon; rather it is likely to involve a process of change.

Most of our knowledge regarding drug use is derived from large-scale quantitative studies, frequently involving cross-sectional and longitudinal quasi-experimental designs. The federal government has developed a number of data sets, which provide drug use indicators. The best known are the National Household Survey on Drug Abuse (NHSDA) and the Monitoring the Future (MTF) project (SAMHSA, 1999; Johnston, O'Malley, & Bachman, 1994, 1999). The NHSDA includes cross-sectional data from nationwide multistage probability samples in the United States. Since 1990, the NHSDA is conducted annually; prior to that date, it was conducted less frequently. The NHSDA is the only study that regularly produces estimates of drug use among noninstitutionalized members of the U.S. population (SAMHSA, 1999). Since 1994, NHSDA has incorporated a limited number of measures to assess problems associated with drug use. The MTF involves sequential cohorts of high school students and also is conducted on an annual basis. Both surveys provide data showing drug trends over time.

The general population surveys are supplemented by institutionally based data systems. The Drug Abuse Warning Network (DAWN) is an ongoing retrospective probability survey conducted annually since 1972. It serves as an early warning system of the nation's drug use. Data are collected from a nonrandom sample in selected metropolitan areas throughout the United States. The study is designed to assess emergency department episodes that are induced by or related to the use of drugs (Abadinsky, 1997). It is important to note that the DAWN data reflect episodes and not individuals (Kandel, 1993). In a single episode, more than one drug may be identified, which will be counted as more than one drug "mention." The DAWN data represent only episodes of drug use among individuals admitted to emergency departments, and may therefore present a biased perspective of the prevalence and incidence of drug use.

The other main institutional data system is the Arrestee Drug Abuse Monitoring (ADAM) program, previously called the Drug Use Forecasting (DUF) project. It involves 35 U.S. jurisdictions (National Institute of Justice, 2000). The ADAM data are collected in central police booking facilities in each of the participating jurisdictions and anonymous survey interviews, combined with the collection of a urine sample, are administered to a convenience sample of recent arrestees.

The Treatment Episode Data Set (TEDS) is an ongoing treatment-based monitoring system, which has been in place since 1989. The TEDS presents an aggregate of substance abuse treatment data that are reported through State Substance Abuse Agency systems, from states receiving federal and state alcohol and/or drug funds for the provision of alcohol and/or drug treatment services. TEDS data primarily reflect drug treatment admissions to publicly funded programs, thereby excluding individuals who seek treatment at privately funded programs. TEDS data also fail to account for intrastate variations due to varying health care payment procedures (SAMHSA, 1998b).

Some additional data sets on drug use are the Worldwide Survey of Substance Abuse and Health Behaviors among Military Personnel, the Survey of Inmates in State and Federal Correctional Facilities, and the Uniform Crime Reporting System. The National Narcotics Intelligence Consumers Committee (NNICC) also issues periodic reports on worldwide illicit drug use. Such reports contain estimates of drug productions, trafficking, availability, and consumption (Abadinsky, 1997). In the United States, the Drug Enforcement Agency (DEA) and High Intensity Drug Trafficking Agencies (HIDTAs) frequently compile similar reports.

These epidemiological data systems provide information on the prevalence and incidence of drug use, thereby allowing for the identification of individuals at risk, e.g., by demographic characteristics and geographical distribution. At the same time, prevalence and incidence data have limitations. The first drawback involves undersampling of important subgroups.

For example, the NHSDA does not include individuals who are homeless or who do not have a permanent address. The MTF study provides limited insight into drug use among school dropouts. The institutionally based studies each represent specific subgroups; for example, drug users who seek care at an emergency room, are arrested, or seek drug treatment (Sterk, Hatch, & Dolan, 1999). In other words, the generalizability of the findings is limited. The sampling bias may explain differences in indicators in the data sets. For example, overall drug use appears to be declining in the population-based surveys; however, morbidity and mortality are increasing among institutional samples.

A second limitation involves the data collection strategies. Whereas the institutional studies include biomedical markers for drug use, the population studies are based on self-reported data. Drug use is an illegal behavior and the responses provided may be subject to reporting bias (Ball, 1967). In addition, the reporting bias is not randomly distributed across the total study population (Mensch & Kandel, 1988).

In addition, the terminology and the time frames used in survey questions should be considered. Respondents might define "average use over the last 30 days" in various ways, raising validity concerns. In addition, the reference point of the last 30 days may not be meaningful to drug users. Also, as is often the case with retrospective responses, the response is likely to be based on self-knowledge and behavioral episodes which provides an answer based on subjective judgment as opposed to the requested ordinal response. The likelihood of incorrect responses increases if the data are self-administered as in the NHSDA and Monitoring the Future project. Respondents may also report never having used a certain drug to skip a lengthy section in the questionnaire (Turner, Lessler, & Gfroerer, 1992).

Clinical Assessments

The main clinical assessment of drug use is derived from the DSM-IV, in which a distinc-tion is made between use, abuse, and dependence using the Substance Abuse Module (SAM). Use typically involves taking at least one (illicit) drug, while abuse includes symptoms such as recurrent use in situations where it presents a physical danger, failure to meet obligations at work, substance-abuse-related legal problems, or recurrent social or interpersonal problems caused by the effects of the drug. Dependence includes physical symptoms such as tolerance or withdrawal, taking larger amounts of drugs or use over a longer period of time than intended, or spending increasing amounts of time seeking, obtaining, and recovering from the effects of drugs. The SAM allows for assessment of patterns of lifetime and current use, abuse, and dependence symptoms.

Ethnographic Studies

Ethnographic research strategies have been used successfully among drug users. The main goal of ethnographic researchers is to study people in their natural setting and to gain an in-depth understanding of everyday phenomena from the subjects' perspective. Qualitative research focuses on the social construction of reality. The main data collection strategies in qualitatively designed studies are participant observation, in-depth interviewing, focus groups or a combination of these (see, for example, Denzin & Lincoln, 1993). Ethnographic studies have provided insight into various aspects of the lives of drug users. These studies have contributed to our understanding of the lives of users, the various social roles and associated behaviors, and the language used among drug users (Preble & Casey, 1969; Agar, 1973; Bourgeois, 1989; Stephens, 1991). Other studies emphasize the unique features of drug-using careers (Faupel, 1991; Waldorf, Reinarman, & Murphy, 1991; Sterk, 1999, 2000). Some researchers focused on the impact of drug use on women's lives (Murphy & Rosenbaum, 1999; Rosenbaum, 1981; Sterk, 1999; Taylor, 1993). Women's drug use also has been studied in the context of their involvement in prostitution (Goldstein, 1979; Williams, 1989; Sterk, 2000) and in the underground economy (Hamid,

1991), including drug sales (Adler, 1985; Inciardi & Pottieyer, 1986). These studies provide us with an insider's perspective on drug use, address the tensions between what people say and what people do, and stress that drug use cannot be viewed as a static social phenomenon.

Linking Sources of Information

Because most epidemiological sources of information include men and women, examining patterns of drug abuse explicitly among women is complex. Quantitative data obtained from institutional systems and survey data disclose information on the distribution of drug use among populations and the population at risk for problems of substance abuse, but they offer little information about the details of drug use patterns, settings of use, and polydrug use (Kandel, 1993).

Frequently, little distinction is made between drug use, abuse and dependence. With the exception of the Epidemiologic Catchment Area study (ECA) (Robins & Regier, 1991), the simultaneous assessment of drug use patterns and drug use disorders has only recently been included in one of the larger population surveys on drug use (NHSDA). Furthermore, some indicators may distort the gender distribution among drug users (Sterk, Dolan, & Hatch, 1999).

Although all sources of quantitative data have provided invaluable information on drug using behavior, data obtained from a single source can be greatly enhanced when supplemented with additional quantitative and qualitative data. The National Institute on Drug Abuse (NIDA) Community Epidemiology Working Group (CEWG) is a surveillance network of U.S. and international researchers who meet semiannually to monitor drug use trends. CEWG combines epidemiological indicators and ethnographic information to assess national and international drug abuse trends, a combination of data sources essential to a reliable and valid assessment of drug use. The inherent limitations to drug use data, coupled with the characteristics of many female drug-using populations, suggest that multiple methodologies on multiple levels (e.g., large and small scale) would be the most effective approach to assessing drug use among women.

Current Epidemiology of Drug Use/Abuse

To provide a summary of female drug use, we present data from the most commonly used sources of drug use information in the United States. Illustrative data are presented in Tables 1 and 2 for the most recently released findings from the 1998 NHSDA. In that year, the annual prevalence rate of any drug use for women was 8.2% as compared to 13.1% among men. Data for past month use show a prevalence rate among women of 4.5 as compared to 8.1 among men (SAMHSA, 1999).

The rates of reported drug use remain higher among men than women, but the gender gap narrows when comparisons are made for the use of legal drugs. For example, the annual prevalence rate for alcohol is 60.0% for women and 68.3% among men; for tobacco, the rate is 28.4 among women and 32.8 among men. Rates of past year heroin use and past month crack cocaine use were equivalent among men and women. Gender differences also vary geographically. For example, the rate of current crack use is equivalent for males and females in the western region of the United States.

Indicators from institutional data systems show a similar gender distribution. According to SAMHSA's Treatment Episode Data Set, males continue to dominate treatment admissions (SAMHSA, 1998b). In the 1998 NHSDA, however, slightly more female than male past year users of an illicit drug reported having received treatment or counseling for alcohol or drug use (SAMHSA, 1999). Data from the Drug Abuse Warning Network (DAWN) for 1998 indicate a rate of 206 per 100,000 population for total drug-related emergency department episodes among women compared to 242 per 100,000 population for men. The ratio of male to female drug abuse deaths according to DAWN 1998 Annual Medical Examiner Data was nearly 3 to 1; 26% of drug abuse deaths in 1998 were among women, with the greatest proportion among women aged 26 to 54 years. According to the National Comorbidity Survey

TABLE 1. Annual Prevalence Rates of the Use of Selected Drugs in 1998 in the General Population, by Age and Sex

| | Percent using in past year | | | | | | | | | |
| | Age 12–17 | | Age 18–25 | | Age 26–34 | | Age 34+ | | Total | |
Substance	M	F	M	F	M	F	M	F	M	F
Alcohol	31.0	32.7	79.3	68.9	77.7	71.5	70.2	59.7	68.3	60.0
Cigarettes	23.6	23.9	50.3	43.9	39.9	33.3	28.6	24.9	32.8	28.4
Marijuana	14.4	13.7	28.1	20.0	13.0	6.5	5.6	2.7	10.8	6.5
Cocaine	1.3	2.0	5.9	3.4	3.6	1.9	1.3	0.5	2.3	1.2
Crack	0.3	0.6	1.0	0.5	0.7	0.7	0.5	0.2	0.6	0.3
Heroin[a]									0.1	0.1
Stimulants	1.0	1.3	2.3	1.4	0.7	0.5	0.6	0.2	0.9	0.5
Hallucinogens	4.0	3.6	8.8	5.6	1.5	0.8	0.2	0.2	2.0	1.3
Inhalants	2.8	3.0	4.6	1.8	0.6	0.4	0.4	[b]	1.3	0.6
Tranquilizer	1.1	1.0	3.4	2.0	1.2	0.9	0.6	0.3	1.1	0.7
Sedative	0.4	0.7	0.7	0.3	0.1	0.1	0.3	0.1	0.3	0.2
Analgesic	3.0	3.1	5.9	2.9	2.4	1.5	1.2	1.0	2.3	1.5
Any psychotherapeutic	3.4	4.0	8.3	4.4	3.6	2.6	1.9	1.3	3.2	2.1
Any illicit drug	16.7	16.0	32.6	22.1	16.2	9.3	7.2	4.0	13.1	8.2
Total (*N*)	6778		7318		4537		6867		25,500	

Source. Office of Applied Studies, Substance Abuse and Mental Health Administration (SAMHSA), National Household Survey on Drug Abuse, 1998.
[a]Only total reported past year use separated by gender.
[b]Low precision; no estimate reported.

TABLE 2. Current (Past Month) Prevalence Rates of the Use of Selected Drugs in 1998 in the General Population, by Age and Sex

| | Percent using in past year | | | | | | | | | |
| | Age 12–17 | | Age 18–25 | | Age 26–34 | | Age 34+ | | Total | |
Substance	M	F	M	F	M	F	M	F	M	F
Alcohol	19.4	18.7	68.2	51.7	67.7	54.2	61.4	45.8	58.7	45.1
Cigarettes	18.7	17.7	45.3	37.8	34.6	30.5	26.9	23.4	29.7	25.7
Marijuana	8.6	7.8	17.2	10.3	8.1	2.9	3.5	1.7	6.7	3.5
Cocaine	0.6	1.0	2.6	1.3	1.4	0.9	0.7	0.2	1.1	0.5
Crack	0.2	0.3	0.4	0.3	0.3	0.3	0.2	0.1	0.2	0.2
Stimulants	0.6	0.6	0.7	0.5	0.3	0.1	0.3	0.1	0.4	0.2
Hallucinogens	2.1	1.6	3.1	2.2	0.7	0.2	0.1	0.2	0.8	0.6
Inhalants	1.0	1.2	1.9	0.3	0.2	[a]	0.1	[a]	0.5	0.2
Tranquilizer	0.2	0.3	1.4	0.6	0.6	0.5	0.1	0.1	0.4	0.2
Sedative	0.1	0.3	0.3	0.1	0.1	[a]	0.1	[a]	0.1	0.1
Analgesic	1.3	1.4	2.4	1.1	0.9	0.8	0.5	0.4	0.9	0.6
Any psychotherapeutic	1.6	1.7	3.6	1.7	1.4	1.2	0.9	0.5	1.4	0.9
Any illicit drug	10.3	9.5	20.5	11.7	9.8	4.3	4.4	2.4	8.1	4.5
Total (*N*)	6778		7318		4537		6867		25,500	

Source. Office of Applied Studies, Substance Abuse and Mental Health Administration (SAMHSA), National Household Survey on Drug Abuse, 1998.
[a]Low precision; no estimate reported.

(NCS), 6% of all women ages 15 to 54 met the criteria for lifetime drug *dependence* (Warner, Kessler, Hughes, Anthony, & Nelson, 1995).

Epidemiologic Profiles of Drug Abuse

Substance abuse affects women of all ages and ethnic backgrounds and those who believe it only affects people of certain racial/ethnic backgrounds or socioeconomic status are proven wrong. Unfortunately, the data to explore racial/ethnic or age comparisons specifically among women who use drugs are scarce.

In the United States, the prevalence of drug use is customarily assessed for Hispanics, non-Hispanic Blacks or African-Americans, and non-Hispanic Whites. Hence, more specific data on ethnicity of other racial groups are generally unavailable. Moreover, the limited sample size of women in most surveys makes it difficult to compare drug use patterns in racial and ethnic subgroups while statistically controlling for important factors such as education, employment and income. Researchers often combine data from multiple population surveys in order to investigate racial/ethnic, gender, and age differences.

Age Differences

The most recent NHSDA recorded the highest past year and past month, or current use for any illicit drug among women between 12 and 25 years old, with the highest rates among those between the ages of 18 and 25 years (Tables 1 and 2). Marijuana remains the most commonly reported illicit drug among women of all ages. The highest, though still very low, rates of women reporting injection drug use were in the 26 to 34 and the 35 and overage brackets (data not shown).

According to the National Comorbidity Survey, 12-month dependence among females in the total sample and among lifetime users was highest among women aged 15 to 24. Lifetime dependence rates were highest among women between 45 and 54 years of age; and

among 12-month users, highest for 35- to 44-year-old women (Warner *et al.*, 1995).

According to the NHSDA, the rate of persons between the ages of 18 and 25 who report current, past month use of any illicit drug has been increasing slightly since 1993 (SAMHSA, 1999). The 1998 percentage rate for young adult women in this age category was 11.7, as compared to 9.6 in 1997. While overall rates of current illicit drug use were lower for women than men, gender differences in the rates of drug use among adolescent users were less pronounced (10.3 for males versus 9.5 for females).

Albeit most surveys indicate a decline in drug use with increasing age, data from various sources continue to reflect the aging of the drug-using population. Age-related maturational patterns are more likely to influence age-specific rates of drug use than lifetime rates (Clayton, Voss, Robbins, & Skinner, 1986; Kandel, 1993). In the most recent NHSDA report, data from 1979 to 1998 are compared for the most commonly used substances. The aging cohort of users is reflected in the 35 and older age category, which has increased from 10% to 32% for any illicit drug use since 1979 (SAMHSA, 1999).

Rates of initiation of marijuana and heroin use among youths are noted to be at historically high levels (Johnston *et al.*, 1999; SAMHSA, 1999). Kandel and colleagues examined National Household survey data from the years 1991, 1992, and 1993. They reported rates of cocaine dependence to be significantly higher among women than men, and that female adolescents were significantly more at risk for becoming dependent on alcohol and marijuana than were women in any other age group (Kandel, Chen, Warner, Kessler, & Grant, 1997). Among adults, rates of nicotine dependence were higher among females, while males were more likely to be dependent on alcohol and marijuana (data not shown).

According to the 1998 NHSDA, drug use rates among adolescent users varied by drug. Rates of current cocaine, crack, and inhalant drug use were slightly higher among young (age 12–17) women than young men. Among adults, rates were consistently higher among men, with the exception of crack use. Annual (past year) and current rates of crack use are equivalent for men and women age 26 to 34.

When considering examining age-related patterns of drug use, it is important to examine the use of licit and illicit substances in terms of their "socially" accepted nature. For example, since the 1960s, marijuana use has gained wide acceptance. In addition, drug experimentation among young adults has recently become somewhat more acceptable.

Finally, "designer" drugs tend to be more accepted than hard drugs such as heroin and cocaine. Recent examples include drugs such as MDMA, ecstasy (3,4-methylenedioxymethamphetamine), or gamma-hydroxybutyrate (GHB). Ethnographic trends suggest that use of these substances is most popular among young adults and that the common perception is that these drugs are not addictive and cause little or no harm.

Racial or Ethnic Differences

According to the 1998 NHSDA, the majority of women who are current illicit drug users are white non-Hispanics (3,796,000 white non-Hispanic women; 499,000 Hispanic women; 704,000 black non-Hispanic women). Yet the rate of current illicit drug use for African-American females (5.2% of the African-American population) remains higher than for white (4.5% of the white non-Hispanic population) and Hispanic females (4.5% of the Hispanic population). Among youth, however, rates of use are roughly comparable for these three ethnic groups (SAMHSA, 1999). The National Comorbidity Survey reported similar findings with regard to lifetime use: Whites were significantly more likely than non-Whites to use drugs at some time in their lives (Warner *et al.*, 1995).

Nonetheless, ethnic differences should be examined according to the specific drug of use. The rate of current psychotherapeutic use of prescription drugs, for example, is highest

among Hispanic women (1.1%) as compared to White or African-American women (0.9% for both groups). On the other hand, the rate of current crack use is highest among African-American women (0.4%) than White (0.1%) or Hispanic (0.2%) women (SAMHSA, 1999).

It had been previously reported that African-American women are more likely to report lower lifetime experience with cocaine than women of other racial/ethnic backgrounds. In addition, African-American and Hispanic women have shown to be more likely to report lower rates of legal drug and marijuana use than White women (Kandel, 1993).

The Office of Applied Statistics examined substance use among racial and ethnic subgroups (SAMHSA, 1998). Groups were defined as Native Americans, Asian/Pacific Islanders, non-Hispanic Blacks, non-Hispanic Whites, and seven groups of Hispanics (Caribbeans, Central Americans, Cubans, Mexicans, Puerto Ricans, South Americans, and other Hispanics). Relative to the total U.S. household population aged 12 and over, Native Americans, Mexicans, Puerto Ricans, and non-Hispanic Blacks had the highest prevalence of illicit drug use as well as heavy cigarette use, alcohol dependence, and the need for illicit drug abuse treatment.

The highest rates of any illicit drug use in the past year were among Native Americans (19.8%); followed by Hispanic Puerto Ricans (13.3%), and non-Hispanic Blacks or African-Americans (13.1%). Hispanic Mexicans (12.7%) and non-Hispanic Whites (11.8%) followed closely behind. Differences between males and females were reported to be generally similar across all racial/ethnic subgroups, with males in each subgroup more likely than females in the same subgroup to use substances, to be dependent on alcohol, and to require treatment for illicit drug abuse (SAMHSA, 1998).

Sexual Orientation

Very few large-scale surveys of drug abuse differentiate among women of different sexual orientations. Nonetheless, evidence of increased prevalence of substance abuse among women reporting same sex contact has been reported (Ryan & Bradford, 1988; McKirnan & Peterson, 1989; Young, Weissman, & Cohen, 1992). Findings from the Epidemiological Study of Health Risk in Lesbians (ESTHER) revealed that for past year substance use, over 25% reported daily cigarette use; nearly 35% weekly or daily alcohol use; approximately 20% reported any marijuana use; 3% reported any cocaine use; and 5% injection drug use in the past year. There were no differences in substance use among lesbians compared to bisexual women. In addition, increasing age was associated with decreased marijuana or cocaine use, and Whites were less likely to use cocaine than African-Americans (Aaron, Markovic, & Danielson, 1999).

Among a group of lesbian/bisexual female youths, Rosario and colleagues (1995) found that 67% reported a history of drug use. Lifetime frequency of substance use suggested more than experimental use and 20% to 41% of the youths sampled endorsed every symptom of abuse.

Cocaine or stimulant use appears to be prevalent among women who self-identify as lesbian or bisexual. According to the National Lesbian Health Care Survey (Ryan & Bradford, 1988), 20% of the respondents reported lifetime use of cocaine. Similarly, stimulant use was shown to be popular (46%) among self-identified lesbians in Kentucky (Skinner, 1994). In a study among predominately bisexual women in New York City, Bevier and colleagues found that women reporting same sex contact were more likely than exclusively heterosexual women to use crack cocaine (37% versus 15%; odds ratio (OR) = 3.3) and to inject drugs (31% versus 7%; OR = 6.3) (Bevier, Chiasson, Hefferman, & Castro, 1995).

Pregnant Women

Approximately half of the women who use illicit drugs are of childbearing age (SAMHSA, 1999), which often has been used as a justification to consider drug use during pregnancy. The NIDA National Pregnancy & Health Survey, conducted in 1992 and published in 1996, provided estimates of licit and illicit substance use during pregnancy by women who gave birth in 1992. The survey indicates that five percent of the approximately 4 million women who gave birth in 1992 used some illicit drug while pregnant. Marijuana and cocaine were the most frequently reported illicit drugs used, with rates of marijuana highest among those under 25 and rates of cocaine higher among those 25 and older. The prevalence of alcohol and cigarette use also was high, and the survey revealed a strong link between cigarette smoking and alcohol use and the use of illicit drugs. Similar to recent NHSDA findings, African-Americans reported the highest usage of any illicit drug (11.3%), followed by Hispanics (4.5%) and Whites (4.4%). On the other hand, the percentage of Whites that used alcohol or cigarettes during pregnancy was higher than the percentage of African-Americans or Hispanics. In terms of the absolute numbers of users in general, most women who used drugs during pregnancy were white (NIDA, 1996).

Recently, Comerford and colleagues (1998) examined drug use among pregnant injection users. The majority (94.4%) had been pregnant at least once, and many had used illicit drugs either alone or in combination with alcohol during any pregnancy (77.4% of African-Americans and 82.5% of whites). In addition, the majority of the women reported using more than one drug. Racial differences were found in terms of the number of live births and therapeutic abortions, with White women having significantly more therapeutic abortions and African-American women having more live births. Zambrana and colleagues (1997) examined the use of alcohol, cigarettes, and illicit drugs before and after pregnancy in a sample of pregnant African-American, Mexican-American, and Mexican immigrant women. Results indicated that African-American women were more likely than women of Mexican origin, and Mexican-American women were more likely than Mexican immigrant women, to report substance use before and during pregnancy.

Although drug use during pregnancy remains a problem in the United States, there is evidence that use among pregnant women remains lower than their counterparts who are not pregnant. In the most recent National Household Survey on Drug Abuse, drug use among pregnant women aged 15 to 44 was compared to women who were not pregnant. Regardless of age, race or ethnicity, marital status, or educational attainment, pregnant women were less likely than nonpregnant women to report illicit drug use or "binge" alcohol use in the past month (SAMHSA, 1999). Higher rates of illicit drug use among younger and unmarried women who were not pregnant were also observed (SAMHSA, 1999). Pregnant African-American women were significantly more likely than their white counterparts to be past month illicit drug users. In comparison, rates of past month illicit drug use did not differ significantly between African-American and White women who were not pregnant (SAMHSA, 1999).

DRUG USE AND ITS IMPACT ON SEXUAL BEHAVIORS

Theoretical Frameworks

A number of psychological and sociological theories have been applied to the study of drug use. Psychological theories—such as psychoanalytic theory, behaviorism/learning theory (cognitive learning in particular)—and sociological theories—such as the stages of drug addiction, anomie, differential association, social control theory, subcultures/cultural deviance theory, and symbolic interactionism (i.e., labeling)—have all been utilized for explanatory models of drug abuse (Abadinsky, 1997). Social theories such as social control theory and cultural deviance theory, as well as gender and social role theories have been used in examining the initiation and persistence of drug use (Kandel & Davies, 1991) and the drug–sex connection (Lucke, 1998; Jadack, Hyde, & Keller, 1995). The use of social-causation theory when examining the association between substance abuse and sociodemographic factors has also been suggested (Dohrenwend *et al.*, 1992).

More recently, our knowledge of drug use has expanded through research on drug-use-related HIV risk behaviors. Theories such as social cognitive or social learning theory (Bandura, 1977; Botvin *et al.*, 1984), the health belief model (Becker & Joseph, 1988), the transtheoretical model of behavior change (Prochaska & DiClemente, 1983), the theory of reasoned action (Fishbein, 1980; Fishbein & Ajzen, 1975), and the empowerment theory (Rappaport, 1981, 1984) have all been applied.

In addition to the above-mentioned theories, several themes have historically been employed in studying women's sexuality as it relates to drug use. Examples of such themes are the introduction or initiation into drug use among women and women's motivations for drug use.

Initiation into Drug Use and Continued Use

Early initiation of drug use has been identified as a strong predictor of later drug abuse (Westherington & Roman, 1998) and women may proceed more rapidly to drug dependence (Hser, Anglin, & McGlothin, 1987). Curiosity and peer acceptance lead many women to experiment with drugs and it is not uncommon for a woman to use her first illicit drug together with a girlfriend or a group of friends. Typically, this requires that at least one of them has access to drugs through a dealer or friend. It is more common, however, for women to be introduced to drugs by a boyfriend or significant other or by a male sex partner (Rosenbaum, 1981; Sterk, 1999). These men already are drug users. Some of them will voluntarily introduce a woman to drugs, while others will not facilitate their girlfriend's use of drugs. Once the female partner has been introduced to drugs, her habit becomes dependent on his access to drugs. Hence, it is not uncommon for women to lose their connection with the drug world once the relationship with the drug-providing male partner fails. Some women will actively seek another male partner who can provide access, while others will develop their own drug connections.

Some women will cease using drugs at this point, while others will continue. The literature on risk and protective factors for continued use is mixed, but those individuals who liked their first high, who have access to drugs, and whose social network supports drugs are most likely to continue using. Subsequent use often is divided in a number of stages, including occasional use, experimental use, continued regular use, maintenance, abuse and dependence. The transition from each stage of use to another has its own unique risk and protective factors (Sterk, 2000). This developmental progression of drug use also leaves room for women who may temporarily stop using and subsequently relapse or who may give up one drug habit, only to substitute another.

After an initial introduction to a drug(s), sustained usage is indicative of traditional sex role differentiation (Rosenbaum, 1981; Sterk, 1999). Drug-promoting relationships can have a profound impact on women's sexuality. Drug use coupled with interactional incompetence in sexual relationships (e.g., not being able to clearly communicate intentions and sexual assertiveness) places many women at risk for sexually transmitted diseases, criminal activities, and sexual victimization (Rosenbaum, 1981; Kane, 1991; Amaro, 1995; Sterk, 1999).

Categories of Drugs

The medical consequences of drug use also depend on the type of drug used. The major drugs can be classified into five categories, according to their effect on the central nervous system (Abadinsky, 1997): (1) depressants, (2) stimulants, (3) hallucinogens, (4) cannabis, and (5) inhalants. Each "type" induces a specific effect in the user, resulting in different acute and chronic medical consequences. Depressants are drugs that depress the central nervous system and reduce pain, and can cause physical and psychological dependence (i.e., withdrawal and craving). Heroin is one of the most frequently used illicit drugs in this category, and is reported to contribute to most overdose deaths in developed countries (Donoghoe et al., 1998).

Heroin has analgesic as well as euphoric properties. Heroin use can depress the respiratory centers in the brain, resulting in respiratory arrest and death if an overdose occurs (Abadinsky, 1997). Other acute effects of opiates include sedation, emotional blunting, dream states, nausea, vomiting, spasms of the ureter and bile duct, impaired thermoregulation, and suppression of sex hormones. Chronic effects include disorders of the hypothalamic and pituitary hormone secretion, constipation, withdrawal cramps, diarrhea, vomiting, and rhinorrhea (Goldstein & Kalant, 1993).

Stimulants include cocaine, amphetamines, methamphetamine, and ecstasy (MDMA, 3,4-methylenedioxymethamphetamine) as well as the more common licit drugs—caffeine and nicotine. These drugs elevate mood by stimulating the central nervous system and have a high potential for abuse and dependence (Abadinsky, 1997). Use of cocaine and amphetamines can result in increased paranoia and aggression, as well as hypertension, cardiac arrhythmia, hyperthermia, and anorexia. Additional chronic effects include paresthesias, stereotypy, seizures, withdrawal depression, chronic rhinitis, and perforation of the nasal septum.

The most common chemically produced hallucinogens include LSD (lysergic acid diethylamide) and PCP (phencyclidine); mescaline, found in the peyote cactus, is a common organic hallucinogen. The increasingly popular drug Ketamine ("K" or "Special K") also falls in this category, and its effects are similar to PCP but with less confusion, irrationality, and violence. Such drugs affect the central nervous system by altering perceptual functions (Abadinsky, 1997). Acute toxicity is often displayed through visual and auditory illusions, hallucinations, and depersonalization (i.e., sympathetic overactivity). Although the risk of addiction has been shown to be quite minimal, chronic effects such as flashbacks, depression, or prolonged psychotic episodes can occur (Goldstein & Kalant, 1993).

Cannabis is most often used in the form of marijuana, and can exhibit characteristics of hallucinogens, depressants, and even stimulants.

Cannabis produces euphoria and relaxation, perceptual and time distortions, and intensifies ordinary sensory experiences (Abadinsky, 1997). Psychomotor impairment is an acute effect of cannabis use. Apathy and mental slowing, impaired memory and learning, and an impaired immune response may occur as a result of long-term use (Goldstein & Kalant, 1993).

Although they are not usually produced with the intention of being applied as a drug, inhalants have been a popular drug of abuse among adolescents (Crider & Rouse, 1988). Inhalants are a diverse group of commonly available chemicals such as glue, paint thinner, hair spray, and nail polish remover. The short-term "high" produced by the rapid adsorption of inhalants into the bloodstream, may be accompanied by sedation, hallucinations, and delusions. Chronic use can result in damage to the brain, liver, and kidneys (Abadinsky, 1997).

Gender differences in the biological effect of many drugs of abuse is likely to significantly influence not only the medical consequences of drug use for women, but also the risk of addiction or dependence as well as drug preference (Levin, Holman, & Mendelson, 1998; Lukas *et al.*, 1996). Women's consumption patterns and absorption rates have been shown to be more variable than men's, and are affected by hormone levels that fluctuate across the menstrual cycle or during pregnancy (Lex, 1991).

Motivations for Drug Use (Sexual Arousal or Enhancement and Self-Medication)

Although the "positive" effects of drugs use (e.g., mood elevation, high, rush, and euphoria) remain motivations for drug use for many women, there are also more specific reasons for using drugs. Researchers have found enhanced sexual experience as a reason for drug use among women (Schafer & Brown, 1991; Wells *et al.*, 1993; Gorman *et al.*, 1999; Taylor, Fulop, & Green, 1999). Taylor and colleagues (1999) examined the link between drug or alcohol use and the occurrence of sexual encounters and specific sexual activities, as well as the deliberate use of drugs or alcohol to affect sex. They found that drugs and alcohol might be used in moderation to deliberately affect sex. Wells and colleagues found that 28% of the women in their study reported occasionally using drugs to enhance sexual behavior or pleasure.

Motivations for drug use, particularly the expected experience or effect, depend on the type of drug one considers using. Certain drugs such as marijuana, ecstasy, amphetamines or cocaine are often seen as sexually enhancing, and may in fact enhance sexual drive or performance when taken in low doses (Abadinsky, 1997). Drugs such as heroin or other opiates have been shown to decrease the desire or pleasure of sex. In examining drug effect expectancies, Schafer and Brown (1991) found relaxation and tension reduction common expectancies of both marijuana and cocaine use, while social and sexual facilitation and generalized arousal were expectancies of marijuana and cocaine, respectively. Flunitrazepam (Rohypnol), as well as other benzodiazepines such as Valium and Xanax, are reportedly used to prolong the effects of alcohol (Calhoun, Wesson, Galloway, & Smith, 1996). Physical and/or sexual arousal has been cited as a primary reason for ecstasy, or MDMA, use (Milkman, & Sunderwirth, 1987; Collin, 1998).

Differences in sexual expectations, arousal or enjoyment may vary according to the duration of drug use as well as the setting of use (Zinberg, 1984). The innocuousness of many illicit substances is a product not only of the pharmacological properties of these substances and the biological or genetic makeup of the individual but also of the cultural context and situations within which they are employed. Social context and the user's expectations can influence a drug's effect (Becker & Joseph, 1988), and is particularly important for first-time or experimental users, regardless of the drug's toxic effect. Context plays a very significant role in the motivation or reasons for drug use among adolescents (Newcomb & Bentler, 1986).

Whether a female user is an adolescent experiencing the pressures that life can bring about at that age, or a woman dealing with current or past physical or psychic trauma, a primary reason for drug use may be to relieve the pressures associated with adverse or uncomfortable life situations. The theory of "self-medication" as a reason for drug use has been proposed by a number of researchers. Gold (1980) proposed that drugs are used in order to increase feelings of power over conflict and to reduce feelings of anxiety. Newcomb and Bentler (1986) proposed the same "self-medication" hypothesis for adolescents dealing with life changes and stressors at that age. Women who have experienced abuse may use drugs to self-medicate.

Frequently, women who use drugs have a history of childhood abuse (Bourgois & Dunlap, 1993; Boyle & Anglin, 1993; Nyamathi et al., 1999; Sterk, 1999). The psychological consequences of sexual victimization (Briere & Runtz, 1993; Zweig, Barber, & Eccles, 1997) may also manifest into the abuse or dependence on alcohol or drugs. For women who have experienced sexual or physical abuse, drug use can serve to facilitate denial of previous physical or sexual abuse experiences by desensitizing them to the sexual acts in which they engage (Sterk, 1999).

There are also functional factors, affecting both drug use and sexual behavior, which must be considered. Many female drug users are involved in prostitution, either to support their habit or as a form of self-medication (Goldstein, 1979; Sterk & Elifson, 1990; Sterk, 2000). These women may also resort to shoplifting or other illegal activities as a way to obtain money for drugs. For a number of women involved in prostitution, drugs may be used to reduce feelings of shame or anxiety associated with having commercial sex.

Drug Use and Sexual Behavior

Illicit drug use, like the use of alcohol, serves as a sexual disinhibitor or aphrodisiac (Abadinsky, 1997). Drug use can therefore affect sexual encounters, sexual activities, as well as the practice of safer sex. However, the co-occurrence of drug use with sex is quite complex. Sexual behaviors that have been associated with drug use include early sexual debut, sex

without condoms, multiple sexual partners, anonymous partners, drug-impaired sex, the exchange of sex for drugs or money, and injection drug using partners (Booth et al., 1993; Cohen et al., 1994; Edlin et al., 1994; Fullilove et al., 1990; Inciardi, 1995). Gender differences in these behaviors have been examined. Sex exchanging has been shown to be more prevalent among female than male drug users (McCoy and Miles, 1992; Elifson et al.,1999), and is reportedly quite prevalent among drug using women (Edlin et al., 1994; Sterk, 1999). Sexual behavior associated with drug use has also been shown to vary according to the type of drug, and the frequency and intensity of use. For example, heroin is known to reduce sexual desires, while stimulants such as cocaine and methamphetamine, at least during the initial stages of use, increase the desire for sex. In addition, the association between crack cocaine and increased sexual activity and high-risk sexual behavior has been frequently demonstrated (Rolfs, Goldberg, & Sharrar, 1990; Chiasson et al., 1991; Des Jarlais et al., 1991; Sterk, 1999; Logan & Leukefeld, 2000). Recent studies have examined the nature of crack and injection drug use and risks associated with different drugs and routes of administration. In a sample of injection drug users, crack smokers, and injection drug users who smoke crack, Booth and colleagues (1993) found that IDUs who also smoked crack used injection drugs more frequently and were more likely to have sex with an IDU, to trade sex for drugs, to use drugs before or during sex, and to have unprotected sex than IDUs who did not smoke crack. Similar studies have reported similar sexual risks among crack and injection drug users (McBride et al., 1992; Wolfe et al., 1992; Williams et al., 1998; Tortu et al., 2000). In addition, sexual risk behaviors of crack smoking and nonsmoking female IDUs has been shown to have a greater association with acquiring HIV than drug risk behaviors alone (Watters et al., 1994).

Differences in sexual behavior by frequency and intensity of drug use have also been revealed. Recently, Hoffman and colleagues (2000) found that risky sexual behavior among

142   KATHERINE P. THEALL *et al.*

women who use crack were more prevalent among those who used crack with the greatest frequency and intensity. In examining the relationship between crack use, alcohol use, drug-impaired sex and HIV risk behaviors, Rasch and colleagues (2000) found similar results. Frequent users exhibited greater risk; frequent female users were more likely to report unsafe sex than their male counterparts. Furthermore, rates of crack-impaired sex were higher for those who used alcohol frequently, with rates nearly as high for those reporting frequent alcohol and only some crack use as opposed to those reporting frequent crack use (Rasch *et al.*, 2000).

The sexual partners of women who use drugs may include their steady partners, non-paying regular partners, and regular and casual paying partners (Sterk, 1999; Sterk *et al.*, 2000). The women's sexual behaviors, including type of sex and use of condoms, varied depending on the type of partner. For example, vaginal sex is most and condom use is least common with steady partners; oral sex and condom use are most common with paying partners. The sexual behavior of drug-using women who have sex with women, or women who self-identify as lesbian has recently been under investigation. Research has also revealed a drug–sex connection among these women. Kral and colleagues (1997) investigated HIV risk behavior among drug (crack cocaine and injection) using women who have sex with women (WSW) in one of the largest epidemiological studies on WSW who also use drugs. Infrequent condom use, sex with men, multiple sex partners, and sex exchanging were found to be common among these women. However, such sexual risks should be examined in terms of sexual identity as sexual behaviors might have a limited connection to sexual identity and instead may function as a survival strategy (Sterk, 1999; Sterk & Elifson, submitted).

Sexual and Reproductive Dysfunction

Female sexual dysfunction or impairment as it relates to drug abuse can be viewed from a number of different perspectives. Dysfunction as a social rather than simply physical connotation may imply a poor selection of partners, or the use of contraceptives. Drug abuse has been shown to influence each of these behaviors, primarily through pharmacologically induced disinhibition (Schafer, Blanchard, & Fals-Stewart, 1994). In a purely physical sense, sexual or reproductive dysfunction has been examined as reasons for drug and/or alcohol use and vice versa.

Lifetime drug dependence and reported drug use have been shown to predict women's gynecological problems, including amenorrhea, anovulation, luteal phase dysfunction, hyperprolactinemia, abnormal secretion of breast milk, spontaneous abortions, as well as decreased libido and decreased sexual arousal (Rosenbaum, 1981; Mello, 1986; Rosen, 1991; Wenzel, Andersen, & Gelberg, 1998; Westherington & Roman, 1998; Sterk, 1999). The reverse has been demonstrated as well. Bush and colleagues (1986) found that reported infertility or pelvic pain preceded increased use of alcohol or drugs among a sample of ob/gyn patients, one third of whom had potential substance abuse problems. Premenstrual dysphoria may also be a possible determinant of increased drug use by women (Mello, 1986). In a longitudinal study of women, Wilsnack and colleagues (1994) found sexual dysfunction to be the strongest predictor of continued problem drinking.

Moreover, sexual dysfunction has been shown to differ according to the type of drug and the route of administration. In a study of sexual behavior among adult heavy users of cocaine (39% female), Macdonald and colleagues found that freebasers and snorters of the drug had similar levels of sexual impairment, while injectors encountered the most sexual dysfunction (Macdonald, Waldorf, Reinarman, & Murphy, 1988). The frequency of amenorrhea, anovulation, luteal phase dysfunction, hyperprolactinema, and spontaneous abortions among women with reported use of cocaine, opiates, or marijuana have been shown to be similar (Lex, 1994).

Drug Use and Pregnancy Outcomes

Drug use during pregnancy can affect the fetus in vastly different ways depending on the drug(s) of exposure. Due to the nature of drug abuse (i.e., polydrug use), a number of factors may affect fetal development. The context of maternal drug use and their social environment are likely to play a key role as well. Research has validated the effect of alcohol and tobacco (Armstrong, McDonald, & Sloan, 1992; Winder, Fenster, Hopkins, & Swan, 1995) on the unborn child, but data on other drugs of abuse remains inconclusive. Researchers have reported that gestational cocaine exposure affects the development of the central nervous system, resulting in decreased head circumference, motor and behavioral problems, among other conditions (Chasnoff et al., 1985; Newald, 1986; Zuckerman et al., 1989). Recently, Ness and colleagues (1999) found that tobacco smoking and cocaine use independently contribute to spontaneous abortion; although an insignificant link between cocaine use and spontaneous abortion has also been demonstrated (Ryan, Ehrlich, & Finnegan, 1987). Premature rupture of membranes, impaired fetal growth, diminished birth weight, preterm and precipitous labor, breech presentation, postpartum hemorrhage, stillbirths, toxemia, and infant withdrawal have all been associated with heroin addiction (Kroll, 1986; Murphy & Rosenbaum, 1999). Marijuana has been shown to interfere with development when used during pregnancy, as well as during the first month of breast-feeding. Use of marijuana as well as other drugs during pregnancy has been shown to result in smaller infants, which can then lead to a number of health problems (Stern, 1984).

Although the consequences of fetal drug exposure have been demonstrated, additional effects due to maternal consequences of drug use may be just as damaging to fetal or childhood development. For example, mental health disorders of parents have been linked to poorer child outcomes independent of drug exposure (Singer et al., 1997). Other problems such as negative role modeling, financial strain, and a lack of attention to children's physical and emotional needs are also likely to play a role in the development of a child. In addition, drug users are less likely to receive prenatal care during pregnancy than are other populations (Funkhouser et al., 1993). Because pregnant users are at risk for anemia, thrombocytopenia, hypertension, and other medical problems (Stern, 1984), prenatal care is important for the health of not only the infant, but the mother's health as well.

A very pressing issue among pregnant female drug users who are infected with HIV or hepatitis C is the transmission of these viruses to the infant. Among the reported cases of pediatric HIV and AIDS cases in the United States, over 45% of both HIV and AIDS cases are due to maternal injection drug use or maternal sex with an injection drug user (CDC, 1999). Maternal infection with hepatitis C has been associated with transmission of HCV to the infant, as well as increased HIV maternal–infant transmission (Hershow et al., 1997).

Drug Use and Victimization

Although findings regarding the link between drug use and violence remain inconclusive, studies have shown that these two behaviors are closely related (DeLaRosa, Lambert, & Gropper, 1990; Maher & Curtis, 1992; Sterk & Elifson, 1990; Sterk, 1999). Violence is seen as a risk factor for substance abuse, while substance abuse can be a risk factor for violence. Many women who use drugs have been the victims of abuse (e.g., sexual victimization, childhood abuse), or have experienced or witnessed the abuse of others. Their drug use may be a form of self-medication to relieve the psychic or physical trauma related to these incidents. Recent data support the hypothesis of a continuum of risk: childhood abuse leading to later domestic violence, leading to an increased risk for drug-using behaviors (Cohen et al., 2000; Thompson et al., 1997; Zierler et al., 1991).

The probability of being a victim of trauma and violence is greatly increased for many female drug users (Rosenbaum, 1981; Sterk, 1999). Violence in the domestic setting, drug-using setting, and community setting is not uncommon in the lives of female users. Domestic violence is common among many women, whether emotional, physical, or sexual; or whether by family members, friends, or strangers (Sterk, 1999). Even among adolescent girls, forced sex has been associated with elevated illegal drug use (Chandy, Blum, & Resnick, 1996). Regardless of the drug-using status of a female user's partner, sexual violence by a partner makes it difficult for many women to exert control over the relationship, which can lead to a lack of competence in the sexual relationship (Rosenbaum, 1981; Sterk, 1999).

The setting where drug use often takes place is characterized by drug-using "highs" and "lows," cravings, and the quest for more drugs (Rosenbaum, 1981; Sterk, 1999). As described by Goldstein (1985), psychopharmacological, economic compulsive, or systemic violence is common among drug users in particular settings where use occurs. Violence is also seen in the communities where many drug-using women reside. Drug use may be a way for women to deal with the social or economic conditions in which they reside or the violent conditions in their drug-using "scene." However, women should not only be viewed as victims of drug-associated violence, but as practicing, independent participants in their own lives. Women's role as perpetrators of violence must also be considered (Hien, 1998; Sterk, 1999).

HIV/AIDS, Hepatitis B and C, and Other Infectious Diseases

Injection drug use has been shown to increase the risk of transmission of HIV and other blood-borne pathogens. AIDS is now the leading cause of death among women aged 15 to 44 years, and approximately two thirds of AIDS cases among women are related to injection drug use (CDC, 1999). Recent research also has shown that the rate of HIV infection among injection drug users is high during the earlier stages of their injection drug use career (Garfein et al., 1996; Neaigus et al., 1998; Nelson et al., 1995). Non-injection-drug users are also at risk for HIV infection, primarily due to their risk associated with sexual behavior. The heterosexual HIV risks associated with sex-for-crack trading is not captured by national data but has shown to be prevalent (Chiasson et al., 1991; Edlin et al., 1994; Sterk, 1988).

The impact of HIV infection among injection drug users has led to renewed interest in the other health problems raised by this population. There are a number of complications associated with injection drug use; effects related to drug toxicity, effects associated with the administration route, and effects associated with social implications of drug dependence can all have deleterious impact on the life of a user (Rosenbaum, 1981). Women who inject drugs often are taught by a male partner how to do so. In addition, it is not uncommon for them to inject themselves after their partner has used the syringe and offers the remainder of the drug in the syringe. This places women at risk for HIV infection, even though many women do not classify using drugs with and immediately after a partner as needle sharing or risky.

In addition to the risk of HIV infection, infection with hepatitis C and B from injection as well as non-injection-drug use has recently received considerable attention. Little is known about hepatitis B (HBV) and C (HCV) among drug users. Researchers have shown unsafe injection drug use to be a major risk behavior for hepatitis B and C (Garfein et al., 1996), with the level of infection for HBV and HCV being highest among new injectors. In examining the prevalence and correlates of viral infections among illicit injection and noninjection drug users, Garfein and colleagues found an overall prevalence of HCV, HBV, and HIV among users who had been injecting for up to six years to be 76.9%, 65.7%, and 20.5%, respectively. Among those injecting for one year or less, rates of HCV, HBV, and HIV were 64.7%, 49.8%, and 13.9%, respectively. Even less is known about HBV and HCV infection among non-injection drug users, although rates of both have been reported in noninjection users as well. Neaigus and colleagues (1998) found that among 398 respondents who never injected drugs, 26% tested positive for hepatitis B and 17% for hepatitis C. No information is available on gender-specific differences.

In discussing the relationship between drug use and HIV, HCV, and HBV, it is important to consider the environment in which drug use takes place. Behaviors that occur in a drug-using environment heighten the risk of infection for a number of infectious diseases. The risk of infection may vary according to the route of administration and the frequency of use. The route of administration has played, and continues to play, a large role in disease transmission. There is recent evidence that hepatitis C can be transmitted through the sharing of straws and pipes (Groopman, 1998).

Tuberculosis and other microbacterial diseases are also a growing problem among intravenous drug users. The association with crack use and sexually transmitted diseases other than HIV is also receiving much attention. An extensive discussion of these infectious diseases among female drug users is beyond the scope of this chapter.

Mental Health

Research has shown drug abuse to be co-morbid with psychiatric disorders at rates higher than in the general population (Tartar & Mezzich, 1992). Rates of anxiety and affective disorders are reportedly higher among women than men (Westherington & Roman, 1998). Psychopathologies that have been mentioned in association with substance abuse/dependence include depression, anxiety, antisocial personality disorder, and post-traumatic stress disorder (Luthar & Rounsaville, 1993). Among female drug users, elevated rates of depression, phobic anxiety, paranoid ideation, antisocial personality disorder, and posttraumatic stress disorder have been identified (Griffin et al., 1989; Singer et al., 1995; Woods et al., 1993).

Elevated rates of suicide among female drug users have also been reported (Lex, 1994).

The link between substance abuse and other psychopathology is unclear and it seems that some people with a predisposing psychiatric disorder initiate drug use as a form of self-medication, while others first take drugs and subsequently develop mental disorders (Westherington & Roman, 1998). Some researchers have suggested that a better understanding of the psychopathology also is important for drug treatment and HIV risk reduction programs (Compton et al., 1995). The link between substance abuse and mental health requires further investigation, especially among women.

Drug Treatment Issues

Despite the prevalence of drug use among women since the 1960s, few studies have focused on women. Consequently, the treatment needs unique to female drug users have received limited attention. Because of the unavailability of female-oriented programs, female drug users often find themselves in drug treatment programs that fail to take their specific circumstances into consideration.

Like drug use, drug treatment has been the topic of heated discussions for more than a century. At the end of the nineteenth century, and during the early decades in the twentieth century, many scientists saw drug use as curable, a view which later shifted to categorizing drug use as a mental health problem or a disease (Musto, 1973). Today, the most common treatment modules for drug habilitation are methadone, involvement in therapeutic communities, outpatient drug-free programs, and detoxification. Whatever the type of treatment, the ultimate goal of therapy is abstinence. Each method, however, varies in the amount of time it takes to achieve abstinence and in the structure of the actual treatment activities.

The nature of the treatment programs often reflects drug trends in society. During the 1960s and 1970s, heroin use dominated the drug market, and drug treatment programs largely served injection heroin users. The two most common treatment modules available to those users were methadone maintenance programs and therapeutic communities (Dole & Nyswander, 1967; Yablonski, 1965). Methadone maintenance programs provide users with a daily dose of methadone enabling them to move from compulsive heroin use to controlled methadone use. The controlled methadone use, in turn, is expected to rehabilitate the users. Frequently, methadone maintenance programs supplement the distribution of methadone with ancillary services such as individual counseling sessions and vocational training. Some methadone maintenance programs also offer medical, financial, and family services. While the original methadone maintenance programs identified maintenance as the ultimate outcome, more recently, programs have shifted to make abstinence their goal. Critics of methadone maintenance programs decry this shift and argue that while heroin use had been replaced with the use of a synthetic opiate, abstinence should be the main goal.

Therapeutic communities (TC) are highly structured residential programs. The program staff often consists of the therapeutic community's own graduates, thereby supporting a self-help approach similar to the one presented in 12-step programs such as Alcoholics Anonymous or Narcotics Anonymous. Synanon, the first TC, was established in 1958, followed by Phoenix House and Daytop Village in the 1960s. Group counseling sessions are central to the treatment plan. To become abstinent, a client resides in the community for an extended period of time from two months to two years. Long-term programs focus on "resocialization," while short-term programs provide their clients with skills to function in society, even when a total resocialization fails to occur.

As the prevalence of other drugs such as amphetamines, cocaine, hallucinogens, and marijuana increased in the 1970s and the subsequent decades, outpatient programs became a popular treatment modality. Centered largely around individual and group counseling sessions, this treatment typically takes place once or twice a week over a six-month time period.

The counseling sessions often include analytic psychotherapy, problem solving, sensitivity groups, and encounter groups. Other services provided by the program may include legal counseling, crisis intervention, assistance in finding housing, employment, and day care, or referral to specified agencies.

Another common treatment involves detoxification, which is a short-term treatment modality with medically supervised withdrawal leading to abstinence. The time period in various detoxification programs ranges between 2 and 21 days. A period between 5 and 7 days is the most common. While undergoing detoxification, patients often receive medications administered through the program to reduce their discomfort from withdrawal. Frequently detoxification programs are hospital based. While the providers' goal is to assist their clients in becoming abstinent, drug users often rely on detoxification programs to solve temporary problems such as an overdose or unintended medical side effects.

Because of the relatively recent emergence of crack cocaine on the drug market, research on the effectiveness of treatment for this drug is limited. The effectiveness of therapeutic and inpatient programs for cocaine users increases with the length of time a patient stays in residence and with a high staff–client ratio (Hubbard *et al.*, 1989). The efficacy of detoxification programs for crack cocaine users appears to be limited. Several medications, such as desipramine, amantadine, and buprenorphine, have been identified as instrumental in the detoxification process (Tennant & Sagherian, 1987; Mello *et al.*, 1980).

Drug treatment increasingly is viewed as an effective strategy to address substance use as well as related health and social problems such as sexually transmitted diseases, including HIV/AIDS, mental health problems, violence and crime. Despite its potential, little attention has been paid to the need for gender-specific substance abuse treatment. Such treatment programs should be for women only, should not be limited to drug use but address all aspects of the women's lives, should provide transitional care, and should help the women reenter mainstream society (Sterk, 1999). For example, while federal and state funds have been made available to develop treatment programs for pregnant and postpartum women, these programs often emphasize the women's reproductive role, while downplaying their other roles and needs. In addition, female drug users have indicated that they prefer programs that are less clinical in nature but are more community based. Some women preferred church-based programs, while others feared these to be influenced by religious beliefs; some women preferred local health centers, yet others viewed these as too clinically oriented; and, again others preferred neighborhood centers, to which some women responded that they preferred keeping their "business" outside the neighborhood (Sterk, Elifson, & Theall, in press).

SUMMARY AND CONCLUSIONS

Female drug users deserve thoughtful consideration, particularly for those with the least resources to either prevent or ameliorate their habit, and the health and social consequences that often accompany their use. The needs of female drug users are different and while considerable attention has been paid to their reproductive role and their risk for HIV and other infectious diseases, a holistic perspective often is lacking. The fact that gender-specific research has gained popularity is a start, but we need to move away from making comparisons between men and women to learning more about female drug users as a unique group. In doing so, we also need to keep in mind that women who use drugs are not a homogeneous group, not only because they may demonstrate various drug use patterns, but also due to the impact of factors such as age, race/ethnicity, sexual orientation, or relationship status.

The focus on the health consequences of drug use among women needs to be expanded as well. Currently, it seems that only those health consequences at the forefront of the public agenda are considered. In the late 1980s to early 1990s it was HIV/AIDS, now we are adding hepatitis B and C. Instead of waiting for the next public health crisis, researchers should begin conducting more comprehensive health research. For example, the potential link between drug use among women and cancer. Serur and colleagues (1995) found that women with cervical cancer who used drugs had poorer survival rates than those who did not use drugs. Another area in which further investigations are needed is mental health. The link between drug use and mental health problems among women is commonly accepted, however, our knowledge of the dynamics involved is extremely limited. In sum, future research is needed to enhance our theoretical understanding of female drug use and its consequences, as well as to apply this knowledge in women-specific prevention and intervention efforts.

REFERENCES

Aaron, D. J., Markovic, N., & Danielson, M. E. (1999). How age, race, education and sexual identity impact the health of lesbian and bisexual women. Presented at the Annual Symposium of the Gay & Lesbian Medical Association, San Diego, CA, August 1999.

Abadinsky, H. (1997). *Drug abuse: An introduction* (3rd ed.). Chicago: Nelson-Hall.

Adler, P.A. (1985). *Wheeling and dealing: An ethnography of an upper-level drug dealing and smuggling community.* New York: Columbia University Press.

Agar, M. (1973) *Ripping and running: A formal ethnography of urban heroin addicts.* New York: Seminar Press. American Psychiatric Association.

Amaro, H. (1995). Love, sex and power: Considering women's realities in HIV prevention. *American Psychologist, 50,* 437–447.

Armstrong, B., McDonald, A., & Sloan, M. (1992). Cigarette, alcohol and coffee consumption and spontaneous abortion. *American Journal of Public Health, 82,* 85–87.

Ball, J. C. (1967). The reliability and validity of interview data obtained from 59 drug addicts. *American Journal of Sociology, 72,* 650–654.

Bandura, A. (1977). *Social learning theory.* Englewood, NJ: Prentice-Hall.

Becker, M. H., & Joseph, J. K. (1988). AIDS and behavioral change to reduce risk: A review. *American Journal of Public Health, 78,* 394–410.

Bevier, P. J., Chiasson, M. A., Heffernan, R. T., & Castro, K. G. (1995). Women at a sexually transmitted disease clinic who reported same-sex contact: Their seroprevalences and risk behaviors. *American Journal of Public Health, 85,* 1366–1371.

Booth, R. E., Watters, J. K., & Chitwood, D. D. (1993). HIV risk-related sex behaviors among injection drug users, crack smokers, and injection drug users who smoke crack. *American Journal of Public Health, 83,* 1144–1149.

Botvin, G. J., Baker, E., Botvin, E. M., Filazzola, B. S., & Millman, R. (1984). Prevention of alcohol misuse through development of personal and social competence. *Journal of Studies on Alcohol, 45,* 550–552.

Bourgeois, P. (1989). Crack in Spanish Harlem: Culture and economy in the inner city. *Anthropology Today, 5,* 6–11.

Bourgeois, P. I., & Dunlap, E. (1993). Exorcising sex for crack: An ethnographic perspective from Harlem. In M. S. Ratner (Ed.), *Crack pipe as a pimp: An ethnographic investigation of sex-for-crack exchanges.* New York: Lexington Books.

Boyle, K., & Anglin, M. D. (1993). To the curb: Sex bartering and drug use among homeless crack users in Los Angeles. In M. Ratner (Ed.), *Crack pipe as a pimp: An ethnographic investigation of sex-for-crack exchanges.* New York: Lexington Books.

Briere, J., & Runtz, M. (1993). Childhood sexual abuse as a precursor to depression and self-destructive behavior in adulthood. *Journal of Traumatic Stress, 8,* 445–459.

Bush, D., McBride, A. B., & Benaventura, L. M. (1986). Chemical dependency in women: The link to ob/gyn problems. *Journal of Psychosocial Nursing and Mental Health Services, 24,* 26–30.

Calhoun, S. R., Wesson, D. R., Galloway, G. O., & Smith, D. E. (1996). Abuse of flunitrazepam (Rohypnol) and other benzoiazepines in Austin and South Texas. *Journal of Psychoactive Drugs, 28,* 183–189.

Centers for Disease Control and Prevention [CDC] (1999). HIV/AIDS Surveillance Report. *Midyear edition, 11,* 1–44.

Chandy, J. M., Blum, R. W., & Resnick, M. D. (1996). Female adolescents with a history of sexual abuse. *Journal of Interpersonal Violence, 11,* 503–517.

Chasnoff, I. J., Burns, W. J., Schnoll, S. H., & Burns, K. A. (1985). Cocaine use in pregnancy. *New England Journal of Medicine, 313,* 666–669.

Chasnoff, I. (1988). Cocaine, pregnancy, and the neonate. *Women and Health, 15,* 23–25.

Chavkin, W., Allen, M. H., & Oberman, M. (1991). Drug abuse and pregnancy: Some questions on public policy, clinical management, and maternal and fetal rights. *Birth, 18:* 107–112.

Chiasson, M. A., Stoneburner, R., Hildebrandt, D., Ewing, W., Telzak, E., & Jaffe, H. (1991). Heterosexual transmission of HIV-1 associated with the use of smokable freebase cocaine (crack). *AIDS, 5,* 1121–1126.

Clayton, R. R., Voss, H. L., Robbins, C., & Skinner, W. F. (1986). Gender differences in drug use: An epidemiological perspective. In B. A. Ray and M. C. Braude (Eds.), *Women and drugs: A new era for research.* Rockville, MD: NIDA.

Cohen, E., Navaline, H., & Metzger, D. (1994). High-risk behaviors for HIV: A comparison between crack-abusing and opioid-abusing African-American women. *Journal of Psychoactive Drugs, 26,* 233–241.

Cohen, M., Deamant, C., Barkan, S., Richardson, J., Young, M., Holman, S., Anastos, K., Cohen, J., & Melrisk, S. (2000). Domestic violence and childhood sexual abuse in HIV-infected women at risk for HIV. *American Journal of Public Health, 90,* 560–566.

Coles, C. (1992). Prenatal alcohol exposure and human development. In M. Miller (Ed.), *Development of the CNS: Effects of alcohol and opiates.* New York: John Wiley.

Collin, M. (1998). *Altered state: The story of ecstasy culture and acid house,* 2d ed. London: Serpent's Tail.

Comerford, M., Chitwood, D. D., McElrath, K., & Taylor, J. (1998). Pregnancy among women with a history of injection drug use. *Drugs & Society, 13,* 177–192.

Compton, W., Cottler, L., Shillington, A., & Price, R. (1995). Is anti-social personality disorder associated with increased HIV risk behaviors in cocaine users? *Drug and Alcohol Dependence, 37,* 37–43.

Crider, R. A., & Rouse, B. A. (1988). *Epidemiology of inhalant abuse: An update.* Rockville, MD: NIDA.

DeLaRosa, M., Lambert, E., & Gropper, B. (1990). *Drugs and violence: Causes, correlations and consequences.* Rockville, MD: NIDA.

Des Jarlais, D. C., Abdul-Quader, A., Minkoff, H., Hoegsberg, B., Landesman, S., & Tross, S. (1991). Crack use and multiple AIDS risk behaviors. *Journal of Acquired Immune Deficiency Syndromes, 4,* 446–447.

Denzin, N. K., & Lincoln, Y. S. (Eds.). (1993). *Handbook of qualitative research.* Thousand Oaks, CA: Sage.

Dohrenwend, B. P., Levav, I., Shrout, P. E., Schwartz, S., Naveh, G., Link, B. G., Skodol, A. E., & Stueve, A. (1992). Socioeconomic status and psychiatric disorders: The causation-selection issue. *Science, 255,* 946–952.

Dole, V. P., & Nyswander, M. (1967). Heroin addiction: A metabolic disease. *Archives of Internal Medicine, 120,* 19–24.

Donoghoe, M., Hall, N., Lopez, A., & Ball, A. (1998). *Opioid overdose: Trends, risk factors, interventions, and priorities for action.* Geneva: WHO.

Edlin, B. R., Erwin, K. L., Faruque, S., McCoy, C. B., Word, C., Serrano, Y., Inciardi, J. A., Bowser, B. P., Schilling, R. F., & Holmberg, S. D. (1994). Intersecting epidemics: Crack cocaine use and HIV infection among inner city young adults. Multicenter Crack Cocaine and HIV Infection Study Team. *New England Journal of Medicine, 24,* 1422–1427.

Elifson, K. W., Boles, J., Darrow, W. W., & Sterk, C. E. (1999). HIV seroprevalence and risk factors among clients of female and male prostitutes. *JAIDS: Journal of Acquired Immune Deficiency Syndromes, 20,* 195–200.

Fagan, J. (1994). Women and drugs revisited: Female participation in the cocaine economy. *Journal of Drug Issues, 24*(1–2): 179–225.

Faupel, C. (1991). *Shooting dope: Career patterns of hard-core heroin users*. Gainsville: University of Florida Press.

Fiddle, S. (1976). Sequences in addiction. *Addictive Diseases: An International Journal, 2*, 4: 553–568.

File, K. (1976). Sex roles and street roles. *International Journal of Addictions, 2*, 553–568.

Fishbein, M. (1980). A theory of reasoned action. Some applications and implications. In H. E. Howe & M. M. Page (Eds.), *Nebraska Symposium on Motivation*, 1979 (pp. 65–116). Lincoln: University of Nebraska Press.

Fishbein, M., & Ajzen, I. (1975). *Belief, attitude, intention, and behavior: An introduction to theory and research*. Reading, MA: Addison-Wesley.

Fullilove, R., Fullilove, M., Bowser, B., & Goss, S. (1990). Risk of sexually transmitted disease among black adolescent crack users in Oakland and San Francisco, Calif. *Journal of the American Medical Association, 263*, 851–855.

Funkhouser, A. W., Butz, A. M., Feng, T. I., McCaul, M. E., & Rosenstein, B. J. (1993). Prenatal care and drug use in pregnant women. *Drug and Alcohol Dependence, 33*, 1–9.

Garcia, A., & Mur, A. (1991). Marijuana and pregnancy: impact on the pregnant woman, the fetus and the newborn infant. *Medicina Clinica, 96*, 106–109.

Garfein, R. S., Vlahov, D., Galai, N., Doherty, M. C., & Nelson, K. E. (1996). Viral infections in short-term injection drug users: The prevalence of the hepatitis C, hepatitis B, human immunodeficiency virus, and human T-lymphotropic viruses. *American Journal of Public Health, 86*, 655–661.

Gold, S. R. (1980). The CAP control theory of drug abuse. In P. J. Letter, M. Sayers, & H. W. Pearson, (Eds.), *Theories on drug abuse: Selected contemporary prospective*. Rockville, MD: NIDA.

Goldstein, P. (1979). *Prostitution and drug use*. Lexington, MA: Lexington Books.

Goldstein, P. J. (1985). The drug violence nexus: A tripartite conceptual framework. *Journal of Drug Issues, 15*, 493–506.

Goldstein, A., & Kalant, H. (1993). In R. Bayer, & G. M. Oppenheimer (Eds.), *Confronting drug policy: Illicit drugs in a free society* (pp. 24–77). New York: Cambridge University Press.

Gorman, E. M., Clark, C. W., Welch, S. P., Nicholson, S., Amato, E., Laughren, L., & Coppedge, K. (1999). Presented at the National HIV Prevention Conference, Aug. 29–Sep. 1 (abstract no. 560).

Griffin, M. L., Weiss, R. S., Mirin, S. M., & Lange, U. (1989). A comparison of male and female cocaine abusers. *Archives of General Psychiatry, 46*, 122–126.

Groopman, J. (1998). The shadow epidemic. *The New Yorker*, May 11, 48–60.

Hershow, R. C., Riester, K. A., Lew, J., Quinn, T. C., Mofenson, L. M., Davenny, K., Landesman, S., Cotton, D., Hanson, I. C., Hillyer, G. V., Tang, H. B., & Thomas, D. L. (1997). Increased vertical transmission of human immunodeficiency virus from hepatitis C virus–coinfected mothers. Women and Infants Transmission Study. *Journal of Infectious Diseases, 176*, 414–420.

Hien, N. M. (1998). Women, violence with intimates, and substance abuse: Relevant theory, empirical findings, and recommendations for future research. *American Journal of Drug and Alcohol Abuse, 24*, 419–438.

Hoffman, J. A., Klein, H., Eber, M., & Crosby, H. (2000). Frequency and intensity of crack use as predictors of women's involvement in HIV-related sexual risk behaviors. *Drug Alcohol Dependence, 58*(3), 227–236.

Hser, Y., Anglin, M. D., & McGlothlin, W. (1987). Sex differences in addict careers. 1. Initiation of use. *American Journal of Drug and Alcohol Abuse, 13*, 37–53.

Hubbard, R. L., Marsden, M. E., Rachal, J. V., Harwood, H. J., Cavanaugh, E. R., & Ginzburg, H. M. (1989). *Drug abuse treatment: A national study of effectiveness*. Chapel Hill, NC: University of North Carolina Press.

Inciardi, J. A., & Pottieger, A. (1986). Drug use and crime among two cohorts of women narcotics users: An empirical assessment. *Journal of Drug Issues, 16*(1), 91–106.

Inciardi, J., Pottieger, D., & Lockwood, A. (1993). *Women and crack cocaine*. New York: Macmillan.

Inciardi, J. A. (1995). Crack, crack house sex, and HIV risk. *Archives of Sexual Behavior, 24*, 249–269.

Jadack, R. A., Hyde, J. S., & Keller, M. L. (1995). Gender and knowledge about HIV, risky sexual behavior, and safer sex practices. *Research in Nursing and Health, 18*, 313–324.

James, J. (1976). Prostitution and addiction: An interdisciplinary approach. *Addictive Disease: An International Journal, 2*, 601–618.

Johnson, B., Goldstein, P., Prebble, E., Schmeidler, J., Lipton, D., Spunt, B., & Miller, T. (1985). *Taking care of business: The economics of crime by heroin users*. Lexington, MA: Lexington Books.

Johnston, L. D., O'Malley, P. M., & Bachman, J. G. (1994). *National survey results on drug use from the Monitoring the Future study, 1975–1993*. Vol. 1. Rockville, MD: National Institute on Drug Abuse.

Johnston, L. D., O'Malley, P. M., & Bachman, J. G. (1999). *Drug trends in 1999 are mixed*. University of Michigan News and Information Services: Ann Arbor (MI). [Online]. Available: http://www.monitoringthefuture.org; accessed 05/30/00.

Kandel, D., & Davies, M. (1991). Friendship networks, intimacy, and illicit drug use in young adulthood: A comparison of two competing theories. *Criminology, 29*, 441–469.

Kandel, D. B. (1993). The social demography of drug use. In R. Bayer and G. M. Oppenheimer (Eds.), *Confronting drug policy: Illicit drugs in a free society* (pp. 24–77). New York: Cambridge University Press.

Kandel, D., Chen, K., Warner, L. A., Kessler, R. C., & Grant, B. (1997). Prevalence and demographic correlates of symptoms of last year dependence on alcohol, nicotine, marijuana and cocaine in the U.S. population. *Drug & Alcohol Dependence, 44*, 11–29.

Kane, S. (1991). HIV, heroin, and heterosexual relations. *Social Science and Medicine, 32*, 1037–1050.

Kearney, M., Murphy, S., & Rosenbaum, M. (1994). Mothering on crack cocaine: A grounded theory analysis. *Social Science and Medicine, 38*, 351–361.

Kral, A. H., Lorvick J., Bluthenthal, R. N., & Watters, J. K. (1997). HIV risk profile of drug-using women who have sex with women in 19 United States cities. *Journal of Acquired Immune Deficiency Syndromes, 16*(3), 211–217.

Kroll, D. (1986). Heroin addiction in pregnancy. *Midwives Chronicle & Nursing Notes*, July, 153–157.

Lieb, J., & Sterk-Elifson, C. (1993). Crack in the cradle: Reproductive decision making among crack cocaine users. *Journal of Contemporary Drug Problems, 12*(4), 687–706.

Levin, J. M., Holman, B. L., & Mendelson, J. H. (1998). Gender differences in cerebral perfusion in cocaine abuse: Technetium-99-m-HMPACO SPECT study of drug abusing women. *Journal of Nuclear Medicine, 35*, 1902–1909.

Lex, B. W. (1991). Some gender differences in alcohol and polysubstance users. *Health Psychology, 10*, 121–132.

Lex, B. W. (1994). Alcohol and other drug abuse among women. *Alcohol Health and Research World, 18*, 212–220.

Logan, T. K., & Leukefeld, C. (2000). Sexual and drug use behaviors among female crack users: A multi-site sample. *Drug and Alcohol Dependence, 58*, 237–245.

Lukas, S. E., Sholar, M., Lundahl, L. H., Lamas, X., Kouri, E., Wines, J. D., Kragie, L., & Mendelson, J. H. (1996). Sex differences in plasma cocaine levels and subjective effects after acute cocaine administration in human volunteers. *Psychopharmacology, 125*, 346–354.

Lucke, J. C. (1998). Gender roles and sexual behavior among young women. *Sex Roles, 39*, 273–297.

Luthar, S., & Rounsaville, B. (1993). Substance misuse and comorbid psychopathology in a high-risk group: A study of siblings of cocaine misusers. *International Journal on Addictions, 28*, 415–434.

Macdonald, P. T., Waldorf, D., Reinarman, C., & Murphy, S. (1988). Heavy cocaine use and sexual behavior. *Journal of Drug Issues, 18*, 437–455.

Maher, L., & Curtis, R. (1992). Women on the edge of crime: Crack cocaine and the changing contexts of street-level sex work in New York City. *Crime, Law, and Social Change, 18*, 221–258.

Maiman, M., Fruchter, R. G., Serur, E., Remy, J. C., Feuer, G., & Boyce, J. G. (1990). Human immunodeficiency virus and cervical neoplasia. *Gynecologic Oncology, 38*, 377–382.

McBride, D. C., Inciardi, J. A., Chitwood, D. D., McCoy, H. V., & the National AIDS Research Consortium (1992). Crack use and correlates of use in a national population of street heroin users. *Journal of Psychoactive Drugs, 24*, 411–416.

McKirnan, D. J., & Peterson, P. L. (1989). Psychosocial and cultural factors in alcohol and drug abuse: An analysis of a homosexual community. *Addictive Behavior, 14*, 555–563.

Mello, N. K. (1986). Drug use patterns and premenstrual dysphoria. In B. A. Ray and M. C. Braude (Eds.), *Women and drugs: A new era for research*. Rockville, MD: NIDA.

Mensch, B. S., & Kandel, D. B. (1988). Do job conditions influence the use of drugs? *Journal of Health and Social Behavior, 29*, 169–184.

Milkman, H. B., & Sunderwirth, S. G. (1987). *Craving for ecstasy: How our passions become addictions and what we can do about them*. San Francisco: Jossey-Bass.

McCoy, V. H., & Miles, C. (1992). A gender comparison of health status among users of crack cocaine. *Journal of Psychoactive Drugs, 24*, 389–397.

Murphy, S., & Rosenbaum, M. (1999). *Pregnant women on drugs: Combating stereotypes and stigma*. New Brunswick, NJ: Rutgers University Press.

Musto, D. F. (1973). *American disease: Origins of narcotic control*. New York: Oxford University Press.

National Institute of Justice (NIJ), (2000). *1999 annual report on drug use among adult and juvenile arrestees*. Washington, DC: NIJ, NCJ 181426.

National Institute on Drug Abuse (NIDA) (1996). *The National Pregnancy and Health Survey—Drug use among women delivering livebirths: 1992*. Rockville, MD: NCADI. Publication No. BKD192.

Neaigus, A., Atillasoy, A., Friedman, S. R., Andrade, X., Miller, M., Ildefonso, G., & Des Jarlais, D. C. (1998). Trends in the noninjected use of heroin and factors associated with the transition to injecting. In J. A. Inciardi & L. D. Harrison (Eds.), *Heroin in the age of crack cocaine* (pp. 131–159). Thousand Oaks, CA: Sage.

Nelson, K. E., Vlahov, D., Solomon, L., Cohn, S., & Munoz, A. (1995). Temporal trends of incident HIV infection in a cohort of injection drug users in Baltimore, Maryland. *Archives of Internal Medicine, 155*, 1305–1311.

Ness, R. B., Grisso, J. A., Hirschinger, N., Markovic, N., Shaw, L. M., Day, N. L., & Kline, J. (1999). Cocaine and tobacco use and the risk of spontaneous abortion. *New England Journal of Medicine, 340*, 333–339.

Newald, I. (1986). Cocaine infants. *Hospitals, 60*, 76.

Newcomb, M. D., & Bentler, P. M. (1986). Cocaine use among adolescents: Longitudinal associations with social context, psychopathology, and use of other substances. *Addictive Behavior, 11*, 263–273.

Nyamathi, A., Bayley, L., Anderson, N., Keenan, C., & Leake, B. (1999). Perceived factors influencing the initiation of drug and alcohol use among homeless women and reported consequences of use. *Women & Health, 29*, 99–114.

Preble, E., & Casey, J. J. (1969). Taking care of business: The heroin user's life on the street. *International Journal of Addictions, 1*, 1–24.

Prochaska, J. O., & DiClemente, C. C. (1983). Stages and

processes of self-change of smoking: Toward an integrative model of change. *Journal of Consulting and Clinical Psychology, 51*, 390–395.

Rappaport, J. (1981). In praise of paradox: A social policy of empowerment over prevention. *American Journal of Community Psychology, 9*, 1–25.

Rappaport, J. (1984). Studies in empowerment: Introduction to the issue. *Prevention in Human Services, 3*, 1–7.

Rasch, R. F. R., Weisen, C. A., MacDonald, B., Wechsberg, W. M., Perrit, R., & Dennis, M. L. (2000). Patterns of HIV risk and alcohol use among African-American crack abusers. *Drug and Alcohol Dependence, 58*, 259–266.

Ratner, M. (1993). *Crack pipe as a pimp.* Lexington: Lexington Books.

Robins, L. N., & Regier, D. S. (1991). *Psychiatric disorders in America: The epidemiological catchment area study.* New York: Free Press.

Rolfs, R. T., Goldberg, M., & Sharrar, R. G. (1990). Risk factors for syphilis: Cocaine use and prostitution. *American Journal of Public Health, 80*, 853–857.

Rosario, M., Hunter, J., & Gwadz, M. (1995). Sexual, alcohol, and drug risk acts of lesbian/bisexual female youths. HIV Infect Women Conference, p S55, Feb. 22–24.

Rosen, R. C. (1991). Alcohol and drug effects on sexual response: Human experimental and clinical studies. *Annual Review of Sex Research, 2*, 119–179.

Rosenbaum, M. (1981). *Women on heroin.* New Brunswick, NJ: Rutgers University Press.

Ryan, C., & Bradford, J. (1988). The national lesbian health care survey: 1988 report. Washington, DC: National Lesbian and Gay Health Foundation.

Ryan, L., Ehrlich, S., & Finnegan, L. (1987). Cocaine abuse in pregnancy: Effects on the fetus and newborn. *Neurotoxicology & Teratology, 9*, 295–299.

Schafer, J., & Brown, S. A. (1991). Marijuana and cocaine effect expectancies and drug use patterns. *Journal of Consulting & Clinical Psychology, 59*, 558–565.

Schafer, J., Blanchard, L., & Fals-Stewart, W. (1994). Drug use and risky sexual behavior. *Psychology of Addictive Behaviors, 8*, 3–7.

Serur, E., Fruchter, R. G., Maiman, M., McGuire, J., Arrastia, C. D., & Gibbon, D. (1995). Age, substance abuse, and survival of patients with cervical carcinoma. *Cancer, 75*, 2530–2538.

Singer, L. T., Farkas, K., Arendt, R., Minnes, S., Yamashita, T., & Kliegman, R. (1995). Postpartum psychological distress in cocaine using mothers. *Journal of Substance Abuse, 7*, 165–174.

Singer, L. T., Arendt, R., Minnes, S., Farkas, J., Coilin, M., & Yamashita, T. (1997). Fetal cocaine exposure and birth outcomes. Biologic and self-report measures. Abstracts of the Fifty Ninth Annual Scientific Meeting, College on Problems of Drug Dependence, 59, 153.

Skinner, W. F. (1994). The prevalence and demographic predictors of illicit and licit drug use among lesbians and gay men. *American Journal of Public Health, 84*, 1307–1310.

Stacy, A. W., & Newcomb, M. D. (1999) Adolescent drug use and adult drug problems in women: Direct, interactive, and mediational effects. *Experimental & Clinical Psychopharmacology, 7*, 160–173.

Stephens, R. C. (1991). *The street addict role.* Albany, NY: State University of New York Press.

Sterk, C. (1988). Cocaine and HIV seropositivity. *Lancet, 1*, 1052–1053.

Sterk C. (1999). *Fast lives: Women who use crack cocaine.* Philadelphia, PA: Temple University Press.

Sterk, C. E. (2000). *Tricking and tripping: Prostitution in the era of AIDS.* Putnam Valley, NY: Social Change Press.

Sterk, C. E., Dolan, K., & Hatch, S. (1999). Epidemiological indicators and ethnographic realities of female cocaine use. *Substance Use and Misuse, 34*, 2055–2070.

Sterk, C., & Elifson, K. (1990). Drug-related violence and street prostitution. In M. De La Rosa, E. Lambert, & B. Gropper (Eds.), *Drugs and violence: Causes, correlations and consequences.* Rockville, MD: NIDA.

Sterk, C. E., & Elifson, K. E. (submitted). Exploring the impact of sexual identity: An ethnographic study among African-American female drug users. *American Journal of Community Psychology.*

Sterk, C., Elifson, K., & Theall, K. (2000). Women and drug treatment experiences: A generational comparison of mothers and daughters. *Journal of Drug Issues, 30*, 839–861.

Stern, L. (1984). Drugs and other substance abuse in pregnancy. In L. Stern (Ed.), *Drug use in pregnancy* (pp. 148–176). Boston: AIDS Health Science Press.

Strauss, A., & Corbin, J. (1990). *Basics of qualitative research: Grounded theory procedures and techniques.* Newbury Park, CA: Sage.

Substance Abuse and Mental Health Services Administration (SAMHSA) (1996). National Household Survey on Drug Abuse: Main Findings 1995, DHHS Pub. No. (SMA) 96–3095.

Substance Abuse and Mental Health Services Administration (SAMHSA) (1997). National Household Survey on Drug Abuse: Main Findings 1996, DHHS Pub. No. (SMA) 98-3200.

Substance Abuse and Mental Health Services Administration (SAMHSA) (1999). National Household Survey on Drug Abuse: Main Findings 1998, DHHS Pub. No. (SMA) 00-3381.

Substance Abuse and Mental Health Services Administration (SAMHSA), National Clearinghouse for Alcohol and Drug Information (NCADI), 1998. *Prevalence of Substance Use among Racial and Ethnic Subgroups in the United States, 1991–1993* [Online]. Available: http://www.samhsa.gov; accessed 5/25/00.

Substance Abuse and Mental Health Services Administration (SMHSA), Drug and Alcohol Services Information System (DASIS), 1998b. *National Admissions to*

Substance Abuse Treatment Services: The Treatment Episode Data Set (TEDS) 1992–1996 [Online]. Available: http://www.samhsa.gov; accessed 5/25/00.

Sutter, A. (1966). The world of the righteous dope fiend. *Issues in Criminology, 2,* 177–182.

Tarter, R. E., & Mezzich, A. C. (1992). Ontogeny of substance abuse: Perspectives and findings. In M. Glantz and R. Pickens (Eds.), *Vulnerability to drug abuse.* Washington, DC: American Psychological Association.

Taylor, A. (1993). *Women heroin injectors.* Oxford: Clarendon Press.

Taylor, J., Fulop, N., & Green, J. (1999). Drink, illicit drugs and unsafe sex in women. *Addiction, 94,* 1209–1218.

Tennant, F. S., & Sagherian, A. A. (1987). Double-blind comparison of amantadine and bromocriptine for ambulatory withdrawal from cocaine dependence. *Archives of Internal Medicine, 147,* 109–112.

Thompson, N. J., Potter, J. S., Sanderson, A., & Maibach, E. W. (1997). The relationship of sexual abuse and HIV risk behaviors among heterosexual adult female STD patients. *Child Abuse and Neglect, 17,* 149–156.

Tortu, S., Beardsley, M., Deren, S., Williams, M., McCoy, H. V., Stark, A., Estrada, A., & Goldstein, M. (2000). HIV infection and patterns of risk among women drug injectors and crack users in low and high seroprevalence sites. *AIDS Care, 12,* 65–76.

Turner, C. F., Lessler, J. T., & Gfroerer, J. C. (1992). Survey measurement of drug use: Methodological studies. National Institute on Drug Abuse. DHHS Pub. No. (ADM) 92-1929.

Waldorf, D., Reinarman, C., & Murphy, S. (1991). *Cocaine changes: The experience of using and quitting.* Philadelphia: Temple University Press.

Warner, L. A., Kessler, R. C., Hughes, M., Anthony, J. C., & Nelson, C. B. (1995). Prevalence and correlates of drug use and dependence in the United States: Results from the national comorbidity survey. *Archives of General Psychiatry, 52,* 219–229.

Watters, J. K., Estilo, M. J., Kral, A. H., & Lorvick, J. J. (1994). HIV infection among female injection drug users recruited in community settings. *Sexually Transmitted Diseases, 21,* 321–328.

Wells, E. A., Calsyn, D. A., Saxon, A. J., & Greenberg, D. M. (1993). Using drugs to facilitate sexual behavior is associated with sexual variety among injection drug users. *Journal of Nervous & Mental Disease, 181,* 626–631.

Wenzel, S. L., Andersen, R., & Gelberg, L. (1998). Homeless women's gynecological symptoms and their use of medical care for symptoms. Abstract Book/Association for Health Services Research, 15, 235.

Westherington, C., & Roman, A. (Eds.) (1998). *Drug addiction research and the health of women.* Rockville, MD: NIDA.

Williams, M. L., Zhao, Z., Freeman, R. C., Elwood, W. N., Rusek, R., Booth, R. E., Dennis, M. L., Fisher, D. G., Rhodes, F., & Weatherby, N. L. (1998). A cluster analysis of not-in-treatment drug users at risk for HIV infection. *American Journal of Drug & Alcohol Abuse, 24,* 199–223.

Williams, T. (1989). *Cocaine kids.* Reading, MA: Addison-Wesley.

Wilsnack, S. C., Wilsnack, R. W., & Hiller-Sturmhoefel, S. (1994). How women drink: Epidemiology of women's drinking and problem drinking. *Alcohol Health and Research World, 18,* 171–181.

Winder, G. C., Fenster, L., Hopkins, B., & Swan, S. H. (1995). The association of moderate maternal and paternal alcohol consumption with birthweight and gestational age. *Epidemiology, 8,* 509–514.

Wolfe, H., Vranizan, K. M., Gorter, R. G., Keffelew, A. S., & Moss, A. R. (1992). Crack use and HIV infection among San Francisco drug users. *Sexually Transmitted Diseases, 19,* 111–114.

Woods, N. S., Eyler, F., Behnke, M., & Conlon, M. (1993). Cocaine use during pregnancy: Maternal depressive symptoms and infant neurobehavior during first month of life. *Infant Behavior and Development, 16,* 83–98.

Yablonsky, L. (1965). *Synanon: The tunnel back.* New York: Macmillan.

Young, R. M., Weissman, G., & Cohen, J. B. (1992). Assessing risk in the absence of information: HIV risk among women injection drug users who have sex with women. *AIDS Public Policy Journal, 7,* 175–183.

Zambrana, R. E., & Scrimshaw, S. C. (1997). Maternal psychosocial factors associated with substance use in Mexican-origin and African-American low-income pregnant women. *Pediatric Nursing, 23,* 253–259.

Zierler, S., Feingold, L., Laufer, D., Velentgas, P., Kantrowitz-Gordon, I., & Mayer, K. (1991). Adult survivors of childhood sexual abuse and subsequent risk of HIV infection. *American Journal of Public Health, 81*(5), 572–575.

Zinberg, N. E. (1984). *Drug, set, and setting: The basis for controlled intoxicant use.* New Haven, CT: Yale University Press.

Zuckerman, B., Frank, D. A., Hingson, R., Amaro, H., Levenson, S., Kayne, H., Parker, S., Vinci, R., Aboagye, K., Fried, L., Cabral, H., Timperi, R., & Bauchner, H. (1989). Effect of maternal marijuana and cocaine use on fetal growth. *New England Journal of Medicine, 320,* 762–768.

Zweig, J. M., Barber, B. L., & Eccles, J. S. (1997). Sexual coercion and well-being in young adulthood. *Journal of Interpersonal Violence, 12,* 291–308.

9

Alcohol Use and Women's Sexual and Reproductive Health

MICHAEL WINDLE and REBECCA C. WINDLE

INTRODUCTION

Recently, over the past 20 years, women's alcohol use and abuse and associated adverse health-related consequences received widespread scientific study. Early myths perpetuated the notion that alcohol problems and alcoholism were principally domains of difficulty for men, and that heavy drinking characterized only a small minority of women. Furthermore, sexual promiscuity and moral corruption were viewed as prominent characteristics among this heavy-drinking female minority, and hence there were few efforts directed toward public health resources and scientific studies to a perceived unsavory minority. Recent research and theoretical perspectives have radically altered this outlook with regard to perceptions of and knowledge about women's alcohol use practices and associated health problems (e.g., Plant, 1997; Wilsnack, Plaud, Wilsnack, & Klassen, 1997a). For example, on the basis of a large, nationally representative sample of adults (age 18 years and older), Grant (1997) reported that 54.7% of women reported using alcohol during their life-

time, 33.9% reported using alcohol in the last 12 months, and 8.4% met clinical diagnostic criteria for an alcohol disorder. Additionally, alcohol use by women has been associated with a range of adverse health-related outcomes, including medical complications (e.g., obstetric and gynecologic problems, breast cancer), sexual dysfunction, risky sexual behavior, and sexual victimization (e.g., Beckman, 1979; Blume, 1991; Cooper, 1992; Longnecker *et al.*, 1995).

An important aim of this chapter is to review research investigating various aspects of the relationship between alcohol use and women's sexual and reproductive health. Cumulative findings from the research literature suggest that, while the detrimental health effects of alcohol are evident in both men and women, for comparable levels of consumption, alcohol appears to have especially adverse health consequences for women. While the mechanisms of these gender-based differences of alcohol's impact on health are not well understood, both biological and sociocultural mechanisms may be involved. For example, as will be discussed subsequently, it is likely that alcohol impacts multiple domains of women's sexual health via its effects on the endocrine system. Also, gender-based differential socialization experiences and cultural belief systems impact the interrelationships between alcohol use and sexual practices (e.g., condom use decisions based on a male

MICHAEL WINDLE and REBECCA C. WINDLE • Department of Psychology, University of Alabama at Birmingham, Birmingham, Alabama 35294-1170.

Handbook of Women's Sexual and Reproductive Health, edited by Wingood and DiClemente. Kluwer Academic / Plenum Publishers, New York, 2002.

dominant model) that, in turn, may influence women's health (e.g., HIV infection rates).

In addition, research has shown that women, relative to men, experience a substantially shorter interval between initial drinking events (e.g., age of drinking onset, age of first intoxication) and later alcohol-related health problems (e.g., alcohol-related liver diseases such as cirrhosis and hepatitis, more rapid neurologic deterioration) (e.g., North, 1996; Randall *et al.*, 1999; Stein & Cyr, 1997). This accelerated progression of alcoholism in women has been referred to as "telescoping" (Piazza, Vrbka, & Yeager, 1989), and such telescoping may be due, in part, to alcohol's more toxic effects on women's organ systems relative to men's. This greater toxicity is associated with gender differences in biological processes that result in women experiencing higher blood alcohol concentrations (BACs) for a longer duration compared to men, even when the same amount of alcohol has been consumed (e.g., Plant, 1997). It is commonly believed that women experience higher BACs because they have a higher percent of body fat, a lower percent of body water, and, therefore, less dilution of alcohol and a smaller volume of distribution (e.g., Gearhart, Beebe, Milhorn, & Meeks, 1991; North, 1996). An additional explanation has been suggested by the research of Frezza *et al.* (1990), who reported that BACs were significantly higher in women than in men when alcohol was administered *orally*, but were more similar when alcohol was administered *intravenously*. To explain this finding, their research indicated lower gastric alcohol dehydrogenase activities in women compared to men, with lower oxidation of alcohol significantly associated with less first pass metabolism of ethanol for women. Frezza *et al.* concluded that the lower first pass metabolism of ethanol increased the systemic bioavailability of alcohol in women.

To better understand how and why alcohol use (even at moderate levels) may have adverse effects on women's sexual and reproductive health, this chapter attempts to cover a broad range of topics, including epidemiology, theory, endocrinology, health outcomes, assessment, and treatment. In addition, where applicable, issues related to gender and ethnic group differences are presented. Because of this breadth of coverage, depth was necessarily sacrificed in many domains, and women's issues related to nonsexual health topics were not covered. The chapter is organized into five sections. First, the assessment and epidemiology of women's drinking is provided to indicate the prevalence and extensiveness of alcohol use and abuse, with consideration given to ethnic and gender group variability. Second, a social-cognitive theoretical perspective on women's drinking and sexual functioning is presented. Third, research related to women's drinking and sexual and reproductive health issues is presented. Fourth, notable assessment and treatment issues are discussed, including the need for assessment of women's heavy drinking and alcohol abuse within the context of primary care settings and the treatment needs of women related to alcohol use and sexual functioning. Finally, we conclude with a chapter summary and a brief discussion of future research directions.

ASSESSMENT AND EPIDEMIOLOGY OF WOMEN'S DRINKING

A variety of different indicators have been used to assess alcohol use among women and men. Large (e.g., national, statewide) epidemiologic studies have commonly collected information pertinent to three domains. The first domain relates to the frequency and quantity of alcohol use (i.e., how often and how much do you usually drink) for specified time windows (e.g., in the last 30 days, in the last year). Typically, these alcohol use data are then used to derive specific quantity–frequency indexes of alcohol use, such as the average amount of ethanol consumed per day, or criteria are established to identify different types of users (e.g., abstainers, moderate drinkers, heavy drinkers). The second domain pertains to alcohol-related problems which consist of adverse social consequences associated with alcohol use (e.g., arrested for drinking and driving, lost job due to drinking, serious conflict with family members due to drinking) and symptoms of alcohol dependence (e.g., drank first thing in the morning, tried to drink less but could not). The third domain concerns the assessment of formal clinical diagnostic criteria to obtain estimates of the incidence and prevalence of alcohol disorders. In large-scale studies, these measures are generally collected via survey self-report methods, or in the case of alcohol disorders, via personal interviews. Epidemiologic findings relevant to these three domains of alcohol assessment are presented below.

Quantity–Frequency

Quantity–frequency based measures are commonly used in epidemiologic studies of alcohol use. Alcohol beverage consumption survey questions are typically asked with regard to the frequency and quantity of use of each of three beverage categories (beer, wine, hard liquor or spirits) for alternative time windows (e.g., last 30 days, last 12 months). Definitions are provided for each beverage such as a 12-ounce can or bottle of beer, a 4-ounce glass of wine, and an ounce of hard liquor. On the basis of the frequency and quantity information, it is possible to derive an index of the average amount of ethanol consumed per day or to derive different drinking categories. For example, Caetano and Clark (1998) identified the following five drinking categories:

- *Frequent heavy drinking*: drinks once a week or more often and has five or more drinks at a sitting at least once a week or more often
- *Frequent drinking*: drinks once a week or more often and may or may not drink five or more drinks at a sitting less than once a week but at least once a year
- *Less frequent drinking*: drinks one to three times a month and may or may not drink five or more drinks at least once a year
- *Infrequent drinking*: drinks less than once a

month but at least once a year and does not drink five or more drinks at a sitting
- *Abstain*: drinks less than once a year or has never drunk

It is important to note that no consensus has been achieved with regard to the "best" definition of drinking categories and that there is considerable variability in the use of terms (e.g., moderate drinker) and operational definitions across studies. Thus, it is important to attend to the associated definitions of drinking categories when evaluating the results of studies linking women's (and men's) alcohol use and health outcomes. Throughout this chapter, efforts are made to provide the drinking definitions associated with given studies.

With regard to lifetime abstention of alcohol, the literature has consistently indicated that women abstain at higher rates than men and that there is variability in abstention rates across different ethnic groups of women. The lifetime rate of abstention for adult women has been estimated at 50% (e.g., Grant, 1997; Wilsnack *et al.*, 1997a). However, on the basis of national data (e.g., Caetano & Clark, 1998; Wilsnack *et al.*, 1997a), white women are significantly less likely to abstain than Hispanic and, especially, black women. For other ethnic groups of women, regional data also indicate different rates of abstention (and, by contrast, of drinking). Gilbert and Collins (1997) reviewed existing data on this topic and reported that among Asian-American groups residing in Los Angeles, Filipino and Chinese women had high rates of abstention (55% and 51%, respectively), as did Korean women (75%), though the rate of abstention for Japanese women was only 27%. Caetano (1988) also reported variation in women's abstention rates among Latino subgroups, with the lowest rates of abstention among Puerto Ricans (33%) and the highest among Cuban-Americans (42%) and Mexican-Americans (46%).

Based on the definitions of drinking status provided previously in this chapter, Caetano and Clark (1998) reported the following 1995 rates of *infrequent/less frequent*, *frequent*, and *frequent heavy drinking*, respectively, for white, black, and Hispanic women: white (41%, 19%, 2%), black (30%, 10%, 5%), Hispanic (31%, 9%, 3%). These data indicate that more white women are frequent drinkers, but that ethnic group differences are small for frequent heavy drinking. In addition, Caetano and Clark reported that in comparison with 1984 prevalence data, the findings in 1995 indicated a decrease in frequent heavy drinking among white women but an increase among black and, to a lesser extent, Hispanic women.

Alcohol Problems

Drinking problems include both adverse social consequences associated with alcohol use (e.g., job problems, spouse problems, problems with friends, police problems) and symptoms of alcohol dependence (e.g., behaviors related to tolerance and withdrawal). Dawson and Grant (1993) used data from current drinkers (with current drinking defined as having consumed at least 12 drinks in the preceding year) in the 1988 National Health Interview Survey Alcohol Supplement to report findings on alcohol problems in the last year. Among current-drinking women, 10.22% reported symptoms of impaired control (e.g., ended up drinking much more than intended), 6.18% reported compulsions (e.g., had a strong urge to drink), 5.55% reported symptoms of withdrawal (e.g., been sick or vomited after drinking, or the morning after), and 4.22% reported symptoms of tolerance (e.g., found that the same amount of alcohol had less effect than before). In a separate national survey, Herd (1997) reported that for drinking women (with drinking defined as any alcohol beverage use in the last year), 9.5% of women indicated alcohol-related health problems and almost 6% reported spouse problems (related to the respondent's drinking). Wilsnack and Wilsnack (1995) reported that higher rates of heavy drinking and associated adverse consequences among women were related to a number of factors, including women lacking social roles or occupying unwanted so-

cial statuses (e.g., unemployed), ethnic minority women experiencing rapid acculturation, and sociodemographic variables (e.g., younger age, cohabiting women). For example, the highest rates of alcohol use and adverse social consequences among women were among those 21–34 years of age and this age span corresponds to a higher rate of never being married. Correlates of never being married among women include a higher percentage of time spent in drinking contexts (e.g., nightclubs and bars) and social settings where there is a higher probability of both alcohol use and adverse consequences associated with such use.

Herd (1997) compared (drinking) Black and White women on adverse drinking consequences (e.g., job problems, spouse problems, health problems) and reported that heavier drinking among White women was associated with higher rates of drinking problems than among Black women. That is, as the frequency of consuming eight or more drinks during the last year increased, the prevalence of drinking problems among White women increased more rapidly, relative to the increase of drinking problems among Black women and men, and of White men. Herd speculated that the social contexts of alcohol consumption for White and Black women may differ such that there is greater tolerance and less stigma associated with drinking among Black, relative to White, women. Such differences may be rooted in a history of more egalitarian gender roles and attitudes among Blacks than Whites. Also, Herd suggested that differences in dietary practices and body weight between the Black and White women may contribute to differential vulnerability to the effects of alcohol on associated adverse consequences.

Alcohol Disorders

Data from the National Comorbidity Study (NCS) provided lifetime prevalence of alcohol disorders for women and men (Kessler *et al.*, 1994). The NCS data were collected from 1990 to 1992 and included participants from ages 15 to 54 years. Consistent with the previous alcohol use data, men had a higher rate of alcohol disorders than women, with a lifetime prevalence of 12.5% for alcohol abuse (without dependence) and 20.1% for alcohol dependence; the corresponding lifetime prevalence for women was 6.4% and 8.2%, respectively; hence, while not as high as men, 14.6% of women met clinical diagnostic criteria for an alcohol disorder. Similar gender differences were indicated in the National Longitudinal Alcohol Epidemiologic Survey (NLAES), which included a nationally representative sample of 42,862 participants from ages 18 and above (Grant, 1997). With regard to lifetime alcohol dependence, the prevalence for men was 18.5% and for women was 8.4%. Further breakdowns of alcohol disorders by gender and ethnic group have yet to be reported for these national epidemiologic studies.

Pregnant Women

On the basis of Behavioral Risk Surveillance System (BRSS) data from 1988 through 1995, Ebrahim *et al.* (1998) analyzed the prevalence of any alcohol use in the last month and "frequent consumption" (defined as at least one binge drinking episode or consumption of at least seven drinks per week in the preceding month) for self-reported pregnant and nonpregnant women. Pregnant women indicated lower levels of alcohol use (14.6%) and frequent consumption (2.1%) relative to nonpregnant women (the respective rates were 52.2% and 15.2%). However, an analysis of historical trend data for pregnant women indicated that relative to 1992, in 1995 there was almost a twofold increase in the prevalence of alcohol use and a fourfold increase in the prevalence of frequent consumption. Characteristics associated with greater alcohol use among pregnant women were a college education, being unmarried, high annual incomes, and smoking.

Similar concerns about drinking during pregnancy were also indicated in the Perinatal Substance Exposure Study (PSES; Noble *et al.*, 1997), which involved an anonymous urine toxicology screening of 29,494 pregnant women admitted for delivery in 202 hospitals in Califor-

nia in 1992. The findings of the PSES indicated a positive alcohol use screening rate of 6.72% at childbirth (this rate exceeds that which has been reported in other studies). The prevalence by ethnic group was African-American (11.58%), Hispanic (6.87%), White (6.05%), Asian and Pacific Islander (5.07%), and Other (4.03%). The findings of the BRSS and the PSES are consistent in identifying high rates of alcohol use among pregnant women.

Adolescents

The previous findings have focused on adult women and their drinking practices. However, it is important to note that there are significant increases in the prevalence of alcohol use and binge drinking among adolescent females (e.g., Windle, 1999). National survey data indicated that over 80% of high school seniors (boys and girls) reported using alcohol at least once in their lifetime (e.g., Johnston, O'Malley, & Bachman, 1996). In addition, over 45% of girls reported drinking alcohol in the last 30 days and over 24% reported binge drinking at least once in the last two weeks. These rates of alcohol use among girls are substantially higher than the lifetime rates reported by adult women and portend numerous health-related issues as these adolescents mature to adulthood. The use of alcohol during adolescence is frequently associated with risky sexual activity and adverse health outcomes (e.g., STDs); hence these interrelated health-risk behaviors are of concern for the future health of women.

A THEORETICAL PERSPECTIVE ON WOMEN'S ALCOHOL USE AND SEXUAL FUNCTIONING

Historically, there has been a pervasive belief in Western culture among both men and women that alcohol is a sexual disinhibitor and enhances sexual pleasure (e.g., Klassen & Wilsnack, 1986; Wilsnack *et al.*, 1997a). Alcohol expectancy research has been an important contributor to our understanding of women's beliefs and expectations about alcohol's facilitative and disinhibiting effects on sexual arousal and functioning (e.g., Crowe & George, 1989). The laboratory-based alcohol expectancy paradigm has provided a useful model that allows researchers to disentangle the pharmacological effects of alcohol on behavior (e.g., alcohol's effects on sexual arousal or aggression) from people's expectancies or beliefs about alcohol's effects on their behavior, with the balanced placebo design (BPD) used as the basic research approach.

Early laboratory-based studies by Wilson and Lawson (1976a, 1976b, 1978) and Malatesta and colleagues (1979, 1982) investigated the relationships among alcohol consumption, alcohol expectancies, and physiological (e.g., vaginal and penile plethysmography) and subjective (e.g., self-report questionnaires) indicators of sexual arousal among college men and women. The findings from these studies suggested that alcohol consumption at moderate or high concentrations had a suppressant effect on physiological measures of sexual arousal and functioning for both sexes (e.g., Malatesta, Pollack, Wilbanks, & Adams, 1979; Malatesta, Pollack, Crotty, & Peacock, 1982; Wilson & Lawson, 1976a, 1978). In addition, the belief or expectation that one had consumed alcohol (independent of whether alcohol was actually consumed) had a facilitative effect on physiologically based sexual arousal for men (at least at lower levels of consumption) but not for women (Wilson & Lawson, 1976a, 1978). However, subjective reports of sexual arousal when consuming alcohol differed by gender. Men reported experiencing less sexual arousal and pleasure at higher BACs, whereas women reported the experience of enhanced sexual arousal and pleasure at higher BACs, even when physiological measures of arousal had decreased (e.g., Malatesta *et al.*, 1982; Wilson & Lawson, 1978). Thus, for women, alcohol seemed to *suppress* physiological sexual arousal but enhance cognitive sexual arousal (Malatesta *et al.*, 1982).

Findings from the above studies provide empirical support for the notion that, for some

men and women, alcohol consumption is closely linked to the perception of enhanced sexual arousal and pleasure. Various explanations have been posited to explain the origins of people's beliefs regarding the alcohol consumption–sexual arousal relationship, including the disinhibition hypothesis of alcohol and social learning theory (Beckman & Ackerman, 1995; Leigh, 1990). Based on a review of the alcohol–sexual behavior literature, Wilson (1981) concluded that a purely physiologically based theory of alcohol disinhibition (i.e., alcohol suppresses inhibitory brain functions, thereby enabling the expression of normally suppressed behaviors) could not adequately account for the nonpharmacologic expectancies observed regarding the association between alcohol use and sexual behavior. Rather, Wilson proposed a social learning theory formulation that emphasized the acquisition and maintenance of alcohol use and sexual behaviors contingent on differential reinforcement, role modeling, and cognitive self-regulatory mechanisms. Accordingly, many of the alcohol and sexuality behaviors observed were not "driven" by sexual impulses that were unconstrained due to alcohol's disinhibiting effects, but to experiential learning and self-regulatory mechanisms.

This more general social–cognitive learning theory framework (e.g., Bussey & Bandura, 1999; Wilson, 1981), guided by gender differences in socialization practices, has served as a broad backdrop for the investigation of gender differences in alcohol use and sexual functioning in women. That is, from an early age onward, there are different sociocultural scripts for males and females with regard to the appropriateness of a broad range of behaviors, including gender appropriate sexual behavior, permissive versus restrictive rules respectively for the consumption of alcohol by men versus women, and differential societal responses to inebriation for men versus women. For example, for men heavy drinking is a more socially sanctioned activity and inebriation is viewed as an acceptable "slip"; for women, heavy drinking or inebriation may be viewed as a sign of immorality or wanton sexuality. Laboratory studies have supported this idea with regard to societal attitudes toward women's drinking. George, Gournic, & McAfee (1988) requested college students to rate vignettes of young women drinking. Students rated a woman drinking alcohol versus a soft drink as "more aggressive and impaired, less socially skillful and more sexually predisposed"; these ratings were even higher if the male in the vignette paid for the drinks. Similarly, Richardson and Campbell (1982) reported findings on ratings of rape scenarios that indicated that both male and female students rated the rapist as less responsible if he was drunk, and the victim as more responsible if she was drunk at the time of the rape. Such societal attitudes may foster the belief or expectancy that women who drink are seeking sexual relations and that sexual aggressors are exempt from responsibility (e.g., Blume, 1991); such beliefs may have serious consequences (e.g., sexual victimization) for women that may impair physical and psychological health (this issue is discussed further in a subsequent section of this chapter).

WOMEN'S DRINKING AND SEXUAL AND REPRODUCTIVE HEALTH ISSUES

Alcohol Use and Sexual Dysfunction

Expectations and beliefs about the facilitative effects of alcohol on sexual functioning may influence the drinking behaviors of some women with sex-related concerns or problems. For example, Leigh (1990) found that women who expected alcohol to decrease their nervousness about sex were more likely to initiate sexual activity when drinking than were women with weaker alcohol expectancies (19% vs. 8%, respectively). In addition, those women who held more negative attitudes about sex (e.g., felt guilty about sexual experiences) and had stronger alcohol expectancies (e.g., a better lover when drinking) reported the highest levels of alcohol consumption during the most recent sexual encounter in which drinking had oc-

curred. These findings were significant after controlling for usual drinking frequency. Thus, women who experienced difficulties related to their sexual behavior (e.g., nervousness or guilt about sexual experiences) may have been motivated to drink during sexual encounters based on expectancies that alcohol would lower their sexual inhibitions and enhance their sexual experiences.

The latter findings by Leigh (1990) raise concerns that some women may be motivated to drink based on beliefs that alcohol will help to alleviate problems related to their sexuality and will enhance their sexual pleasure; such cognitively based drinking motivations may contribute to the development or continuation of alcohol-related problems or alcohol disorders. Although existing studies have not addressed this specific issue, research has indicated significant associations between heavy and abusive levels of drinking and sexual dysfunction among women (Beckman, 1979; Klassen & Wilsnack, 1986). However, while studies have indicated such an association, they have not addressed the issue of causality, nor have they shed light on the potential mechanisms linking these behaviors. A possible explanation postulated by Wilsnack, Klassen, Schur, & Wilsnack (1991) was that a reciprocal relationship may best explain the alcohol abuse–sexual dysfunction association seen among some women. That is, problem-drinking women who experience sexual dysfunction and who believe that alcohol lowers sexual inhibitions and enhances sexual pleasure may self-medicate with alcohol based on their existing belief system. However, because heavier alcohol use dampens physiologically based sexual arousal, women may find themselves in a negative cycle in which they drink to improve sexual functioning but they experience less physiological arousal due to their alcohol consumption. While this explanation is speculative, it nevertheless points to the need for future research that identifies variables that mediate the relationship between abusive drinking and sexual dysfunction in women. Research on women's alcohol consumption, alcohol expectancies, and sexual behaviors suggests that investigating the mediational effects of alcohol-related expectations is a fruitful avenue of inquiry. Positive findings from such research could provide direction for cognitively and informationally based intervention efforts with heavy and problem-drinking women who experience sexual dysfunctions.

Alcohol Use and Sexual Victimization

The extant literature suggests that alcohol use and sexual victimization are related in at least two ways, and that both have adverse impacts on women's physical and psychological health and well-being. First, childhood sexual abuse is a common antecedent to alcoholism in women, and sexual victimization among females is higher in families with paternal alcoholism relative to families without paternal alcoholism (Windle, Windle, Scheidt, & Miller, 1995). Thus, heavy alcohol use by others (e.g., male family members) may contribute to increased risk for the sexual victimization of females who are not drinking. Second, personal drinking by women in some contexts (e.g., in bars, at fraternity parties) may increase risk for sexual victimization via miscommunication and stereotyping about women and drinking (Blume, 1991).

With regard to the link between sexual victimization in childhood and alcohol disorders in adult women, there have been consistent findings that childhood sexual abuse occurs with a high frequency among women with alcohol disorders and alcohol problems (e.g., Miller, Downs, Gondoli, & Keil, 1987; Windle et al., 1995). Windle et al. reported a prevalence of 49% for childhood sexual abuse among a sample of 321 women in alcohol treatment inpatient settings in New York State. With a national sample of women, Wilsnack (1991) reported that twice as many problem drinkers as nonproblem drinkers had at least one incident of sexual abuse prior to age 18 years. Prior sexual abuse was also prospectively associated with the onset of problem drinking at a five-year follow-up. Of those women who had not been problem drinkers in 1981, 51% of those with a history of sexual abuse reported one or more alcohol prob-

lems in 1986; by contrast, of those women who had not been problem drinkers in 1981 and did not have a history of sexual abuse, only 19% reported one or more alcohol problems in 1986.

The adult correlates and potential adverse health consequences for women who have been sexually abused in childhood are multiple, including higher rates of alcohol and other substance abuse disorders, psychiatric disorders, and sexual dysfunction (e.g., Hurley, 1991; Wilsnack, Vogeltanz, Klassen, & Harris, 1997; Windle et al., 1995). The findings of Wilsnack et al. (1997b) indicated that childhood sexual abuse was associated both with higher levels of alcohol abuse (e.g., more drinking problems, more alcohol dependence symptoms) and indicators of sexual dysfunction (e.g., pain that prevented sexual intercourse). The findings by Windle et al. also revealed that those alcoholic women who reported childhood sexual abuse were more likely to have co-occurring psychiatric disorders (e.g., anxiety disorders) and to have attempted suicide than those alcoholic women who did not report sexual abuse in childhood. Hurley's (1991) review of women, alcohol, and incest concluded that incest-surviving alcoholic women, relative to nonincest alcoholic women, reported more problems with sexual dysfunction, including lack of sexual interest, lack of orgasm, and lack of sexual arousal or pleasure. Collectively, these findings strongly support the health-impairing role of childhood sexual abuse on adult women's alcohol use and sexual health.

In addition to childhood sexual abuse, victimization associated with alcohol use among women occurs with high frequency in adulthood, especially young adulthood. For instance, it has been estimated that alcohol use by the perpetrator, the victim, or both is associated with at least 50% of rapes in adulthood (e.g., Koss, Gidycz, & Wisniewski, 1987). Furthermore, serious problems associated with acquaintance rape and sexual assault on college campuses have been identified, with alcohol use a common feature of these episodes (e.g., Abbey, Ross, & McDuffie, 1994). In a nationally representative study of over 3000 women students from 32 colleges in the United States,

Koss *et al.* (1987) reported that 74% of the perpetrators and 55% of the victims had been consuming alcohol prior to the sexual assault or rape; higher levels of alcohol use were more likely associated with rape than with other nonpenetrative sexually coercive activities. Similarly, the findings of Abbey *et al.* with a large sample of college women ($n = 1160$) and men ($n = 814$) showed that 30% of men who reported raping a woman indicated the use of alcohol at the time of the incident, and 29% of the women reporting being raped indicated the use of alcohol at the time of the incident. The relationship between alcohol use and sexual victimization of women may be due, in part, to biased societal beliefs that link women's alcohol use to greater sexual availability and responsivity (Blume, 1991; George *et al.*, 1988).

The consequences of rape and sexual assault on women's health are multiple, ranging from physical injury and organ damage to severe psychological trauma and chronic mental health conditions (e.g., posttraumatic stress disorder, major depressive disorder). Restricting our discussion to alcohol abuse as an unhealthy outcome, Kilpatrick, Edmonds, & Seymour (1992) reported a concurrent and prospective association between rape and alcohol problems among women. In 1990, Kilpatrick *et al.* conducted a national telephone survey about violent victimization with 4008 adult women. Among those rape victims with posttraumatic stress disorder, 20.1% reported two or more major alcohol-related problems relative to 1.5% of the women who had not been raped. Follow-up findings with the full sample of women also indicated that violent victimization was much more likely to predict subsequent alcohol dependence than vice versa. Hence, with regard to temporal ordering, violent victimization was much more likely to precede than to follow alcohol dependence among women.

Alcohol Use and Risky Sexual Behaviors

A commonly held belief in our culture is that alcohol use disinhibits many behaviors that may, in turn, influence levels of sexual forwardness and risky sexual activities (e.g., noncondom use), and enhance pleasurable aspects of sexual encounters. Systematic studies have revealed a relatively consistent positive association between higher levels of drinking and higher engagement in sexually risky activities, such as unprotected sexual intercourse and multiple sexual partners (e.g., Caetano & Hines, 1995; Cooper, 1992). However, critical reviews of this literature (e.g., Cooper, 1992; Leigh & Stall, 1993) have identified a number of difficulties in making causal connections based on these bivariate associations. For example, these bivariate association studies have not demonstrated that alcohol was used by one or both partners at the time of these risky sexual activities, or whether these two activities (i.e., alcohol use and sexual encounters) were temporally independent events. Also, issues pertinent to whether a third variable (e.g., sensation seeking) may account for the positive association between alcohol use and risky sex were not examined and excluded as a possible cause of the association.

Recent studies have been directed away from more global association studies to an event (or "incident") based approach (e.g., Graves & Hines, 1997; Scheidt & Windle, 1996). These studies typically focus on the use of alcohol by one or both partners in relation to an identified sexual episode, such as most recent sexual incident, or first sexual incident. On the basis of national survey data and with reference to the most recent encounter with a new sexual partner, Graves and Hines reported that, for women, alcohol use during the sexual encounter predicted a failure to use a condom. This relationship was stronger for Whites and Blacks, as Hispanic women were more likely to use protection even if they consumed alcohol in the sexual encounter. Using a large sample of women in alcohol treatment centers and with reference to the last sexual encounter prior to entry to treatment, the findings of Scheidt and Windle indicated that alcohol use in the sexual encounter yielded a fivefold increase in the likelihood that the sex partner was a nonprimary partner; knowledge of the sexual history and current serostatus of nonprimary partners are typically unknown to women and thus may pose increased risk for sexually transmitted diseases, including HIV.

Not all studies using the event-based approach have supported the association between alcohol use and risky behavior within the sexual episode (e.g., Leigh & Stall, 1993). Furthermore, in the discussion of results by both Graves and Hines (1997) and Scheidt and Windle (1996), there was a recognition of the multiple additional personal (e.g., sexual history) and situational influences that impact risky behavior outcomes. Based on the current data, there is little evidence to argue that alcohol use is a prominent cause of sexually risky behavior, though as a defining feature of some social situations (e.g., with a new partner in a sex-facilitative context), it may be a contributing factor or cue for sexually risky behavior.

Alcohol Use and Endocrine Functioning

Alcohol use has been implicated in the etiology of menstrual cycle irregularities and disorders via its effects on endocrine functioning. Among premenopausal women, both moderate (e.g., three to four drinks per day) and abusive levels of alcohol use are associated with a number of menstrual cycle disorders, including amenorrhea, anovulation, luteal phase dysfunction, and hyperprolactinemia (e.g., Becker, Tønnesen, Kaas-Claesson, & Gluud, 1989; Gearhart et al., 1991; Mello, Mendelson, & Teoh, 1989; Wilsnack, Klassen, & Wilsnack, 1984). The alcohol use–menstrual disorder relationship is dose-dependent, such that the probability of menstrual cycle disorders increases with higher levels of alcohol consumption (Mello et al., 1989; Wilsnack et al., 1984).

While the particular mechanisms by which alcohol impacts endocrine functioning and thus contributes to menstrual irregularities and disorders are not known, alcohol's effects on the endocrine system are both multiple and complex (Gearhart et al., 1991; Mello et al., 1989; Van Thiel, Tarter, Rosenblum, & Gavaler, 1989). Mello et al. reviewed literature suggestive of alcohol's effects on various neuroendocrine systems and hormones—including the hypothalamic–pituitary–adrenal–gonadal axis—and potential pathways by which alcohol impacts such systems. For example, alcohol consumption may contribute to anovulation by increasing levels of estradiol, which, in turn, could result in suppression of follicle stimulating hormone (FSH), which is essential for normal follicular development and maturation. Similarly, the high rates of amenorrhea (complete cessation of menses) found in alcoholic women could be due to alcohol suppressing the release of luteinizing-hormone-releasing hormone (LHRH), or to alcohol-induced stimulation of prolactin or corticotropin-releasing factor (CRF), either one of which could, in turn, suppress gonadotropin secretory activity. These explanations remain speculative (Mello et al., 1989), and future research is needed that more clearly explicates alcohol's effects on endocrine functioning.

Alcohol's effects on endocrine system functioning are not limited to premenopausal women. Associations between moderate and heavy levels of alcohol consumption and increases in circulating levels of estrogen (such as estradiol and estrone) have been found in postmenopausal women (as well as premenopausal women) (e.g., Gavaler, 1991; Reichman et al., 1993; Van Thiel et al., 1989). Alcohol may increase estrogen levels in postmenopausal women by stimulating the production of androgens, which are then converted to estrogen (Gavaler, 1991). The alcohol–estrogen relationship is meaningful when considered in the context that increases in levels of plasma estrogen may be an important mediating factor in the relationship between alcohol consumption and breast cancer (e.g., Longnecker et al., 1995; Zhang et al., 1999). Although beyond the scope of this chapter, there is some support for a dose-response relationship between women's alcohol use and breast cancer, though uncertainty remains regarding the specific biological mechanism(s) underlying this relationship and the precise alcohol use cut-point that confers high risk (see Longnecker et al., 1995; Smith-Warner et al., 1998; Zhang et al., 1999).

Alcohol Use and Infertility

A number of studies have investigated the risk of infertility in women as a function of varying levels of alcohol consumption (e.g., light, moderate, heavy), after controlling for potentially confounding variables (e.g., smoking, caffeine consumption, history of menstrual disturbances). The findings of these studies have been mixed, with some indicating no significant associations between alcohol use and infertility (e.g., Curtis, Savitz, & Arbuckle, 1997; Joesoef, Beral, Aral, Rolfs, & Cramer, 1993; Olsen, Bolumar, Boldsen, Bisanti, & The European Study Group on Infertility and Subfecundity, 1997), and others suggesting that even light to moderate amounts of alcohol significantly increase the risk for infertility (e.g., Grodstein, Goldman, & Cramer, 1994; Hakim, Gray, & Zacur, 1998; Jensen et al., 1998). However, as described below, differences in research design and the timing of assessments may partially account for these discrepant findings.

Three of the studies that found no increased risk of infertility based on levels of alcohol consumption (Curtis et al., 1997; Joesoef et al., 1993; Olsen et al., 1997) requested subjects to retrospectively report on their "time to conception" (i.e., the time from when they began trying to conceive until conception) and their alcohol use around the time they were trying to conceive. The time interval between the occurrence of these events and the study interview sometimes spanned many years. Thus, inaccurate retrospective recall may have biased study findings. In addition, if alcohol has more proximal effects on at least some factors affecting fertility (e.g., current alcohol use affecting hormone levels; e.g., Reichman et al., 1993), then it would be essential to investigate the correspondence in time of alcohol use and infertility. For example, it would be essential to know if heavy alcohol use was occurring simultaneously with difficulties in conceiving. None of the above-mentioned studies tested for this proximal relationship.

In contrast, prospective studies by Hakim et al. (1998) and Jensen et al. (1998) found a significant decreasing trend in the probability of conception with higher levels of alcohol consumption. Hakim et al. studied women across a two-year period (or until pregnancy), collecting data monthly on average daily alcohol use during the previous 30-day period and assaying daily urine specimens for ovulation and pregnancy. They found an inverse relationship between alcohol consumption and the probability of conception, such that increasing levels of alcohol use were associated with a lower probability of conception, after controlling for potentially confounding variables. Likewise, Jensen et al. collected monthly self-reports on alcohol use and conception across a six-month period. They too reported that increasing levels of alcohol consumption were related to a lower probability of conception. In both these studies, light to moderate drinking levels were related to a lower probability of conception, although the patterns of drinking (e.g., binge drinking) were not assessed. Thus, it is not known if patterns of heavier episodic drinking (such as binge drinking) were more closely related to infertility, or if steady, lighter patterns of alcohol use characterized those women with lower incidences of conception. Nevertheless, these studies are important because they collected data on alcohol use that was temporally proximal to menstrual cycles in which conception could have occurred (i.e., sexual intercourse occurred in the absence of birth control), thus providing stronger evidence for the adverse impact that light to moderate alcohol use may have on women's ability to conceive.

Finally, Grodstein et al. (1994) collected alcohol use data on a clinic sample of women diagnosed with fertility disorders, including ovulatory factor, tubal disease, cervical factor, endometriosis, and idiopathic infertility. In multiple logistic regression analyses (controlling for several potentially confounding variables), varying levels of alcohol consumption were used to predict each disorder. Results indicated that moderate (i.e., one drink or less per day) and heavier levels of use (i.e., more than one drink per day) significantly increased the risk for both ovulatory factor and endometriosis. The authors indicated that both these disorders are hormone-associated fertility disorders, suggesting that one pathway by which alcohol may impact women's fertility is via its influence on endocrine functioning.

Alcohol Use, Fetal Development, and Pregnancy Outcomes

Heavy maternal alcohol consumption during pregnancy adversely affects the developing fetus (e.g., fetal growth retardation, central nervous system dysfunction) and is associated with poor birth outcomes (e.g., fetal alcohol syndrome, infant mortality). Wilsnack *et al.* (1984) reported that, in a general population sample of women, those who were heavy drinkers (i.e., drank six or more drinks per day at least three times per week) were more likely to report having had a miscarriage or still birth relative to women who drank at lower levels. In a review of the literature, Abel (1997) reported on animal studies which indicated that BACs at approximately 200 mg/dl or higher produced spontaneous abortions in nonhuman primates and dogs. According to Abel, in order to achieve a similar BAC in humans, a pregnant woman weighing 120 pounds would have to drink about eight drinks in a 3-hour period. Heavy alcohol consumption during pregnancy appears to be an important (but not sufficient) condition to produce Fetal Alcohol Syndrome (FAS) and Fetal Alcohol Effects (FAE) (Abel & Hannigan, 1995). FAS is the leading cause of mental retardation in Western countries, and is characterized by pre- and postnatal somatic growth deficiencies (e.g., deficits in height, weight, and head circumference), central nervous system dysfunction (e.g., brain anomalies such as microcephaly), and distinctive facial abnormalities (e.g., short palpebral fissures, diminished to absent philtrum) (e.g., West, Perrotta, & Erickson, 1998).

The effects of *heavy* alcohol consumption during pregnancy are well-recognized; however, the relationship between *low to moderate* levels of alcohol use and adverse fetal and birth outcomes is less clear. For example, in his review of the literature, Abel (1997) indicated that studies conducted in North America (the United States and Canada) consistently show significant associations between low to moderate levels of alcohol use and spontaneous abortion, but that such consistency is not reported for studies conducted in Europe and Australia. The disparate findings reported by Cavallo, Russo, Zotti, Camerlengo, & Ruggenini (1995) and Windham, Von Behren, Fenster, Schaefer, & Swan (1997) support this conclusion. Cavallo *et al.* reported on findings from a study conducted in Torino, Italy, which showed that varying levels of daily alcohol use (i.e., no use, one daily drink, ≥ 2 daily drinks) did not confer significantly increased risk for spontaneous abortion, after controlling for potentially confounding variables (e.g., age, occupational status, coffee consumption, cigarette use). In contrast, Windham *et al.* (1997) reported data from a prospective study of pregnant women recruited from a large prepaid health plan in California. Results from logistic regression analyses (controlling for maternal age, prior spontaneous abortion, gestational age at interview, and cigarette and caffeine consumption) indicated that consumption of more than three drinks per week during the first trimester conferred a greater than twofold increased risk (OR = 2.3) for spontaneous abortion. In addition, the risk for spontaneous abortion among women consuming ≥ 3.5 drinks per week was higher in the first trimester relative to the second trimester, and was highest during the first 10 weeks of pregnancy.

Abel (1997) suggested that other variables associated with both alcohol use and spontaneous abortion (e.g., poverty, undernutrition, poor health status) were responsible for the alcohol use–spontaneous abortion relationship found in North American studies. While Windham *et al.* (1997) did control for some variables that are associated with spontaneous abortion, they unfortunately did not control for socioeconomic variables. However, their sample of women was selected from members of a large prepaid health plan and thus had access to health care services, suggesting that they may have been a relatively low-risk sample with regard to socioeconomic variables. An important aspect of the Windham *et al.* study is that it identified a period in the pregnancy process (i.e., first trimester) in which the developing fetus may be more vulnerable to the toxic effects of alcohol and thus at increased risk for spontaneous abortion.

In addition to alcohol's association with spontaneous abortions, other studies conducted in the United States have found relationships between low-to-moderate alcohol use (e.g., three to five drinks per week) and fetal deaths, intrauterine growth retardation, low birthweight (i.e., <2500 g), and infant deaths (e.g., Shu, Hatch, Mills, Clemens, & Susser, 1995; Windham, Fenster, Hopkins, & Swan, 1995). The results from these studies continued to be significant after controlling for influential variables (e.g., race, parity, income, maternal smoking, caffeine consumption). These studies are important because they suggest that even low-to-moderate levels of alcohol use can have adverse effects on the developing fetus and on birth outcomes.

Thus, it appears that the teratogenic effects of alcohol on the developing fetus are evident even at relatively low levels of consumption, and these effects may be especially potent early in pregnancy (although alcohol's deleterious effects on central nervous system development occur throughout pregnancy; West *et al.*, 1998). The specific pathways leading from maternal alcohol use to adverse fetal and birth outcomes are not clear. However, Abel and Hannigan (1995) proposed a model in which permissive factors (e.g., low SES, drinking patterns such as binge drinking, cigarette use) facilitate the existence of provocative factors (e.g., poor nutritional status, increased stress, high BACs, products of tobacco smoke); in turn, permissive and provocative factors interact with alcohol use to contribute to fetal hypoxia and free radical formation. Hypoxia and free radical oxidative stress are hypothesized to be important factors contributing to fetal growth retar-

dation, central nervous system disturbance, and other alcohol-related fetal anomalies and birth defects. With regard to fetal hypoxia, Abel and Hannigan suggested that even low levels of ethanol can constrict umbilical cord arteries, and that high BACs (such as those that may be seen with binge drinking) can collapse umbilical vasculature.

WOMEN'S ALCOHOL USE: HEALTH CARE AND TREATMENT ISSUES

A number of important issues arise in medical health settings related to both the identification of, and appropriate intervention with, women who have drinking problems. Many of these issues have not been systematically addressed in health care communities due to historical influences (e.g., beliefs that alcoholism was a "man's disease") and to current cost-cutting, managed health care practices that may not accommodate the comprehensive needs of women with serious alcohol problems or an alcohol disorder. As the prior information in this chapter attests, there are some significant gender differences in the impact of alcohol use on women's health that merit increased attention. As such, this section discusses several health care and treatment issues that may facilitate greater identification and treatment referral of women with alcohol problems and disorders.

Identification of Alcohol Disorders among Women in Primary Health Care Settings

The potentially serious health consequences of heavy and abusive alcohol use for women (e.g., endocrine dysfunction, fertility disorders, alcohol-related liver cirrhosis), and of maternal alcohol use for the unborn child (e.g., FAS, low birthweight, fetal death), suggest the need for aggressive alcohol screening procedures by health care professionals (e.g., primary care physicians), especially those who specialize in the treatment of women (e.g., obstetricians, gynecologists). Yet, the majority of women with alcohol disorders and problems attending primary health care settings go undetected by their physicians (Chang et al., 1998; North, 1996; Stein & Cyr, 1997).

A contributing factor to the lack of identification of alcohol problems among women in health care settings pertains to whether salient symptoms for alcohol problems are identical for women and for men. It has been widely acknowledged that the current symptoms and criteria for alcohol disorders have evolved from clinicians' experiences based on male alcoholic patients, with little or no reference to the drinking patterns, circumstances surrounding drinking, and alcohol problems encountered by women. As such, some of the symptoms may be inadvertently confounded with sex-role-related activities that may be disproportionately enacted by men rather than women (e.g., Dawson & Grant, 1993). For example, more men are in the labor force than women; hence losing a job due to drinking is (everything else held constant) more probable for men than for women. Similarly, higher levels of physical violence are more prominent among men than women, independent of alcohol use; therefore, a symptom based on physical fighting while drinking is more probable among men than women. Women with alcohol problems are more likely than men to present with comorbid affective conditions (e.g., depressive and anxiety disorders) and to have problems in sexual, gynecologic, and reproductive domains.

A practical implication of such gender differences in the expression of alcohol-related symptoms is that health care professionals may be less likely to identify female patients with alcohol disorders or problems because they do not recognize symptoms that are more specific to women (North, 1996; Stein & Cyr, 1997). Research efforts are needed to more closely identify alcohol-related symptoms in women, and health care professionals need to be educated about these symptoms for early identification and treatment. Reliable and valid brief screening instruments that could easily be administered in health care settings do exist for

the identification of women with alcohol problems and include the CAGE, TWEAK, Brief Michigan Alcoholism Screening Test (BMAST), T-ACE, and Alcohol Use Disorders Identification Test (AUDIT) (Bradley, Boyd-Wickizer, Powell, & Burman, 1998). In recent comparisons of various screening measures, the AUDIT and the TWEAK appeared to be the most sensitive in identifying women with potential alcohol-related problems or disorders, and both instruments performed well with racially diverse groups of women (Bradley et al., 1998; Chang et al., 1998; Steinbauer, Cantor, Holzer, & Volk, 1998).

Once a positive screen has been confirmed, health care providers have several options available to them. For instance, Cloud et al. (1997) proposed that women should be informed about the adverse health consequences associated with heavy alcohol consumption, such as gynecologic and reproductive dysfunction. Pregnant women should be advised to abstain from alcohol use during pregnancy. Women who are of childbearing age and who are abusing alcohol need to be informed about the teratogenic effects of alcohol on the fetus, with a suggestion for the use of effective birth control methods until a time when the patient is no longer abusing alcohol. Finally, health care providers should be prepared to make treatment referrals if brief intervention efforts are not effective.

Women's Alcohol and Substance Abuse Treatment Needs

Over the past several decades, there has been an increasing recognition that pregnant and parenting women in treatment for alcohol and substance abuse problems have unique treatment needs that (typically) differ from those of men, including the need for child care availability, health care services (e.g., obstetric and gynecologic services), and parenting and vocational skills training (e.g., Stein & Cyr, 1997). Fortunately, expanded, specialized treatment services for women became more readily available from the mid-1980s to the mid-1990s, in part, because of Congressional allocation of funds for the development of demonstration programs for pregnant and parenting substance abusers (Howell, Heiser, & Harrington, 1999; Schmidt & Weisner, 1995; Stein & Cyr, 1997). Based on preliminary findings of a limited number of evaluation studies, these programs appear to have demonstrated some success in the treatment of alcohol and substance disorders among women due, in part, to longer retention of clients in treatment (Howell *et al.*, 1999).

However, while forward strides have been made in alcohol and substance abuse treatment services for women, there nevertheless remains a shortage of programs that comprehensively address women's multiple treatment needs (Howell *et al.*, 1999). Furthermore, a recent report by Chavkin, Breitbart, Elman, and Wise (1998) raised concerns about continued federal and state support for such programs. Based on data collected in both 1992 and 1995 from state directors regarding treatment services for pregnant substance using women, Chavkin *et al.* found that (a) from 1992 to 1995 there had been an initial positive trend toward increased services; (b) across time there was a shift toward Medicaid managed care, which tended to translate into fewer treatment choices for women; and (c) there was a movement away from federal funding and control toward greater local control and reduced funding of services. The authors concluded that there appeared to be a shift toward reduced treatment services for women, this after an expansion in such services during the 1980s and early 1990s.

In addition to meeting the comprehensive needs of pregnant and parenting women in alcohol and substance abuse treatment, attention to at least three other issues is required for a more comprehensive treatment approach to the sexual and reproductive health needs of women with alcohol problems or disorders. First, an additional focus on the counseling of women with alcohol problems who have experienced sexual victimization is quite important. As reported in a previous section of this chapter, childhood and adult sexual abuse and victimization events occur at high rates among alcoholic women. Nelson-Zlupko, Kauffman, and

Dore (1995) stated that traditional substance abuse programs frequently encourage clients to divulge secrets, with such confessions presumably resulting in a cathartic or "cleansing" effect for the substance abuser. For alcoholic women with a history of sexual victimization, these types of exercises may be therapeutically counterproductive and lead to a feeling of revictimization. Hence, alcohol treatment programs must be sensitive to the therapeutic needs of women with histories of sexual victimization. Roesler and Dafler (1993) suggested that consumption of alcohol and other substances serves as a coping mechanism for substance abusers who experienced childhood sexual abuse and, therefore, these clients must be taught alternative, constructive coping skills to replace their reliance on substances.

Second, heavy and abusive alcohol use and sexual dysfunction are co-occurring problems among a number of women (Beckman, 1979; Klassen & Wilsnack, 1986), and each may reciprocally influence the other as women attempt to self-medicate sexual problems with alcohol, and, in turn, alcohol exerts a suppressant effect on sexual arousal and functioning (Wilsnack *et al.*, 1991). Thus, an additional treatment focus is the education of health care providers, mental health counselors, and patients regarding the interrelationships between heavy alcohol use and sexual dysfunction. In addition, the collection and use of alcohol-related patient information as part of a standard intake interview protocol would provide useful treatment information for physicians, other health care professionals, and counselors in both general medical settings and alcohol treatment settings.

A third area that requires additional focus is the increased awareness and knowledge of the interrelationships among alcohol use, risky sexual behaviors, STDs and HIV, and reproductive problems with heavy drinking and alcoholic teenagers and young adults. Although the more impulsive, immediate satisfaction orientation of many of these youth can make intervention success difficult, knowledge about the potential sexual and reproductive health risks related to current alcohol use and sexual behavior would be an important component of alcohol and substance abuse treatment programs. In addition, counseling young people about these issues within primary health care settings and STD clinics could provide an avenue of effective information dissemination with this potentially hard-to-reach group.

The above discussion is premised on the idea that health care providers and counselors can serve the function of "frontline" professionals to identify women with alcohol problems and disorders and make appropriate referrals for treatment. For women with access to health care facilities, such a system, if implemented, would work effectively. However, for poor women and women of color who do not have ready access to health care services, alternative avenues of identification and referral are needed. Rouse, Carter, and Rodriguez-Andrew (1995) suggested that community health care centers, neighborhood community centers, and churches are useful resources to develop outreach programs to effectively reach disadvantaged women with needed information regarding alcohol and substance abuse treatment services.

CONCLUSIONS

In contrast to prior "male only" myths about alcohol use and serious alcohol problems, many women experience a broad range of health problems related to alcohol use. These problems range from conception and the intrauterine environment, to child and adolescent nonconsensual and risky sexual activity, to adult obstetric and gynecologic problems, to premature death and mortality (e.g., via alcoholic liver cirrhosis, alcohol-related fatal automobile crashes). A particularly startling finding in the literature has been the telescoping effect whereby there is a more rapid progression of the impact of alcohol on organ systems and alcohol-related medical conditions for women relative to men. Furthermore, societal perceptions of

women's drinking may pose increased risk for victimization by male sexual aggressors such that women's psychological and physical health may be compromised. These health risks are especially important given that epidemiologic trends indicate an increase in the number of adolescent and young adult women drinking and the number of women drinking heavily. Because much of our existing knowledge about alcohol use and alcoholism has stemmed from research on men, our knowledge of the correlates, causes, and consequences of heavy alcohol use among women is less extensive.

Of the existing literature on women and alcohol use, it is evident that there are important biological and psychosocial role differences between women and men that have a critical bearing on the etiology, time course, prevention, and treatment of alcohol disorders among women, and that sexual health is a key domain of inquiry. Future research is needed regarding the assessment and diagnosis of alcohol disorders in women, and more fully explicated causal linkages and mechanisms for the alcohol–sexual health associations identified in this chapter. These include systematic studies of the precise mechanisms linking alcohol use to endocrine system functioning, and of psychosocial and cognitive processes underlying alcohol expectancies and stereotyped beliefs about women's drinking and sexuality. Greater attention also needs to be focused on theoretical articulation to account for these interrelationships between alcohol use and sexual health among women, and to the observed gender differences in these relations. Finally, much greater consideration must be given to providing primary, secondary, and tertiary interventions for women to effectively treat alcohol disorders and the sexual and reproductive problems that may accompany the abuse of alcohol.

ACKNOWLEDGMENT. The authors' efforts on this chapter were supported in part by the National Institute on Alcohol Abuse and Alcoholism Grant No. R37-AA07861 awarded to Michael Windle.

REFERENCES

Abbey, A., Ross, L. T., & McDuffie, D. (1994). Alcohol's role in sexual assault. In R. R. Watson (Ed.), *Drug and alcohol abuse reviews: Vol. 5. Addictive behavior in women* (pp. 97–123). Totowa, NJ: Humana.

Abel, E. L. (1997). Maternal alcohol consumption and spontaneous abortion. *Alcohol & Alcoholism, 32,* 211–219.

Abel, E. L., & Hannigan, J. H. (1995). Maternal risk factors in fetal alcohol syndrome: Provocative and permissive influences. *Neurotoxicology and Teratology, 17,* 445–462.

Becker, U., Tønnesen, H., Kaas-Claesson, N., & Gluud, C. (1989). Menstrual disturbances and fertility in chronic alcoholic women. *Drug and Alcohol Dependence, 24,* 75–82.

Beckman, L. J. (1979). Reported effects of alcohol on the sexual feelings and behavior of women alcoholics and nonalcoholics. *Journal of Studies on Alcohol, 40,* 272–282.

Beckman, L. J., & Ackerman, K. T. (1995). Women, alcohol, and sexuality. In M. Galanter (Ed.), *Recent developments in alcoholism, Vol. 12: Women and alcoholism* (pp. 267–285). New York: Plenum Press.

Blume, S. B. (1991). Sexuality and stigma: The alcoholic woman. *Alcohol Health & Research World, 15,* 139–146.

Bradley, K. A., Boyd-Wickizer, J., Powell, S. H., & Burman, M. L. (1998). Alcohol screening questionnaires in women: A critical review. *Journal of the American Medical Association, 280,* 166–171.

Bussey, K., & Bandura, A. (1999). Social cognitive theory of gender development and differentiation. *Psychological Review, 106,* 676–713.

Caetano, R. (1988). Alcohol use among Hispanic groups in the United States. *American Journal of Drug and Alcohol Abuse, 14,* 293–308.

Caetano, R., & Clark, C. L. (1998). Trends in alcohol consumption patterns among Whites, Blacks and Hispanics: 1984 and 1995. *Journal of Studies on Alcohol, 59,* 659–668.

Caetano, R., & Hines, A. M. (1995). Alcohol, sexual practices, and risk of AIDS among Blacks, Hispanics, and Whites. *Journal of Acquired Immune Deficiency Syndromes and Human Retrovirology, 10,* 554–561.

Cavallo, F., Russo, R., Zotti, C., Camerlengo, A., & Ruggenini, A. M. (1995). Moderate alcohol consumption and spontaneous abortion. *Alcohol & Alcoholism, 30,* 195–201.

Chang, G., Wilkins-Haug, L., Berman, S., Goetz, M. A., Behr, H., & Hiley, A. (1998). Alcohol use and pregnancy: Improving identification. *Obstetrics & Gynecology, 91,* 892–898.

Chavkin, W., Breitbart, V., Elman, D., & Wise, P. H. (1998). National survey of the states: Policies and practices regarding drug-using pregnant women. *American Journal of Public Health, 88,* 117–119.

Cloud, S. J., Baker, K. M., DePersio, S. R., DeCoster, E. C., Lorenz, R. R., & The PRAMS Working Group (1997). Alcohol consumption among Oklahoma women: Before and during pregnancy. *Journal of the Oklahoma State Medical Association, 90,* 10–17.

Cooper, M. L. (1992). Alcohol and increased behavioral risk for AIDS. *Alcohol Health & Research World, 16,* 64–72.

Crowe, L. C., & George, W. H. (1989). Alcohol and human sexuality: Review and integration. *Psychological Bulletin, 105,* 374–386.

Curtis, K. M., Savitz, D. A., & Arbuckle, T. E. (1997). Effects of cigarette smoking, caffeine consumption, and alcohol intake on fecundability. *American Journal of Epidemiology, 146,* 32–41.

Dawson, D. A., & Grant, B. F. (1993). Gender effects in diagnosing alcohol abuse and dependence. *Journal of Clinical Psychology, 49,* 298–307.

Ebrahim, S. H., Luman, E. T., Floyd, R. L., Murphy, C. C., Bennett, E. M., & Boyle, C. A. (1998). Alcohol consumption by pregnant women in the United States during 1988–1995. *Obstetrics & Gynecology, 92,* 187–192.

Frezza, M., di Padova, C., Pozzato, G., Terpin, M., Baraona, E., & Lieber, C. S. (1990). High blood alcohol levels in women: The role of decreased gastric alcohol dehydrogenase activity and first-pass metabolism. *The New England Journal of Medicine, 322,* 95–99.

Gavaler, J. S. (1991). Effects of alcohol on female endocrine function. *Alcohol Health & Research World, 15,* 104–109.

Gearhart, J. G., Beebe, D. K., Milhorn, H. T., & Meeks, G. R. (1991). Alcoholism in women. *American Family Physician, 44,* 907–913.

George, W. H., Gournic, S. J., & McAfee, M. P. (1988). Perceptions of postdrinking female sexuality: Effects of gender, beverage choice, and drink payment. *Journal of Applied Social Psychology, 18,* 1295–1317.

Gilbert, M. J., & Collins, R. L. (1997). Ethnic variation in women's and men's drinking. In R. W. Wilsnack & S. C. Wilsnack (Eds.), *Gender and alcohol: Individual and social perspectives* (pp. 357–378). New Brunswick, NJ: Rutgers Center of Alcohol Studies.

Grant, B. F. (1997). Prevalence and correlates of alcohol use and DSM-IV alcohol dependence in the United States: Results of the National Longitudinal Alcohol Epidemiologic Survey. *Journal of Studies on Alcohol, 58,* 464–473.

Graves, K. L., & Hines, A. M. (1997). Ethnic differences in the association between alcohol and risky sexual behavior with a new partner: An event-based analysis. *AIDS Education and Prevention, 9,* 219–237.

Grodstein, F., Goldman, M. B., & Cramer, D. W. (1994). Infertility in women and moderate alcohol use. *American Journal of Public Health, 84,* 1429–1432.

Hakim, R. B., Gray, R. H., & Zacur, H. (1998). Alcohol and caffeine consumption and decreased fertility. *Fertility and Sterility, 70,* 632–637.

Herd, D. (1997). Sex ratios of drinking patterns and problems among Blacks and Whites: Results from a national survey. *Journal of Studies on Alcohol, 58,* 75–82.

Howell, E. M., Heiser, N., & Harrington, M. (1999). A review of recent findings on substance abuse treatment for pregnant women. *Journal of Substance Abuse Treatment, 16*, 195–219.

Hurley, D. L. (1991). Women, alcohol and incest: An analytical review. *Journal of Studies on Alcohol, 52*, 253–268.

Jensen, T. K., Hjollund, N. H. I., Henriksen, T. B., Scheike, T., Kolstad, H., Giwercman, A., Ernst, E., Bonde, J. P., Skakkebaek, N. E., & Olsen, J. (1998). Does moderate alcohol consumption affect fertility? Follow up study among couples planning first pregnancy. *British Medical Journal, 317*, 505–510.

Joesoef, M. R., Beral, V., Aral, S. O., Rolfs, R. T., & Cramer, D. W. (1993). Fertility and use of cigarettes, alcohol, marijuana, and cocaine. *Annals of Epidemiology, 3*, 592–594.

Johnston, L. D., O'Malley, P. M., & Bachman, J. G. (1996). *National survey results on drug use from the Monitoring the Future Study, 1975–1994: Vol. 1. Secondary school students*. Rockville, MD: National Institute of Drug Abuse.

Kessler, R. C., McGonagle, K. A., Zhao, S., Nelson, C. B., Hughes, M., Eshleman, S., Wittchen, H.-U., & Kendler, K. S. (1994). Lifetime and 12-month prevalence of DSM-III-R psychiatric disorders in the United States: Results from the National Comorbidity Study. *Archives of General Psychiatry, 51*, 8–19.

Kilpatrick, D. G., Edmonds, C. N., & Seymour, A. K. (1992). *Rape in America: A report to the nation*. Arlington, VA: National Victim Center.

Klassen, A. D., & Wilsnack, S. C. (1986). Sexual experience and drinking among women in a U.S. national survey. *Archives of Sexual Behavior, 15*, 363–392.

Koss, M. P., Gidycz, C. A., & Wisniewski, N. (1987). The scope of rape: Incidence and prevalence of sexual aggression and victimization in a national sample of higher education students. *Journal of Consulting and Clinical Psychology, 55*, 162–170.

Leigh, B. C. (1990). The relationship of sex-related alcohol expectancies to alcohol consumption and sexual behavior. *British Journal of Addiction, 85*, 919–928.

Leigh, B. C., & Stall, R. (1993). Substance use and risky sexual behavior for exposure to HIV: Issues in methodology, interpretation, and prevention. *American Psychologist, 48*, 1035–1345.

Longnecker, M. P., Newcomb, P. A., Mittendorf, R., Greenberg, E. R., Clapp, R. W., Bogdan, G. F., Baron, J., MacMahon, B., & Willett, W. C. (1995). Risk of breast cancer in relation to lifetime alcohol consumption. *Journal of the National Cancer Institute, 87*, 923–929.

Malatesta, V. J., Pollack, R. H., Crotty, T. D., & Peacock, L. J. (1982). Acute alcohol intoxication and female orgasmic response. *The Journal of Sex Research, 18*, 1–17.

Malatesta, V. J., Pollack, R. H., Wilbanks, W. A., & Adams, H. E. (1979). Alcohol effects on the orgasmic-ejaculatory response in human males. *The Journal of Sex Research, 15*, 101–107.

Mello, N. K., Mendelson, J. H., & Teoh, S. K. (1989). Neuroendocrine consequences of alcohol abuse in women. *Annals of the New York Academy of Sciences, 562*, 211–240.

Miller, B. A., Downs, W. R., Gondoli, W. R., & Keil, A. (1987). Role of childhood sexual abuse in the development of alcoholism in women. *Violence and Victims, 2*, 157–172.

Nelson-Zlupko, L., Kauffman, E., & Dore, M. M. (1995). Gender differences in drug addiction and treatment: Implications for social work intervention with substance-abusing women. *Social Work, 40*, 45–54.

Noble, A., Vega, W. A., Kolody, B., Porter, P., Hwang, J., Merk, G. A., & Bole, A. (1997). Prenatal substance abuse in California: Findings from the Perinatal Substance Exposure Study. *Journal of Psychoactive Drugs, 29*, 43–53.

North. C. S. (1996). Alcoholism in women: More common— and serious—than you might think. *Postgraduate Medicine, 100*, 221–233.

Olsen, J., Bolumar, F., Boldsen, J., Bisanti, L., & The European Study Group on Infertility and Subfecundity (1997). Does moderate alcohol intake reduce fecundability? A European multicenter study on infertility and subfecundity. *Alcoholism: Clinical and Experimental Research, 21*, 206–212.

Piazza, N. J., Vrbka, J. L., & Yeager, R. D. (1989). Telescoping of alcoholism in women alcoholics. *The International Journal of the Addictions, 24*, 19–28.

Plant, M. (1997). *Women and alcohol: Contemporary and historical perspectives*. New York: Free Association Press.

Randall, C. L., Roberts, J. S., Del Boca, F. K., Carroll, K. M., Connors, G. J., & Mattson, M. E. (1999). Telescoping of landmark events associated with drinking: A gender comparison. *Journal of Studies on Alcohol, 60*, 252–260.

Reichman, M. E., Judd, J. T., Longcope, C., Schatzkin, A., Clevidence, B. A., Nair, P. P., Campbell, W. S., & Taylor, P. R. (1993). Effects of alcohol consumption on plasma and urinary hormone concentrations in premenopausal women. *Journal of the National Cancer Institute, 85*, 722–727.

Richardson, D., & Campbell, J. L. (1982). The effect of alcohol on attributions of blame for rape. *Personality and Social Psychology Bulletin, 8*, 468–476.

Roesler, T. A., & Dafler, C. E. (1993). Chemical dissociation in adults sexually victimized as children: Alcohol and drug use in adult survivors. *Journal of Substance Abuse Treatment, 10*, 537–543.

Rouse, B. A., Carter, J. H., & Rodriguez-Andrew, S. (1995). Race/ethnicity and other sociocultural influences on alcoholism treatment for women. In M. Galanter (Ed.), *Recent developments in alcoholism, Vol. 12: Women and alcoholism* (pp. 343–367). New York: Plenum Press.

Scheidt, D. M., & Windle, M. (1996). Individual and situational markers of condom use and sex with nonprimary partners among alcoholic inpatients: Findings from the ATRISK study. *Health Psychology, 15*, 185–192.

Schmidt, L., & Weisner, C. (1995). The emergence of problem-drinking women as a special population in need of treatment. In M. Galanter (Ed.), *Recent developments in alcoholism, Vol. 12: Women and alcoholism* (pp. 309–334). New York: Plenum Press.

Shu, X. O., Hatch, M. C., Mills, J., Clemens, J., & Susser, M. (1995). Maternal smoking, alcohol drinking, caffeine consumption, and fetal growth: Results from a prospective study. *Epidemiology, 6*, 115–120.

Smith-Warner, S. A., Spiegelman, D., Yaun, S-S., van den Brandt, P. A., Folsom, A. R., Goldbohm, A., Graham, S., Holmberg, L., Howe, G. R., Marshall, J. R., Miller, A. B., Potter, J. D., Speizer, F. E., Willett, W. C., Wolk, A., & Hunter, D. J. (1998). Alcohol and breast cancer in women: A pooled analysis of cohort studies. *Journal of the American Medical Association, 279*, 535–540.

Stein, M. D., & Cyr, M. G. (1997). Women and substance abuse. *Medical Clinics of North America, 81*, 979–998.

Steinbauer, J. R., Cantor, S. B., Holzer, III, C. E., & Volk, R. J. (1998). Ethnic and sex bias in primary care screening tests for alcohol use disorders. *Annals of Internal Medicine, 129*, 353–362.

Van Thiel, D. H., Tarter, R. E., Rosenblum, E., & Gavaler, J. S. (1989). Ethanol, its metabolism and gonadal effects: Does sex make a difference? *Advances in Alcohol and Substance Abuse, 7*, 131–169.

West, J. R., Perrotta, D. M., & Erickson, C. K. (1998). Fetal alcohol syndrome: A review for Texas physicians. *Texas Medicine, 94*, 61–67.

Wilsnack, S. C. (1991). Sexuality and women's drinking: Findings from a U.S. national study. *Alcohol Health & Research World, 15*, 147–150.

Wilsnack, S. C., & Wilsnack, R. W. (1995). Drinking and problem drinking in US women: Patterns and recent trends. In M. Galanter (Ed.), *Recent developments in alcoholism, Vol. 12. Alcoholism and women* (pp. 29–60). New York: Plenum Press.

Wilsnack, S. C., Klassen, A. D., & Wilsnack, R. W. (1984). Drinking and reproductive dysfunction among women in a 1981 national survey. *Alcoholism: Clinical and Experimental Research, 8*, 451–458.

Wilsnack, S. C., Klassen, A. D., Schur, B. E., & Wilsnack, R. W. (1991). Predicting onset and chronicity of women's problem drinking: A five-year longitudinal analysis. *American Journal of Public Health, 81*, 305–318.

Wilsnack, S. C., Plaud, J. J., Wilsnack, R. W., & Klassen, A. D. (1997a). Sexuality, gender, and alcohol use. In R. W. Wilsnack & S. C. Wilsnack (Eds.), *Gender and alcohol: Individual and social perspectives* (pp. 250–288). New Brunswick, NJ: Rutgers Center of Alcohol Studies.

Wilsnack, S. C., Vogeltanz, N. D., Klassen, A. D., & Harris, T. R. (1997b). Childhood sexual abuse and women's substance abuse: National survey findings. *Journal of Studies on Alcohol, 58*, 264–271.

Wilson, G. T. (1981). The effects of alcohol on human sexual behavior. *Advances in Substance Abuse, 2*, 1–40.

Wilson, G. T., & Lawson, D. M. (1976a). Expectancies, alcohol, and sexual arousal in male social drinkers. *Journal of Abnormal Psychology, 85*, 587–594.

Wilson, G. T., & Lawson, D. M. (1976b). Effects of alcohol on sexual arousal in women. *Journal of Abnormal Psychology, 85*, 489–497.

Wilson, G. T., & Lawson, D. M. (1978). Expectancies, alcohol, and sexual arousal in women. *Journal of Abnormal Psychology, 87*, 358–367.

Windham, G. C., Fenster, L., Hopkins, B., & Swan, S. H. (1995). The association of moderate maternal and paternal alcohol consumption with birthweight and gestational age. *Epidemiology, 6*, 591–597.

Windham, G. C., Von Behren, J., Fenster, L., Schaefer, C., & Swan, S. H. (1997). Moderate maternal alcohol consumption and risk of spontaneous abortion. *Epidemiology, 8*, 509–514.

Windle, M. (1999). Alcohol use among adolescents. Thousand Oaks, CA: Sage.

Windle, M., Windle, R. C., Scheidt, D. M., & Miller, G. B. (1995). Physical and sexual abuse and associated mental disorders among alcoholic inpatients. *American Journal of Psychiatry, 152*, 1322–1328.

Zhang, Y., Kreger, B. E., Dorgan, J. F., Splansky, G. L., Cupples, L. A., & Ellison, R. C. (1999). Alcohol consumption and risk of breast cancer: The Framingham Study revisited. *American Journal of Epidemiology, 149*, 93–101.

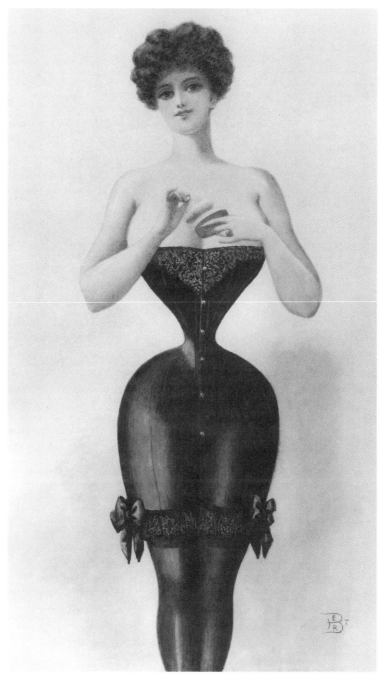

"The Ideal Corseted Figure," by Bert, early 20th c., watercolor (A001 B536). (Reproduced with permission of the Kinsey Institute for Research in Sex, Gender, and Reproduction.) This picture depicts a woman in a corset. An hourglass figure was considered ideal for a beautiful woman at the turn of the century—here the artist has exaggerated the tight lacing of the corset to create an impossibly tiny waist that contrasts with the full curves of woman's hips and bust. The phenomenon of molding the shape of women's bodies with extremely tight corsets was condemned in the late 19th century as a result of the discomfort and unhealthiness associated with the use of the popular undergarment.

II

Epidemiologic, Psychological, Prevention, and Policy Issues in Women's Sexual and Reproductive Health

10

Women's Body Images

THOMAS F. CASH

INTRODUCTION

The psychology of physical appearance is organized around two perspectives—the "outside view" and the "inside view" (Cash, 1990). The first perspective considers how attributes of human appearance, such as physical attractiveness, height, weight, hair color, etc., influence social perceptions, cognitions, and behaviors. From this viewpoint, researchers study appearance stereotyping and seek to understand whether people who differ vis-à-vis certain physical characteristics receive different social treatments and outcomes (Bull & Rumsey, 1988; Cash, 1990; Jackson, 1992). The second perspective is the self-view of one's appearance, which defines the construct of "body image" (Cash & Pruzinsky, 1990, in press; Thompson, Heinberg, Altabe, & Tantleff-Dunn, 1999). Here, researchers examine the roles that persons' perceptions of and attitudes toward their own appearance play in their psychological and social functioning.

Despite humanistic wishes to the contrary, physical appearance can exert both subtle and profound effects on human relations, from the bedroom to the boardroom. Moreover, many of these effects are stronger for women's than men's appearance (Feingold, 1990; Jackson, 1992). Notwithstanding the importance of this "outside view," I believe that the "inside view" has even greater psychosocial significance (Cash, 1990). People's experiences of their own bodily appearance are often very different from how others see and evaluate them. Good looks do not guarantee a subjectively favorable body image; conversely, a plain or even homely appearance is not necessarily associated with a negative body image. A negative body image, however, often portends greater psychosocial adversity than does physical unattractiveness.

This chapter describes and discusses the relationship of body image with various facets of psychological functioning. Because women clearly have more difficulties with body acceptance than men do, the focus here is on women's body-image experiences, (Cash & Pruzinsky, 1990, in press; Jackson, 1992; Feingold & Mazzella, 1998; Muth & Cash, 1997). Much of the current popular and professional discourse about body image concerns its association with eating disorders, such as anorexia nervosa and bulimia nervosa. However, this chapter explores body image as a multidimensional concept in a manner that includes and transcends its role in the eating disorders. The chapter considers the scientific assessment of body image, its psychosocial correlates and consequences, and a model of dysfunctional body-image development. Finally, the chapter delineates a structured therapeutic

THOMAS F. CASH • Department of Psychology, Old Dominion University, Norfolk, Virginia 23529-0267.

Handbook of Women's Sexual and Reproductive Health, edited by Wingood and DiClemente. Kluwer Academic / Plenum Publishers, New York, 2002.

program that combines cognitive and behavioral interventions to promote positive body-image changes.

DEFINING AND ASSESSING THE BODY-IMAGE CONSTRUCT

The study of body image originated at the turn of the twentieth century when physicians could not understand the causes of certain neurological patients' strange bodily sensations. From 1914 to 1940, Schilder shifted the focus from neurological phenomena to the attitudes and feelings patients had about their bodies (Fisher, 1990). At the same time, psychoanalytic professionals expanded Freud's psychosexual theory to understand patients' perceptions of the body as the "boundary" between themselves and their external world (Fisher, 1986).

In recent decades, a clinical and scientific interest in body image has flourished, largely in response to the increasing prevalence of eating disorders. Body image is now regarded as a multidimensional construct consisting of two key components: *perception* and *attitude* (Cash & Pruzinsky, 1990, in press; Thompson, 1996; Thompson *et al.*, 1999). The perceptual facet of body image typically pertains to the extent to which an individual is able to judge his or her body size accurately. Scientists have developed instruments to measure individuals' degree of body-size distortion, whether based on perceptions of the whole body or discrete areas of the body (Cash & Deagle, 1997; Thompson, 1996; Thompson *et al.*, 1999). These assessments range from simple figure drawings or silhouettes to elaborate video technologies that permit persons' to adjust projected images of their own body to convey their body percepts. However, key limitations of these perceptual assessments involve (1) the sometimes poor convergence across different perceptual methods, and (2) the exclusion of self-perceived attributes other than body size (e.g., facial features, height, hair, etc.).

Body-image attitudes are typically assessed by self-report questionnaires that measure people's beliefs and feelings about their physical attributes. Thompson and his colleagues (1999) provide an extensive listing of these instruments. For example, well validated and widely used measures of body satisfaction are the Body Cathexis Scale (Secord & Jourard, 1953), the Body Esteem Scale (Franzoi & Shields, 1984), the Body Dissatisfaction subscale of the Eating Disorders Inventory-2 (Garner, 1991), and the Body Shape Questionnaire (Cooper, Taylor, Cooper, & Fairburn, 1987). The first two questionnaires examine feelings about specific body parts, areas, and functions. The latter two measures focus specifically on concerns about weight and shape (i.e., being fat). Another more comprehensive instrument is the Multidimensional Body-Self Relations Questionnaire (MBSRQ), which contains multiple subscales to measure particular attitudes toward one's appearance, physical fitness, and bodily health (Brown, Cash, & Mikulka, 1990; Cash, 1994a). The MBSRQ reflects the fact that attitudinal body image consists of at least two relatively distinct components (Cash, 1994b)—evaluation/affect and investment.

Body-image evaluation refers to one's level of body satisfaction or dissatisfaction and evaluative thoughts or beliefs about one's body (e.g., appearance). The degree of body satisfaction (or dissatisfaction) depends on the degree of congruence (or discrepancy) between self-views of the body or body parts and one's personal physical ideals (Cash & Szymanski, 1995; Keeton, Cash, & Brown, 1990; Szymanski & Cash, 1995). The Body-Image Ideals Questionnaire assesses this self-ideal discrepancy dimension of the construct (Cash & Szymanski, 1995; Szymanski & Cash, 1995).

Body-image affect refers to the emotional experiences that result from these body-image appraisals. When a person evaluates his or her appearance unfavorably in some specific situational context, dysphoric emotions (e.g., anxiety, dejection, shame, disgust) may result. The Situational Inventory of Body-Image Dysphoria (Cash, 1994d) measures how often persons experience negative body-image emotions in each of 48 situations (e.g., looking in the mirror, exercising, having sex, weighing, interacting with attractive people, etc.).

Finally, *body-image investment* refers to the extent to which one's attention, thoughts, and actions focus on one's own looks, including how much one relies on physical appearance to define one's sense of self. Exemplary assessments of this facet of body image include the following: (1) the Appearance Orientation subscale of the MBSRQ (Cash, 1994a), (2) the Appearance Schemas Inventory (Cash & Labarge, 1996), which taps dysfunctional body-image investment, and (3) the Sociocultural Attitudes Towards Appearance Questionnaire-Revised (Thompson *et al.*, 1999), which measures the awareness and internalization of societal standards of physical attractiveness.

THE PREVALENCE OF BODY-IMAGE DISCONTENT

Large-sample survey research confirms that negative body-image experiences are commonplace in America. Indeed, their prevalence has increased over several decades. From a national *Psychology Today* magazine survey using the MBSRQ, Cash and his colleagues (1986) sampled 2000 individuals to represent the United States population vis-à-vis age and gender distributions. The results revealed that 38% of women and 34% of men were dissatisfied with their overall appearance. Although most respondents were content with their face and height, body weight and shape were clear sources of discontent. In another national survey in 1993 (Cash & Henry, 1995), 48% of American women reported dissatisfaction with overall appearance, in addition to a preoccupation with being or becoming overweight. Garner's 1997 *Psychology Today* magazine survey determined that 56% of the women and 43% of the men evaluated their overall appearance negatively. Eighty-nine percent of the women wanted to lose weight, and 15% reported that they would sacrifice five years of their life to do so. Attesting to growing body-image problems among American women, a recent meta-analysis of 222 body-image studies from the past 50 years found a widening gender gap in body image, with continual increases in women's discontent (Feingold & Mazzella, 1998).

These and other surveys confirm significant gender differences in body satisfaction, especially among young people (Drewnowski & Yee, 1987; Pliner, Chaiken, & Flett, 1990). However, differences extend beyond the body-image satisfaction and dissatisfaction. Muth and Cash (1997) investigated body-image evaluation, investment, and affect among college women and men. Relative to men, women reported greater self-ideal discrepancies, more cognitive and behavioral investment in their physical appearance, and more frequent negative body-image affect. Thus, dissatisfaction with and distress about their looks are more common among women, who are more invested in their appearance as a source of self-definition. Furthermore, gender differences in body-image evaluation appear to be greatest during adolescence and early adulthood, when females are especially vulnerable to body-image disturbances (Cash *et al.*, 1986; Feingold & Mazzella, 1998; Pliner *et al.*, 1990). Although Garner (1997) did not observe greater discontent among young people in his survey, he noted the ironic fact that with increasing body weight among older groups, women's body dissatisfaction did not worsen. Perhaps aging brings a shift in values and a more secure identity that permits divestment of youthful appearance standards.

Body-image concerns are not restricted to the United States. Surveys conducted in other nations, such as England, Australia, and Sweden, reveal that girls and women report substantial levels of body dissatisfaction, especially related to worries about weight/shape (Thompson *et al.*, 1999). In addition to age and gender differences, race is relevant to body satisfaction. In general, African-American women hold more favorable body images than do Caucasian or Hispanic women. For example, Black college women's self-evaluations were more positive both with respect to global appearance and to weight-related satisfaction (Rucker & Cash, 1992). Because a thin female body size is idealized less within African-American culture, they may experience less of a self-ideal discrepancy, even at heavier body weights (Parker *et al.*, 1995). Relative to Caucasian women, they also have a higher threshold for perceiving a body as "fat" (Rucker & Cash, 1992). Cash and Henry's (1995) national survey found Black women to be more satisfied with their looks and less preoccupied with weight and dieting than their White and Hispanic counterparts.

Body-image experiences may also differ due to sexual orientation, yet the research findings are clearer for men than for women. Beren, Hayden, Wilfley, and Grilo (1996) found that gay men had a more negative body image than heterosexual men did. Other studies confirm this difference between gay and heterosexual men (Finch, 1991; French, Story, Remafedi, Resnick, & Blum, 1996; Silberstein, Mishkind, Striegel-Moore, Timko, & Rodin, 1989). Moreover, several studies observed higher levels of appearance investment among gay versus heterosexual men (Finch, 1991; Gettelman & Thompson, 1993; Siever, 1994; Wagenbach, 1997). Among women, some studies revealed no difference in body satisfaction between lesbians and heterosexuals (Beren *et al.* 1996; Striegel-Moore, Tucker, & Hsu, 1990; Wagenbach, 1997). Other studies found that lesbians reported a more favorable body image (Finch, 1991; Herzog, Newman, Yeh, & Warshaw, 1992; Siever, 1994).

THE DEVELOPMENT OF A NEGATIVE BODY IMAGE

According to a cognitive social learning perspective, body image develops as a complex function of various historical and concurrent influences (Cash, 1995b, 1996, 1997; Cash & Grant, 1996). Historical factors pertain to early socialization about the meaning of physical appearance and one's experiences, especially interpersonal experiences during childhood and adolescence, concerning one's body. As a result of these events, individuals acquire basic body-image attitudes that, in turn, serve to predis-

pose how they perceive, interpret, and react to current life events.

Media Influences

American culture's emphasis on beauty and thinness as standards for women permeates all levels of media (Fallon, 1990; Rumble & Cash, 1999; Thompson *et al.*, 1999; Wooley, 1994). The widespread dissemination of these cultural expectations fuels the drive for the "ideal female shape" in girls and women. This quest to achieve the societal standard is so prevalent that it has been referred to as a "normative" process (Rodin, Silberstein, & Striegel-Moore, 1985).

Complicating women's desires to resemble media images of feminine attractiveness is the fact that these standards have changed over time (Fallon, 1990; Heinberg, 1996; Mazur, 1986). Garner and his colleagues (1980) observed that the early 1970s brought a transition of body ideals from a voluptuous to a more lean, angular body type. The researchers examined the evolution of norms of weight and shape among *Playboy* models and contestants of the Miss America beauty pageant, finding that the average weight of both groups of women had significantly decreased over two decades. Both models and pageant contestants weighed significantly less than the average American woman, and pageant winners were thinner than their competitors. Miss America contestants from 1979 to 1988 weighed between 13% and 19% less than the "normal" weight for women their height (Wiseman, Gray, Mosimann, & Ahren, 1992). Moreover, during the 30-year period from 1959 to 1989, there was a growing prevalence of women's magazine articles focusing on weight-loss dieting and exercise (Wiseman *et al.*, 1992). Television advertising has similarly increased its emphasis on weight-loss products and services (Wiseman, Gunning, & Gray, 1993).

Research has demonstrated associations between exposure to these media images and women's body dissatisfaction. The more a woman internalizes such beauty standards, the greater the likelihood that she will feel dissatisfied with her own appearance (Stice, Schupak-Neuberg, Shaw, & Stein, 1994; Stormer & Thompson, 1996). Media messages of the beauty ideal are particularly damaging to women who are highly invested in their looks or who view their bodies negatively. For example, Irving (1990) found that, when exposed to slides depicting thin models, women with bulimic symptoms reported significantly lower levels of self-esteem and weight satisfaction than they did after viewing slides of normal or overweight women. Even among women with subclinical levels of body-image disturbance, the media's portrayal of the "thin and toned" standard has been shown to have a negative effect on body acceptance (Heinberg & Thompson, 1995). This adverse impact occurs in two ways. First, the messages encourage girls to adopt these extreme standards as their own. Second, continued exposure to these "ideal images" engenders social-comparison processes (Stormer & Thompson, 1996). The images are a recurrent reminder to the appearance-invested, body-dissatisfied individual that she is a failure in relation to the standard.

Familial Influences

Expectations, opinions, and verbal or nonverbal messages within the family also contribute to the formation of body image. Parental role modeling conveys the extent to which physical appearance is valued within the family, establishing a yardstick by which the child measures himself or herself. Highly-appearance-invested mothers who value and engage in dieting behavior or engender family competition based on physical attractiveness may promote a negative body image in their daughters (Striegel-Moore, Silberstein, & Rodin, 1986). Rozin and Fallon (1988) have noted a correspondence between the degree of body dissatisfaction and weight/dieting concerns of mothers and their college-aged daughters. Rieves and Cash (1996) also observed that daughters' perceptions of their mothers' body satisfaction, weight preoc-

cupation, and investment in appearance correlated with their own.

The attractiveness of one's siblings may affect body-image development. Having a more attractive sibling may contribute to a less favorable body image, just as having a less attractive sibling may have the opposite effect (Rieves & Cash, 1996). Siblings often represent a social-comparison standard for self-evaluations of one's physical appearance. Siblings, especially brothers, are also frequent perpetrators of appearance-related teasing (Cash, 1995a; Rieves & Cash, 1996). Thus, family members are powerful agents of socialization about the meaning and acceptability of one's physical characteristics.

Appearance Teasing

Appearance teasing is a common occurrence in childhood and adolescence (Shapiro, Baumeister, & Kessler, 1991), and for many persons, such interpersonal ridicule by peers predisposes body dissatisfaction. Correlational evidence confirms a relationship between prior appearance teasing and the existence of a negative body image in adulthood (Cash, 1995a; Cash et al., 1986; Grilo, Wilfley, Brownell, & Rodin, 1994; Rieves & Cash, 1996; Thompson et al., 1999). Such experiences may play a causal role in faulty body-image development and in the emergence of eating disturbances (Thompson & Heinberg, 1993). In addition to teasing, explicit or subtle criticisms about one's appearance may be seen as feedback that one's looks are socially unacceptable (Rieves & Cash, 1996).

Pubescent Changes

Pubertal maturation during adolescence, a period marked by rapid physical change, can influence body-image development. For girls, puberty often begins around 9 to 10 years of age and brings with it adipose weight gain in the hips, abdomen, and breasts (Papalia & Olds, 1992). At about 12 years old, boys enter puberty and experience a broadening of the shoulders, changes in voice, and body growth with increased muscularity. Puberty seems to affect the body images of boys and girls differently. Because boys' physical changes bring them closer to society's standard of "masculinity," they evaluate their looks more positively (Striegel-Moore et al., 1986). However, girls' pubertal weight and shape changes may be experienced as a movement away from society's thinness ideal, resulting in increased dieting efforts and weight dissatisfaction (Attie & Brooks-Gunn, 1989). Furthermore, among girls with early pubertal development and boys with late development, there may be a negative impact on body image and self-esteem (Alsaker, 1992; Brooks-Gunn & Warren, 1985; Thompson et al., 1999).

Body Weight and Obesity

Given society's emphasis on thinness and its prejudice and discrimination against fat persons, it is not surprising that overweight or obese children, teenagers, and adults often struggle with issues of body image and social acceptance (Cash & Roy, 1999; Friedman & Brownell, 1995; Gortmaker, Must, Perrin, Sobal, & Dietz, 1993; Hoover, 1984; Milkewicz & Cash, 2000). Obesity affects females' body-image attitudes more than it does males (Cash & Hicks, 1990; Cash & Roy, 1999; Tiggermann & Rothblum, 1988). Surveys consistently reveal that most women, even average-weight women want to lose weight. Men who desire a different weight are divided between those who want to lose and those who want to gain (Cash et al., 1986; Drewnowski & Yee, 1987; Heatherton, Nichols, Mahamedi, & Keel, 1995).

The age of onset of obesity has been hypothesized to exert differential effects on adult body image. Stunkard and Burt (1967) proposed that juvenile-onset obesity leads to greater body-image disparagement than does adult-onset obesity and maintained that such discontent may persist even after weight loss. Cash, Counts, and Huffine (1990) tested the latter proposition by comparing formerly overweight women with currently overweight and normal weight participants. Formerly overweight women continued to perceive themselves as too fat. They were nearly as dissatisfied with their appearance and

anxious about their weight as were currently overweight women and more than the women who had never been overweight. Termed "phantom fat," the experience of being heavy may persist as a body-image vulnerability even after weight loss. Milkewicz and Cash (2000) similarly observed vestigial body-image effects among formerly overweight or obese women. One determinant of this vulnerability may be the extent of one's weight-related experiences of social stigmatization (Cash & Roy, 1999; Grilo et al., 1994; Milkewicz & Cash, 2000).

Sexual Abuse

Does a history of sexual abuse predispose individuals to a negative body image? In 1990, Rosen observed that the evidence was lacking to support a relationship. Garner's (1997) body-image survey indicated that 23% of women said sexual abuse had adversely affected their body image during childhood or adolescence. Moreover, 30% of women who were extremely dissatisfied with their bodies reported that sexual abuse was an important determinant of body-image difficulties, compared to only 13% of the women who were extremely dissatisfied with their bodies. Albeit provocative, these data are hardly definitive. In a more recent review of the research evidence on this question, Thompson and his colleagues (1999) concluded that "the findings on the role of sexual abuse and body image are conflictual" (p. 237). Much of the inconsistency in the literature pertains to the variability in how sexual abuse is defined and measured. A comparison of "abused" and "nonabused" groups is too simplistic, as it ignores the nature, timing, and duration of the experiences. The causal pathway from sexual abuse to body-image dysfunction is not apt to be a direct one; rather the pathway may depend upon psychological factors "such as self-criticism, control, shame, internalization, and projection" (Thompson et al., 1999, p. 242).

Pregnancy

Pregnancy is truly a body-changing experience. How does it affect body image? Surprisingly, researchers have largely ignored this question. Although Garner's (1997) survey results indicated that about one-third of women felt that pregnancy provoked negative body-image experiences, it is not clear that they described only actual and not anticipated experiences. Davies and Wardle (1994) found more body satisfaction and less weight concern among pregnant than nonpregnant women. However, body-image concerns during pregnancy may be especially salient for teenagers (Sternberg & Blinn, 1993) and for very-weight-conscious or eating-disordered women (Fahy & O'Donoghue, 1991). Perhaps pregnancy constitutes a period of "suspended reality" for most women, in which the weight gain is expected and acceptable. The postpartum period, on the other hand, is the "return to reality" that brings concerns about body weight and shape (Davies & Wardle, 1994; Stein & Fairburn, 1996).

The Role of Gender Attitudes

A cognitive social learning perspective suggests several personality factors that may serve as either diatheses or buffers in the development of a negative body image (Cash, 1995b, 1996, 1997; Cash & Grant, 1996). For example, poor self-esteem, public self-consciousness, and high levels of appearance investment (or "appearance schematicity") may be predisposing factors. One could also hypothesize that having more traditional gender-role attitudes and values might foster greater appearance investment and body dissatisfaction. However, recent research has found that a link between body image and gender-role attitudes exists only with respect to ideology about male–female social relations (Cash, Ancis, & Strachan, 1997). Regardless of their degree of feminist identity, women who endorsed traditional gender attitudes in their social relationships with men were more invested in their appearance, had internalized cultural standards of beauty, and held more maladaptive assumptions about their looks. Women who espouse traditional feminine role enactment in male–female relations exhibit greater eating disturbance (Cash, Strachan, & Roy, 1997). Moreover, believing

that it is their "feminine duty to be what men want," women not only put their body image in jeopardy, they also are more apt to view other women ambivalently, as their "beauty competitors" (Cash, Roy, & Strachan, 1997).

PROXIMAL BODY-IMAGE PROCESSES

Having considered the historical contexts—the developmental, social, and intrapersonal factors—related to the acquisition of negative body-image attitudes, let's consider how such attitudes function within the context of everyday life. According to a cognitive-behavioral perspective (Cash, 1995b, 1996; Cash & Grant, 1996), specific situational cues or events activate cognitive processing of information about and self-appraisals of one's appearance. Such cognitive activity is especially salient among individuals who are highly invested in (or schematic for) physical appearance. The precipitating events may entail, for example, body exposure, social scrutiny, social comparisons, wearing certain clothing, weighing, exercising, mood states, remarks by others, and so forth. The self-appraisals often focus on perceived discrepancies from personal or interpersonal appearance ideals and expectations. The internal dialogues that ensue involve affect-laden automatic thoughts, inferences, interpretations, and conclusions about one's looks. Due to problematic body-image attitudes and assumptions, these inner dialogues are habitual, distorted, and dysphoric.

Subsequently, to manage or cope with these distressing body-image thoughts and emotions, persons may engage in defensive, self-regulating actions. Such adjustive efforts include avoidant and body-concealment behaviors, appearance-correcting rituals, social reassurance-seeking, and compensatory strategies. These maneuvers actually serve to maintain body-image problems via negative reinforcement, as they enable the individual temporarily to escape, reduce, or regulate body-image discomfort.

BODY-IMAGE DISORDERS

Body-image problems may be viewed as falling on a continuum, ranging from mild dissatisfaction to clinical pathology (Cash, 1997; Thompson *et al.*, 1999). For many people, their negative thoughts and feelings about their appearance are merely annoying and are transient. For others, their chronic preoccupation and distress greatly undermine their quality of life. When a negative body image reaches a critical level of severity, it may contribute to several disorders included in the *Diagnostic and Statistical Manual of Mental Disorders* (4th ed., American Psychiatric Association, 2000). For example, body-image disturbance is a central diagnostic criterion for body dysmorphic disorder (BDD) as well as certain eating disorders.

Body Dysmorphic Disorder

This disorder of "imagined ugliness" entails relentless preoccupation with a perceived defect or minor flaw in one's appearance (Phillips, 1996). For individuals with BDD, the obsessive worry and compulsive appearance checking significantly disrupt functioning, particularly participation in social interactions. BDD involves both perceptual and attitudinal body-image disturbances. Individuals who have no discernible physical flaw perceive one to exist, and those who do exhibit a minor defect see it as much more noticeable and "uglier" than objective observers. People with BDD rigidly adhere to distorted thoughts and maladaptive assumptions related to their perceived defect (Rosen, 1995). Although they typically recognize the exaggerated nature of their complaints, their feelings of unattractiveness are profound. They feel continually embarrassed and repulsive to others. Behavioral manifestations of BDD include avoidance of social situations, grooming to hide the perceived defect, recurrent appearance-checking rituals, and efforts to repair their looks, including the pursuit of plastic surgery.

Eating Disorders and Disturbances

For some individuals, being unhappy with their weight or body shape entails drastically

Ashley: A Case of Body Dysmorphic Disorder

Ashley is a 24-year-old college student whom most people would consider to be quite attractive. She is tall, slender, and shapely, with bright eyes and a warm smile. However, these are not the features she sees. Several times each day, for a total of about two hours, Ashley anxiously scrutinizes her face in the mirror. She zooms in on three tiny "scars" on her jaw and chin. Although she "knows" these are practically invisible to others, she feels that they "ruin" her looks. Sometimes she picks at them, reddening her complexion and causing her to feel even more self-conscious. Ashley is also convinced that her hair is getting thin and that her "huge forehead" makes her "stupid looking." Applying concealing make-up and brushing and re-brushing her hair adds another couple of hours to her daily grooming rituals. Once she musters enough courage to leave her house and go to school, she is sidetracked by compulsive visits to restrooms in order to check her hair and face in the mirror. Rather than walk into class a few minutes late and risk others noticing her, she will skip class. Ashley describes her preoccupation with her appearance as exhausting, leaving her feeling depressed and helpless most of the time. Her primary care physician put her on an anti-depressant medication. Ashley has seen four different psychotherapists over the past five years but dropped out each time after only a few sessions "because they just didn't understand."

‑‑‑ ‑ ‑‑

altered eating behaviors. Indeed, a negative body image is a cardinal feature of eating disorders, such as anorexia and bulimia nervosa (Bruch, 1962). A multitude of studies have documented both attitudinal and perceptual body-image disturbances among eating-disordered patients (see Cash & Brown, 1987; Cash & Deagle, 1997; Cash & Strachan, 1999; Rosen, 1990; Thompson et al., 1999). This research further suggests that the severity of body-image disturbance may determine the severity of eating-disordered symptoms and that body-image dysfunctions serve as predisposing, precipitating, and maintaining causes of eating disorders.

What exactly is the nature of the body-image difficulties in the eating disorders? Is it perceptual distortion (body-size overestimation) or attitudinal disturbance (Cash & Brown, 1987; Hsu & Sobkiewicz, 1991)? To shed light on this question, Cash and Deagle (1997) conducted a meta-analysis of 66 investigations of perceptual and attitudinal body image among patients with anorexia nervosa or bulimia nervosa. Relative to "normal" controls, eating disordered women exhibited greater body dissatisfaction and perceptual body-size distortion.

Effect sizes for perceptual distortion were moderate (from .61 to .64) among women with eating disorders relative to control participants. However, body dissatisfaction measures yielded consistently larger effect sizes (from 1.10 to 1.13). Thus, women with clinical eating disorders experience attitudinal body dissatisfaction more than they overestimate their body size. Although anorexics and bulimics' perceptual distortions were comparable, bulimics clearly had more negative body-image evaluations than did anorexics.

Seldom have researchers examined the investment (or schematicity) dimension of body-image attitudes among persons with eating disorders. This neglect is surprising in view of the fact that overinvestment in appearance, thinness, and body shape for defining self-worth may be a central and distinctive feature of eating disorders (see Cash & Deagle, 1997). In addition to negative body-image evaluations, excessive body-image investment is associated with greater eating disturbance among quasi- and nonclinical samples (Brown, Cash, & Lewis, 1989; Cash, 1991b; Cash & Labarge, 1996; Cash, Strachan, & Roy, 1997; Cash & Szymanski, 1995; Szymanski & Cash, 1995).

Kimberly: A Case of Bulimia Nervosa

Kimberly is in her first year of college at a small private liberal arts school several hundred miles from home. During high school she dieted often, in hopes of getting her weight down from 135 to 115 pounds, which she felt would be perfect for her height of 5'6". She says she was always a "chubby kid" and was teased about her weight by her brothers and some classmates. A year ago, she began to binge about once a week on ice cream, cookies, and potato chips. Afterwards she would force herself to vomit and would not eat anything for at least a day. Now at 129 pounds, she says feels really fat and especially despises her stomach, hips, and thighs. She always wears loose clothing to hide her body shape. She nervously weighs herself several times a day. Her bedside table is piled with beauty magazines, depicting the thin models with whom she compares herself until she is too depressed to look at them anymore. Due to her physical self-consciousness, Kimberly avoids the gym and will not dress or undress in front of her roommate. She also hides her binge-purge episodes, which have now increased to four or five per week. Kimberly hates her body and her secret eating disorder. "Tomorrow," she tells herself, "I'm going to stop bingeing and barfing, go on a diet, and get it together." But she's made this decision dozens of times before.

BODY-IMAGE DISCONTENT: SELF-ESTEEM, DEPRESSION, AND ANXIETY

Most people with a negative body image have neither BDD nor a clinical eating disorder. Still, whether as cause and/or consequence, a negative body image is associated with a range of difficulties in psychosocial functioning.

Body-image attitudes and self-esteem are interdependent (Cash & Pruzinsky, 1990, in press). Children, teenagers, or adults who feel negatively about their appearance typically report lower self-esteem, including social self-esteem (e.g., Ben-Tovim, Walker, Murray, & Chin, 1990; Cash & Labarge, 1996; Mable, Balance, & Galgan, 1986; McCaulay, Mintz, & Glenn, 1988; Mendelson & White, 1982; Pliner *et al.*, 1990; Rosen & Ross, 1967). Put simply, if one dislikes one's body, it is difficult to like oneself.

Depression has also been linked to body-image discontent. Marsella, Shizuru, Brennan, and Kameoka (1981) demonstrated that, regardless of age and gender, depressed individuals had increased levels of body dissatisfaction. Noles, Cash, and Winstead (1985) found that depressed college students reported less body satisfaction and rated their own attractiveness less favorably than did their nondepressed peers. Cash and Szymanski (1995) assessed college women's self-ideal discrepancies of body image and their degree of investment in these ideals. Women with greater self-ideal discrepancies and higher appearance investment reported more symptoms of depression. Cash and Labarge (1996) also observed dysfunctional body-image schemas were related to higher levels of depression.

To feel that one's physical appearance is personally unacceptable may lead one to believe that it is also socially unacceptable and that others view one more negatively. Thus, a negative body image could lead to more discomfort in interpersonal relations. Cash and his colleagues (Cash & Labarge, 1996; Cash & Szymanski, 1995) found that women with greater physical self-ideal discrepancies and with more

Janet: A Typical Case of Body Dissatisfaction

In her life of 34 years, Janet cannot recall ever truly liking her looks, especially since adolescence. She's always wished she could be thinner and prettier. She believes that if she had been more attractive as a teenager, she would have been more popular, with more friends and dates. From time to time, she goes on some "new and improved" diet and starts an exercise regimen to lose a few pounds. She changes her hairstyle and hair color every year or so, and she has a weakness for new clothes and cosmetics that promise to make her feel more attractive. Yet before long, Janet's familiar feelings of being plain and fat return. Everyday situations, such as going to the pool or exercise class, parties, or clothing stores, readily become a "body-image minefield." She compares herself to "the beauty queens," mentally reviews and denigrates her own looks, and feels hopeless. When she's stressed about work or in a bad mood for some other reason, she "takes it out on her appearance" and feels particularly "fat and ugly." Although her body image definitely gets her down at times, she's not clinically depressed. Her body-image discontent engenders social discomfort, yet not to the extent of social phobia. While she doesn't have an eating disorder per se, her yo-yo diets aren't especially health promoting. Her displeasure with her appearance undermines her self-esteem—contributing to her sense that she's not quite as good as other women. Body dissatisfaction needlessly lowers Janet's quality of life.

psychological investment in their looks reported significantly higher levels of social-evaluative anxiety.

BODY IMAGE AND SEXUAL FUNCTIONING

Does body image influence the quantity and quality of sexual experiences? It is certainly reasonable to expect an affirmative answer to this question. After all, sexual intimacy entails exposing one's body—"the naked truth"—to another person. The body-concealing adornments and apparel are stripped away for a partner to see and feel the body as it really is. Sex means taking a social-evaluative risk. Of course, the opposite question could also be posed: Does sex affect body image? Whether one's sexual experiences are positive or negative could shape one's own body-image evaluations. Body-image acceptance might be enhanced by the receipt of sexual pleasure and by feeling that the partner is excited by and enjoys one's body.

Regardless of the causal direction(s) in the relationship, the research literature clearly supports a link between body image and the quantity and quality of sexual activities. Large-scale body-image surveys (Berscheid, Walster, & Bohrnstedt, 1973; Cash et al., 1986; Garner, 1997) confirm this conclusion. Other investigators have found that, for both genders, body-image discontent is related to reports of fewer sexual partners, fewer sexual behaviors, more sexual problems, and lower sexual dissatisfaction (e.g., Cash, Beskin, & Yamamiya, 2001; Hangen & Cash, 1991; Schiavi, Karstaedt, Schreiner-Engel, & Mandeli, 1992; Young, 1980). Hangen and Cash (1991) found that body-dissatisfied women reported lower rates of orgasm and more sexually dysfunctional experiences in general.

One mediating process whereby a poor body image could interfere with sexual pleasure and performance is "spectatoring" (Masters & Johnson, 1970), or anxious self-focus on one's physical appearance during sex (Barlow, 1986). Indeed, during sexual activity, persons with generally negative body-image attitudes are more likely to attend to those physical attributes they dislike, worry about their partner's perceptions, and try to hide or camouflage those body areas (Cash et al., 2001; Hangen & Cash, 1991). Hangen and Cash (1991) developed a psychometrically sound measure of these processes, the Body Exposure during Sexual Activities Questionnaire (BESAQ). In a series of studies (Hangen & Cash, 1991; Cash et al., 2001), sexually active individuals who scored high on the BESAQ reported less frequency and variety in their sexual experiences, less sexual satisfaction, and (for women) less frequent orgasms during sex.

Another process whereby a negative body image might interfere with sexual activities and experiences is the projection of one's own feelings about one's body onto the partner's attitudes. Recent research on couples indicates a moderately strong correlation between one's own body image and assumptions about how a partner views one's looks (Rieves & Cash, 1999). This study also found that, for both sexes, these assumptions are often quite inaccurate and are usually less favorable than how partners actually feel. Women and men with a more negative body image underestimated partners' attitudes to a greater degree. Body image was positively related to sexual satisfaction for women but not for men. Perceived partner evaluations correlated significantly with sexual satisfaction for both sexes. Although the partner's actual evaluation of one's looks was unrelated to one's own sexual satisfaction, women who liked their partner's appearance more were more sexually satisfied.

Collectively these findings underscore the importance of body image and associated projective assumptions in sexual satisfaction. This process might also include misattributions based on body image, such as assuming one's appearance is at fault if the partner seems sexually disinterested or exhibits arousal or orgasmic difficulties. Body dissatisfaction and distorted assumptions about partners' perceptions may lead to self-conscious discomfort and avoidance of body exposure during sex, which

Tanya: A Case of Sexual Difficulties

Tanya finally divorced after a troubled marriage of 22 years. She hadn't had sex for the last 8 years of her marriage, due to her alcoholic husband's complete lack of interest. She had always felt that he might have been more interested if she somehow looked sexier. Reluctantly, at the age of 46, she started dating again by answering ads in a singles' magazine. She found that the men would go out with her once or twice before they either stopped calling or made it clear that they wanted a sexual relationship. Earlier in her life she had really enjoyed sex, but now she isn't sure. She feels like "damaged goods," not as sexy, youthful, or firm as she was years ago. The thought of a man seeing her naked makes Tanya extremely uncomfortable. So she avoided the experience until she met Larry, who seems very loving and accepting. Despite his positive, nonjudgmental attitude, Tanya always keeps the lights off during sex and prefers to keep her nightgown on. When he touches her breasts or stomach, she feels intensely self-conscious and quickly moves his hands. Her mind overflows with self-critical ruminations about her physical imperfections and what Larry might be thinking about them. She cannot relax, and an orgasm seems out of the question. She worries about how long it will take before Larry gets bored with her and sees her as unappealing. So now Tanya is having second thoughts about a relationship. "Maybe," she laments, "I'm just too old for this."

may compromise pleasure and performance. Recognizing the likely reciprocal relationship between body image and sex, a good sexual relationship may enhance feelings of body acceptance.

BODY-IMAGE CHANGE

Dieting and Weight Loss

Given the prevalence of weight dissatisfaction among the majority of women in our society, it is no surprise that dieting to lose weight is so commonplace, even among those who are not obese (Brownell & Rodin, 1994; Cash & Roy, 1999; Garner, 1997). Does weight loss effectively improve body image? Remarkably few weight-loss studies have assessed body image—an unfortunate fact that reveals the incorrectly presumed irrelevance of body image as a motive and goal of weight loss.

Some investigations do confirm that better body satisfaction may result from "success-

ful" weight loss. Two studies observed body-image improvements among severely obese patients who lost considerable weight as the result of gastrointestinal surgery (Adami *et al.* 1994; Stunkard & Wadden 1992). In one longitudinal study of a commercial very-low-calorie-diet program, Cash (1994c) found that program completers lowered their weight by an average of 24% and reported substantial improvements in body satisfaction.

Similarly, in a large-sample, 24-week diet-and-exercise treatment of obesity, Foster and his colleagues (1997) found that significant body-image improvements accompanied the mean 19.4-kg weight reduction. Body-image changes were not linearly related to the amount of weight loss. Nevertheless, both Cash (1994c) and Foster *et al.* (1997) documented that a partial regaining of weight at follow-up produced a modest but significant erosion of the body-image gains. Diminished body satisfaction is one of the most frequent "side effects" of regaining weight in obesity treatment programs (see Cash & Roy, 1999).

The substantial weight regains in such programs and the poor long-term maintenance of weight loss (Brownell, 1992; Garner & Wooley, 1991; Grilo, 1996; Wadden, 1993; Wilson, 1994) call into question the durability of their efficacy in promoting body acceptance. Cash and Roy (1999) have argued that by ignoring the personal and social meanings of body weight, programs and practitioners may unwittingly contribute to clients' maladaptive equation of fatness, failure, and body-image disparagement. Reflecting the previously discussed "phantom fat" phenomenon, the ups and downs of recurrent dieting may fuel a vulnerable, weight-based body image. Indeed, obese people with a history of such dieting have a more negative body image (Foster et al., 1997).

In 1992, the National Institutes of Health recommended a shift from the traditional dieting treatments and concluded that "approaches that can produce health benefits independently of weight loss may be the best way to improve the physical and psychological health of Americans seeking to lose weight" (p. 947). An emerging perspective recognizes the necessity of addressing body-image issues in their own right, whether as a component of weight-management interventions or a needed alternative to weight reduction, particularly for individuals who are poor candidates for weight-loss regimens (Brownell & Rodin 1994; Cash & Roy, 1999; Foster et al., 1997; Rosen & Cash, 1995).

Physical Exercise

Physical exercise is another common means by which people try to enhance body appearance and manage weight (McDonald & Thompson, 1992; Moore, 1993; Novy & Cash, 1995). Some studies indicate that individuals who exercise regularly report better body satisfaction (e.g., Cash et al., 1986; McDonald & Thompson, 1992; Tucker 1982). However, Davis and Cowles (1991) concluded that the frequency of exercise among women and older men was not associated with their body satisfaction. Of course, such studies do not permit causal inferences about the effectiveness of exercise in improving body image. Women's motivations for exercise may focus as much or more on appearance and weight management as on fitness and health enhancement or stress management (Cash, Novy, & Grant, 1994; Garner, 1997; Novy & Cash, 1995). Women's negative body-image concerns, especially about weight, shape, or muscularity, may serve to motivate increased exercise behaviors (Cash et al., 1994). Thus, more exercise may not facilitate body satisfaction if the exercise does not help them achieve an idealized slender physique (Davis & Cowles, 1991).

Experimental and quasi-experimental investigations do suggest that regular physical exercise can produce favorable changes in body image and other aspects of well-being for both sexes (Kirkcaldy & Shephard, 1990). For example, in one controlled study of body-dissatisfied women, Fisher and Thompson (1994) found that a combination of aerobic exercise and weight training was as effective in improving body image as was short-term cognitive-behavioral body-image therapy, relative to untreated controls. Koff and Bauman (1997) observed body-image gains for women who enrolled in either a fitness class or a wellness class, but not for participants in a sports-skills class. Hensley and Cash (1995) examined the body-image effects of a 13-week aerobic exercise program for college women. Compared to a matched but sedentary control group, exercisers not only enhanced their cardiorespiratory fitness but they also improved body image, without weight changes. These improvements were sustained 10 weeks later among women who continued regular exercise. Williams and Cash (2001) evaluated the body image over the course of a six-week circuit-weight training program. Relative to a matched control sample, exercisers (mostly women) reported improvements in body image, physique anxiety, and physical self-efficacy, as well as gains in upper and lower body strength. Similarly, Tucker and his colleagues (Tucker & Maxwell, 1992; Tucker & Mortell, 1993) observed body-image benefits among college women and middle-aged women who participated in weight training programs.

In sum, although physical exercise can sometimes promote a favorable body image, exercise is not always adaptive. Compulsive physical activity may reflect a desperate struggle to control one's body weight and appearance (Rodin, 1992; Yates, 1991), including a compensatory pattern associated with binge eating (American Psychiatric Association, 2000).

COGNITIVE-BEHAVIORAL BODY-IMAGE THERAPY

Because a negative body image is a widespread problem that may impair the quality of life, professionals have developed a variety of psychotherapeutic treatments for this problem (Cash & Pruzinsky, 1990, in press; Rosen, 1997; Thompson *et al.*, 1999). Among these therapies, cognitive-behavioral treatment (CBT) has emerged as an effective, empirically sound intervention (Cash, 1996; Cash & Grant, 1996). CBT has proven efficacy as individual therapy (Butters & Cash, 1987; Dworkin & Kerr, 1987), group therapy (Fisher & Thompson, 1994; Grant & Cash, 1995; Rosen *et al.*, 1989, 1990), and a self-help modality (Cash & Lavallee, 1997; Grant & Cash, 1995; Lavallee & Cash, 1997; Strachan & Cash, 1999). Cash's CBT program for a negative body image has gone through four generations of development. The first was a treatment manual from the seminal study by Butters and Cash (1987). The second version was Cash's (1991b) published audiotape program available to mental health practitioners, *Body-Image Therapy: A Program for Self-Directed Change*, which includes four one-hour cassettes, a client manual, and a clinician's manual. In the third version of the program, Cash (1995b) expanded its contents into a self-help book for the public, entitled *What Do You See When You Look in the Mirror?: Helping Yourself to a Positive Body Image*. The most recent refinement of the program, based on empirical data and client feedback, is *The Body Image Workbook: An 8-Step Program for Learning to Like Your Looks* (Cash, 1997). It is presented in a user-friendly format and contains over 40 "Self-Discovery

Helpsheets" and "Helpsheets for Change." The elements of this version of the program are summarized as follows:

The *Workbook*'s introduction elucidates the nature of body-image problems and gives an overview of the program, including evidence of its effectiveness. Problems that require professional assistance are discussed (e.g., BDD, eating disorders, clinical depression).

Step 1 involves taking baseline assessments with a series of scientific measures of various facets of body image. Using interpretations provided for the assessment profile, participants then set specific goals for body-image change.

Step 2 is a psychoeducational facet of the program, detailing information on the nature of body image and the causes of a negative body image. The self-discovery process also includes mirror-exposure activities and an autobiographical summary of participants' own body-image development. Using a "Body-Image Diary," participants learn how to monitor their current body-image experiences by attending to and recording the triggers of distress and the effects that these activating events have on their thought processes ("Private Body Talk"), emotions, and subsequent behaviors. This diary is used systematically throughout the program.

Step 3 teaches "Body and Mind Relaxation," which integrates muscle relaxation, diaphragmatic breathing, mental imagery, and positive self-talk to develop skills for managing dysphoric body-image emotions. These skills are applied in body-image desensitization exercises to increase body-image comfort.

Step 4 identifies 10 dysfunctional "appearance assumptions"—beliefs or schemas about appearance that impact daily body-image experiences. Examples of these problematic assumptions are: "Physically attractive people have it all." "If I could look just as I wish, my life would be much happier." "If people know how I really look, they would like me less." "I should do whatever I can to always look my best." "The only way I could ever like my looks would be to change them." Participants learn to become cognizant of the operation of these core assumptions in daily life and to question and refute them.

Step 5 enables participants to identify cognitive distortions in their Private Body Talk and offers strategies for modifying them. Such distortions include comparing one's appearance to more attractive persons, thinking of one's looks in dichotomous extremes (e.g., fat or thin, ugly or good-looking), and arbitrarily blaming one's appearance for life's disappointments or difficulties. Participants expand their body-image diary to incorporate cognitive restructuring exercises in correcting their distortions and observing the consequences.

Step 6 delineates specific behavioral strategies to alter avoidant behaviors related to a poor body image—avoiding certain activities (e.g., exercising, going without make-up, or having sex), situations (e.g., the beach), or people (e.g., attractive women) that might provoke self-consciousness and body-image distress. Participants also target and modify "appearance-preoccupied rituals," such as repeated mirror checking or excessive grooming regimens.

Step 7 applies the metaphor of interpersonal relationship satisfaction (i.e., a good friendship or marriage) to engender a proactive, positive relationship with one's body. Participants engage in prescribed activities for body-image affirmation and enhancement—for example, pleasurable and reinforcing activities vis-à-vis physical fitness and health, sensate pleasure, and grooming for enjoyment instead of for concealment or repair.

Step 8 concludes the program by having persons retake the body-image assessments and receive feedback about their attained changes. Participants then set goals for further changes. From a perspective of relapse prevention, they learn to identify and prepare for situations that place their body image at risk, especially difficult interpersonal situations.

As previously cited, numerous studies attest to the effectiveness of body-image CBT conducted as individual therapy, group therapy, and self-administered treatment. Outcomes not only reflect body-image improvements, but they also reveal a generalization of positive ef-

fects to self-esteem, social functioning, sexual experiences, depressive symptoms, and eating pathology. Although most treatment studies were carried out with extremely-body-dissatisfied college women, further evidence confirms the efficacy of body-image CBT with obese persons (Rosen, Orosan, & Reiter, 1995) and individuals with BDD (Rosen, 1995; Rosen, Reiter, & Orosan, 1995).

CONCLUSIONS

The quality of our embodied lives can be enhanced or diminished by the views we hold of our own physical appearance. In this society and others, many women invest their self-worth in the size and appearance of their body's conformity to exacting cultural standards of beauty. Women are at substantial risk for body-image difficulties and disorders. Body-image discontent can impair self-esteem, emotional health, social well-being, eating behaviors, and sexual experiences. The continued pursuit of scientific knowledge concerning the development, prevention, and treatment of body-image problems is of paramount importance.

REFERENCES

Adami, G. F., Gandolfo, P., Campostano, A., Bauer, B., Cocchi, F., & Scopinaro, N. (1994). Eating Disorder Inventory in the assessment of psychosocial status in obese patients prior to and at long term following biliopancreatic diversion for obesity. *International Journal of Eating Disorders, 15*, 165–274.

Alsaker, F. D. (1992). Pubertal timing, overweight, and psychological adjustment. *Journal of Early Adolescence, 12*, 396–419.

American Psychiatric Association. (2000). *Diagnostic and statistical manual of mental disorders* (4th ed.). Washington, DC: Author.

Attie, I., & Brooks-Gunn, J. (1989). Development of eating problems in adolescent girls: A longitudinal study. *Developmental Psychology, 25*, 70–79.

Barlow, D. H. (1986). Causes of sexual dysfunction: The role of anxiety and cognitive interference. *Journal of Consulting and Clinical Psychology, 54*, 140–148.

Ben-Tovim, D., Walker, M. K., Murray, H., & Chin, G. (1990). Body size estimates: Body image or body attitude measures? *International Journal of Eating Disorders*, 9, 57–67.

Beren, S. E., Hayden, H. A., Wilfley, D. E., & Grilo, C. M. (1996). The influence of sexual orientation on body dissatisfaction in adult men and women. *International Journal of Eating Disorders*, 20, 135–141.

Berscheid, E., Walster, E., & Bohrnstedt, G. (November, 1973). The happy American body: A survey report. *Psychology Today*, 7, 119–131.

Brooks-Gunn, J., & Warren, M. P. (1985). The effects of delayed menarche in different contexts: Dance and non-dance students. *Journal of Youth and Adolescence*, 14, 285–300.

Brown, T. A., Cash, T. F., & Lewis, R. J. (1989). Body-image disturbances in adolescent female binge-purgers: A brief report of the results of a national survey in the U.S.A. *Journal of Child Psychology and Psychiatry*, 30, 605–613.

Brown, T. A., Cash, T. F., & Mikulka, P. J. (1990). Attitudinal body-image assessment: Factor analysis of the body-self relations questionnaire. *Journal of Personality Assessment*, 55, 135–144.

Brownell, K. D. (1992). Relapse and the treatment of obesity. In T. A. Wadden & T. B. Van Itallie (Eds.), *The treatment of severe obesity by diet and lifestyle modification* (pp. 437–445). New York: Guilford Press.

Brownell, K. D., & Rodin, J. (1994). The dieting maelstrom: Is it possible and advisable to lose weight? *American Psychologist*, 49, 781–791.

Bruch, H. (1962). Perceptual and conceptual disturbances in anorexia nervosa. *Psychosomatic Medicine*, 24, 187–194.

Bull, R., & Rumsey, N. (1988). *The social psychology of facial appearance*. New York: Springer-Verlag.

Butters, J. W., & Cash, T. F. (1987). Cognitive-behavioral treatment of women's body-image dissatisfaction. *Journal of Consulting and Clinical Psychology*, 55, 889–897.

Cash, T. F. (1990). The psychology of physical appearance: Aesthetics, attributes, and images. In T. F. Cash & T. Pruzinsky (Eds.), *Body images: Development, deviance, and change* (pp. 51–79). New York: Guilford Press.

Cash, T. F. (1991a). Binge-eating and body images among the obese: A further evaluation. *Journal of Social Behavior and Personality*, 6, 367–376.

Cash, T. F. (1991b). *Body-image therapy: A program for self-directed change*. New York: Guilford Publications.

Cash, T. F. (1994a). *A users' manual for the Multidimensional Body-Self Relations Questionnaire*. Available from the author, Old Dominion University, Norfolk, VA. Updated manual (2000) available from the author at www.body-image.com.

Cash, T. F. (1994b). Body-image attitudes: Evaluation, investment, and affect. *Perceptual and Motor Skills*, 78, 1168–1170.

Cash, T. F. (1994c). Body image and weight changes in a multisite, comprehensive very-low-calorie diet program. *Behavior Therapy*, 25, 239–254.

Cash, T. F. (1994d). The Situational Inventory of Body-

Image Dysphoria: Contextual assessment of a negative body image. *The Behavior Therapist*, 17, 133–134.

Cash, T. F. (1995a). Developmental teasing about physical appearance: Retrospective descriptions and relationships with body image. *Social Behavior and Personality*, 23, 123–130.

Cash, T. F. (1995b). *What do you see when you look in the mirror?: Helping yourself to a positive body image*. New York: Bantam.

Cash, T. F. (1996). The treatment of body image disturbances. In J. K. Thompson (Ed.), *Body image, eating disorders, and obesity* (pp. 83–107). Washington, DC: American Psychological Association.

Cash, T. F. (1997). *The body image workbook: An 8-step program for learning to like your looks*. Oakland, CA: New Harbinger.

Cash, T. F., Ancis, J. R., & Strachan, M. D. (1997). Gender attitudes, feminist identity, and body images among college women. *Sex Roles*, 36, 433–447.

Cash, T. F., Beskin, C., & Yamamiya, Y. (2001, July). *Body image and sexual functioning in a college population*. Poster presented at the World Congress of Behavioral and Cognitive Therapies, Vancouver, Canada.

Cash, T. F., & Brown, T. A. (1987). Body image in anorexia nervosa and bulimia nervosa: A review of the literature. *Behavior Modification*, 11, 487–521.

Cash, T. F., Counts, B., & Huffine, C. E. (1990). Current and vestigial effects of overweight among women: Fear of fat, attitudinal body image, and eating behaviors. *Journal of Psychopathology and Behavioral Assessment*, 12, 157–167.

Cash, T. F., & Deagle, E. A. (1997). The nature and extent of body-image disturbances in anorexia nervosa and bulimia nervosa: A meta-analysis. *International Journal of Eating Disorders*, 21, 2–19.

Cash, T. F., & Grant, J. R. (1996). Cognitive-behavioral treatment of body-image disturbances. In V. B. Van Hasselt & M. Hersen (Eds.), *Sourcebook of psychological treatment manuals for adult disorders* (pp. 567–614). New York: Plenum.

Cash, T. F., & Henry, P. E. (1995). Women's body images: The results of a national survey in the U.S.A. *Sex Roles*, 33, 19–28.

Cash, T. F., & Hicks, K. L. (1990). Being fat versus thinking fat: Relationships with body image, eating behaviors, and well-being. *Cognitive Therapy and Research*, 14, 327–341.

Cash, T. F., & Labarge, A. S. (1996). Development of the Appearance Schemas Inventory: A new cognitive body-image assessment. *Cognitive Therapy and Research*, 20, 37–50.

Cash, T. F., & Lavallee, D. M. (1997). Cognitive-behavioral body-image therapy: Extended evidence of the efficacy of a self-directed program. *Journal of Rational-Emotive and Cognitive-Behavior Therapy*, 15, 281–294.

Cash, T. F., Novy, P. L., & Grant, J. R. (1994). Why do women exercise? Factor analysis and further validation of the reasons for exercise inventory. *Perceptual and Motor Skills*, 78, 539–544.

Cash, T. F., & Pruzinsky, T. (Eds.). (1990). *Body images: Development, deviance, and change.* New York: Guilford Press.

Cash, T. F., & Pruzinsky, T. (Eds.). (in press). *Body images: A handbook of theory, research, and clinical practice.* New York: Guilford Press.

Cash, T. F, & Roy, R. E. (1999). Pounds of flesh: Weight, gender, and body images. In J. Sobal & D. Maurer (Eds.), *Interpreting weight: The social management of fatness and thinness* (pp. 209–228). Hawthorne, NY: Aldine de Gruyter.

Cash, T. F., Roy, R. E., & Strachan, M. D. (1997, May). *How physical appearance affects relations among women: Implications for women's body images.* Poster presented at the convention of the American Psychological Society, Washington DC.

Cash, T. F., & Strachan, M. D. (1999). Body images, eating disorders, and beyond. In R. Lemberg (Ed.), *Eating disorders: A reference sourcebook* (pp. 27–36). Phoenix, AZ: Oryx Press.

Cash, T. F., Strachan, M. D., & Roy, R. E. (1997, May). *Women's attitudes about male–female relations: Relevance to body-image and eating disturbances.* Poster session presented at the convention of the American Psychological Society, Washington, DC.

Cash, T. F., & Szymanski, M. L. (1995). The development and validation of the Body-Image Ideals Questionnaire. *Journal of Personality Assessment, 64,* 466–477.

Cash, T. F., Winstead, B. A., & Janda, L. H. (1986, April). The great American shape-up. *Psychology Today, 20,* 30–37.

Cooper, P. J., Taylor, M. J., Cooper, Z., & Fairburn, C. G. (1987). The development and validation of the Body Shape Questionnaire. *International Journal of Eating Disorders, 6,* 485–494.

Davies, K., & Wardle, J. (1994). Body image and dieting in pregnancy. *Journal of Psychosomatic Research, 38,* 787–799.

Davis, C., & Cowles, M. (1991). Body image and exercise: A study of relationships and comparisons between physically active men and women. *Sex Roles, 25,* 33–44.

Drewnowski, A., & Yee, D. K. (1987). Men and body image: Are males satisfied with their body weight? *Psychosomatic Medicine, 49,* 626–634.

Dworkin, S. H., & Kerr, B. A. (1987). Comparison of interventions for women experiencing body image problems. *Journal of Counseling Psychology, 34,* 136–140.

Fahy, T. A., & O'Donoghue, G. (1991). Eating disorders in pregnancy. *Psychological Medicine, 21,* 577–580.

Fallon, A. E. (1990). Culture in the mirror: Sociocultural determinant of body image. In T. F. Cash & T. Pruzinsky (Eds.), *Body images: Development, deviance, and change* (pp. 80–105). New York: Guilford Press.

Feingold, A. (1990). Gender differences on the effect of physical attractiveness on romantic partner attraction: A comparison across five research paradigms. *Journal of Personality and Social Psychology, 59,* 981–993.

Feingold, A., & Mazzella, R. (1998). Gender differences in body image are increasing. *Psychological Science, 9,* 190–195.

Finch, C. B., Jr. (1991). *Sexual orientation, body image, and sexual functioning.* Unpublished master's thesis, Old Dominion University, Norfolk, VA.

Fisher, E., & Thompson, J. K. (1994). A comparative evaluation of cognitive-behavioral therapy (CBT) versus exercise therapy (ET) for the treatment of body image disturbance. *Behavior Modification, 18,* 171–185.

Fisher, S. (1986). *Development and structure of the body image* (vols. 1 & 2). Hillsdale, NJ: Erlbaum.

Fisher, S. (1990). The evolution of psychological concepts about the body. In T. F. Cash & T. Pruzinsky (Eds.), *Body images: Development, deviance, and change* (pp. 3–20). New York: Guilford Press.

Foster, G. D., Wadden, T. A., & Vogt, R. A. (1997). Body image in obese women before, during, and after weight loss treatment. *Health Psychology, 16,* 226–229.

Franzoi, S. L., & Shields, S. A. (1984). The body-esteem scale: Multidimensional structure and sex differences in a college population. *Journal of Personality Assessment, 48,* 173–178.

French, F. A., Story, M., Remafedi. G., Resnick, M. D., & Blum, R. W. (1996). Sexual orientation and prevalence of body dissatisfaction and eating disordered behaviors: A population-based study of adolescents. *International Journal of Eating Disorders, 19,* 119–126.

Friedman, M. A., & Brownell, K. D. (1995). Psychological correlates of obesity: Moving to the next research generation. *Psychological Bulletin, 117,* 3–20.

Garner, D. M. (1991). *Eating Disorder Inventory-2: Professional manual.* Odessa, FL: Psychological Assessment Resources.

Garner, D. M. (1997, January/February). The 1997 body image survey results. *Psychology Today, 30–44,* 75–80, 84.

Garner, D. M., Garfinkel, P. E., Schwartz, D., & Thompson, M. (1980). Cultural expectations of thinness in women. *Psychological Reports, 47,* 483–491.

Garner, D. M., & Wooley, S. C. (1991). Confronting the failure of behavioral and dietary treatments for obesity. *Clinical Psychology Review, 11,* 729–780.

Gettleman, T. E., & Thompson, J. K. (1993). Actual differences and stereotypical perceptions in body image and eating disturbance: A comparison of male and female heterosexual and homosexual samples. *Sex Roles, 29,* 545–561.

Gortmaker, S. L., Must, A., Perrin, J. M., Sobol, A. M., & Deitz, W. H. (1993). Social and economic consequences of overweight in adolescence and young adulthood. *New England Journal of Medicine, 329,* 1008–1012.

Grant, J. R., & Cash, T. F. (1995). Cognitive-behavioral body-image therapy: Comparative efficacy of group and modest contact treatments. *Behavior Therapy, 26,* 69–84.

Grilo, C. M. (1996). Treatment of obesity: An integrative model. In J. K. Thompson (Ed.), *Body image, eating disorders, and obesity: An integrative guide for assessment and treatment* (pp. 389–423). Washington, DC: American Psychological Association.

Grilo, C. M., Wilfley, D. E., Brownell, K. D., & Rodin, J. (1994). Teasing, body image, and self-esteem in a clinical sample of obese women. *Addictive Behaviors, 19*, 443–450.

Hangen, J. D., & Cash, T. F. (1991, November). *Body-image attitudes and sexual functioning in a college population.* Paper presented at the convention of the Association for Advancement of Behavior Therapy, New York.

Heatherton, T. F., Nichols, P., Mahamedi, F., & Keel, P. (1995). Body weight, dieting, and eating disorder symptoms among college students, 1982 to 1992. *American Journal of Psychiatry, 152*, 1623–1629.

Heinberg, L. J. (1996). Theories of body image disturbance: Perceptual, developmental, and sociocultural factors. In J. K. Thompson (Ed.), *Body image, eating disorders, and obesity* (pp. 27–47). Washington, DC: American Psychological Association.

Heinberg, L. J., & Thompson, J. K. (1995). Body image and televised images of thinness and attractiveness: A controlled laboratory investigation. *Journal of Social and Clinical Psychology, 14*, 325–338.

Hensley, S. L., & Cash, T. F. (1995, November). *The effects of aerobic exercise on state and trait body image and physical fitness among college women.* Paper presented at the conference of the Association for Advancement of Behavior Therapy, Washington, DC.

Herzog, D. B., Newman, K. L., Yeh, C. J., & Warshaw, M. (1992). Body image satisfaction in homosexual and heterosexual women. *International Journal of Eating Disorders, 11*, 391–396.

Hoover, M. L. (1984). The self-image of overweight adolescent females: A review of the literature. *Maternal Child Nursing Journal, 13*, 135–137.

Hsu, L. K. G., & Sobkiewicz, T. A. (1991). Body image disturbance: Time to abandon the concept for eating disorders? *International Journal of Eating Disorders, 10*, 15–30.

Irving, L. M. (1990). Mirror images: Effects of the standard of beauty on the self- and body-esteem of women exhibiting varying levels of bulimic symptoms. *Journal of Social and Clinical Psychology, 9*, 230–242.

Jackson, L. A. (1992). *Physical appearance and gender: Sociobiological and sociocultural perspectives.* Albany, NY: SUNY Press.

Keeton, W. P., Cash, T. F., & Brown, T. A. (1990). Body image or body images?: Comparative, multidimensional assessment among college students. *Journal of Personality Assessment, 54*, 213–230.

Kirkcaldy, B. D., & Shephard, R. J. (1990). Therapeutic implications of exercise. *International Journal of Sport Psychology, 21*, 165–184.

Koff, E., & Bauman, C. L. (1997). Effects of wellness, fitness, and sports skills programs on body image and lifestyle behaviors. *Perceptual and Motor Skills, 84*, 555–562.

Lavallee, D. M., & Cash, T. F. (1997, November). *The comparative efficacy of two cognitive-behavioral self-help programs for a negative body image.* Poster presented at the convention of the Association for Advancement of Behavior Therapy, Miami Beach.

Mable, H. M., Balance, W. D. G., Galgan, R. J. (1986). Body-image distortion and dissatisfaction in university students. *Perceptual and Motor Skills, 63*, 907–911.

Marsella, A. J., Shizuru, L., Brennan, J., & Kameoka, V. (1981). Depression and body image satisfaction. *Journal of Cross-Cultural Psychology, 12*, 360–371.

Masters, W., & Johnson, V. (1970). *Human sexual inadequacy.* Boston: Little, Brown.

Mazur, A. (1986). U.S. trends in feminine beauty and overadaptation. *Journal of Sex Research, 22*, 281–303.

McCaulay, M., Mintz, L., & Glenn, A. A. (1988). Body image, self-esteem, and depression-proneness: Closing the gender gap. *Sex Roles, 18*, 381–391.

McDonald, K., & Thompson, J. K. (1992). Eating disturbance, body image dissatisfaction, and reasons for exercising: Gender differences and correlational findings. *International Journal of Eating Disorders, 11*, 289–292.

Mendelson, B. K., & White, D. R. (1982). Relation between body-esteem and self-esteem of obese and normal children. *Perceptual and Motor Skills, 54*, 899–905.

Milkewicz, N., & Cash, T. F. (2000, November). *Dismantling the heterogeneity of obesity: Determinants of body images and psychosocial functioning.* Poster presented at the convention of the Association for Advancement of Behavior Therapy, New Orleans.

Moore, K. A. (1993). The effect of exercise on body image, self-esteem, and mood. *Mental Health in Australia, 5*, 38–40.

Muth, J. L., & Cash, T. F. (1997). Body-image attitudes: What difference does gender make? *Journal of Applied Social Psychology, 27*, 1438–1452.

National Institutes of Health (NIH), Technology Assessment Conference Panel (1992). Methods for voluntary weight loss and control. *Annals of Internal Medicine, 116*, 942–949.

Noles, S. W., Cash, T. F., Winstead, B. A. (1985). Body image, physical attractiveness, and depression. *Journal of Consulting and Clinical Psychology, 53*, 88–94.

Novy, P. L., & Cash, T. F. (1995). *Exercise patterns and motivations of college men and women: Factor analysis and further validation of the Reasons for Exercise Inventory.* Paper presented at the conference of the American Psychological Society, Washington, DC.

Papalia, D. E., & Olds, S. W. (1992). *Human development* (5th ed.). New York: McGraw-Hill.

Parker, S., Nichter, M., Nichter, M., Vuckovic, N., Sims, C., & Ritenbaugh, C. (1995). Body image and weight concerns among African American and white adolescent females: Differences that make a difference. *Human Organization, 54*, 103–114.

Phillips, K. A. (1996). *The broken mirror: Understanding and treating body dysmorphic disorder.* New York: Oxford University Press.

Pliner, P., Chaiken, S., & Flett, G. L. (1990). Gender differences in concern with body weight and physical appearance over the life span. *Personality and Social Psychology Bulletin, 16,* 263–273.

Rieves, L., & Cash, T. F. (1996). Social developmental factors and women's body-image attitudes. *Journal of Social Behavior and Personality, 11,* 63–78.

Rieves, L. C., & Cash, T. F. (1999). *Do you see what I see?: A study of actual and perceived physical appearance attitudes in romantic relationships.* Unpublished manuscript, Old Dominion University, Norfolk, VA.

Rodin, J. (1992). *Body traps.* New York: William Morrow.

Rodin, J., Silberstein, L., & Striegel-Moore, R. (1985). Women and weight: A normative discontent. *Nebraska Symposium on Motivation, 32,* 267–307.

Rosen, G. M., & Ross, A. O. (1967). Relationship of body image to self-concept. *Journal of Consulting and Clinical Psychology, 32,* 100.

Rosen, J. C. (1990). Body-image disturbance in eating disorders. In T. F. Cash & T. Pruzinsky (Eds.), *Body images: Development, deviance, and change* (pp. 190–216). New York: Guilford Press.

Rosen, J. C. (1995). The nature of body dysmorphic disorder and treatment with cognitive behavior therapy. *Cognitive and Behavioral Practice, 2,* 143–166.

Rosen, J. C. (1997). Cognitive-behavioral body image therapy. In D. M. Garner & P. E. Garfinkel (Eds.), *Handbook of treatment for eating disorders* (2nd ed.) (pp. 188–201). New York: Guilford Press.

Rosen, J. C., Cado, S., Silberg, N. T., Srebnik, D., & Wendt, S. (1990). Cognitive behavior therapy with and without size perception training for women with body image disturbance. *Behavior Therapy, 21,* 481–498.

Rosen, J. C., & Cash, T. F. (1995). Learning to have a better body image. *Weight Control Digest, 5,* 409 & 412–416.

Rosen, J. C., Orosan, P., & Reiter, J. (1995). Cognitive behavior therapy for negative body image in obese women. *Behavior Therapy, 26,* 25–42.

Rosen, J. C., Reiter, J., & Orosan, P. (1995). Cognitive-behavioral body image therapy for body dysmorphic disorder. *Journal of Consulting and Clinical Psychology, 63,* 263–269.

Rosen, J. C., Saltzberg, E., & Srebnik, D. (1989). Cognitive behavior therapy for negative body image. *Behavior Therapy, 20,* 393–404.

Rozin, P., & Fallon, A. (1988). Body image, attitudes to weight, and misperceptions of figure preferences of the opposite sex: A comparison of men and women in two generations. *Journal of Abnormal Psychology, 97,* 342–345.

Rucker, C. E., & Cash, T. F. (1992). Body images, body-size perceptions, and eating behaviors among African-American and White college women. *International Journal of Eating Disorders, 12,* 291–299.

Rumble, A., & Cash, T. F. (1999). *Beauty versus the beast: Images of good and evil in children's animation films.* Unpublished manuscript, Old Dominion University, Norfolk, VA.

Schiavi, R., Karstaedt, A., Schreiner-Engel, P., & Mandeli, J. (1992). Psychometric characteristics of individuals with sexual dysfunction and their partners. *Journal of Sex and Marital Therapy, 18,* 219–230.

Secord, P. F., & Jourard, S. M. (1953). The appraisal of body-cathexis: Body-cathexis and the self. *Journal of Consulting Psychology, 17,* 343–347.

Shapiro, J. P., Baumeister, R. F., & Kessler, J. W. (1991). A three component model of children's teasing: Aggression, humor, and ambiguity. *Journal of Social and Clinical Psychology, 10,* 459–472.

Silberstein, L. R., Mishkind, M. E., Striegel-Moore, R. H., Timko, C., & Rodin, J. (1989). Men and their bodies: A comparison of homosexual and heterosexual men. *Psychosomatic Medicine, 51,* 337–346.

Siever, M. D. (1994). Sexual orientation and gender as factors in socioculturally acquired vulnerability to body dissatisfaction and eating disorders. *Journal of Consulting and Clinical Psychology, 62,* 252–260.

Stein, A., & Fairburn, C. G. (1996). Eating habits and attitudes in the postpartum period. *Psychosomatic Medicine, 58,* 321–325.

Sternberg, L., & Blinn, L. (1993). Feelings about self and body image during adolescent pregnancy. *Families in Society, 74,* 282–290.

Stice, E., Schupak-Neuberg, E., Shaw, H., & Stein, R. (1994). Relation of media exposure to eating disorder symptomatology: An examination of mediating mechanisms. *Journal of Abnormal Psychology, 103,* 836–840.

Stormer, S. M., & Thompson, J. K. (1996). Explanations of body image disturbance: A test of maturational status, negative verbal commentary, social comparison, and sociocultural hypotheses. *International Journal of Eating Disorders, 19,* 193–202.

Strachan, M. D., & Cash, T. F. (1999, June). *Cognitive-behavioral self-help for a negative body image: A components analysis.* Poster presented at the convention of the American Psychological Society, Denver, CO.

Striegel-Moore, R. H., Silberstein, L. R., & Rodin, J. (1986). Toward an understanding of risk factors for bulimia. *American Psychologist, 41,* 246–263.

Striegel-Moore, R. H., Tucker, N., & Hsu, J. (1990). Body image dissatisfaction and disordered eating in lesbian college students. *International Journal of Eating Disorders, 9,* 493–500.

Stunkard, A., & Burt, V. (1967). Obesity and the body image: II. Age at onset of disturbances in the body image. *American Journal of Psychiatry, 123,* 1443–1447.

Stunkard, A. J., & Wadden, T. A. (1992). Psychological aspects of severe obesity. *American Journal of Clinical Nutrition, 55,* 524S–532S.

Szymanski, M. L., & Cash, T. F. (1995). Body-image disturbance and self-discrepancy theory: Expansion of the body-image ideals questionnaire. *Journal of Social and Clinical Psychology, 14*, 134–146.

Thompson, J. K. (1996). Assessing body image disturbance: Measures, methodology, and implementation. In J. K. Thompson (Ed.), *Body image, eating disorders, and obesity* (pp. 49–82). Washington, DC: American Psychological Association.

Thompson, J. K., & Heinberg, L. J. (1993). Preliminary test of two hypotheses of body image disturbance. *International Journal of Eating Disorders, 14*, 59–63.

Thompson, J. K., Heinberg, L. J., Altabe, M., & Tantleff-Dunn, S. (1999). *Exacting beauty: Theory, assessment, and treatment of body image disturbance.* Washington, DC: American Psychological Association.

Tiggemann, M., & Rothblum, E. D. (1988). Gender differences in social consequences of perceived overweight in the United States and Australia. *Sex Roles, 18*, 75–86.

Tucker, L. A. (1982). Effect of a weight-training program on the self-concepts of college males. *Perceptual and Motor Skills, 54*, 1055–1061.

Tucker, L. A., & Maxwell, K. (1992). Effects of weight training on the emotional well-being and body image of females: Predictors of greatest benefit. *American Journal of Health Promotion, 6*, 338–344.

Tucker, L. A., & Mortell, R. (1993). Comparison of the effects of walking and weight training programs on body image in middle-aged women: An experimental study. *American Journal of Health Promotion, 8*, 34–42.

Wadden, T. A. (1993). Treatment of obesity by moderate and severe caloric restriction: Results of clinical research trials. *Annals of Internal Medicine, 119*, 688–693.

Wagenbach, P. M. (1997). *Relationship between body image, sexual orientation, and gay identity.* Unpublished doctoral dissertation, Virginia Consortium Program in Clinical Psychology, Virginia Beach, VA.

Williams, P., & Cash, T. F. (2001). The effects of a circuit weight training program on the body images of college students. *International Journal of Eating Disorders, 30*, 75–82.

Wilson, G. T. (1994). Behavioral treatment of obesity: Thirty years and counting. *Advances in Behaviour Research and Therapy, 16*, 31–75.

Wiseman, C. V., Gunning, F. M., & Gray, J. J. (1993). Increasing pressure to be thin: 19 years of diet products in television commercials. *Eating Disorders: The Journal of Treatment and Prevention, 1*, 52–61.

Wiseman, C. V., Gray, J. J., Mosimann, J. E., & Ahren, A. H. (1992). Cultural expectations of thinness in women: An update. *International Journal of Eating Disorders, 11*, 85–89.

Wooley, O. W. (1994). … and man created "woman": Representations of women's bodies in Western culture. In P. Fallon, M. A. Katzman, & S. C. Wooley (Eds.), *Feminist perspectives on eating disorders* (pp. 17–52). New York: Guilford Press.

Yates, A. (1991). *Compulsive exercise and the eating disorders: Toward an integrated theory of activity.* New York: Brunner/Mazel.

Young, M. (1980). Body image and females' sexual behavior. *Perceptual and Motor Skills, 50*, 425–426.

11

Sexual Abuse

GAIL E. WYATT, JENNIFER VARGAS CARMONA,
TAMRA BURNS LOEB, ARMIDA AYALA,
and DOROTHY CHIN

INTRODUCTION

At first glance, Mrs. Green presented complaints similar to many other women. After being a "no-show" at other doctors' offices, Mrs. Green finally kept an appointment with an obstetrician–gynecologist (OB-GYN). Her complaints ranged from extended and boring waiting room delays and discourteous medical staff to the difficulty and expense of parking. She also perceived doctors as incompetent, who could not seem to find out what ailed her. Nobody could diagnose the basis for her pelvic pain, the menstrual problems that she had for years and the discomfort she experienced during intercourse. One of the reasons that finally brought her to the doctor was to get some sleeping and diet pills, since she rarely had time to exercise and lose the "baby fat" that she gained during pregnancy.

Her sexual history revealed that she was currently married and using birth control. However, she often forgot and doubled up on the pills, or would just give her body a "rest" and did not take them at all. Before her marriage eight months ago, she had dated many men with whom she had both unprotected vaginal, oral and anal sex and had some "lost weekends" partying with drugs and alcohol. Once, she woke up and found semen around her vagina. While she suspected that someone had taken advantage of her, she had no idea who that someone would have been. Regardless of the trauma of being violated by an unknown person, she considered her past sexual exploits necessary in order to discover her sexuality. She wanted to find a partner with whom she could have a good sex life. Mrs. Green

GAIL E. WYATT, JENNIFER VARGAS CARMONA,
TAMRA BURNS LOEB, ARMIDA AYALA, and
DOROTHY CHIN • Department of Psychiatry and Biobehavioral Sciences, University of California at Los Angeles, Los Angeles, California 90024-1759.

Handbook of Women's Sexual and Reproductive Health, edited by Wingood and DiClemente. Kluwer Academic / Plenum Publishers, New York, 2002.

had been pregnant three times: one pregnancy resulted in the birth of her five-year-old son, and the others ended in abortions.

Sex with her husband had always been painful. She had difficulty becoming aroused before intercourse, and was often not lubricated. She also complained to her husband that he was "too rough" and had yet to experience an orgasm. He had become so frustrated that he rarely initiated sex and when he did, he tried to ignore her complaints, feeling that he was entitled to sex with his wife.

Her health history revealed that Mrs. Green smoked cigarettes, and used marijuana for years, but cut back while pregnant, and drank "mostly on the weekends." However, she was plagued with persistent headaches and had trouble sleeping. As a result, she was often tired and couldn't get out of bed, symptoms she attributed to having a young and active son and "too many things to do."

When asked about her family, Mrs. Green admitted that she was not close to her mother and older sister. She had not spoken to her father for years. He had sexually abused her over a period of two years. When she finally told her mother and sister, both advised her against telling anyone else.

Mrs. Green had attempted to manage her abdominal and menstrual problems with over-the-counter remedies, which rarely helped. She also reported having a history of recurrent bladder infections for which no current remedies alleviated. She admitted that she has not received regular care from an OB-GYN or general practitioner. Even when she was pregnant with her son, she only saw a doctor "when she knew something was wrong." Her lack of consistent care was now bothering her. Recently, she had been informed that one of her past sexual partners had died of AIDS. She had not disclosed her fears to her husband, and was reluctant to ask her physician to test her for HIV. Instead, she chose to put the matter out of her mind and to have sex less frequently with her husband. Her reasoning was that with fewer sexual contacts, he probably would not get infected, even if she were HIV positive. She never considered the possibility that her son might have been exposed to HIV.

While none of the problems that Mrs. Green presented are unique, these characteristics are not usually associated with a history of child sexual abuse or the physical, sexual and psychological effects that sometimes occur in the aftermath. This chapter will describe the prevalence and circumstances of sexual abuse before and since the age of 18 and the associated sexual, gynecological, health, and specifically, the reproductive problems that can increase risks for lasting effects on women's psychological well-being. The meanings ascribed to abuse experiences which may vary according to cultural definitions and beliefs will be discussed to better understand the needs of women from diverse cultural backgrounds. Programs and issues regarding primary and secondary prevention, health policy implications and suggestions for future research will also be discussed.

It is important to acknowledge that women's health has a ripple effect. What happens to their bodies can set a template for risks that they will continue to encounter. The health and well-being of their children and their ability to take care of themselves and others can also be compromised. For the purposes of this chapter, we adapt a developmental approach to understanding sexual abuse. Previous research has documented that experiences that occur in early life are associated with revictimization (Wyatt, 1991.) Thus, this chapter will cover the spectrum of incidents and their potential effects in adulthood as well.

EPIDEMIOLOGY

Prevalence of Child Sexual Abuse

Clinical and community samples reveal that one in three African-American, European-American, and Latina women report at least one incident of sexual abuse prior to age 18. Approximately 30 percent of women with sexual abuse histories report two or more incidents (Romero, Wyatt, Loeb, Carmona, & Solis, 1999; Wyatt, Loeb, Ganz, & Desmond, 1997). Higher rates of sexual revictimization, which is associated with negative sexual outcomes, have also been noted among women with child abuse histories (Johnsen & Harlow, 1996; Urquiza & Goodlin-Jones, 1994; Wyatt, Guthrie, & Notgrass, 1992). Women with histories of abuse as children and as adults have greater psychological distress and more physical symptoms than those who report abuse only as a child or as an adult (McCauley *et al.*, 1997). Experiencing two or more incidents of child sexual abuse in childhood is predictive of a risky pattern of behavior, including engaging in early first intercourse, perceiving first intercourse negatively, having more sexual partners, being less satisfied with sexual relationships, and having greater numbers of unintended pregnancies in adulthood (Wyatt, Ganz, & Loeb, 1998).

Circumstances of Child Sexual Abuse

In one community sample, over half of the women reported very severe abuse incidents, including attempted or completed oral sex, anal sex, or rape, and digital penetration. African-American and European-American women (approximately 75%) reported higher rates of very severe abuse than Latina women (over 50%). Among African-American and European-American breast cancer survivors, approximately 15–20% of women reported incidents which were physically violent (Ganz, Wyatt, Loeb, & Desmond, 2000). Despite the severity of abuse incidents, the majority of women do not disclose the sexual abuse incident(s) to anyone (Wyatt & Loeb, 1997; Romero, Wyatt, Loeb,

Carmona, & Solis, 1998; Wyatt, Loeb, Romero, Solis & Carmona, 1998; Romero, Wyatt, Loeb, Carmona & Solis, 1999). Rates of nondisclosure over time do not appear to differ by ethnicity (Wyatt, Loeb, Ganz, & Desmond, 2000).

Many women report sexual abuse at the hands of a family member. More than a third of African-American and European-American women, and almost half of Latinas reported interfamilial abuse (Wyatt & Loeb, 1997; Wyatt, Loeb, Romero, Solis & Carmona, 1998; Wyatt, Loeb, Ganz, & Desmond, 2000). In one study, four Latinas reported marrying their alleged perpetrator; three of whom described being forced or pressured to marry by their families of origin (Romero, Wyatt, Loeb, Carmona, & Solis, 1999). This pattern stems from a lack of education of parents and health professionals regarding the potential lasting effects. A coercive sexual relationship can negatively influence women's sexual, reproductive and psychological health. Approximately one third to one half of women report lasting effects of abuse incidents (Wyatt & Loeb, 1997; Romero, Wyatt, Loeb, Carmona, & Solis, 1998; Wyatt, Loeb, Romero, Solis, & Carmona, 1998; Wyatt, Loeb, Ganz, & Desmond, 2000).

Nationally, incidents that were reported provide a different perspective. In 1993, The U.S. Department of Health and Human Services (1999) estimates that over 217,000 children were sexually abused under the Harm Standard (i.e., demonstrated harm has been suffered). For this estimate, sexual abuse included a wide range of behaviors, including exposure, inappropriate fondling, genital molestation, intrusion, and unspecified sexual molestation. Females were more likely to be the targets of child sexual abuse than males, and perpetrators were male in 75% of the child sexual abuse cases. Child sexual abuse cases made up approximately 13% of all substantiated or indicated cases of child abuse and neglect (U.S. Department of Health and Human Services, 1999).

Variations in CSA Definitions

Each state in the United States has statutes identifying the kind of sexual acts that are considered to be illegal with minors, and variations in these statutes require a careful examination of state provisions, along with the penalty for such crimes. Likewise, definitions of sexual abuse tend not to be uniform in research. Some do not include any definition of the types of experiences that are considered to be abusive. Others vary on the upper age limit of childhood: Some have used age 14 (Briere & Runtz, 1986), and others age 16 (Finkelhor, 1979). Russell (1983) and Wyatt (1985) used age 17, in accordance with the legal age of adulthood in the United States. Differences in criteria have implications for treatment of survivors. Interventions for girls in early adolescence will differ for those who are in late adolescence or early adulthood. The severity of the abuse may also influence the scope and depth of treatment needed. Finally, decisions about child welfare will also be affected by the age of the victims for the duration of these incidents.

Definitions also vary on the age difference between the perpetrator and the victim. For example, a 5-year age span between victims up to age 12 and perpetrators, and 10 years between adolescents and their perpetrators is sometimes used to ensure data collection of incidents with coercion between younger victims and their adult perpetrators (Finkelhor, 1979). In another study, the definition of abusive experiences during adolescence by perpetrators who were not related to victims (extrafamilial abuse) was limited to incidents of completed or attempted forcible rape (Russell, 1983). Wyatt's definition of abuse differentiated between childhood and adolescent victims on the issue of consent.

Child Safety

The National Institute of Justice (1997) reports that the level of intervention needed is usually decided by individual case workers, or in very severe cases, the courts. Child safety may be achieved by removing the child from the home, short or long-term placement, short-term intensive in-home assessment and service provision to the family and the child, or providing the child and his or her family with access to long-term community-based services. Interventions strive to achieve three potentially conflicting aims, including ensuring the child is safe, preserving the child's family, and providing a means of permanent placement of the child.

Historical Trends

Even though studies of the population reporting sexual abuse during childhood (prevalence rates) date back to 1929 in the United States (Hamilton, 1929; Landis & Bolles, 1940), most of the research on child sexual abuse and its effects have been conducted in the last 20 years. Coincidentally, early case studies of human sexual behavior were also just beginning in the 1920s and 1930s (Davis, 1929; Dickinson, 1933; Hamilton, 1929, 1936; Landis & Bolles, 1940; Terman *et al.*, 1938). Studies of the human sexual experience in clinical and nonclinical samples have proliferated ever since. Much of the research, however, has been conducted as if these were two distinct areas of study; consensual and nonconsensual sexual experiences. Indeed, few studies include sexual abuse as one of the experiences that could or should be reported within the context of sexual history taking. Likewise, few studies of child sexual abuse examine the specific effects on other sexual practices.

Sexual Abuse across the Decades

In 1994, incidents involving body contact reported by a community sample of African-American and European-American women were compared to incidents obtained from women with similar demographic characteristics from comparable data. Although no significant difference in prevalence rates was noted over the ten year period, women were more likely to report experiencing very severe abuse (attempted or completed oral sex, anal sex, or rape, and digital penetration) in 1994 than in 1984. The odds of European-American women not disclosing child sexual abuse were five times greater in 1994 than in 1984 (Wyatt, Loeb, Romero, Solis, & Carmona, 1998). The findings further suggested that incidents of abuse may be becoming more severe (Wyatt, Loeb, Ganz, & Desmond, 2000), also reported that African-American women age 50 and older experienced less abuse that was penetrative than those under the age of 50 (Wyatt, Loeb, Ganz, & Desmond, 2000). Those results confirm that sexual abuse may be more intrusive for younger rather than older women.

Issues of Consent

Incidents involving a victim 12 years or younger are included as sexual abuse, regardless of the victim's consent, because children cannot understand sex-related incidents in which they are being asked to participate. Incidents occurring with victims ages 13 to 17 that were non-consensual and involved coercion, regardless of the age of the perpetrator were also included, in order to examine the prevalence of peer abuse by adolescent perpetrators. Much more attention has been given to definitions of abuse among female victims–male perpetrators rather than male victims–female perpetrators dyads. It is also important to acknowledge that females can be sexually aggressive (Risin & Koss, 1987). A national study of the prevalence of sexual abuse among male college students used *any* one of the following criteria for sexual abuse: (a) if there was a significant age discrepancy between the child and another person: (i.e., five or more years older for boys under 12, eight or more years older for boys 13 and older); (b) if some form of coercion was used to obtain the participation of the victims (with candy, money, threats, or physical force); or (c) if the other person was a care giver or an authority figure, including baby-sitters, members of the family, or teachers.

Variations by Sample

Variations in definitions of child sexual abuse will clearly influence prevalence rates (Wyatt & Peters, 1986). Similarly, prevalence rates also tend to vary according to the type of sample used (Wyatt & Peters, 1986). Studies using college student samples usually report low prevalence rates, whereas studies using clinical samples report moderate levels, and community samples report the highest rates (Wyatt & Peters, 1986).

Child Sexual Abuse

Sexual abuse is defined by federal legislation and may vary by state. The U.S. Department of Health and Human Services, National Center on Child Abuse and Neglect (1997), provides the following definition for sexual abuse from the Child Abuse Prevention and Treatment Act (CAPTA), 1996 (Public Law 104-235, Section 111; 42 U.S.C. 5105g) "the employment, use, persuasion, inducement, enticement, or coercion of any child to engage in, or assist any other person to engage in, any sexually explicit conduct or simulation of such conduct for the purpose of producing a visual depiction of such conduct; the rape, and in cases of caretaker or inter-familial relationships, statutory rape, molestation, prostitution, or other forms of sexual exploitation of children, or incest with children." Acts of child sexual abuse may include fondling, oral copulation, intercourse, sodomy, exhibitionism, and exploitation through prostitution or pornography (Damon, Todd, & MacFarlane, 1986; U.S. Department of Health and Human Services, National Center on Child Abuse and Neglect, 1997).

Personal Definitions of Abuse

A further key factor influencing prevalence rates is the preparedness to disclose information about sexual abuse to the interviewer. Researchers who use direct interview methods or who include a history of sexual abuse within the context of a broader sexual history have found that many people will answer "no" to a general screening question about abuse for a variety of reasons (e.g., see Shearer & Herbert, 1987). These reasons are directly and indirectly related to how incidents are defined and how victims attribute their involvement in them. First, survivors of sexual abuse do not tend to organize their sexual experiences into those that were consensual and nonconsensual. Consequently, when asked about experiences that occurred "against their will," what they often describe may not meet the researchers' or health care provider's definition. If they consented to participate in a sexual activity, regardless of the degree of physical or psychological coercion involved, survivors may themselves not consider these incidents as meeting the definitions of sexual abuse. Similarly, it is sometimes difficult for survivors to perceive their experiences as abusive if no physical force was used, or if the incident was described as a "game," or "as a way to teach them about sex," or if they experienced sexual pleasure from it. Incidents involving family members that spent time with victims and with whom they had nonsexual relationships in addition to sexual victimization may not be perceived as abusive by a survivor. This is particularly the case when victims may not have had other nurturing adults in their lives and who perceived their perpetrators as "the only person who cared about me." In these cases, victims often feel that sex with the perpetrator was an even exchange for affection, attention and acceptance. Thus, abuse survivors will evaluate whether their experiences meet or do not meet the criteria of abuse depending on how they became involved, who the perpetrator was, the perceived benefits of the relationship, whether force was used, and whether they blamed themselves for the sexual acts. Incidents where victims blamed themselves for having been victimized may involve a high degree of coercion or force, but if they were told that they were the "seductress or seductor," they may not consider the incident to be anyone's fault other than their own. Therefore, they may not define the incident as "sexual abuse." There are also well-known instances where victims fear the consequences of their disclosure and are unwilling to take the risk of hurting themselves and other family members. They may also be reluctant to be identified as the person who caused the family to dissolve the financial support to be

jeopardized when the perpetrator is separated from the family (Wyatt, 1985, 1990). Interviewers or therapists often find themselves discussing each incident with survivors in order to examine their criteria and to compare them with research-based criteria as well as legal definitions of sexual abuse. Potential survivors of child sexual abuse may not understand that some of their experiences are considered to be such and that perceptions, attributions, and coping strategies that result from the abuse might have influence on later sexual functioning.

Adult Sexual Abuse

Forcible rape is defined as "the carnal knowledge of a female forcibly and against her will. Included are rapes by force and attempts or assaults to rape" (Maguire & Pastore, 1996). Official statistics regarding sexual abuse are compiled by the U.S. Department of Justice. These data reflect only those assaults that are reported to law enforcement officials. As most women do not report sexual assaults to the police, these statistics underrepresent the true incidents of sexual assault in the United States. It is estimated that over 100,000 forcible rapes were reported to the police in 1994 (Maguire & Pastore, 1996).

Most women are sexually assaulted by intimate partners (Koss, Goodman, Browne, Fitzgerald, Keita, & Russo, 1994). Fewer than one in three rapes and sexual assaults were reported to law enforcement officials in 1996 (U.S. Department of Justice, 1997); the most likely explanation for this underreporting stems from the perpetrator being a known person or loved one. According to Maguire and Pastore (1996), approximately 28% of perpetrators of rape are the victims' husbands or boyfriends, 35% are acquaintances, and 5% are relatives.

SEXUAL ABUSE AND ITS EFFECTS

Most survivors of child sexual abuse have difficulty in identifying how some of these experiences may affect their reproductive sexual and psychological health because they tend not to receive psychological treatment when incidents occur. Thus, like Mrs. Green, when they are seen in health care centers of the etiology, their behaviors are not fully understood. Health care professionals are often equally as uninformed about the cluster of behaviors characteristic of survivors of sexual abuse. Consequently, patient and health providers often do not take a thorough sexual history, or establish the necessary rapport needed to engage a survivor in conversation about the need to obtain psychological treatment before more problems with sexual or reproductive aspects of their health occur.

Among the most pervasive effects of sexual victimization are the behaviors and arousal patterns that survivors use to adapt to their consensual practices, and the impaired decision-making about sexual behaviors and relationships.

The Dynamics of Sexual Abuse

One of the most widely accepted models describing effects of child sexual abuse on survivors is the Traumagenic Dynamics Model of Child Sexual Abuse by David Finkelhor and Angela Brown (1985). It describes four dynamics: (1) traumatic sexualization, (2) betrayal, (3) stigmatization, and (4) powerlessness.

1. *Traumatic sexualization* refers to the manner in which a child's sexuality is shaped in "developmentally inappropriate and interpersonally dysfunctional ways" (Finkelhor, 1982). Children learn about sexual arousal, sexual practices, and how to use sex as a means to an end through their victimization experiences. They are, however, often traumatized from sexual contact and exhibit patterns of sex avoidance years later.

2. *Betrayal* refers to the feelings that arise immediately or years later that someone in whom they trusted or had a relationship with has harmed them. They may also feel betrayed by nonoffending parents or other adults who do not protect them from victimization.

3. *Stigmatization* involves negative messages that victims perceive about themselves as a result of having been victimized. For example, one woman considered herself "tarnished" because she was no longer a virgin before marriage. Other survivors recalled that they withdrew from peers in childhood because they had knowledge about sex that they could not share with anyone, lest their friends become aware of the sexual relationship in which they were involved. In essence, victims become stigmatized because their knowledge and experiences are no longer age-appropriate and are distorted as a result of sexual victimization. They often feel different from other people.

4. *Powerlessness* refers to the victim losing or never developing the ability to control the experiences that they encounter: They are forced and often threatened to engage in activities against their will. Similarly, they often have fears about their survival. As a victim, they perceive that they are powerless to protect themselves and to survive except at the will of another.

The effects of sexual abuse can be long-lasting because someone controls (1) when a victim has contact; (2) where the incident will occur; (3) the level of sexual arousal as well as the perpetrator's own; (4) whether force or coercion is used; (5) how long these incidents continue; and (6) whether the victim or perpetrator discloses sexual contact.

While not all under a perpetrator's control, victims are often convinced that the power to alter any aspect of sexual encounters is totally within the control of the perpetrator. Repeated incidents only further confirm that decisions about sex and the circumstances are best made by the powerful partner. However, healthy sexual decision-making may elude a survivor. Even when victims identify with perpetrators and become sexually aggressive sexual partners in other relationships, they often do not develop healthy decision making skills that allow for the consequences of sexual contact to be considered. Thus, they may be revictimized in future encounters and be unable to understand their own sexual needs to negotiate with partners.

They may also victimize other partners and not allow them to make decisions in their own best interest—the same dynamics that emerged from their own abuse (Wyatt, 1997).

LONG-TERM EFFECTS OF CHILD SEXUAL ABUSE

Physical Health Effects

Depending on the severity of past experiences, incidents of child sexual abuse can impact women's health years later. Poor subjective health and medical problems, including somatization disorder, gastrointestinal complaints, pain syndromes, pelvic pain, gynecological complaints, asthma, labile hypertension, eating disorders, and vague neurologic symptoms are associated with a history of sexual abuse (Bolen, 1993; Cunningham, Pearce, & Pearce, 1988; Golding, Cooper, & George, 1997; Laws & Golding, 1996; Springs & Friedrich, 1992). Similar to Mrs. Green, these women are more likely to seek help for digestive and reproductive system complaints, compared to nonabused women (Cunningham, Pearce, & Pearce, 1988).

Women with histories of CSA may also ignore various body signals and symptoms (Briere, 1992). Traumatic experiences may cumulatively increase the likelihood of developing chronic pelvic pain or other somatic symptoms (Schei & Bakketeig, 1989; Schei, 1990a, 1990b; Heise, Moore, & Toubia, 1995). Women tend not to voluntarily disclose a history of abuse to their physician (Springs & Friedrich, 1992). A history of abuse may also affect efforts to develop coping skills or management of pain. Incidents of sexual abuse are often associated with low self esteem and with it, perceptions of limited resourcefulness and beliefs that pain is due to external factors (Toomey, Seville, Mann, & Abashian, 1995).

Women's health care service utilization is often affected by a history of abuse. Compared to nonabused women, women with histories of abuse are more likely to use the emergency room for their pain symptoms, and to have greater numbers of hospital admissions and surgical procedures in adulthood (Toomey, Seville, Mann, & Abashian, 1995; Salmon & Calderbank, 1996). Consequently, women with these histories may have sporadic health care and medical records that are not kept at one hospital. Thus, one unsuspecting professional may actually encourage an abuse survivor to miss appointments because they can find nothing wrong, and, like Mrs. Green, assume that not discussing the issues will minimize the problems and the symptoms they experience.

Psychological Well-being

While short term effects may vary depending on the resilience of the child (Wrobel *et al.*, 1996), there are many aspects of these incidents that can disturb a sense of well-being, particularly if they are ongoing.

Long term psychosocial effects of child abuse include low self-esteem, passivity, and negative self-evaluations such as, "I am not very friendly," "I am not a good sex partner" (Classen, 1995; Romans, Martin, & Mullen, 1996; Briere, 1992; Smith, 1992). Cognitive distortions that may result from more severe incidents of sexual abuse, particularly among those who are poor and undereducated, may pose a particular threat to HIV infected women, because women may assume that they have limited options in a wide range of circumstances (Briere, 1992). Possibly as a means to avoid negative, intrusive images of or associations with the abuse, women abused as children are more likely to have past or current alcohol problems, and engage in substance use (McCauley *et al.*, 1997). Women with abuse histories also may experience increased levels of depressive and anxious symptoms (Gorcey, Santiago & McCall-Perez, 1986; Boudewyn & Liem, 1995). They may also mutilate themselves (e.g., arm or leg markings or self-induced tattoos), have suicidal ideation or attempts (Briere, 1992; Boudewyn & Liem, 1995), report posttraumatic stress symptoms, and dissociate or depersonalize painful events (Maltz, 1988; Briere, Cotman, Harris, & Smiljanich, 1992; Briere, 1992).

Negative Sexual Outcomes

There is also much about past sexual experiences in childhood or adolescence which are learned. Like Mrs. Green, decisions about contraceptive use were not consistent with her sexual activity, resulting in unintended outcomes such as pregnancy and abortion. While unprotected sex may result in unintended pregnancy, STD infection and HIV infection may direct outcomes of child sexual abuse (Wyatt, 1988; Heise, Moore, & Toubra, 1995; Lodico & DiClemente, 1994).

Experiences of trauma and coercion can often restrict a woman's ability to make independent decisions about the timing and circumstances of sex, resulting in patterns of risk taking that may be repeated in the future (Wyatt, 1997; Wyatt et al., 1997). Negative sexual outcomes which have been associated with child sexual abuse include early onset of sexual activity, an inability to distinguish between sex as a means to an end, or affectionate versus sexual behavior (Donalson, Whalen, & Anastas, 1989; Brown & Finkelhor, 1986; Riggs, Alario, & McHorney, 1990). Prostitution (Widom & Kuhns, 1996), compromised contraceptive decision making, the inability to refuse unwanted sex (Johnsen & Harlow, 1996; Heise, Moore, & Toubia, 1995), and high risk sexual activity have also been associated with histories of abuse (Handwerker, 1993, Lodico & DiClemente, 1994; Alexander & Lupfer, 1987, Wyatt, Newcomb & Riederle, 1993).

Interpersonal Relationships

Mrs. Green's sexual difficulties with her husband also extended to interpersonal problems. Women often experience intimacy disturbances, including communication skills deficits (Smith, 1992), a fear and distrust of sexual partners, and power imbalances in relationships (Gorcey, Santiago, & McCall-Perez, 1986; Mennen & Pearlmutter, 1993). Some women, who have been abused years earlier may avoid men who resembled their perpetrators (Wyatt & Mickey, 1987). Histories of sexual abuse also

have been associated with loneliness, and less general satisfaction with and less use of their social support system (Gibson & Hartshorne, 1996; Rhodes, Ebert, & Myers, 1993).

Interpersonal problems may also result from or contribute to sexual difficulties or sexual distress (Briere & Runtz, 1988; Fromuth, 1986). For example, African-American and European-American women who reported incidents of attempted or completed intercourse and oral sex (before age 18) were also more likely to report problems in their adult sexual functioning. In particular, they were likely to avoid engaging in the sexual behaviors such as intercourse, oral and anal sex, that was forced upon them when they were victimized (Wyatt, 1990). Abuse victims seeking therapy, and others not seeking therapy, were compared to a matched control group of women in their perceptions of being sexually "well adjusted." Although the latter two groups did not differ in this respect, women seeking therapy reported fewer orgasms, less sexual responsiveness, and less sexual satisfaction (Jackson et al., 1990).

Sexual Dysfunction in CSA Survivors

Several studies have identified sexual dysfunction in survivors of child sexual abuse. Like Mrs. Green, these are not uncommon problems. One study reported an avoidance of sex among sexual abuse survivors, more commonly labeled as "being frigid" (McGuire & Wagner, 1978). In other studies (e.g., Gagnon, 1965), women however, had no difficulty reaching orgasm through intercourse. Women have been described as rarely initiating sex and having difficulty in touching and caressing their partner or being caressed. They have also reported feelings of disgust and revulsion about their own and partner's body and only enjoyed sexual contact with penetration (McGuire & Wagner, 1978, p. 12). However, penetrative sexual abuse is also specifically linked to female sexual dysfunction (Sarwer & Durlak, 1996). Sexual problems found in child sexual abuse survivors include sexual dysfunction, compulsive sexual behavior, fear of sex, and conditioned negative reactions to sex (Classen, 1995; Gorcey, Santiago, & McCall-Perez, 1986; Maltz, 1988; Wyatt, 1990; Smith, 1992).

In a review of long term effects of sexual trauma (Shearer & Herbert, 1987), women who were sexual abuse survivors were described as experiencing an aversion to sex, being anorgasmic, and having vaginismus. They also reported either having difficulties in trusting men or being overly trusting of them. These are problems attributed to untreated traumatic sexual experiences that professionals can help victims to overcome. Similarly, Gold, Hughes, and Swingle (1986) compared women who were sexually abused as children to female cohorts who did not report abuse and found that abuse survivors reported more negative sex symptoms, fewer positive responses to sexual initiation, and less sexual satisfaction.

While few researchers have examined sexual dysfunction in men, a small case study of 11 men, some of whom were abused in childhood by female perpetrators, described difficulty with attaining erections, fear and guilt about sexual pleasure, as well as an avoidance of a disclosure of sexual needs (Sarrel & Masters, 1982). There is also little information about survivors of sexual abuse and their partners, male or female, who may also have these histories. More research is needed to better understand the reproductive health histories of couples with histories of early sexual trauma (Wyatt, 1997).

CSA, HIV Risks, and Psychiatric Comorbidity

Child sexual abuse has been linked to substance use and psychiatric disorders (Amaro *et al.*, 1999a, p. 268). As mentioned earlier, women often use alcohol and drugs for temporary relief to cope with anxiety, depression, or upsetting memories caused by the child sexual abuse (Perez, Kennedy, & Fullilove, 1995, p. 87; Kilpatrick, 1987). Recent data indicate that women substance users have reported higher rates of sexual abuse than men and acute effects of drugs and alcohol. These effects include

memory of painful events, provision of expressing painful affect that might otherwise be inhibited, and avoidance from developing healthy social networks, anxiety, and depression (Briere, 1992; Brady *et al.*, 1993; NIDA, 1994: Rohsenow *et al.*, 1998; Wallen, 1998). Close collaboration among health care providers and substance abuse treatment centers is critical for the comprehensive care of women who have dual diagnosis of drug and alcohol abuse and psychiatric disorders as a result of CSA.

Mental health service providers and researchers have not fully addressed the unique treatment needs of women who use drugs, have histories of child sexual abuse, and are living with HIV/AIDS (Daley & Argeriou, 1997; Blumenthal, 1998; Perez *et al.*, 1995; Amaro *et al.*, 1999b; Wyatt *et al.*, 1999). There are few studies that address issues of drug addiction, HIV, and child sexual abuse among women (Perez *et al.*, 1995; Amaro *et al.*, 1999b; Wyatt *et al.*, 1999) Long-term biological, psychological, and social consequences of alcohol and drug addiction vary across gender. Compared to men, women are more affected by the consequences of addiction by morbidity and mortality, socioeconomic status, treatment needs, family roles, and comorbidity factors (i.e. suicide, HIV, sexual dysfunction, depression, anxiety), which are critical for treatment outcomes (Amaro *et al.*, 1999b; Palacios *et al.*, 1999; Jarvis & Copeland, 1997; Gil-Rivas *et al.*, 1997; Wilsnack *et al.*, 1997; McCauley *et al.*, 1997: Moncrief *et al.*, 1996).

CSA and HIV Risks

Higher rates of childhood sexual abuse are found in drug user samples than in the general population (Miller & Paone, 1998). Kilpatrick *et al.* (1992) found that history of sexual abuse was associated with cocaine use among women. Several studies have found links between sexual abuse and trading sex for drugs among women (Miller & Paone, 1998). Fleming *et al.* (1998) found that childhood sexual abuse was not related to alcohol abuse in a mother perceived as cold and uncaring, who had an alcohol-abusing partner, and who believed alcohol was sexually disinhibiting. This suggests that the relationship between sexual abuse and substance abuse may depend in part on significant cofactors.

The relationship between drug use, HIV, and child sexual abuse is mediated by many of the long-term sequeale of sexual abuse that increase risk-taking behaviors (Miller, 1999; Kilpatrick et al., 1997; Bravant et al., 1997). For example, drug addicted women have an increased reliance on drug use as a coping mechanism for their sexual abuse. This increases risk-taking behaviors for HIV because women may be more likely to have sex under the influence of drugs and not use barrier methods of protection. Women who use drugs also report having limited social networks (i.e., network membership type, social support). The lack of social resources increases their vulnerability for HIV risk exposure because they lack the support to maintain risk-reduction behaviors (Miller, 1999; Medrano et al., 1999; Goldberg, 1995; Walker, 1999).

These findings suggest that abuse can play a central role in the type of interventions or treatment outcomes targeted for drug using women who are survivors of CSA, and are living with HIV. Thus, it is important for service providers to take detailed histories of CSA. It is also important for service providers to take detailed histories of drug abuse and sexual abuse and to increase their coordination with substance abuse and sexual abuse programs, and related mental and health services for HIV infected populations. Women's social networks need to be better informed about the characteristics of many abuse survivors in order to lower the influence or risk exposure opportunities and increase social support. For example, service providers might suggest that drug-addicted women limit their association with active drug-using peers. For some individuals, replacing their drug-using reference group with 12 step groups can produce better treatment outcomes and avoid relapse. The time of the intervention is also crucial for better outcomes since studies suggest that adolescence is a crucial time for the influence of sexual abuse experiences on substance abuse. This type of abuse is more likely to occur more among women early in life (Jarvis et al., 1998).

Cultural Factors and Sexual Abuse

The lack of reported ethnic differences in the prevalence of child sexual abuse among African-American, Latina, and European-American women suggests that there are most likely few, if any, cultures in the Western world that condone sexual contact between a child and an adult. We know less about the prevalence of sexual abuse in Asian/Pacific Islander and American Indian communities, but the incest taboo operates within these cultures, as well. Correlates of ethnicity (i.e., socioeconomic status, and family environment) have more to do with how families and individuals cope with abuse than its occurrence with an ethnic family. How families respond to these incidents once it is uncovered may be influenced by the beliefs of families about how the disclosure will affect the family and how the legal system will treat both the victim and perpetrator.

Sexuality comprises underlying values and attitudes as well as behaviors, and it is an aspect of the self that is inextricable from one's particular cultural framework. As such, cultural values pervade all aspects of sexual abuse. For example, cultural stereotypes or expectations may influence the abuse experience itself, whether and to whom the experience is disclosed, and the treatment and well-being of the victim.

The existence and influence of sexual stereotypes, particularly of ethnic minorities, have been discussed at length (e.g., Wyatt, 1990, 1997). For example, the myths surrounding African-American sexuality have long been documented (Goldstein, 1948; Bell, 1970; Deckard, 1975, Wyatt, 1997). African-American men and women have been variously depicted as being anatomically different, hypersexual, sexually aggressive and promiscuous, undergoing earlier sexual development, possessing more "primitive" sexual knowledge, and engaging in more premarital sex than other ethnocultural groups (Wyatt, 1982). Thus, given the pervasiveness of these stereotypes, African-American victims of sexual abuse may encounter legal and health professionals who perceive consent to have sexual contact when none was given (Wyatt, 1990). Furthermore, they may encounter overt discrimination as they seek treatment, further compounding the trauma of abuse. Victims themselves are not necessarily immune to the influence of these negative stereotypes having incorporated these images into their own sexuality. They may attribute the abuse to their own behavior, thinking that they are somehow "at fault" for what happened. Thus, health professionals who work with CSA survivors need to be aware of the cultural context and stereotypes in which abuse occurs, and to be cognizant of their personal biases and those of the larger society in order to avoid doubly victimizing survivors.

For other cultural groups, values proscribing sexuality and the discussion of sex have important implications on abuse outcomes as well. For example, some Asian/Pacific Islander (A/PI) groups perceive sex and sexuality to be a highly private—and perhaps taboo—topic, not to be openly acknowledged or discussed (Gock, 1994; Chin, 1999; Chin & Kroesen, 1999). Therefore, the experience of sexual abuse is highly stigmatizing, conferring shame to the victim. Victims may be highly motivated to hide the abuse. In cases of incest, barriers to disclosure may be even stronger, as A/PI cultures tend to emphasize a collectivistic cultural orientation which place the interests of the family over the interests of the individual (Triandis, 1995). For Latino Americans, cultural values may operate in a similar fashion. A cherished value among Latinos is familism (Amaro, 1995; Simoni *et al.*, 1995), which stresses the importance and unity of the family above the individual. As with A/PI Americans, abuse by a family member is likely to place the victim in the painful bind of having to choose between loyalty to the family and disclosing the abuse. In some cases, disclosure may bring about rejection and ostracization of the victim by the family. Thus, cultural values that complicate the abuse, disclosure, and treatment process must

be addressed in order to achieve the best health outcomes for survivors.

Aside from their cultural values, the social context in which Latinas or other recently immigrated groups experience child sexual abuse is influenced by several factors including acculturation, immigration status, and relationship with the host community in the US. For example, nondisclosure of child sexual abuse among Latinas may be dependent on the response from legal institutions that are perceived as unsympathetic (i.e., the Immigration and Naturalization System (INS), police, and social workers). Health professionals need to identify both the cultural (i.e., nondisclosure, forced marriage) and sociostructural (i.e., immigration status, distrust of legal institutions) circumstances to appropriately assess the effects of the family and community in their response to sexual abuse.

Child abuse among Asian/Pacific Islander immigrant families appears to be influenced by five social and cultural factors: (1) traumas in the home country, especially among refugees; (2) differences in child rearing practices; (3) visibility to welfare professionals; (4) lack of continuity of social support; and (5) difficulties coping with cultural conflicts (Ima & Hohm, 1991). These factors appear to exacerbate family conflict which then may escalate to abuse. Physical abuse appears to be more common and sexual abuse less common among A/PI groups compared to other ethnic groups (Ima & Hohm, 1991). More research is needed on other ethnic groups in order to fully understand how culture influences the aftermath of sexual abuse across the life course.

HEALTH CARE SETTINGS

Women with abuse histories are more likely to report pain and other health symptoms than nonabused cohorts. Compared to nonabused women, women with abuse histories are more likely to use the emergency room for their pain symptoms, and have a greater number of hospital admissions and surgical procedures in adulthood (Toomey, Seville, Mann, & Abashian, 1995; Salmon & Calderbank, 1996).

Given the variety of physical symptoms and medical conditions associated with early childhood sexual abuse, nurses, physicians, and other health professionals need to understand how trauma impacts women's sexual, physical, and emotional health. This would increase our knowledge of how trauma can exacerbate health related symptoms or conditions.

Assessment procedures also need to include questions of early experiences of trauma. Further, given that women rarely disclose histories of abuse to their physicians (Springs & Freidrich, 1992), health care providers need the tools for gathering such important information. Further, if an abuse survivor does disclose past abuse in a medical setting, this may be the first time the individual discloses which may necessitate referrals to therapeutic support services.

PRIMARY PREVENTION OF SEXUAL ABUSE

Efforts to prevent sexual abuse for children usually include teaching individuals about their rights to sexual ownership, and appropriate behavior between children and adults. Their rights and responsibility to decide about when and with whom you have sexual contact are also emphasized. However, while these incidents are common, the burden for preventing abuse is often placed on victims and not perpetrators. It is important to remember that primary prevention programs target young children with the goal of developing a fairly sophisticated decision making ability, they are creating expectations and skills that some adults do not have. Most children do not have fact-based discussions about sex with parents and conversations about potential or real incidents are even more difficult (Wyatt, 1997). In many cultures, it is also perceived as inappropriate for adults and children to discuss sex, because sex is not something that children, adolescents, or single individuals need to know about until marriage (Wyatt, 1997). The ability to differentiate with

whom children should have physical or sexual contact and be able, regardless of their relationship or feelings about that person, to separate appropriate from inappropriate touch is also not easily achieved. These are very complicated instructions that have to be applied across a wide variety of occasions and often confuse and frighten children. For example, one parent requested a psychiatric evaluation for her child because of his fear of adults. The parents had a large extended family and on many occasions children were expected to greet adults and children with affection. However, the child had recently completed a "good and bad touch" program in an elementary school. The program attempted to help children understand that there are parts of their bodies like their genitals that few people should touch. As a consequence of the program, however, this child was afraid of hugging or sitting on the lap of relatives. Some of his cousins were aggressive in their play and the child considered touch football as a "bad touch" because he always got hurt. However, the parents became annoyed with his repeated trips into the house to "tell on" someone, when in these situations, the parents expected the child to take care of these situations himself.

These are sometimes subtle nuances of social interactions that are better understood with age. However, prevention programs target young children, and rightly so. The prevalence of sexual abuse challenges health professionals to imbed prevention messages into all developmentally appropriate information for children. We can only hope that it is better to overprepare and modify children's understanding of bad touch than to leave them unprepared for possible incidents that may occur, even in the family context.

The need to protect children and offer them tools for self-protection is motivating schools to offer sexual abuse prevention to children. Evaluations of these programs will help to better identify what aspects still need finetuning and incorporate the most recent findings about how to minimize the sexual abuse and exploitation of children. Mrs. Green did not have any such information offered to her when she was being abused by her father. Had sexual abuse prevention been offered by the schools, she might have disclosed the incidents to a teacher or another adult and the aftermath of abuse might have taken a very different turn.

SECONDARY PREVENTION STRATEGIES

According to the National Institute of Justice (1997), the following are intervention goals for victims of child abuse and neglect: (1) to protect the future welfare of the victim by preventing further abuse through the provision of emergency services, out-of-home placement, or intensive in-home services; (2) to address specific psychological, physical, developmental, or cognitive damage resulting from the abuse by referring the child to providers of psychological counseling, therapeutic day care, cognitive-behavioral skills-building programs, or academic assistance; or (3) to cultivate or reinforce potential protective factors that may help the victim overcome the harmful effects of abuse, such as promoting attachment to a nonabusive adult, positive school experiences, better academic performance, a supportive relationship with nonabusing parent or sibling, or a stabilized living arrangement.

These goals should be implemented in programs for abuse survivors with acknowledgment that educational, and recreational institution resources, therapeutic relationships, and families should work in tandem to create an environment conducive to healing from abuse.

A history of sexual abuse may affect interventions that patients receive. Because abuse reduces perceptions of resourcefulness and is associated with the belief that pain is due to external factors, interventions that involve coping skills training or management of pain are needed (Laws & Golding, 1996).

Treatment of Child Sexual Abuse

Along with primary prevention of child sexual abuse, intervention efforts include secondary prevention for high-risk families and tertiary prevention for children who have experienced sexual abuse. The U.S. Department of Health and Human Services, National Center on Child Abuse and Neglect, 1997, identifies the following aspects for secondary prevention: parent education, substance abuse programs for families with young children, respite care, and family resource centers that provide information and referral services.

Tertiary prevention includes intervention programs for children and families that have experienced sexual abuse. Various treatment modalities include individual treatment for the child, perpetrator, and nonoffending parent, family treatment, and group treatment. Treatment approaches can include behavior therapy, play therapy, and psychoanalytic/psychodynamic approaches. Because the impact of sexual abuse varies with the child and family, it is essential to conduct a comprehensive assessment that identifies the severity of the sexual abuse, the impact on the child and family, the family dynamics, as well as the child's perception of the abuse (Walker, Bonner, & Kaufman, 1988).

Treatment phases range from crisis intervention, short-term therapy, and long-term therapy. Treatment goals are often aimed at addressing the sexual abuse as well as focusing on self-image, increasing the child's ability to trust, learning boundaries, and increasing a sense of security (Long, 1986). Resulting from the sequelae of sexual abuse, 10 general treatment issues summarized by Long address "the damaged goods syndrome, guilt, fear, depression, low self-esteem and social skills, anger and hostility, inability to trust, blurred role boundaries and role confusion, pseudomaturity and failure to complete developmental tasks, self-mastery and control." Five specific treatment issues address the "importance of teaming with the child's mother, inappropriate attachment behavior, infant regressive behavior, need for body contact and body awareness, and need for education on feelings" (pp. 226–231).

Waterman *et al.* (1986), recommends a multimodal, multidisciplinary approach to the treatment of sexual abuse. Specialized training is necessary to gain the expertise for professionals to effectively work with children and families who are victims of sexual abuse. It is also essential that the professional interface with medical, legal, law enforcement, and mental health agencies.

PSYCHOLOGICAL SEQUELAE AND SECONDARY PREVENTION

At first glance, Mrs. Green had a history that some might interpret as sexually irresponsible. Indeed, much of her past and current sexual behaviors and decision making increased both her and her partner's risks for unintended outcomes including STDs and HIV. However, sexual and drug-related risk taking as well as depressive symptomatology can have more than one etiology. Sexual abuse has not been well understood among professionals who develop interventions for unintended pregnancy, STDs and HIV/AIDS. Further, intervention models such as Twelve Step Programs sometimes have too limited an approach for a recovering substance abuser, with histories of child sexual abuse. The basic problem is that many of these programs are not well integrated. For women, an unintended pregnancy, an STD or HIV may be the result of unprotected sexual intercourse. Consequently, it is important to integrate these prevention messages into one program and to recognize all of the factors influencing these unwanted outcomes, including sexual abuse (Bolen, 1993).

Clinical Treatment

Intake procedures for mental health settings must also include extensive sexual health histories and traumatic experiences. Assessment protocols in clinical settings need comprehensive medical histories to identify trauma-related symptoms that have been attributed to physiological causes, as well as an understanding of health care utilization.

Clinical treatment settings including family planning clinics need referrals and resources for health promotion when working with victims of child sexual abuse. Given the potentially extensive psychosocial impact of CSA, treatment typically involves individual and/or group treatment. Clinicians have advocated group psychotherapy as the treatment of choice or as an adjunct to individual treatment (Cahill, Llewelyn, & Pearson, 1991) because the group format decreases isolation and stigmatization for survivors (Lundberg-Love, 1990). Group treatment is effective in decreasing depression and increasing self-esteem (Brooke, 1995; Richter, Snider, & Gorey, 1997). Improvement has also been noted for locus of control, sexual problems, self-esteem, trauma symptoms, and psychological distress (Hazzard, Rogers, & Angert, 1993). Groups typically focus on cognitive and affective mastering of various themes related to sexual abuse, including shame, anger, sadness, guilt, anxiety, and connecting trauma with current family or intimate relationships (Cole & Barney, 1987). In addition, by developing an understanding of dissociation and triggers of PTSD, including flashbacks, group members are better able to identify how CSA has impacted their emotional functioning, as well as sexual behaviors. Peer modeling related to disclosing past experiences and ways of managing trigger of PTSD offers validation and support for group members, decreases a sense of isolation, and increases feelings of group cohesion (Cole & Barney, 1987; Armsworth, 1989). These well-established components of sexual abuse interventions should be coupled with successful elements of health education, including family planning and HIV interventions, in order to more comprehensively address the compounded health risks for women with abuse histories. By focusing on the linkage between early sexual trauma and physical, reproductive and emotional health, survivors of sexual abuse can gain insight into the long-term impact of their early experiences.

Health Policy Implications: Social and Psychological Perspectives

Sexual abuse is not yet perceived as a public health problem. Many people do not understand its effect on the social fabric of our lives. Sex is one of the most intimate experiences in life and to be forced into sexual contact without consent or full knowledge of the experiences or its consequences can often expose children and adults to trauma that can have immediate and lasting effects. Unfortunately, instead of working to refine the disclosure of these incidents and the consistency of recalling past events, some have focused solely on the accuracy of disclosures and the consequent memory performance errors.

The prevalence and trauma of sexual abuse, most of which is not disclosed and for which little or no psychological treatment is sought, has somehow emerged second to the accuracy of the disclosure and whether the effects are as severe as research has demonstrated. Indeed, there are still a substantial proportion of people in the health professional community who feel that sexual abuse, especially childhood incidents, do not always have the severe impact on psychological adjustment than has been reported in the past (Rind *et al.*, 1998). It is important to evaluate the quality of the research and the representation of the sample used in research before disregarding the impact of these incidents. While they may not be the sole predictor of health problems, they make a significant contribution to problems later in life, especially if the contact involves penetration and is perpetrated by a family member (Wyatt, Newcomb, Reiderle, 1993).

Worst still, survivors of sexual abuse, regardless of whether incidents occurred before or since age 19, are often overlooked in the health care system. Like Mrs. Green, they are often perceived as highly irritable, demanding individuals who are impatient and critical of professionals who are overburdened with too many patients and inadequate staff to provide services. Health care is often complicated because survivors of sexual abuse often are not able to identify the etiology of the symptoms they present and are subsequently misdiagnosed or mistreated. Consequently, funds for health care are often misspent on emergency room visits, and potential patients often receive erratic or inconsistent care from a variety of professionals who see them once or too infrequently to develop a comprehensive understanding of the problems

and the treatment that can help them. Further, the mental health system is often equally as unprepared for patients who present physical symptoms for psychological problems. Not being able to get up in the morning, sleeping or eating problems, pelvic pain, or inorgasmia are too often the signals of sexual trauma that should be evaluated in order to rule in or out the possibility that these types of experiences have occurred. Given that when incidents occur before 18, they are more likely to reoccur, particularly if no treatment is received, early identification of sexual abuse can minimize the likelihood of a reoccurrence and also minimize health-related and psychological problems that can result. As a society we can develop policy to facilitate prevention or pay later by witnessing the escalation of health care for problems that ail us.

CONCLUSIONS

While the focus of research and treatment on sexual abuse has concentrated on the victim, given that someone known to the victim perpetrates most incidents, our focus needs to broaden on several levels. First, we need statewide, general public health-related campaigns focusing on individual rights and sexual and violence prevention. This issue has recently received attention because of gun control debates and increasing rates of violence by children. However, violence prevention should be ongoing within a developmental perspective. That is, prevention messages for young children should consider that the message itself could be confusing and frightening. The example of the mother who brought her child for an evaluation because of his fear of close contact illustrates how too much information conveyed to young children does not necessarily increase awareness of the central issues that children can understand and control. Prevention messages for middle school children and early adolescence can increase in complexity. Messages for older teens should also include more aggressive methods of reporting perpetrators. However, all children need a safety plan, or people who are identified by the family as persons who can be called if they do not feel safe. Safe places or houses also need to be identified in neighborhoods for children who walk or play in the community. Youth of all ages should have safety cards including emergency phone numbers. Strategies like these also need to be evaluated for their efficacy in reducing attempted or completed incidents of sexual violence.

In the future, the second level of research needs to focus on perpetrators of these incidents and should include a variety of individuals ranging in demographic characteristics, in a variety of settings. There is still too little information about the factors that motivate male or female perpetrators to commit acts of sexual abuse, whether they are convicted for these acts or not. We also need to better understand the factors in our society that reinforce the perpetration of more than one act, or serial patterns of abuse of specific populations such as the elderly, developmentally disabled, or the mentally ill. Further, we need more research on incarcerated populations and law enforcement employees. Some of those who are trained to protect the rights of others are often the ones who violate those rights. We need to understand the factors that promote the violation of those rights and develop effective primary prevention programs for those populations.

In order to conduct this research, we also need guidance from federal agencies regarding protection of confidentiality. It is very difficult to conduct research of this nature and report incidents of abuse at the same time. It would be very helpful to have more conferences and policies on these issues so that researchers and clinicians can share their strategies of retaining confidentiality and reporting cases of sexual abuse to protect research participants and patients.

The third level of research should involve couples and families, individuals who live in a context where abuse has occurred. Most programs address individual safety, whereas programs for physical battery are more likely to be designed for couples. The issue of who is the target for intervention often has to do with the

age of the victim. With CSA, opportunities to reconstitute the family in cases of incest depend on the severity of the abuse and the conviction of family members. Reunification can be quite protracted, and in many cases, inappropriate. Research is needed with families where members outside as well as inside of the family have perpetrated incidents, in order to better understand how family dynamics can help to minimize or increase the lasting psychological effects of CSA.

We also need more research on couples where, at one time in the relationship, one partner reports marital rape. There is very little research that identifies how survivors of abuse cope when they are currently still in relationships with persons who have sexually assaulted them (Russell, 1982). In some cases, both partners have abuse histories which appear to increase the likelihood that one or both partners will abuse each other in the current relationship. Because many couples do not wish to end the relationship with single or repeated incidents of abuse, it is important to identify the effects of these incidents on the partners, children and on the family as a unit.

Finally, given our multiethnic, diverse society, we still need more research on adequate samples of ethnic and cultural groups, men and women with different sexual orientations, and religious beliefs. In order to minimize sexual abuse, we need both a national and international consensus on how a society should define abuse and the rights of individuals, regardless of age, gender, religious, political views, sexual orientation or other beliefs. We need to document how the effects of sexual abuse impact the quality of life, as well as the psychological, sexual and reproductive health. It is quite possible that a cost analysis of treatment for psychological, sexual and reproductive problems and disease transmission may help to stimulate policy that minimizes the occurrence of sexual abuse and promotes the recognition that individual rights need to include control over one's body and mind. Those rights are basic to our humanity and the legacy we leave for those to follow.

ACKNOWLEDGMENTS.   This manuscript was supported by Grant #MH54965 and Grant #AI28697. Requests for reprints should be sent to first author at: University of California Los Angeles, Department of Psychiatry and Bio-behavioral Sciences, 760 Westwood Plaza, C8-871C, Los Angeles, California 90095. The author wishes to thank Douglas Longshore, Ph.D., for his assistance, Sunil Obediah for literature research, and Annette Abeyta for manuscript preparation.

REFERENCES

Alexander, P. C., & Lupfer, S. L. (1987). Family characteristics and long-term consequences associated with sexual abuse. *Archives of Sexual Behavior*, 16(3), 235–245.

Amaro, H. (1995). Love, sex, and power: Considering women's realities in HIV prevention. *American Psychologist*, 50, 437–447.

Amaro, H., Nieves, R., Johannes, S. W., & Cabeza, N. M. L. (1999). Substance abuse treatment: Critical issues of child sexual abuse: Changes across a decade. *Child Abuse & Neglect. Jan.* 23(1), 45–60.

Amaro, H., Nieves, R., Sergut Wolde, J., & Lobult Cabeza, N. M. (1999). Substance abuse treatment: Critical issues and challenges in treatment for Latinas. *Hispanic Journal of Behavioral Sciences*, 21(3), 266–282.

Armsworth, M. W. (1989). Therapy of incest survivors: Abuse or support? *Child Abuse & Neglect*, 13(4), 549–562.

Bell, A. (1970) Black sexuality: Fact and fantasy. In R. Staples (Ed.), *The Black family: Essays and studies* (pp. 77–80). Belmont, CA: Wadsworth.

Blumenthal, S. (1998). Women and substance abuse: A new national focus. In *National Institute of Drug Abuse, Drug Addiction Research and the Health of Women* (NIH Publication No. 98-4290, pp. 13–32). Rockville, MD: U.S. Department of Health and Human Services, National Institutes of Health.

Bolen, J. D. (1993). The impact of sexual abuse on women's health. *Psychiatric Annals*, 23 (8), 446–453.

Boudewyn, A. C., & Liem, J. H. (1995). Childhood sexual abuse as a precursor to depression and self-destructive behavior in adulthood. *Journal of Traumatic Stress*, 8(3), 445–459.

Brady, K. T., Grice, D. E., Dustan, K., & Randall, C. (1993). The relationship between substance abuse and bipolar disorder. *Journal of Clinical Psychiatry*, 56 (Suppl. 3), 19–24.

Bravant, S., Forsyth, C. J., & LeBlanc, J. B. (1997). Child sexual trauma and substance misuse: A pilot study. *Substance Use & Misuse*, 32(10), 1417–1431.

Briere, J., & Runtz, M. (1986). Suicidal thought and behaviors in former sexual abuse victims. *Canadian Journal of Behavioral Science, Oct.* 18(4), 413–423.

Briere, J., & Runtz, M. (1988). Symptomatology associated with childhood sexual victimization in a nonclinical adult sample. *Child Abuse and Neglect*, 12, 51–59.

Briere, J., Cotman, A., Harris, K., & Smiljanich, K. (1992). The trauma symptoms inventory: Preliminary data on reliability and validity. Paper presented at the annual meeting of the American Psychological Association, Washington, DC.

Briere, J. N. (1992). *Child abuse trauma: Theory and treatment of the lasting effects*. Newbury Park: Sage.

Brooke, S. L. (1995). Art therapy: An approach to working with sexual abuse survivors. Special issue: *Sexual Abuse. Arts in Psychotherapy*, 22(5), 447–466.

Brown, A., & Finkelhor, D. (1986). The impact of child sexual abuse: A review of the research. *Psychological Bulletin*, 99(1), 66–77.

Cahill, C., Llewelyn, S. P., & Pearson, C. (1991). Treatment of sexual abuse that occurred in childhood: A review. *British Journal of Clinical Psychology, Feb.* 30(1), 1–12.

Chin, D., & Kroesen, K. W. (1999). Disclosure of HIV infection among Asian/Pacific Islander American women: Cultural stigma and support. *Cultural Diversity and Ethnic Minority Psychology*, 5(3), 222–235.

Chin, D. (1999). HIV-related sexual risk assessment among Asian/Pacific Islander American women: An inductive model. *Social Science & Medicine, Jul.* 49(2), 241–278.

Classen, C. (1995). Introduction. In C. Classen & I. D. Yalom (Eds.), *Treating women molested in childhood* (pp. xiii–xxxii). San Francisco: Jossey-Bass.

Cole, C. H., & Barney, E. E. (1987). Safeguards and the therapeutic window: A group treatment strategy for adult incest survivors. *American Journal of Orthopsychiatry, Oct.* 57(4), 601–609.

Cunningham, J., Pearce, T., & Pearce, P. (1988). Childhood sexual abuse and medical complaints in adult women. *Journal of Interpersonal Violence*, 3(2), 131–144.

Daley, M., & Argeriou, M. (1997). Characteristics and treatment needs of sexually abused pregnant women in drug rehabilitation: The Massachusetts MOTHERS Project. *Journal of Substance Abuse Treatment, Mar.–Apr.* 14(2), 191–196.

Damon, L., Todd, J., & MacFarlane, K. (1987). Treatment issues with sexually abused young children. *Child Welfare*, 66(2), 125–137.

Davis, K. B. (1929). *Factors in the sex life of twenty-two hundred women* (p. 430). New York: Harper.

Deckard, B. S. (1975). *The women's movement: Political, socioeconomic, and psychological issues*. New York: Harper and Row.

Dickinson, R. L. (1933). *Human sex anatomy* (pp. xiv, 145). Baltimore: Williams & Wilkins.

Donalson, P. E., Whalen, M. H., & Anastas, J. W. (1989). Teen pregnancy and sexual abuse: Exploring the connection. *Smith College Studies in Social Work*, 59(3), 289.

Finkelhor, D. S. (1979). *Sexual victimized children and their families*. University of New Hampshire, Dissertation Abstracts International. May. 39 (11-A): pp. 7006–7007.

Finkelhor, D. (1982). Sexual abuse, A sociological perspective. *Child Abuse & Neglect*, 6, 95–102.

Finkelhor, D., & Brown A. (1985). The traumatic impact of child sexual abuse: A conceptualization. *American Journal of Orthopsychiatry*, Oct., 55(4), 530–541.

Fleming, J., Mullen, P. E., Sibthorpe, B., Attewell R., & Bammer, G. (1998). The relationship between childhood sexual abuse and alcohol abuse in women—a case control study. *Addiction*, 93(12), 1787–1798.

Fromuth, M. E., (1986). The relationship of childhood sexual abuse with later psychological and sexual adjustment in a sample of college women. *Childhood Abuse and Neglect*, 10(1), 5–15.

Gibson, R. L., & Hartshorne, T. S. (1996). Childhood sexual abuse and adult loneliness and network orientation. *Child Abuse and Neglect*, 20(11), 1087–1093.

Gil-Rivas, V., Fiorentine, R., Anglin, D., & Taylor, E. (1997). Sexual and physical abuse: Do they compromise drug treatment outcomes? *Journal of Substance Abuse Treatment*, Jul.–Aug. 14(4), 351–358.

Gock, T. S. (1994). Acquired Immunodeficiency syndrome. In N. W. S. Zane, D. T. Takeuchi, & K. N. J. Young (Eds.), *Confronting critical issues of Asian/Pacific Islanders* (pp. 247–265). London: Sage.

Gold, S. N., Hughes, D. M., & Swingle, J. M. (1996). Characteristics of childhood sexual abuse among female survivors in therapy. *Child Abuse and Neglect*, 20(4), 323–335.

Goldberg, M. E. (1995). Substance-abuse women: false stereotypes and real needs. *Social Work*, 40(6), 789–798.

Golding, J. M., Cooper, M. L., & George, L. K. (1997). Sexual assault history and health perceptions: Seven general population studies. *Health Psychology*, 16(5), 417–425.

Goldstein, M. (1948). *The roots of prejudice against the Negro in the United States*. Boston: Boston University Press.

Gorcey, M., Santiago, J. M., & McCall-Perez, F. (1986). Psychological consequences for women sexually abused in childhood. *Social Psychiatry*, 21, 129–133.

Hamilton, G. V. (1929) *A research in marriage*. New York: Albert & Charles Boni.

Hamilton, G. V. (1936). Can personality be measured? *Journal of Social Psychology*, 7, 358–363.

Handwerker, P. (1993). Gender power differences between parents and high-risk behavior by their children: AIDS/STD risk factors extend to a prior generation. *Journal of Women's Health*, 2(3), 301.

Hazzard, A., Rogers, J. H., & Angert, L. (1993). Factors affecting group therapy outcome for adult sexual survivors. *International Journal of Group Psychotherapy*, Oct. 43(4), 453–468.

Heise, L., Moore, K., & Toubia, N. (1995). *Sexual coercion and reproductive health: A focus on research*. New York: The Population Council.

Ima, K., & Hohm, C. F. (1991). Child maltreatment among Asian and Pacific islander refugees and immigrants: The San Diego case. *Journal of Interpersonal Violence*, 6(30), 267–285.

Jackson, J. L., Calhoun, K. S., Amick, A. E., Madderer, H. M., *et al.* (19900. Young adult women who report childhood intrafamilial sexual abuse: Subsequent adjustment. *Archives of Sexual Behavior*, 19(3), 211–221.

Jarvis, T. J., & Copeland, J. (1997). Child sexual abuse as a predicator of psychiatric co-morbidity and its implications for drug and alcohol treatment. *Drug & Alcohol Dependence*, Dec. 49, 61–69.

Jarvis, T. J, Copeland, J., & Walton, L. (1998). Exploring the nature of the relationship between child sexual abuse and substance use among women. *Addiction*, 93(6), 865–875.

Johnsen, L. W., & Harlow, L. L. (1996). Childhood sexual abuse linked with adult substance use, victimization, and AIDS risk. *AIDS Education and Prevention*, 8(1), 44–57.

Kilpatrick, A. C. (1987). Childhood sexual experiences: Problems and issues in studying long-range effects. *Journal of Sex Research*, 23(2), 173–196.

Kilpatrick, A. C. (1992). Long-range effects of child and adolescent sexual experiences: Myths, mores, and menaces. Hillsdale, NJ: Erlbaum.

Kilpatrick, D. G., Acierno, R., Resnick H. S., Sauders B. E., & Best C. L. (1997). A two–year longitudinal analysis of the relationships between violent assault and substance abuse in women. *Journal of Consulting and Clinical Psychology*, 65(5), 834–847.

Koss, M. P., Goodman, L. A., Browne, A., Fitzgerald, L. F., Keita, G. P., & Russo, N. F. (1994). No safe haven: Male violence against women at home, at work, and in the community. Washington, DC: American Psychological Association.

Landis C., & Bolles, M. M. (1940). Psychosexual immaturity. *Journal of Abnormal & Social Psychology*, 35, 449–452.

Laws, A., & Golding, J. M. (1996). Sexual assault history and eating disorder symptoms among European American, Hispanic, and African American women and men. *American Journal of Public Health*, 86(4), 579–582.

Lodico, M. A., & DiClemente, R. J. (1994). The association between childhood sexual abuse and prevalence of HIV-related risk behaviors. *Clinical Pediatrics*, XX, 498–502.

Long, S. (1986). Guidelines for treating young children. In K. MacFarlane, J. Waterman, S. Conerly, L. Damon, M. Durfee, & S. Long (Eds.), *Sexual abuse of young children* (Chapter 12). New York: Guilford Press.

Lundberg-Love, P. K. (1990). Childhood sexual abuse and psychobiology: A commentary. *Journal of Child Sexual Abuse*, 1(2), 109–111.

Maguire, K., & Pastore, A. L. (1996). Sourcebook of criminal and justice statistics 1995. U.S. Department of

Justice, Bureau of Justice Statistics. Washington DC: USGPO.

Maltz, W. (1988). Identifying and treating the sexual repercussions of incest: A couple's therapy approach. *Journal of Sex and Marital Therapy*, 14(2), 142–170.

McCauley, J., Kern, D., Kolodner, K., Dill, L., Schroeder, A. F., DeChant, H. K., Ryden, J., Derogatis, L. R., & Bass, E. B. (1997). Clinical characteristics of women with a history of childhood abuse. *Journal of the American Medical Association*, 277(17), 1362–1368.

McGuire, L. S., & Wagner, N. N. (1978). Sexual dysfunction in women who were molested as children: One response pattern and suggestions for treatment. *Journal of Sex and Marital Therapy*, 4(1), 11–15.

Medrano, M. A., Desmond, D. P., Zule, William, A., & Hatch, J. P. (1999). Histories of childhood trauma and the effects on risky HIV behaviors in a sample of women drug users. *American Journal of Drug & Alcohol Abuse, Nov. 25* (4), 593–606.

Mennen, F. E., & Pearlmutter, L. (1993). Detecting childhood sexual abuse in couples therapy. *Families in Society*, 74(2), 74–83.

Miller, M. (1999). A model to explain the relationship between sexual abuse and HIV risk among women. *AIDS Care*, 11(1), 3–20.

Miller, M., & Paone, D. (1998). Social network characteristics as mediators in the relationship between sexual abuse and HIV risk. *Social Science & Medicine, Sep.* 47(6), 765–777.

Moncrief, J., Drummond, D. C., Candy, B., Checinski, K., & Farmer, R. (1996). Sexual abuse in people with alcohol problems. A study of the prevalence of sexual abuse and its relationship to drinking behavior. *British Journal of Psychiatry*, 169(3), 355–60.

National Crime Victimization Survey. Bureau of Justice Statistics. U.S. Department of Justice, 1997.

National Institute of Justice (1997). Child Abuse Intervention Strategic Planning Meeting Background Papers. Cambridge: MA: Abt Associates.

National Institute on Drug Abuse (1994). Women and Drug Use. (NIH Publication No. 94-3732). Rockville, MD: U.S. Department of Health and Human Services, National Institutes of Health).

Nationality data set, U.S. Department of Health and Human Services (1993). SETS version 1.22a [Hyattsville, MD]: U.S. Dept. of Health and Human Services: Public Health Service: Centers for Disease Control and Prevention: National Center for Health Statistics.

Palacios, W. R., Urman, C. F., Newel, R, & Hamilton, N. (1999). Developing a sociological framework for dually diagnosed women. *Journal of Substance Abuse Treatment*, 17 (1–2), 91–102.

Perez, B., Kennedy, G., & Fullilove, M. T. (1995). Childhood sexual abuse and AIDS: Issues and interventions. In Ann O'Leary & Lorette Sweet Jemmott (Eds.), *Women at risk: Issues in the primary prevention of AIDS* (pp. 83–101). New York: Plenum Press.

Rhodes, J. E., Ebert, L., & Myers, A. B. (1993). Sexual victimization in young pregnant and parenting, African-American women: Psychological and social outcomes. *Violence & Victims, Sum.8*(2), 153–163.

Richter, N. L., Snider, E., & Gorey, K. M. (1997). Group work intervention with female survivors of childhood sexual abuse. *Research on Social Work Practice, Jan.* 7(1), 53–69.

Riggs, A., Alario, A. J., & McHorney, C. (1990). Health risk behaviors and attempted suicide in adolescents who report prior maltreatment, *Journal of Pediatrics*, 116(5), 815.

Rind, B., Tromovitch, P., & Bauserman, R. (1998). A meta-analytic examination of assumed properties of child sexual abuse using college samples. *Psychological Bulletin, Jul. 124*(1), 22–53.

Risin, L., & Koss, M. P. (1987). The sexual abuse of boys: Prevalence and descriptive characteristics of childhood victimization. *Journal of Interpersonal Violence, Sep. 2*(3), 309–323.

Rohsenow, D. J., Corbett, R., & Devine, D. (1988). Molested as children: A hidden contribution to substance abuse. *Journal of Substance Abuse Treatment*, 5, 13–18.

Romans, S. E., Martin, J., & Mullen, P. (1996). Women's self-esteem: A community study of women who report and do not report childhood sexual abuse. *British Journal of Psychiatry*, 169(6), 696–704.

Romero, G. J., Wyatt, G. E., Loeb, T. B., Carmona, J. V., & Solis, B. M. (1999). The prevalence and circumstances of child sexual abuse among Latina women. *Hispanic Journal of Behavioral Sciences, Aug. 21*(3), 351–365.

Russell, D. (1983). The incidents and prevalence of intrafamilial and extrafamilial sexual abuse of female children. *Child Abuse & Neglect*, 7(2), 133–146.

Russell, D. F. H. (1982). *Rape in marriage*. New York: Macmillan.

Salmon, P., & Calderbank, S. (1996). The relationship of childhood physical and sexual abuse to adult illness behavior. *Journal of Psychosomatic Research*, 40(3), 329–336.

Sarrel, P. M., & Masaters, W. H. (1982). Sexual molestation of men by women. *Archives of Sexual Behavior*, 11(2), 117–131.

Sarwer, D. B., & Durlak, J. A. (1996). Childhood sexual abuse as a predictor of adult female sexual dysfunction: A study of couples seeking sex therapy. *Child Abuse and Neglect*, 20(10), 963–972.

Schei, B., & Bakketeig, L. S. (1989). Gynecological impact of sexual and physical abuse by spouse: A random sample of Norwegian women. *British Journal of Obstetrics and Gynecology*, 96, 1379–1383.

Schei, B. (1990a). Prevalence of sexual abuse history in a random sample of Norwegian women. *Scandinavian Social Medicine*, 18(63).

Schei, B. (1990b). Psychosocial factors in pelvic pain: A controlled study of women living in physically abusive relationships. *Acta Obstetrica et Gynecologica Scandinavica*, 69(67).

Shearer, S. L., & Herbert, C.A. (1987). Long term effects of unresolved sexual trauma [published erratum appears in *American Family Physician* 1988 Jan; 37(1):44] *American Family Physician, Oct. 36*(4), 169–175.

Simoni, J. M., Mason, H. R. C., Marks, G., Ruiz, M. S., Reed, D., & Richardson, J. L. (1995). Women's self-disclosure of HIV infection: Rates, reasons, and reactions. *Journal of Consulting and Clinical Psychology, 63*, 474–478.

Smith, G. (1992). The unbearable traumatogenic past: Child sexual abuse. In V. P. Varma (Ed.), *The secret life of vulnerable children* (pp. 130–156). Florence, KY: Taylor & Francis/Routledge.

Springs, F. E., & Friedrich, W. N. (1992). Health risk behaviors and medical sequelae of childhood sexual abuse. *Mayo Clinic Proceedings, 67*, 527–532.

Stalking and domestic violence: The third annual report to Congress under the Violence Against Women Act. Washington, DC: Violence Against Women Grants Office, Office of Justice Programs, U.S. Department of Justice, 1998. iii, 67 p.; 28 cm.

Terman, L. M, Buttenwieser, P., Ferguson, L. W., Johnson, W. B., & Wilson, D. P. (1938). *Psychological factors in marital happiness.* NY: McGraw-Hill.

Toomey, T. C., Seville, J. L., Mann, J. D., Abashian, S. W. (1995). Relationship of sexual and physical abuse to pain description, coping, psychological distress and health-care utilization in a chronic pain sample. *Clinical Journal of Pain, 11*(4), 307–315.

Triandis, H. (1995). *Individualism and collectivism.* Boulder, CO: Westview Press.

U.S. Department of Health and Human Services, Administration on Children, Youth, and Families (1999). *Child maltreatment 1997: Reports from the states to the National Child Abuse and Neglect Data System.* Washington, DC: U.S. Government Printing Office.

U.S. Department of Health and Human Services, National Center on Child Abuse and Neglect (1997). *Child maltreatment 1995: Reports from the states to the national child abuse and neglect data system.* Washington, DC: National Clearinghouse on Child Abuse and Neglect Information.

Urquiza, A. J., & Goodlin-Jones, B. L. (1994). Child sexual abuse and adult revictimization with women of color. *Violence & Victims, 9*(3), 223–232.

Violence Against Women. Bureau of Justice Statistics. U.S. Department of Justice, 1994.

Walker, E. C., Bonner, B. L., & Kaufman, K. L. (1988). *The physically and sexually abused child: Evaluation and treatment.* New York: Pergamon Press

Walker, L. E. (1999). Psychology and domestic violence around the world. *American Psychologist, Jan. 54*(1), 21–29.

Wallen, J. (1998). Need for services research on treatment for drug abuse in women. In *National Institute on Drug Abuse, Drug Addiction Research and the Health of Women* (NIH publication No. 98-4290 (pp. 229–236). Rock-

ville, MD: U.S. Department of Health and Human Services, National Institutes of Health.

Waterman, J., MacFarlane, K., Conerly, S., Damon, L., Durfee, M., & Long, S. (1986). Challenges for the future. In K. MacFarlane, J. Waterman, S. Conerly, L. Damon, M. Durfee, & S. Long (Eds.), *Sexual abuse of young children* (Chapter 15). New York: Guilford Press.

Widom, C. S., & Kuhns, J. B. (1996). Childhood victimization and subsequent risk for promiscuity, prostitution, and teenage pregnancy: A prospective study. *American Journal of Public Health, 86*(11), 1607–1612.

Wilsnack, S. C., Vogeltanz, N. D., Klassen, A. D., & Harris, R. (1997). Childhood sexual abuse and women's substance abuse: National survey finding. *Journal of Studies on Alcohol, May 58*(3), 264–271.

Wrobel, G. M., Ayers-Lopez, S., Grotevent, H. D., McRoy, R. G., & Friedrick, M. (1996) Openness in adoption and the level of child participation. *Child Development, Oct, 67*(5), 2358–2374. (UI: 97174518) Medline.

Wyatt, G. E., (1982). Identifying stereotypes of African-American sexuality and their impact upon sexual behavior. In B. A. Bass, G. E. Wyatt, & G. J. Powell (Eds.). *The Afro-American Family assessment, treatment and research issues* (pp. 333–346). New York: Grune and Stratton.

Wyatt, G. E. (1985). The sexual abuse of Afro-American and White-American women in childhood. *Child Abuse & Neglect, 9*(4), 507–519.

Wyatt, G. E. (1988). The relationship between child sexual abuse and adolescent sexual functioning in Afro-American and European American women. *Annals of the New York Academy of Sciences, 528*, 111–122.

Wyatt, G. E. (1990). Sexual abuse of ethnic minority children: Identifying dimensions of victimization. *Professional Psychology: Research and Practice, 21*(5), 338–343.

Wyatt, G. E. (1991). Child sexual abuse and its effects on sexual functioning. In J. Bancroft (Ed.), *Annual review of sex research* (pp. 249–266). Lake Mills, IA: The Society for the Scientific Study of Sex.

Wyatt, G. E. (1997). *Stolen women: Reclaiming our sexuality, taking back our lives.* New York: Wiley.

Wyatt, G., Newcomb, M. D., & Riederle, M. H. (1993). *Sexual abuse and consensual sex: Women's developmental patterns and outcomes.* Newbury Park, CA: Sage.

Wyatt, G. E., & Loeb, T. B. (1997). The prevalence, circumstances, and later consequences of child sexual abuse. National Institute of Justice Child Abuse Intervention Strategic Planning Meeting Background Papers. Cambridge, MA: Abt Associates.

Wyatt, G. E., & Mickey R. M. (1987). Ameliorating the effects of child sexual abuse. An exploratory study of support by parents and others. *Journal of Interpersonal Violence, Dec. 2*(4), 403–414.

Wyatt, G. E., & Peters, S. D. (1986). Issues in the definition of child sexual abuse in prevalence research. *Child Abuse & Neglect, 10*(2), 241–251.

Wyatt, G. E., Guthrie, D., & Notgrass, C. M. (1992).

Differential effects of women's child sexual abuse and subsequent revictimization. *Journal of Consulting & Clinical Psychology*, *60*(2), 167–173.

Wyatt, G. E., Loeb, T. B., Romero, G., Solis, B., & Carmona, J. V. (1998). The prevalence and circumstances of child sexual abuse: Changes across a decade. *Child Abuse & Neglect*, *23*(1), 45–60.

Wyatt, G. E., Tucker, M. B., Romero, G. J., Carmona, J. V., Newcomb, M. D., Wayment, H. A., Loeb, T. B., Solis, B. M., & Mitchell-Jernan, C. (1997). Adapting a comprehensive approach to African American women's sexual risk taking. *Journal of Health Education*, *28*(6), 52–60.

Wyatt, G. E., Loeb, T. B., Ganz, P., & Desmond (2000). *The prevalence and circumstances of child sexual abuse among breast cancer survivors: Relationship to high-risk sexual behaviors*. Manuscript submitted for publication.

12

Chronic Pelvic Pain

ANDREA J. RAPIN and MELINDA L. MORGAN

INTRODUCTION

In a gendered social environment, the mores regarding a woman's body powerfully influence the medical care she will receive. Women who suffer from pain that arises from the pelvic cavity and the perineum comprise a group whose medical care historically has been inadequate. Because the etiology of chronic pelvic pain (CPP) is often unidentifiable, the disorder is a perplexing and frustrating condition for patients and for providers. Often the severity of pain is not proportional to the degree of pelvic pathology. Women with long-standing pelvic pain frequently have limited social support systems and may experience financial hardship and subsequent loss of medical insurance due to impaired occupational functioning. Other sequelae include decreased physical activity, impaired social relations, altered family roles, depression, and accompanying vegetative signs such as sleep and appetite dysregulation.

Pelvic pain patients often have had poor outcomes with traditionally successful medical treatments and multiple unsuccessful surgeries for pain. It is estimated that $2.8 billion are spent annually on diagnosis and treatment of chronic pain (Wenof and Perry, 1999). Such expenditures contribute to the rising costs of health care and significantly impact society. The emotional cost is significant as well, in that women may feel their pain has been "invalidated" if a work-up reveals no obvious organic pathologies. They may have been told directly or by implication that the pain is "all in their head." Women with chronic pelvic pain, as with other chronic painful conditions, may become irritable, depressed and somatically focused, because they have endured the pain for an extended length of time with no hope for relief. Marital relations may be disrupted as there is typically dyspareunia (pain with sexual activity) and the loss or deterioration of physical and emotional intimacy. Likewise CPP patients are often perceived negatively by medical professionals, due to the difficulty in treating the disorder and possible demands for narcotic pain medications (Self et al., 1998).

DEFINITION AND EPIDEMIOLOGY

Definition

Pain that emanates from the generalized pelvic region (below the umbilicus and above

ANDREA J. RAPKIN • Department of Obstetrics and Gynecology, Center for the Health Sciences, UCLA School of Medicine, Los Angeles, California 90095-1740. MELINDA L. MORGAN • Department of Psychiatry, UCLA Neuropsychiatric Institute and Hospital, Los Angeles, California 90095.

Handbook of Women's Sexual and Reproductive Health, edited by Wingood and DiClemente. Kluwer Academic / Plenum Publishers, New York, 2002.

the groin) can be acute or chronic. Acute pain is characterized by sudden onset and short course, whereas chronic pelvic pain is pain that lasts for more than six months. This chapter will focus on chronic pelvic pain because acute pain typically has an identifiable cause that responds to appropriate medical or surgical treatment, whereas chronic pelvic pain is far more complex. Acute pain is likely caused by infection, rupture or obstruction of a vicsus or release of an irritating fluid into the peritoneal cavity such as blood, pus, or the contents of an ovarian cyst. In the case of chronic pelvic pain, an initiating event may not be apparent or there may have been a triggering event such as a surgical procedure, but the pain persists long after adequate healing. This may occur because of changes in the threshold for signaling of pain in peripheral tissues or the central nervous system. Over time, in the course of reacting to chronic pain, abdominal and pelvic floor muscles may become tense and develop tender or "trigger" points. Other systems innervated by the same nerves as the reproductive organs including the urinary tract and the bowel may also become involved. Even the overlying connective tissues and skin in the surrounding areas may be affected. This secondary "referred pain" process may become the predominant problem, obscuring the original pain process, particularly when there is no identifiable primary pathology. Therefore, the factors that initiated the painful condition are likely to be different from factors maintaining the pain.

Prevalence of Chronic Pelvic Pain

Pelvic pain is one of the most common complaints among women seeing gynecologists in outpatient settings. The prevalence of a disorder in the general population is often difficult to determine because the data are collected and analyzed in different manners. Reiter (1990) is often cited when discussing prevalence of chronic pain, indicating that CPP is responsible for 12% of hysterectomies, 40% of laparoscopies, and 15–40% of all secondary and tertiary outpatient gynecological visits. Collett (1998) in-

dicated that CPP accounts for 10% of outpatient consultations, 40% of laparoscopies, and 10–12% of the hysterectomies in the United Kingdom accounting for 70,000 procedures annually. Milburn, Reiter, and Rhomberg (1993) estimate that 10% of outpatient consultations are because of CPP and one third of laparoscopies are performed because of the syndrome. Walker and Shaw (1993) report that 38% of patients in their research reported chronic pelvic pain (persisting more than six months) at some point in their lives.

Prevalence rates for subtypes of CPP also vary. The literature reports widely discrepant rates of CPP in women with visible organic pathology versus those without obvious pathology (CPPWOP). For instance, Savidge and Slade (1997) report a range of 8% to 88% of positive finding such as adhesions or endometriosis at the time of laparoscopy. Gillibrand (1981) reports that in 63% of women having laparoscopies, no visible pathology was found. Hodgkiss and Watson (1994) also report 60% rate of negative laparoscopy findings. According to Wenof and Perry (1999), 61% of women suffering from CPP do not have a diagnosis.

Conversely, several other studies have reported that there is a larger proportion of laparoscopies that do reveal obvious pathology as opposed to those that do not. For instance, Rosenthal et al. (1984) identified pathology in 75% of their sample. Reiter, Gambone, and Johnson (1991) indicate a physical cause in two thirds of CPP cases. Vercellini et al. (1996) report positive laparoscopy findings in approximately 60% of cases in adolescent women. Until such time as a clear understanding of the pathophysiology of CPP with standardized definitions and methodologies for the diagnosis of CPP, prevalence rates will remain unclear. However, the important issue is the large number of patients suffering and the inadequate attention that has been given to this group of women.

Pathophysiology of CPP

The neural mechanisms underlying the transmission of chronic pain from the internal organs are not known. There are two types of nerves innervating the pelvis: visceral and somatic. The visceral nerves carry afferent impulses or sensations from intraabdominal organs such as the bowel, bladder, ureter, rectum, uterus, ovary, and fallopian tubes, whereas the somatic nerves innervate superficial tissues such as the skin and muscle of the abdominal wall and pelvis, external genitals, as well as the perineum (Cervero & Tattersall, 1986). Visceral and somatic nerves synapse on the same second order neuron in the dorsal horn of the spinal cord and in this way have an influence on each other. The pain from the viscera is poorly localizable but is often "referred" or felt in the area of muscle or skin receiving its nerve supply from the same segment or region of the spinal cord (dermatome). This convergence, when visceral and somatic neurons project onto the same neurons in the dorsal horn of the spinal cord, is most likely responsible for the sensation of referred pain. When visceral nerves are stimulated, this "referred" pain will be perceived in areas of the abdominal wall, pelvic muscles, and superficial tissues. Specific areas of tenderness develop at those sites of referral and area termed tender or "trigger points." Hence, referred visceral pain is experienced at a site other than the region affected by the pathological process. It is postulated that even after the original visceral stimulation has resolved, the referred pain may persist. Additionally in a susceptible individual, visceral injury can lead to altered thresholds for signaling such that previously nonpainful stimuli are now perceived as painful. This change in sensation is the focus of much current research and entails altered processing at the level of the spinal cord and brain.

Theoretical Constructs of Pain Perception

The neurophysiology of the perception of pain is a nascent area of research, but there is information on the psychology of pain and this has led to theoretical constructs on pain perception. Pain stimulates an organism to initiate activity aimed at stopping the painful sensation. If the pain continues over time, it is ac-

companied by physiologic, behavioral, and affective responses that differ from those of a brief acute signal. The traditional theory of pain perception, the Cartesian or somatic theory, posits that specific neurons carry pain signals from the site of damage to the spinal cord directly to the brain cortex (Jacob, 1997). Many health care providers still adhere to this theory, such that they have firm ideas about how much pain should accompany given conditions (Jacob, 1997). If the patient deviates from the norm, this may influence the provider's response to the patient.

A newer, more comprehensive theory, was the gate control theory developed by Melzack and Wall (1965). This model postulated that rather than following a fixed route, the signal is modified (intensified, reduced, or blocked) within the central nervous system. In other words, the spinal cord functions as a "gate" through which the signal must pass before the signal is transmitted to the brain. Should the gates be altered by a painful stimulus from the periphery, they may remain "open" even after tissue damage is controlled. The pain will remain (be perceived) despite treating the originating cause. This type of pain is called neuropathic pain (Wenof and Perry, 1999).

A third theory of pain perception is the diathesis stress theory which integrates neurobiological and psychological factors (Kerns and Jacob, 1995). This model suggests that there may be a predisposing, genetic proclivity that increases the risk of developing a pattern of chronic pain. The predisposing factor exists within a social context which may also influence the perception of pain. Kerns and Jacob (1995) give an example of a person who has always been active, who suffers a back injury. If she is instructed to maintain strict bed rest, tolerating such inactivity may be very stressful. The stress may lead to increased muscle tension, anxiety, worry, insomnia, and cognitive distortions of her prognosis. Another illustration of the diathesis stress model can be seen in a person who has a genetic predisposition for depression who also has a history of physical or sexual abuse. This patient may have low self-esteem and deficits in ego strengths. She may delay seeking help and depression may increase her perception of pain. A situation that could have been addressed early thus becomes a chronic pain problem. Furthermore, purely neuro-physiological processes may lead to a chronic pain response to a trauma or surgical procedure. For example some patients develop severe pain after amputation of a limb termed "phantom limb pain," while others do not (Devore, 1997). An interesting discussion of neuroplasticity and pain is found in a book written for lay audiences called *Phantoms in the Brain* (Ramachardran, 1998).

Differential Diagnosis of CPP

The differential diagnosis of chronic pelvic pain focusing on those factors in the pelvis are listed in Table 1. Although detailed description of the epidemiology, pathophysiology, and treatment of these conditions is beyond the scope of this chapter, many thorough reviews exist (Steege, *et al.*, 1993; Ling, 1993; Rocker, 1990; Rapkin,

TABLE 1. Differential Diagnoses of Chronic Pelvic Pain

I. Gynecologic
  A. Noncyclic
    1. Adhesions
    2. Endometriosis
    3. Salpingo-oophoritis
      a. Acute
      b. Subacute
    4. Ovarian remnant syndrome
    5. Pelvic congestion syndrome (varicosities)
    6. Ovarian neoplasms
    7. Pelvic relaxation
    8. Residual ovary syndrome
  B. Cyclic
    1. Primary dysmenorrhea
    2. Secondary dysmenorrhea
      a. Imperforate hymen
      b. Transverse vaginal septum
      c. Cervical stenosis
      d. Uterine anomalies (congenital malformation, bicornuate uterus, blind uterine horn)
      e. Intrauterine synechiae (Asherman's syndrome)
      f. Endometrial polyps
      g. Uterine leiomyomas
      h. Adenomyosis
      i. Pelvic congestion syndrome (varicosities)
      j. Endometriosis
    3. Atypical cyclic
      a. Endometriosis
      a. Adenomyosis
      a. Ovariant remnant syndrome
      a. Chronic functional cyst formation
II. Gastrointestinal
  A. Irritable bowel syndrome
  B. Ulcerative colitis
  C. Granulomatous colitis (Crohn disease)
  D. Carcinoma
  E. Infectious diarrhea
  F. Recurrent partial small bowel obstruction

II. Gastrointestinal (*cont.*)
  G. Diverticulitis
  H. Hernia
  I. Abdominal angina
  J. Recurrent appendiceal colic
III. Genitourinary
  A. Recurrent or relapsing cystourethritis
  B. Urethral syndrome
  C. Interstitial cystitis
  D. Ureteral diverticuli or polyps
  E. Carcinoma of the bladder
  F. Ureteral obstruction
  G. Pelvic kidney
IV. Neurologic
  A. Nerve entrapment syndrome
  B. Neuroma
  C. Trigger points
V. Musculoskeletal
  A. Low back pain syndrome
    1. Congenital anomalies
    2. Scoliosis and kyphosis
    3. Spondylolysis
    4. Spinal injuries
    5. Inflammation
    6. Tumors
    7. Osteoporosis
    8. Degenerative changes
    9. Coccydynia
  B. Myofascial syndrome
  C. Fibromyalgia
  D. Pelvic floor muscle tension myalgia
VI. Systemic
  A. Acute intermittent porphyria
  B. Abdominal migraine
  C. Systemic lupus erythematosus
  D. Lymphoma
  E. Neurofibromatosis

in press). Women with CPP complain of lower abdominal pain either diffuse or localizable to the right or left lower quadrants or both, often radiating to the hips, thighs, or back. The pain can be dull and aching or sharp, throbbing, and stabbing. Pain levels are usually described as at least 7 out of 10 (if zero is no pain and 10 is the most severe pain imaginable). The pain may be confined to certain activities such as exercise, intercourse, or daily activities of living but may also occur at rest or be limited to certain times of the month such as premenstrually or menstrually. Very often there is pain with sexual arousal and it increases with penetration. Gastrointestinal symptoms such as pain with bowel movements, diarrhea, constipation, bloating, and gas may be present, and often there is increased pain with a full bowel and full bladder. Urinary symptoms can accompany CPP symptoms, including urinary frequency and sometimes pain with urination. Most women have tried aspirin and acetaminophen-containing products as well as nonsteroidal anti-inflammatory agents without relief. They may be receiving a narcotic prescription from their physician but it is rarely enough to control the pain.

BEHAVIORAL AND PSYCHOLOGICAL CORRELATES

The signal from the afferent nerves transmitting the sensation of pain is distinct from the accompanying suffering and subsequent behavioral, social, and psychological responses. As pain persists over time, the potential to affect behavior increases. Sexual/physical abuse, family and marital interactions, cultural background, severe anxiety or depression, and drug dependence have all been correlated with increased chronicity and poor treatment outcomes in women with pelvic pain.

Sexual and Physical Abuse

An interest in the correlation between sexual/physical abuse and CPP has become prominent in the last two decades. The litera-

ture is equivocal, but suggests that women with CPP have a higher prevalence of abuse, either physical or sexual, than women without pain or with nonpelvic pain. Ehlert (1999) found a higher prevalence of sexual abuse in women with CPP-WOP than controls. Rapkin et al. (1990) found significantly more physical abuse in women with pelvic pain compared with women with other painful conditions. Reiter et al. (1991) concluded that previous sexual abuse is a significant predisposing risk for non-somatic chronic pelvic pain. Toomey et al. (1993) did not find differences between abused and nonabused women with CPP with respect to demographics, pain description, or functional interference; however, the abused group perceived less life control, more punishing responses to pain, and higher levels of somatization and global distress. At this point, it is clear that many women with CPP have a history of physical and/or sexual abuse or violence. The evidence suggests that a history of abuse increases the risk for somatization, greater utilization of medical services, and probably CPP.

Marital and Family Interaction

Marital interaction also affects chronic pain. Flor (1989) found that perceived pain and activity levels of patients were affected by spousal reinforcement of overt expressions of pain. Kerns et al. (1990) reported pain-contingent responses from spouses accounted for a significant proportion of variance in perceived pain severity. He indicated that a higher level of spouse solicitousness predicted greater severity of pain. Turk (1992) also studied the importance of spouses' responses to communication of pain from the patient.

Likewise, the family environment is a critical component of how health-related beliefs and behaviors are learned. Some people may not have been taught to respond overtly to pain, whereas others may have lived in an environment that as soon as any member was feeling pain he or she was taken immediately to the hospital. Women are often fearful that pain signals pathology which could be morbid or lead to loss of reproductive potential. Baker & Symonds (1992) noted that women with CPP often have resolution of pain after being apprised of normal laparoscopic findings. Kerns and Payne (1996) discusses the importance of understanding transactional family functions in order to appreciate the perpetuation of the chronic pain experience. Also the expectation of women's beliefs about pain, her ability to control the pain, stress, mood, and pending disability influence how pain is perceived. Attitudes and action of health care providers may also affect whether patients "doctor shop" and therefore lose the benefit of continuity of care.

Cultural Background

People from different cultural backgrounds may express pain differently. Stoicism may be highly valued in certain cultures, whereas other cultures may encourage emotional expression of distress (Bates *et al.*, 1993). In the United States, value is placed on stoicism, therefore if pain is emotionally communicated, mainstream health care providers may see the patient as exaggerating the intensity of her pain. Also in the United States, there is a tendency to deny the adverse physical consequences of emotional or environmental stress. Zola (1966, 1973), in earlier studies, reported that even when the diagnosis was held constant, people of different ethnic backgrounds presented with differing complaints. Bates (1987) and Bates and Edwards (1992) studied biocultural variability to pain responses and linked social learning within ethnocultural groups, in conjunction with prior pain experiences, to inhibitory and cognitive control of pain. In another study, Bates, Rankin-Hill, and Sanchez-Ayendez (1997) looked at the role of cultural and ethnic factors that influence the chronic pain experience. They found the best predictors of variation in pain intensity were ethnic group affiliation and perception of locus of control. Grace (1998) concludes that mind–body dualism contributes to patient stress and alienation, whereas a mind–body integration approach contributed to more supportive patient–provider relationships and less treatment related stress.

Psychological Correlates

Lack of obvious organic pathology in women with CPP has led to speculation of psychological correlates of the condition. The role of psychological factors in the etiology of CPP has long been debated. Early studies such as Gidro-Frank, Kerns, & Taylor (1960) report a very high incidence of psychiatric illness in women with pelvic pain. Renaer and Guzinski (1978) note that some practitioners do not even accept the existence of CPPWOP and view it as a form of neurosis.

On a more rational note, Rudy, Kerns, and Turk (1988) found that the existence of pain was not sufficient in and of itself to develop psychiatric disorders, in particular depression. If level of life interference and self control were affected, the patient was more likely to develop depression secondary to the chronic pain. Savidge and Slade (1997) reviewed the literature on psychological correlates of chronic pelvic pain and concluded that there are higher rates of distress and psychopathology for women with CPP (both with and without organic pathology) than women without pain. However, they are careful to point out that these findings are common in people suffering from *other* kinds of chronic pain as well. Within the CPP population, they report that there is inconclusive evidence to suggest psychopathological differences in women with CPPWOP versus women with identifiable pathology. Pearce (1987) found no differences between women with or without identifiable pathology in mood and personality variables. Even when studies document an association between emotional disturbance and chronic pain, causality cannot be inferred. It is difficult to discern whether one's psychological profile can lead to experiencing and reporting more pain, or that living with chronic pain leads to emotional upheaval and disturbance.

Grace (1998) reviewed the debate in the literature as to whether chronic pelvic pain is psychogenic or not and concluded that one must look beyond a mind–body dualism. The reader is also referred to the comprehensive reviews of the literature by Fry *et al.* (1996a,b) and Savidge and Slade (1997). The overall impression from these reviews is that psychological, sociological, and behavioral correlates are heterogeneous in the chronic pain population and that women with CPP do not fit a specific profile that distinguishes them from other groups.

VIGNETTES

The following vignettes portray several of the long-term psychological sequelae of pelvic pain. The stories of these women illustrate the diverse presentation, wide domain of impact, and varied outcomes of chronic pelvic pain.

PAIN REDUCTION, INTERVENTION, TREATMENT, AND PREVENTION

The broad array of symptoms and nonspecificity of etiology makes treatment of chronic pelvic pain both challenging and frustrating. Because the nervous system incorpo-

rates the mind and the body, pain must be treated in both psychic and somatic arenas in order to achieve effective responses. Various disciplines are brought into the treatment arena because of the multiple organ systems and environmental factors involved in CPP. Treatment takes a gradual and extended course. Unfortunately, insurance carriers and family members and even the patient may falter and give up hope on multidisciplinary management. If framed as pain management and reduction and achieving an improved quality of life rather than total elimination of pain, prognosis is good.

Physical Evaluation

A complete history and physical exam should be conducted with particular attention to the abdomen, back, vagina, and urethrovesicle, including a bimanual, rectovaginal, and pelvic neurological exam. Various maneuvers are performed to determine the visceral and somatic pain components as well as areas of referred pain or trigger points. An attempt

Vignette 1

Megan was 30 years old when she began to experience nonspecific pelvic pain intermittently throughout the month. Her physician said, "not to worry, that some women are just more sensitive about their bodies than others." The pain typically would remit on the first day of her menstrual cycle. Even though the menstrual cramps were painful, they were bearable compared to the midcycle pain. She got married and had two children. She did not experience pain during the pregnancies or while lactating. However after the second baby was weaned, the pain returned and was worse than before. Sometimes she needed to come home from work; sometimes she vomited; other times she slept. Her husband began to be annoyed and said that she had the pain to get back at him because he had lost his job. He resented taking on more of the child care and household responsibilities when Megan was not well. When not in pain, Megan was high functioning and productive. A laparoscopy revealed a small amount of endometriosis which was removed. The doctor told her that she shouldn't have any more pain. Unfortunately, she continued to have pain and was told there was nothing more that could be done for her. Her husband was convinced now that the pain was all in her head. She started to believe that there was in fact something wrong with her mind and therefore did not seek further medical treatment. She and her husband separated and Megan resigned herself to living with the pain.

Vignette 2

Linda, now a 47-year-old married woman with one child, began her periods at 11 years old and from the first cycle had extreme pain accompanied by vomiting and heavy bleeding. Her periods were regular from the outset, as was the pain. During her late teens, she began to have mid-cycle pain and she could not use tampons because it made the cramping worse. Linda sought help from a physician at 21 and was told, "it's all in your head." In her thirties, the pain became worse; there was no pattern now, it occurred throughout the cycle. She began to use birth control pills which provided only minimal relief with the cramps. She had two D & C's and a laparoscopy. No identifiable pathology was found. By this time, her sleeping was interrupted by the pain, her social and emotional function were impaired, and her mood was depressed. She felt that everything was "tumbling out of control." Finally Linda was referred to a pain management clinic and a gynecologist specializing in pelvic pain. She was diagnosed with myofascial pain. She was injected with anesthesia at the trigger points and was given a low-dose antidepressant. She sees a physical therapist two times a week who specializes in pelvic pain. She does daily exercises at home and was trained in relaxation and visualization techniques. She attends a support group for women with chronic pelvic pain. The pain has been significantly reduced and Linda has had as many as five consecutive days without pain.

should be made to reproduce and thus localize the patient's pain. The patient should be given a daily pain diary to note the episodes and intensity of pain, as well as mood symptoms, stressful life events and family interactions. Pain that increases in intensity with menses can be more easily treated with hormonal suppression or even surgical approaches. Lab tests include urinalysis and culture, complete blood count, cervical cultures, Pap smear, and stool culture if diarrhea is present. Other appropriate imaging studies should be conducted of gastrointestinal, genitourinary, or musculoskeletal systems as needed. If abnormalities are found,

Vignette 3

Susan is a 41-year-old married professional woman. Her pain began six years ago and was too severe for her to continue working. She saw a variety of clinicians: a family physician, a rheumatologist, a gynecologist, an oncologist, a physical therapist. Pain medication, even narcotics, was not useful. She tried steroid cream, oral contraceptives, and antidepressants. Susan had multiple medical procedures: laparoscopies, a biopsy of the vulva, removal of a fibroid tumor. She felt the doctors were becoming impatient with her. She went on disability. She felt criticized and discounted. She was told "if *we* just think about things right, *we* might not have this pain." She hated going to the doctor and would often leave crying. Up until six years ago, Susan was a fully functioning, productive member of society, living a satisfying life. Eventually she was referred to a pain clinic that used a multidisciplinary approach. With the integrated approach, she has had some reduction in pain; however, she has not been able to return to full-time work and impairment remains in family and social functioning.

appropriate treatments should be initiated. Evaluation may require laparoscopy to visualize the pelvic organs. If trigger points are identified, trigger point injections with local anesthetics should be administered and may need to be repeated weekly or biweekly. The patient should be evaluated by a physical therapist and a mental health clinician skilled in treating pelvic pain.

Mental Health Evaluation

Pain management entails reducing suffering while optimizing functioning. The mental health practitioner should assess the pain complaint, the impact of the pain on life circumstances, and the patient's coping strategies. Measures of subjective report should be accompanied with behavioral assessment. The patient may experience a downward spiral of events that lead her to feel a loss of control and to become depressed. Feelings of helplessness and depression may compound the situation in that they may inhibit her from engaging in events and social interactions that are likely to generate an elevation in mood. New skills can be taught based on a cognitive behavioral approach identifying cognitive distortions, and adjusting perception. Cognitive behavioral stress reduction techniques can raise the pain threshold such that more pain input is needed in order to perceive the sensation as pain (Keefe et al., 1992). It is important to enhance opportunities for the patient to gain control of her pain and her environment. This may be particularly important if past or present trauma and abuse impact current functioning. If past sexual abuse is impacting current function, psychotherapy is indicated. Pelvic pain may affect sexual function, which may also have repercussions on self-esteem, mood, and quality of life. A careful sexual history should be taken. If there is a history of dyspareunia, there should be further exploration of how the pain has impacted the marital relationship.

Relaxation training, visualization, and biofeedback can be an important component of pain management. Reducing muscle tension may facilitate a reduction in the pain condition. The patient also learns to redirect her attention away from the pain. Relaxation should be utilized early on in treatment. As women become more adept at identifying muscular tension, they will be able to incorporate this into their coping repertoire.

Attending a support group for women with chronic pelvic pain may be particularly helpful. Group members can exchange information and by listening to the experiences of each other, they are likely to feel less isolated. Peer support and feedback can be extremely helpful. Research has shown that group work is particularly effective with people who are learning to cope with stress, marital difficulties, and assertiveness issues (Zastrow, 1998). Because referral to a mental health specialist may be met with resistance/denial, the patient must be assured that the medical practitioner is not discounting the reality of the pain, rather that CPP is a dynamic interaction of the several features of the psyche, nervous system, and body. The physician should also assure the patient that she will remain an active participant in her health care.

Multidisciplinary Pain Management

Because chronic pelvic pain is often refractory to traditional approaches, an interdisciplinary pain management program is advocated for treating patients with CPP. This approach involves integrating the mind–body paradigm while utilizing a team of health care practitioners of varying disciplines. Communication is essential between the gynecologist, the mental health practitioner, the physical therapist, the dietitian, and any other practitioners involved. Multidisciplinary pain management has been shown to reduce pain by at least 50% in 85% of the participants (Kames et al., 1990). Other studies have also had positive results (Reiter et al., 1991; Milburn et al., 1993; Gambone, 1990). A randomized, controlled study found the multidisciplinary approach (combining gynecological, dietary, psychosocial, and physical therapy treatment) more effective than traditional (medical and surgical) management (Peters, 1991).

Treatment modalities: Components of a multidisciplinary approach may include

- Pharmacological approaches to increase pain threshold utilizing low doses of tricyclic antidepressants, anticonvulsants, and sodium channel blockers
- Medication to relieve pain including nonsteroidal anti-inflammatory agents and long acting narcotics (use of narcotics should be guided with a narcotics "contract")
- Hormonal agents such as birth control pills, progestins or gonadotropin releasing agents to suppress menses if pain occurs in concert with menstrual periods or premenstrually
- Antidepressants if depression is identified
- Local anesthetic nerve blocks and trigger point injections if indicated
- Surgery, possibly including laparoscopy, presacral neurectomy (removal of the nerves supplying the uterus), hernia repair, treatment of endometriosis or adhesions or hysterectomy as indicated
- Physical therapy for abdominal, back, and pelvic floor muscles
- Psychosocial intervention to reduce stress and instruction in cognitive pain reduction techniques
- Psychotherapy as indicated for history of abuse, marital discord, or depression
- Alternative medicine such as chiropractic treatment, acupuncture, and hypnosis

The reader is referred to several comprehensive references for further details (Steege *et al.*, 1998; Ling, 1993; Rapkin, in press). Outcome research has reported successful treatment with these methods, but there is a lack of controlled studies to document that treatment was better than placebo or that treatment effects endured over time.

FINANCIAL IMPACT AND HEALTH CARE POLICY

The exact fiscal impact of CPP is difficult to estimate; however, Mathias *et al.* (1996) report that more than $881.5 million are spent annually on outpatient visits in the United States alone. The impact of the disorder on society, however, cannot be confined to the amount spent on diagnoses and treatment but also on opportunity cost. A 45% reduction in work productivity in women with CPP has been reported by Mathias and colleagues (1996) as well as a 15% increase in time lost from work. Wenof (1997) reports that 25% of women with CPP remain in bed for an average of 2.6 days per month and that 58% must cut down on their usual activity one or more days a month. Wenof (1997) indicates that $2.8 billion are spent for diagnosis and treatment. If 16% of a large sample of the general population report CPP (Schlaff, 1997), it is reasonable to assume that a disproportionate number of health care dollars are consumed in dealing with the disorder. Obviously it is more cost effective if the patient is diagnosed and treated early in the course of the disorder.

Carter (1999) presents a cost analysis of laparoscopy versus gonadotropin releasing hormone (GnHR) agonist therapy. He suggests that using a GnRH agonist, which suppresses ovarian function, menses, and endometriosis, as a diagnostic/therapeutic tool represents a 46% savings over the cost of initial laparoscopy to rule out endometriosis.

Women's perceptions must be addressed as an integral part of health policy aimed at treating women. Women's health care experience in regard to chronic pelvic pain has often not been satisfactory. Grace (1995b) reports the following themes that were frequently brought up by women in focus groups in a qualitative study: receiving a patronizing attitude from medical professionals and getting the sense of not being taken seriously, a history of poor health care (not getting referred to gynecologists for their pelvic pain), not receiving adequate information regarding a diagnosis or surgery, inadequate information about options to surgery, incomplete information about side effects of medication and being told "it's all in your head."

CONCLUSIONS

In order to improve the outcome for women in their medical encounter for treatment of chronic pelvic pain, an integrative approach is needed. A multidisciplinary approach to women's health care is based on the concept that many organ systems are involved in the production of symptoms; thus it is sensible that a team of providers from different fields would be best suited to provide treatment for the CPP patient.

There is a need to deconstruct the dichotomy of CPP being either a physiological or psychological problem as this creates a barrier to effective diagnosis and treatment. Pain need not be an inevitable part of being a woman; however, a "medical voice" concerned primarily with determining tissue damage and disease processes is likely to silence a woman (Grace, 1995a). Conversely, due to cultural contingencies, many women do not want to accept the role of the central nervous system (spinal cord and brain) in the production of pain. They may not understand the concept of modulation of pain signals in the peripheral and central nervous system and may feel they are being told the pain is psychological.

A supportive health care team is essential. If there is a specific treatable physiological problem underlying the pain, the problem is located and treated; however, when the problem is chronic and involves all levels of the neuraxis, the treatment approach is long term and comprehensive. The patient must be listened to and supported throughout the course of treatment. She should be educated about her pain and its implications and she should be encouraged to take an active role in her treatment.

REFERENCES

Baker, P. N., & Symonds, E. M. (1992). The resolution of chronic pelvic pain after normal laparoscopy findings. *American Journal of Obstetrics & Gynecology*, *166*, 835–836.

Bates, M. S., Edwards, W. T., & Anderson, K. O. (1993). Ethnocultural influences on variation in chronic pain perception. *Pain*, *52*, 101–112.

Bates, M. S. (1987). Ethnicity and pain: A biocultural model. *Social Science and Medicine*, *24*(1), 47–50.

Bates, M. S., & Edwards, W. T. (1992). Ethnic variations in the chronic pain experience. *Ethnic Disease*, *2*, 63–83.

Bates, M. S., Rankin-Hill, L., & Sanchez-Ayendez, M. (1997). The effects of the cultural context of health care on treatment of and response to chronic pain and illness. *Social Science and Medicine*, *5*(9), 1433–1447.

Carter, J. E. (1995). Cost effective management of women with chronic pelvic pain. *Keio Journal of Medicine*, *44*, 96.

Carter, J. E. (1999). *Chronic pelvic pain diagnosis and management*, OBGYN.net/english/pubs/features/carter/cpp/

Cervero, F., & Tattersall, J. E. (1986). Somatic and visceral sensory integration in the thoracic spinal cord. In F. Cerver & J. Morrison (Eds.), *Visceral sensation* (pp. 21–36). New York: Elsevier Science.

Collett, B. J., Cordle, C. J., Stewart, C. R., & Jagger, C. (1998). A comparative study of women with chronic pelvic pain, chronic non-pelvic pain and those with no history of pain attending general practitioners. *British Journal of Obstetrics and Gynecology*, *105*(1), 87–92.

Devore, M. (1997). Phantom pain as an expression of referred and neuropathic pain. In R. Z. Sherman (Ed.) *Phantom pain*. New York: Plenum Press.

Ehlert, Ulrike, Heim, C., & Hellhammer, D. H. (1999). Chronic pelvic pain as a somatoform disorder. *Psychotherapy and Psychosomatics*, *68*(2), 87–94.

Flor, H., Turk, D. C., & Rudy, T. E. (1989). Relationship of pain impact and significant other reinforcement of pain behaviors; the mediating role of gender, marital status, and marital satisfaction. *Pain*, *38*, 45–50.

Fry, R. P., Crisp, A. H., & Beard, R. W. (1996a). Sociopsychological factors in chronic pelvic pain: A review. *Journal of Psychosomatic Research*, *42*, 1–15.

Fry, R. P., Beard, R. W., Crisp, A. H., & McGuigan, S. (1996b). Sociopsychological factors in women with chronic pelvic pain with and without pelvic venous congestion. *Journal of Psychosomatic Research*, *42*(1), 71–85.

Gambone, J. C., & Reiter, R. C. (1990). Nonsurgical management of chronic pelvic pain: A multidisciplinary approach. *Clinical Obstetrics and Gynecology*, *33*, 643–661.

Gidro-Frank, L., Kerns, R. D., & Taylor, H. C. (1960). Pelvic pain and female identity: A survey of emotional factors in 40 patients. *American Journal of Obstetrics and Gynecology*, *79*, 1184–1202.

Gillibrand, P. N. (1981). Investigation of pelvic pain. Communication at the scientific meeting on chronic pelvic pain—a gynecological headache. Royal College of Obstetricians and Gynaecologists: London, May 1981.

Grace, M. M. (1998). Mind/body dualism in medicine: The case of chronic pelvic pain without organic pathology:

A critical review of the literature. *International Journal of Health Services, 28*(1), 127–151.

Grace, V. M. (1995a). Problems women patients experience in the medical encounter for chronic pelvic pain: A new Zealand study. *Health Care for Women International, 16*(6), 509–519.

Grace, V. M. (1995b). Problems of communication, diagnosis and treatment experience by women using the New Zealand health services for chronic pelvic pain: A quantitative analysis. *Health Care for Women International, 16*(6), 521–535.

Hodgkiss, A. D., & Watson, J. P. (1994). Psychiatric morbidity and illness behavior in women with chronic pelvic pain. *Journal of Psychosomatic Research, 38*(1), 3–9.

Jacob, M. C. (1997). Psychological issues. In *An integrated approach to the management of chronic pelvic pain*. A monograph developed following a scientific symposium at the American College of Obstetricians and Gynecologists annual meeting. Killingworth, CT: Pharmedica Press.

Kames, L. D., Rapkin, A. J., Naliboff, B. D., Afifi, S., & Ferrer-Brechner, T. (1990). Effectiveness of an interdisciplinary pain management program for the treatment of chronic pelvic pain. *Pain, 41*, 41–46.

Keefe, F. J., Dunsmore, J., & Burnett, R. (1992). Behavioral and cognitive behavioral approaches to chronic pain: Recent advances and future direction. *Journal of Consulting and Clinical Psychology, 60*, 528–536.

Kerns, R. D., & Payne, A. (1996). Treating families of chronic pain patients. In R. J. Gatchel, & D. C. Turk (Eds.), *Psychological approaches to pain management: A practitioner's handbook* (pp. 283–304). New York: Guilford Press.

Kerns, R. D., & Jacob, M. C. (1995). Toward an integrative diathesis-stress model of chronic pain. In A. J. Goreczny (Ed.), *Handbook of health and rehabilitation psychology* (pp. 325–340). New York: Plenum Press.

Kerns, R. D., Southwick, S., & Giller, E. L. (1991). The relationship between reports of pain-relevant social interaction and expressions of pain and affective distress. *Behavioral Therapy, 22*, 101–111.

Kerns, R. D., Haythornthwaite, J., Southwick, S., & Geller, E. L. (1990). The role of marital interaction in chronic pain and depressive symptom severity. *Journal of Psychosomatic Research, 34*, 401–408.

Ling, F. W. (Ed.) (1993). Contemporary management of chronic pelvic pain. *Obstetrics and Gynecology Clinics of North America, 20*(4).

Mathias, S. D., Kuppermann, M., Liberman, R. F., Lipschutz, R. C., & Steege, J. F. (1996). Chronic pelvic pain: Prevalence, health related quality of life and economic correlates. *Obstetrics and Gynecology, 87*, 321–327.

Melzack, R., & Wall, P. D. (1965). Pain mechanisms: a new theory. *Science, 150*, 971–979.

Milburn, A., Reiter, R. C., & Rhomberg, A. T. (1993). Multidisciplinary approach to chronic pelvic pain. *Obstetrics and Gynecology Clinics of North America, 20*, 643–641).

Pearce, S. (1987). The concept of psychogenic pain: A psychological investigation of women with pelvic pain. *Current Psychology: Research and Reviews, 6*(3), 219–228.

Peters, A., Van Dorst, E., Jellis, B., VanZuuren, E., Hermans, J., & Trimbos, J. B. (1991). A randomized clinical trial to compare two different approaches in women with chronic pelvic pain. *Obstetrics and Gynecology, 77*, 740–744.

Ramachardran, V. S. with Blakely, S. (1998). *Phantoms in the brain*. New York: William Morrow.

Rapkin, A. J. (in press). Chronic pelvic pain . In P. Wall and R. Melzack (Eds.), *Textbook of pain* (3rd ed.). New York: Churchill Livingstone.

Rapkin, A. J., Kames, L. D., Darke, L. L., Stampler, F. M., & Naliboff, B. D. (1990). History of physical and sexual abuse in women with chronic pelvic pain. *Obstetrics and Gynecology, 76*, 92–96.

Reiter, R. C., Gambone, J. C., & Johnson, S. R. (1991). Availability of a multi disciplinary pelvic pain clinic and frequency of hysterectomy for pelvic pain. *Journal of Psychosomatic Obstetrical Gynecology, 12*, 109–116.

Reiter, R. C., Shakerin, L. R., Gambone, J. C., Milburn, A. K. (1991). Correlation between sexual abuse and somatization in women with somatic and nonsomatic chronic pelvic pain. *American Journal of Obstetrics and Gynecology, 165*, 104–109.

Renaer, M., & Guzinski, G. M. (1978). Pain in gynecologic practice. *Pain, 5*, 305–331.

Rosenthal, R. H., Ling, F. W., Rosenthal, T. L., McNeeley, S. G. (1984). Chronic pelvic pain: Psychological features and laparoscopic findings. *Psychosomatics, 25*, 833–841.

Rudy, T. E., Kerns, R. D., & Turk, D. C. (1988). Chronic pain and depression: Toward a cognitive-behavioral mediation model. *Pain, 35*, 129–140.

Savidge, C. J., & Slade, P. (1997). Psychological aspects of chronic pelvic pain. *Journal of Psychosomatic Research, 42*(5), 433–444.

Schlaff, W. D. (1997). Treatment approaches. In *An integrated approach to the management of chronic pelvic pain*. Killingworth, CT: Pharmedica Press.

Steege, J. F., Metzger, D. A., & Levy, B. S. (Eds.) (1998). *Chronic pelvic pain—an integrated approach*. Philadelphia: W. B. Saunders.

Steege, J. F., Stout, A. L., & Somkuti, S. G. (1993). Chronic pelvic pain in women: Toward an integrative model. *Journal of Psychosomatic and Obstetrical Gynecology, 12*, 3–30.

Self, S. A., van Vult, M., & Stones, W. (1998). Chronic gynecological pain: An exploration of medical attitudes. *Pain, 77*, 215–225.

Toomey, T. C., Hernandez, J. T., Gittelman, D. F., Hulka, J. F. (1993). Relationship of sexual and physical abuse to pain and psychological assessment variables in chronic pain patients. *Pain, 53*, 105–109.

Turk, D. C., Kerns, R. D., & Rosenberg, R. (1992). Effects of marital interaction on chronic pain and disability: Examining the down side of social support. *Rehabilitation Psychology, 37*(4), 259–274.

Walker, K. G., & Shaw, R. W. (1993). Gonadotropin-releasing hormone analogues for the treatment of endometriosis: long-term follow-up. *Fertility and Sterility, 59,* 511–515.

Wenof, M., & Perry, C. P. (1999). *Understanding the principles of chronic pelvic pain, a patient education booklet.* International Pelvic Pain Society. www.pelvicpain.org.

Vercellini, P., Trespidi, L., De Giorgi, O., Cortesi, I., Parazzini, F., & Crosignane, P. G. (1996). Endometriosis and pelvic pain: Relating to disease stage and localization. *Fertility and Sterility, 65,* 299–304.

Zastrow, C. (1998). *Social work with groups.* Chicago: Nelson Hall.

Zola, I. K. (1973). Pathways to the doctor—from person to patient. *Social Science and Medicine, 7,* 677–689.

Zola, I. K. (1966). Culture and symptoms—an analysis of patients' presenting complaints. *American Sociological Review, 31,* 615–630.

13

Adolescent Pregnancy

LAURIE SCHWAB ZABIN and KATHLEEN M. CARDONA

INTRODUCTION

Over the past several decades, there has been considerable debate over youthful sexual onset, pregnancy, and childbearing. In the course of these debates, as in most issues of demographic significance, issues arise of ethics and morality, of health and medicine, of politics and economics, of family and the social order. Each area of concern has implications from the most personal dimension of individual choice, through the couple, the family and the neighborhood, to the larger dimension of the nation and—with its implications for populations at large—the world. Because of the complexity of the issues that are raised in these debates, it is not surprising that positions become extreme and stereotyped. These positions are often reflective, not of teenagers' dilemmas nor of pregnancy itself; in the context of the community as a whole, adolescents become not a metaphor for social change but a target. And despite all the public discourse, their own problems and their very real needs are misconstrued and often ignored.

In the current chapter, we will first address the epidemiology of adolescent sexual behavior and fertility in the United States, focusing on the question: What, if anything, has changed—and what are the implications of those changes for the health and welfare of the young men and, more especially, the young women involved? We will address the degree to which certain subgroups, based on age, ethnic identity, social, economic, or educational status, are differentially involved in sexual behaviors, and differentially affected by them. We will suggest many alternative definitions of the problem; and, because each definition has so powerful an effect on how the nation intervenes, we ask: Are the sequelae attributed to that catchall commonly referred to as "adolescent pregnancy" in fact the sequelae of early sexual onset, of unprotected sex, of pregnancy, of childbearing, or of childrearing? Or are they the consequences of preexisting structural conditions which were, in fact, causes and not effects?

We then consider the implications of contraception and reproductive health services for the teenager, including questions of availability, accessibility, usage, and their effects on behavior, health, and well-being. We discuss the implications of program and program design and propose characteristics of programs which can best be expected to postpone or prevent unintended pregnancy and childbearing among the young or, in their presence, to ameliorate their effects.

LAURIE SCHWAB ZABIN and KATHLEEN M. CARDONA • Department of Population and Family Health Sciences, Johns Hopkins School of Hygiene and Public Health, Baltimore, Maryland 21205.

Handbook of Women's Sexual and Reproductive Health, edited by Wingood and DiClemente. Kluwer Academic / Plenum Publishers, New York, 2002.

EPIDEMIOLOGY

Adolescent childbearing encompasses a variety of social and demographic processes; those interested in the epidemiology of adolescent fertility must therefore examine each of its underlying rates and measures individually to truly comprehend the composition of the adolescent fertility rate. For example, different components of fertility (e.g., frequency of coitus and frequency of conception) might be moving in opposite directions, causing changes in the overall fertility rate that are not intuitively apparent (Hayes, 1987c). Aggregate figures, such as pregnancy and birthrates among all teenagers, can only be understood in the context of the larger picture. Basing programs and policies solely on the adolescent fertility rate is inadequate, and may be counterproductive; to make effective decisions, all demographic components must be accurately assessed.

The Size of the Adolescent Population

The size of the teenage population, relative to the overall population in the United States, has an influence on adolescent pregnancies and births. The absolute number and proportion of teenagers in the population change over the years, which has an effect on the total numbers of births to the age group as well as the proportion of all births contributed by them. Even within the 15- to 19-year-old population, the age balance affects overall rates because birth and pregnancy rates are much higher in the older teen years. Although the teenage population in the United States had been decreasing between 1976 and 1992, it began to increase thereafter and is expected to continue growing through the next decade.

The composition of the teenage population also changes with time. It is becoming more likely that a teenager will be a member of a minority group; Black youth made up 16% of the teen population and Hispanics 14% in 1997 (U.S. Census Bureau, 1998). In some urban areas, these subgroups are and/or will be in the majority in the near future. The overall level of teenage childbearing will be affected as these proportions rise, to the extent that the fertility rates of these groups differ from that of the white majority.

Births to Teenagers

The number of births to 15- to 19-year-olds has been declining in the United States. In 1972, there were 616,280 births to women 15 to 19 years old (Moore, Wenk, Hofferth, & Hayes, 1987); by 1998 that number had decreased to 484,975, with 9481 of those births to girls younger than age 15 (Ventura, Mathews, & Curtain, 1999). Births to teenagers aged 15–19, as a proportion of all births has also decreased, from 19% in 1972 to 12% in 1998 (Moore et al., 1987; Ventura et al., 1999). These trends are a result of both a reduction in the teenage birth rate and an increase in the overall U.S. birthrate as the "baby boom" generation reached their thirties and began having children (Ventura, Taffel, Mosher, Wilson, & Henshaw, 1995).

The birthrate to teenagers as a whole declined from the early 1970s to the late 1980s; it then peaked in 1991 but fell again to the lowest level since 1987 (Henshaw, 1999). In 1972, there were 61.7 births per 1000 females 15–19 years old, in 1986, 50.2 births per 1000, and, in 1991, 62.1 (Henshaw, 1999). A preliminary estimate of the birthrate for U.S. teenagers in 1998 was 51.1 per 1000, a rapid 18% decline from 1991 (Ventura et al., 1999).

There is wide variation by ethnic group in the demographic effect of births to teenagers. Nearly 22% of births in the Black population and 21% among native Americans are to teenagers, while only 5% of births to Asian/Pacific Islander women are to teens; nationally, 12.5% of all births are to teenagers (Martin, Smith, Mathews, & Ventura, 1999). For all women aged 15–19, the birth rate is 51.1 per thousand, but among Black Americans this rate is 85.3 per 1000, and among Hispanic teens the rate is even higher, at 93.7 per 1000 (Ventura et al., 1999). Given these differences, it would appear that an adolescent's risk of conception and birth is affected by environmental, socioeconomic, and cultural conditions in her immediate and greater community.

Pregnancies among Teenagers

Over the last decade, the pregnancy rate among teenagers has decreased along with the birthrate. The chance of a teenage girl becoming pregnant has steadily decreased from its peak in 1990, from 117 to 97 per 1000 in 1996, a 17% decline (Alan Guttmacher Institute [AGI], 1999b; Henshaw, 1999). While some of this decline is due to a decrease in sexual activity among teens, it is estimated that 80% is a result of more effective contraceptive use (AGI, 1999a). Historically, the pregnancy rate for teenagers aged 15–19 increased in the 1970s, and stabilized in the early 1980s before significantly increasing in the late 1980s (AGI, 1999b). The magnitude of the change in the pregnancy rate for adolescents has differed by race; among Black teens, it declined more than 20% between 1990 and 1996, while for White teens it declined by only 16% over the same time period (AGI, 1999b).

Although the adolescent pregnancy rate has significantly declined over the past decades, there are still nearly 1 million pregnancies among United States teenagers (Henshaw, 1999). The majority of these pregnancies are unintended; for unmarried teens, 90% were not planning to become pregnant (Henshaw, 1998). Given this fact, it is not surprising that an estimated 30% of teens terminate their pregnancy with elective abortion; just more than half of their pregnancies result in a live birth, and approximately 14% end in miscarriage (Henshaw, 1999). Overall, it has been estimated that 25% of all young women experience a pregnancy by age 18, and half will become pregnant by age 21 (AGI, 1994).

Sexual Activity

Researchers most often classify a teen as "sexually active" if she or he has had vaginal intercourse at least once. As a means of quan-

tifying pregnancy risk, this definition of sexual activity is problematic; it does not take into account numerous other factors (e.g., frequency of intercourse, number of partners) necessary to accurately assess an individual's level of sexual contact (Zabin & Hayward, 1993). Because it can be assessed with a single question that is relatively easy to answer and analyze, research has relied heavily upon it. When using it as a measure of pregnancy risk, however, it is an imperfect measure; for example, many teens do not have sexual intercourse on a regular basis and therefore the risk for these teens is overstated.

Our knowledge about sexual activity among teenagers has grown over the last half of the century. In the late 1940s and early 1950s, Kinsey et al. conducted the first nonprobability surveys of sexual activity in the United States (Kinsey, Pomeroy, & Martin, 1948; Kinsey, Pomeroy, Martin, & Gebhard, 1953). From these surveys, they estimated that between 1938 and 1950, only 7% of White females had experienced intercourse by age 16. In the 1970s, Zelnik and Kantner (1973, 1977, 1980) conducted landmark studies of adolescent sexual behavior; their findings showed marked change over the course of one decade. In 1971, 27.6% of never-married females ages 15–19 had experienced intercourse, but by 1979 that proportion had grown to 46.0%. Rates of sexual activity among teenagers continued to increase through the 80s; according to data from the National Survey of Family Growth (NSFG), the proportion of 15- to 19-year-old women who had ever experienced intercourse increased from 47% in 1982 to 53% in 1988 (Singh & Darroch, 1999). The proportion of adolescents sexually active appears to have stabilized: the 1995 NSFG findings show 52% of women aged 15–19 ever having had intercourse (Singh & Darroch, 1999).

Rates of sexual activity vary by race and ethnicity, although the gap has narrowed over the past two decades. In 1971, 30% more Black teenagers than White teenagers were sexually active (Zelnik & Kantner, 1980). By 1995, the differential between Whites and non-Hispanic Blacks had narrowed to only 10 percentage points (Singh & Darroch, 1999). Race, in this case, is largely used as a proxy for socioeconomic disadvantage. However, increases in rates of sexual activity among young women have occurred almost entirely in the White, nonpoor population, while there has been little change in the Black population; as a result, socioeconomic measures in these two groups have moved closer together (Forrest & Singh, 1990; Singh & Darroch, 1999).

Contraceptive Use

Contraceptive use is measured by researchers in a number of ways. Distinguishing between ever and never use is one way; contraceptive use at first intercourse is often cited as a measure of preparedness for sexual onset, while determining use at last intercourse—a random event—is a proxy for consistency of method use. However it is measured, contraceptive use among American women increased dramatically as more options became available and accessibility improved. Through the 1960s and 1970s, method use at first intercourse remained stable, at approximately 44–47%. In the early 1980s this proportion increased to 59%, and to 76% in the 1990s (Mosher & McNally, 1991; Abma, Chandra, Mosher, Peterson, & Piccinino, 1997). This marked increase is attributable to the increasing use of condoms during the 1980s and 1990s. Before 1980, 18% of women stated that, at first intercourse, their partner had used a condom, whereas in 1990–1995 this figure was 54%. The proportion of women who used other methods at first intercourse has declined slightly from the high levels of the mid-1980s, and one quarter of women remain unprotected at this event (Abma et al., 1997).

In 1982, 71% of sexually active 15- to 19-year-old women indicated that they used contraception; this proportion increased to 84% in 1995 (Abma et al., 1997). Teenagers who use contraception most often report use of the pill (44%), but condom use is a close second at 37% (Abma et al., 1997). There are racial and ethnic

differences in contraceptive use as well. At first intercourse, 83% of White women under age 20 reported using a contraceptive; this figure is 72% for Black teens and only 53% for Hispanic women (Abma et al., 1997). Black women ages 15-19 report the highest level of contraceptive use, 86% at last intercourse; the proportion of White teens who used contraception at last intercourse is just slightly lower, but again Hispanic teens lag behind, at 74% (Abma et al., 1997). The increase in condom use is dramatic in all groups, but greatest among non-Hispanic Black teens: the proportion reporting the condom as their current contraceptive method rose from 13% to 38% between 1982 and 1995, compared to a rise from 23% to 36% among non-Hispanic White teens (Piccinino & Mosher, 1998).

Contraceptive use by teens has clearly improved from rates of the late 1970s. Much of this improvement has stemmed from an increased use of the condom at first intercourse, largely due to education and concerns about HIV and other sexually transmitted diseases. That condom use has generally replaced nonuse rather than medical contraception is indicated by the small decline in the use of other female methods, an encouraging trend. Increased condom use by teenagers appears to have affected the risk of pregnancy early in a young woman's sexual career. In the late 1970s, Zabin et al. (1979) found that adolescent women are at high risk of unintended pregnancy in the months following first intercourse, partly because of poor contraceptive practice but also because of a delay in the first visit to a family planning provider. Recent analyses of the 1995 NSFG data have shown that, although the median interval to that visit increased from 16.7 months in 1982 to 21.9 months in 1995, there was a decline over the same time period in the percentage of women experiencing an unintended pregnancy during the interval (Finer & Zabin, 1998). This occurred even as a larger proportion of women waited until after initiating intercourse to see a provider, and as the median age of first sexual intercourse declined. Increased condom use—probably as a result of increased public education about AIDS and pregnancy—is the most plausible explanation for this reduction in unintended pregnancy (Finer & Zabin, 1998).

CORRELATES

As the foregoing epidemiological discussion suggests, adolescent childbearing involves a series of steps; it is not a single event but the end of a process which leads from virginity to parenthood. The correlates of these steps may not all be the same. Some of the behavioral and social factors associated with early sexual onset may, indeed, be similar to those associated with childbearing, but others may differ. Similarly, some of the decisions that young people make in the course of that process—to engage or not engage in sexual contact, to contracept or not to contracept, to bear or not to bear a child—are conscious, and some may be made by default. In each case, whether conscious or not, those decisions are based on a value structure and a knowledge structure which undergird young people's calculus of choice. Long histories of biological, familial, environmental and cultural influences have helped to form the subjective perceptions and objective assessments they make of the world in which they live.

In the model proposed here, we show a historical environment—formed by community, school, family, and peers—as having a direct effect on the personal characteristics a young person brings to the decision to engage or not to engage in sexual contact (see Figure 1). Similarly, developmental and biological characteristics, on a more individual basis, have a strong effect on the young person at the moment of adolescence. That historic dynamic relating internal and external influences has been taking place since birth, and will continue into the future. Decisions made in adolescence, then, are a product of a past history and a current environment. How these factors interact has been explained theoretically in many

different ways, each with more or less emphasis on individual, family, social, and community factors.

Individual Factors and Self-Concept

An individual's biological characteristics, primarily age of physical maturity, will have a strong effect on the timing of sexual onset; this will necessarily affect age at first childbearing. Age of physical maturation (menarche or nocturnal emission) in young women and men is associated with age at sexual debut (Udry, 1979; Udry & Cliquet, 1982); this relationship is strongest in the early years of adolescence, but attenuates with increasing age as normative pressures become more important than the purely physical effects of maturation (Zabin, Hirsch, Smith, & Hardy, 1986). The relationship between biological development and behaviors that lead to childbearing are both direct, due to hormonal changes, and indirect: physical development affects the way the teen is perceived by others, peers and adults, and by herself (Smith, 1989). The younger the age at physical maturity, the greater discrepancy we would expect between cognitive, emotional, and social development and the adolescent's physical status. This potentially places a very young woman who is physically able to bear a child at considerable risk; she has probably not yet completed critical developmental tasks of her own childhood.

The status of a teen's psychosocial development—her ability to make rational decisions and perceive risks—will impact her sexual, contraceptive, and childbearing behaviors. Early adolescence is marked by egocentrism and a sense of invincibility and an assumption, however detailed her knowledge about conception, that "pregnancy won't happen to me." As the adolescent ages, there is a change in the perception of "self" relative to "others," and a greater understanding of the consequences of his/her own behaviors (Elkind, 1975). That low internalization of risk may be the reason for the typically lower levels of contraceptive use by

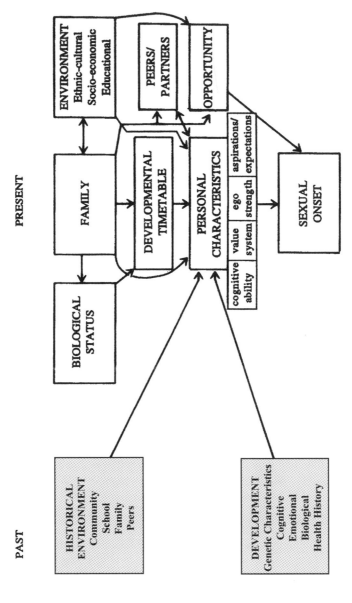

Figure 1. Model depicting influences upon the onset of coitus and interactions between them (Hardy & Zabin, 1991).

girls at early ages of first coitus (Zabin *et al.*, 1979); hence the finding that even a six-month delay in sexual onset would reduce the pregnancy rate to teens by 20% (Moore, Snyder, & Daly, 1991).

Other emotional and psychological variables may also play an important role in the occurrence of adolescent pregnancy. Hanson finds that teens with strong control over their lives have decreased chances of out-of-wedlock childbearing (Hanson, Myers, & Ginsburg, 1987). Associated with the concept of self-image is the current focus on self-esteem as a correlate of early parenting. As Hayes (1987d) points out, there is no clear data to establish that relationship, although girls' puberty and self-esteem appear linked (Hogan, Astone, & Kitagawa, 1985). Relationships between psychological constructs and early parenting are of particular importance when seeking positive factors with which to strengthen resilience to stress (Hamburg, 1986; Rutter, 1990).

There is considerable evidence that early childbearing is associated with lower aspirations and expectations for the future (Abrahamse, Morrison, & Waite, 1988a). Such a world view can be seen as a realistic adaptation to circumstances many youth must confront (Brewster, 1994a, b; Burton, 1990; Moore, Miller, Glei, & Morrison, 1995; Moore, Simms, & Betsey, 1986). As we will see when we address the role of the community; this view also supports an "opportunity cost" model of childbearing which suggests that a girl with fewer economic and occupational opportunities may believe she has little to lose by having a child (Miller & Moore, 1990). The same has been found for boys (Hanson, Morrison, & Ginsburg, 1989). A lack of future vision might then weaken the intention to avoid pregnancy (Plotnick, 1992), and Zabin, Hirsch, and Emerson (1989) have shown that ambivalence towards parenthood is associated with rates of childbearing as high as those among young women who claim, unequivocally, to want to conceive. Thus, low self-esteem may not be a wholly individual weakness that can be altered with individual interventions; it is also a social characteristic which only a real

and perceived change in opportunity structure can effectively address (Zabin, 1994).

Clustering of Risk Behaviors

The idea that adolescent problem behaviors may be clustered has relevance to adolescent pregnancy and childbearing, even though sexual onset and parenthood are problematic not because they are inherently wrong but because they depart from a normative ordering of these behaviors in the life course (Dragastin & Elder, 1975; Jessor & Jessor, 1977). There is considerable literature showing the clustering of early sexual onset with problem behavior (Dryfoos, 1990; Elliott & Morse, 1989; Ensminger, 1990; Rosenbaum & Kandel, 1990; Zabin, Hardy, Smith, & Hirsch, 1986), but less that focuses specifically on pregnancy and childbearing. Assessing determinants of early childbearing in an analysis of High School and Beyond's cohort of tenth graders in 1980, who were followed for six years, Abrahamse *et al.* (1988a,b) identify problem behaviors such as unexcused absences from school as risk factors for adolescent childbearing. They find that, among Blacks, low academic achievers tend to have lower future aspirations, which are associated with childbearing. Among Whites, too, low-ability women are more likely to become mothers, adjusting for an array of background characteristics. Such findings are similar to Hanson *et al.* (1987) as well as Hogan and Kitagawa (1985), who examine pregnancy, as opposed to childbearing. Young men at risk of becoming teen fathers are also more likely to have academic and behavioral problems in school and negative attitudes about their future (Hanson *et al.*, 1989). A long tradition of work in life course theory as well as problem behavior (Dragastin & Elder, 1975; Elliott & Morse, 1989; Jessor & Jessor, 1977) suggests that longitudinal analysis of relationships between cognitive and social development and delinquency, drug use, sexual activity, and pregnancy may confirm that problem behaviors occur well before the teen years. It may be, then, that these problem behaviors could act as "red flags," signaling the need for individual intervention early in the developmental process, in time to prevent sexual risk-taking and subsequent pregnancy and childbearing.

The Family Environment

Many characteristics of the individual have roots within the family. For example, family attributes such as low socioeconomic status and female headship have significant effects, increasing the likelihood that a black teen becomes a single mother (Abrahamse et al., 1988a; Bumpass & McLanahan, 1989; Duncan & Hoffman, 1990; Furstenberg, Levine, & Brooks-Gunn, 1990; Hogan & Kitagawa, 1985; Wu & Martinson, 1993) or a single father (Robbins, Kaplan, & Martin, 1985). Those with sisters who are teen mothers are at increased risk of early pregnancy (Hogan & Kitagawa, 1985). Unmarried parents, a larger number of siblings, and low educational level of the adolescent's mother are associated with early childbearing (Ahn, 1994; Cooksey, 1994; Hogan & Kitagawa, 1985; Lewis & Ventura, 1990; McLanahan & Bumpass, 1988; Miller, 1995; Rodgers, Rowe, & Harris, 1992). Religious identification (of the individual or family) (i.e., commitment to religion rather than denomination) can discourage both premarital sex and abortion, with opposite effects on childbearing (Abrahamse et al., 1988a).

Household structure has also been shown to play an important role in a child's life. Coresidence with grandparents or other extended kin (Astone & Washington, 1994) can have a stabilizing effect, while excessive transiency in and out of the home, whether or not the movement involves the child's parent(s), can have strong negative effects (Zabin, Wong, Weinick, & Emerson, 1992). Wu and Martinson (1993) describe adolescent childbearing as a response to stresses from family disruptions and other childhood events; Zabin et al. (1992) have found a large amount of transiency typical of the inner-city homes of young women who bear children in adolescence. Clearly, then, the best family environment for a child begins with a close and stable relationship with an adult in the household, someone caring and attentive, whether this be a parent, grandparent, other family member or other adult (Kellam, Ensminger, & Turner, 1977; Kellam, Adams, Brown et al., 1982; McLanahan, 1983, 1985). Werner (1985, 1986) suggests that a relationship of this type "protects" children living in socially disadvantaged environments, who might otherwise be vulnerable to negative influences. Ideally, this relationship would exist in a setting with sufficient resources to prevent chronic stress from eroding the family, while promoting the health and learning of children, an environment less likely to exist for children in deprivation.

The environment created by current and historical household factors clearly influences the behavior of the child; these factors include parents, household structure, stability, health, educational level, participation in the workforce, income level, religious affiliation, access to health care, timing of first birth to the mother, and parenting style. The strength of these influences varies over the life course: they may have differing effects at different points in time. During infancy and early childhood, the family has the strongest influence on the child's development, and all outside influences are filtered through the protective layer formed by the family (Hardy & Zabin, 1991). As the child grows to adolescence and young adulthood, family influence gradually loses its dominance as school, peer and the community effects become more important to the increasingly independent child. In a stable family environment, the influence of the family will continue to be substantial even as the child ages, but this may not be the case in nonintact, single parent families. Children in these families may be more frequently unsupervised, allowing peer and community influence a greater role in determining adolescent social development, with possible deleterious effects.

School and Peer Influence

Problem behaviors, even when seen as "individual effects," may relate to the individual in the school context. Disciplinary problems in school, class cutting, and absenteeism were indexed in a scale highly associated with the willingness to become a single mother, independent of background variables (Abrahamse et al., 1988b). A relationship between a loose attachment to school and adolescent parenthood is increasingly clear; problems with school often precede fertility among those who leave school prematurely (Upchurch & McCarthy, 1990). However, the causal relationships between education and fertility are probably not unidirectional (Rindfuss, Bumpass, & St. John, 1980; Marini, 1984); this is true among males who become fathers as well (Marsiglio, 1987). Furthermore, there has been little attention to how that loose attachment is related to achievement and inborn abilities determined before a particular school environment has its effects.

While peers are also a part of the larger community in which the adolescent lives, the influence of peers more often occurs over the course of the child's school career. One study using the female subset of the High School and Beyond data set combines responses of schoolmates to estimate a "peer environment," a measure of acceptance of teen motherhood. A bivariate association reveals a correlation between a school environment and teen motherhood, although in multivariate models the effect is significant only for whites (Abrahamse et al., 1988a). Using the male subset, Hanson et al. found that peer influence significantly impacted the likelihood of fathering a child; when peers placed a high value on education, the chance of a teen male fathering a child decreased by 16% (Hanson et al., 1989). The importance of the value system or youth culture within a particular school for the adolescent who is acculturated there has been well demonstrated (Coleman, 1961), and other literature elucidates the relative strength of hormonal and peer influence (Smith, Udry, & Morris, 1985; Udry, Billy, Morris, Groff, & Raj, 1985; Billy & Udry, 1985; Udry, Talbert, & Morris, 1986).

Community Factors

The community in which the adolescent lives has the potential to act as either a positive or negative influence on social development and adolescent pregnancy. The community can af-

fect the developing adolescent indirectly through characteristics such as housing quality and density, lack of privacy, opportunities for employment, day care, and transportation, which have their main effects on the family and its available resources. Of more direct influence are the quality of education, recreation and medical care, and other resources which affect the adolescent's motivation and expectations for future employment and family formation (Hardy & Zabin, 1991).

The community may play a positive role in the development of its adolescents, especially if it has such resources as sports, library and recreation programs, scouting, Boys and Girls Clubs, volunteer work, mentoring programs, and church-related activities. Participation in community activities in which adolescents have the opportunity to interact with positive adult role models, activities that encourage personal responsibility and growth, can be "protective"; it can discourage behaviors that may lead to early pregnancy not only by allowing teens to explore the world around them in a positive manner but also by filling the critical after-school hours.

If the community is lacking strong social institutions, and the family is unable to counteract these effects, community characteristics such as drug abuse, delinquency and crime can act as negative influences, especially in adolescence when school, peer, and community influence increase. Crane (1991) describes the extreme case of this influence in his "epidemic theory" of neighborhoods, which states that at some point as neighborhood quality declines, the numbers of social problems will explode at an increasing rate. His study found a strong association between declining neighborhood quality and rising rates of school dropout and teen childbearing.

Development of Interventions

Based on the many factors associated with adolescent pregnancy and childbearing mentioned in this section are opportunities for the development of primary prevention interventions. The design of successful interventions depends in part on the theoretical interpretation of how these various factors predispose to risk. For example, a developmental framework suggests that interventions should focus earlier than the high school years, on the period prior to adolescence. Early intervention would provide many benefits. Those who physically mature early can be supported to help them make rational choices about sexual intercourse and contraceptive use even while cognitively and emotionally immature. If clustered problem behaviors are addressed by intervention early in the developmental process, adolescent sexual risk-taking and subsequent pregnancy and childbearing might be avoided. And all children could be exposed to programs which promote self-esteem and high expectations for the future, since these appear to be important individual determinants of a willingness to conceive.

Potential interventions related to family, school/peer, and community could have overlapping effects; strengthening community resources could benefit individuals, families, schools, and neighborhoods. Interventions that promote communication between parents and children could serve to bolster weak family relationships, giving the adolescent the supportive environment that is needed for strong emotional development. And improved access to reproductive health services could assist families and adolescents alike. The following section addresses interventions that have worked and identify further avenues for primary prevention of adolescent pregnancy.

PRIMARY PREVENTION

Because adolescent childbearing is the culmination of a series of steps, primary prevention can be focused anywhere along a decision path which leads from sexual onset to childbearing. It can be aimed at influencing the young person's decisions with regard to sexual onset versus abstinence, contracepted versus unprotected sexual contact, pregnancy outcome, parenthood versus adoption, and then, in the context of secondary prevention, the same cycle of decisions once again. To ignore any step in this process is to waste an important opportunity to enhance an adolescent's trajectory toward a successful life course.

Preventive interventions have traditionally been divided into three separate modalities:

1. Educational initiatives designed to affect knowledge and/or attitudes and values with respect to sexual behaviors and reproductive health
2. Medical or clinical initiatives which provide individual counseling and services in the broad fields of family planning and reproductive health
3. Wide-ranging comprehensive initiatives which seek to enhance life skills and life options

The last category may include programs as diverse as community services, mentoring, tutoring, and job training. These programs are based on the assumption that by improving a young person's chances for future achievement, his or her decisions relative to current sexual behaviors may be impacted and intercourse, pregnancy, and parenthood delayed.

Clearly, programs in these three areas would require totally different approaches toward their evaluation, and lend themselves in greater or lesser degree to outcome measurement. Only a fraction of all teen pregnancy prevention programs have been evaluated in a rigorous manner, with results published in peer-reviewed journals. In recent years, several attempts have been made to survey the field of pregnancy prevention in the United States, to reach some conclusions about the effectiveness of programs in each of these categories. This section reviews this current literature to identify characteristics of primary prevention interventions that have proven effective.

Programs that Work

What have we learned from the many teen pregnancy interventions implemented in communities throughout the United States? How do we know what efforts might be worth repeating, and which approaches should be retired? Even among specific programs, what works in one community may not work in another; therefore, it is beneficial to look at the characteristics of programs that work instead of individual programs in their entirety. Because so few programs have been appropriately evaluated, and even fewer have shown positive effects on adolescent sexual behaviors, it might be reasonable to start with what we know does not work in pregnancy prevention programs. Philliber and Namerow (1995) in their literature review conclude that no single intervention will be helpful for all teens and at all ages/stages of adolescence. They also suggest that stand-alone interventions—contraceptive access, abstinence-only, or sexual education classes—have not been shown to impact teen pregnancy rates; however, these elements in concert with one another are part of many successful multi-faceted programs (Philliber & Namerow, 1995), and contraceptive access has measurable preventive effects.

Kirby et al. (1994) reviewed 16 studies of specific school-based adolescent pregnancy prevention programs; they included abstinence-only, sexuality, and HIV education and education plus reproductive health service models. The authors found insufficient evidence that abstinence-only programs actually delayed the onset of intercourse or affected other behaviors. They also could not determine from published studies if school-based or -linked reproductive health services had a significant impact on pregnancy or birthrates. As for sexuality and HIV education programs, four of eight programs reviewed increased contraceptive use among participating students. These four programs are Postponing Sexual Involvement (Howard & McCabe, 1990), Reducing the Risk (Kirby, Barth, Leland, & Fetro, 1991), AIDS Prevention for Adolescents in School (Walter & Vaughn, 1993), and a curriculum designed by Schinke et al. (1981). The authors identified six characteristics these four programs had in common: (1) a focus on reducing specific risky sexual behaviors that could lead to pregnancy; (2) a grounding in social learning theories; (3) the

use of experiential activities to personalize the provision of information on avoiding the risks of unprotected sex; (4) addressing social and/or media pressures to engage in sexual behaviors through activities; (5) an emphasis on age-appropriate individual values and group norms against unprotected sexual activity; (6) opportunities to model and practice effective communication (negotiation and refusal) skills. These common characteristics provide a strong base upon which to build new pregnancy prevention programs.

In their excellent review of education and/or training programs for adolescents, Frost and Forrest (1995) chose five programs which were designed to impact either the initiation of sexual activity, contraceptive use or pregnancy/birth rates and were scientifically evaluated with control groups. These programs are Postponing Sexual Involvement (Howard & McCabe, 1990, 1992), Reducing the Risk (Barth, Leland, Kirby, & Fetro, 1992; Kirby et al., 1991), School/Community Program (Vincent, Clearie, & Schluchter, 1987; Koo, Dunteman, George, Green, & Vincent, 1994), Self-Center (Zabin, 1992; Zabin et al., 1988; Hardy & Zabin, 1991), and Teen Talk (Eisen & Zellman, 1992; Eisen, Zellman, & McAlister, 1990). All five programs promoted abstinence as an effective way to prevent pregnancy and encouraged teens to delay initiation of sexual intercourse. Unlike abstinence-only curricula, these programs also offered life skills training along with sexuality and contraceptive education; four programs also provided either indirect or direct contraceptive access. These additional program components are important; as has been noted in other reviews, programs that focus solely on abstinence have little to offer those who have already initiated intercourse (Philliber & Namerow, 1995). Sexually active teens need information about choosing and using contraception to prevent unintended pregnancies. And there has been no evidence that access to contraception increases sexual activity or encourages initiation of sexual intercourse (Kirby et al., 1994); they may, indeed, delay or reduce sexual activity.

Frost and Forrest concluded that these

programs were effective in changing the behavior of their participants; many teenagers delayed initiation of sexual intercourse, and those who were sexually active were more likely to use contraception as a result of the program. The authors also found that there was no significant change in the pregnancy rates for participants in three of the programs compared to teens in the control groups. However, two showed significantly lower pregnancy rates, the Self-Center and School/Community Programs. These two programs were similar in that they both combined education components (abstinence, life skills, sex and contraceptive education) with contraceptive access provided by program staff either on site or nearby. They suggest that the other programs might, indeed, have impacted the teen pregnancy rates in the longer term: decreased sexual activity and consistent contraceptive use by an increased number of teenagers over a longer period of time than the studies' follow-up period might ultimately cause a decline in teen pregnancy rates to the individuals enrolled.

The authors also point out that programs focusing on younger teens are most effective in reducing the rate of sexual initiation, while the effect on older teens is more likely to be an increase in contraceptive use. Most of these interventions were implemented in low-income areas with mostly Black adolescents; it is therefore unclear how teens from different cultural groups or higher socioeconomic status might respond to these same programs. With that caveat, these five evaluated programs are models that have worked and could be used in other communities to decrease adolescent pregnancy through education, training, and services.

Using a more liberal set of inclusion criteria, Philliber and Namerow (1995; also Philliber, 1996) reviewed the results of 17 pregnancy prevention programs. To be included in their review, interventions had to have caused behavior changes in teen participants, and evaluations had to include a control or comparison group. Causing changes in knowledge or attitudes about sexuality and contraception was not enough to be included. Program types in their

review included curriculum or education, life options, contraceptive distribution, combinations of the previous three types, comprehensive (deal with the whole teenager, not just sexuality related issues), and early childhood intervention. They found only modest behavioral changes among participants in the 17 programs, but found similarities across these "successful" programs. These characteristics are (1) allowing for the creation of meaningful relationships with adults who are involved with the program; (2) skill-building educational components, not just didactic provision of information; (3) using volunteering and paid internships to introduce teens to the world of work; and (4) addressing the importance of peer influence by teaching skills to confront peer pressure (Philliber, 1996). Another valuable characteristic is the provision of support over a long enough period and with a consistent enough staff so that trust can be developed and maintained; this is critical as at-risk teens may not have enough adult support in their homes, and programs of this nature often act as surrogate families. Also, the inclusion of educational or job related services to increase young people's ability to provide for their own futures, or at the very least, to motivate and assist young men and women to access such services, is important in providing life options to the participants.

Franklin et al. (1997) conducted a meta-analysis of 32 outcome studies of adolescent pregnancy prevention interventions. The method they used for inclusion was less rigorous/more inclusive than either Philliber or Frost and Forrest, as can be evidenced by the large number of studies selected; the primary difference is that studies did not need to have a control or comparison group for inclusion. They propose that these pregnancy prevention programs did not have an effect on the sexual activity of the teens in the studies; this is in contrast to Frost and Forrest (1995), who found that the five programs they reviewed did delay initiation of sexual intercourse among program participants. However, Franklin et al. found that programs had a stronger effect on the reduction of adolescent pregnancy rates than did Frost and Forrest.

The meta-analysis also showed that teens participating in these prevention programs increased their use of contraceptives. Contraceptive use improved more among participants in community-based than school-based programs; clinic-based services were more effective in influencing contraceptive behavior than nonclinical programs. The meta-analysis identified contraceptive programs as the most effective at changing adolescent sexual behaviors.

Common Threads

The characteristics of effective primary prevention programs reported in the preceding reviews should be taken into consideration when designing new interventions to reduce the incidence of adolescent pregnancy. However, we have identified additional aspects of programs that work that might also be addressed. First, successful programs need to reach young people in time to strengthen their attachment to school and in time to help them avoid a first pregnancy. This means that programs cannot begin in high school; they must begin in middle school or even earlier to build a strong bond with school and reinforce the belief that learning is key to the future. Programs for any age group should be cognizant of and adapted to the developmental, cognitive, and emotional stages of their clients. Children will tune out messages that are not stage-appropriate.

Program activities and objectives should build on the strengths of the young people and families they serve, providing tools to adolescents and their families to negotiate in their day-to-day environments. And interventions must be culturally sensitive and acceptable to the community; ideally, the early stages of planning an intervention should include members of the community whenever possible, to determine their own neighborhood needs. Listening to parents, other adults, and teens both before and during implementation is the best way to design or adapt an existing intervention so that it is seen as a positive influence within the community.

Important physical attributes of successful programs are that they are close to where young people are or congregate, whether this be in schools, community centers, or shopping malls. Even if programs are conveniently located, they need to find ways to provide a psychological bridge to or between services (outreach, shared staff, supportive referral, etc.). Programs should also be free to ensure access by all teens, and teens need to know that what is said to program staff, and services provided, are confidential.

What types of services would "ideal" interventions offer? They would be a combination of educational and clinical/social services across the childhood and adolescent years. They would provide young people with early, comprehensive information on reproduction and sexual health in the context of their basic biological education. In late childhood and into adolescence, they would help young people to define their goals and vision for the future, and to make appropriate connections between their actions today and aspirations for tomorrow. In adolescence, they would provide a range of services to meet reproductive health needs, including contraceptive and other reproductive health services, abortion, prenatal and postnatal care—or, if not provide them, to legitimate them and facilitate young people's access in each of these areas. Programs would actively include males, giving boys and young men opportunities to learn, to participate and to be responsible partners. Ideally, they would have some impact on the family and/or community (neighborhood, school, etc.) within which individual adolescents must make their way.

Limitations of Primary Prevention Research

Research on the primary prevention of adolescent pregnancy has been limited to date because the vast majority of local interventions have not been evaluated and published in peer-reviewed journals; there is not a large body of data with which to work. Many interventions are described only anecdotally in newsletters and other limited circulation publications without data. But even when surveying the peer-reviewed literature, the data presented are not what is really needed. For example, for their meta-analysis of adolescent pregnancy prevention programs, Franklin *et al.* (1997) searched the peer-reviewed literature across family/social sciences, psychology, medicine, nursing, and education for articles published through 1995. They found more than 500 references on the topic and ended with only 32 studies for their analysis; nonetheless, most of these published accounts of interventions did not include outcome measures, and of the remaining sample many evaluated knowledge or attitudes rather than behavioral effects.

Assessing behaviors among participants both before and after interventions is the gold standard of program evaluation. Evaluations are even stronger when conducted with both treatment and control groups; as stated previously, Frost and Forrest (1995) found only five published studies of programs that involved comparison of program participants and controls. With different evaluation standards for published studies of prevention programs, it becomes difficult to combine or survey results across studies to determine the "best" model. To determine what works, funders need to require rigorous evaluation and include evaluation in the funding plan so that the knowledge base on primary prevention programs can be broadened.

Summary

Based on studies and reviews published in peer-reviewed journals, a handful of effective programs for the primary prevention of adolescent pregnancy have been identified. Aspects of programs that work have been characterized based on the literature and anecdotal evidence; these common characteristics should be taken into consideration when designing new interventions to reduce the incidence of adolescent pregnancy. To broaden the field of primary prevention research, more programs must carry out evaluations of their interventions, preferably measuring participant behaviors—both sexual and contraceptive—before and after exposure

to the program. Grant-making organizations need to require evaluation and provide funds for this important aspect of primary prevention so that program planners can truly determine what works.

PSYCHOSOCIAL SEQUELAE AND SECONDARY PREVENTION

The goal of primary prevention interventions with adolescents is to either delay initiation of sexual intercourse or to encourage behaviors that are likely to prevent the occurrence of pregnancy. When pregnancy and subsequent childbearing does occur, however, there are potential psychological, social, economic, and fertility effects on the adolescent that can be both immediate and long lasting. The pregnant and parenting adolescent is vulnerable both because adolescence is a period of psychological and physical development, and because many pregnant teens come from socioeconomically disadvantaged backgrounds. Pregnancy during this life phase, then, requires both social and medical supports beyond those available to most adult women if maternal and child outcomes are to be optimized. This section will discuss the potential long-term psychosocial sequelae of adolescent pregnancy and childbearing, and then review the literature on effective secondary prevention programs designed to improve the health of pregnant adolescents.

Long-Term Psychosocial and Economic Sequelae

There are many potential sequelae of pregnancy and childbearing for the adolescent. These often life-altering events have been shown to affect the teen's psychological development and well-being, educational/economic status, long-term family formation, spacing of births, and completed fertility. While these effects of pregnancy and childbearing may occur to some degree for all women, not just for teens, it seems that because the pregnant and/or parenting adolescent has not completed her biological and emotional development nor her educational tasks, the effects may be stronger and more far-reaching. It should be made clear, however, that the consequences we describe here cannot be attributed to adolescent *pregnancy* as so often is the case, but to *childbearing*; no negative consequences of terminated pregnancy have been demonstrated.

During adolescence, the teen is developing a sense of self outside of the family unit within which the child has been acculturated. Growing contact and socialization with peers is an important part of this development. Pregnancy and childbearing interrupts this normative process through which the adolescent forms her identity, and can lead to an inability to complete the developmental tasks of adolescence, hence a stunting of appropriate psychological development (Coley & Chase-Lansdale, 1998). While continued residence with the maternal family can be beneficial for the development of the teenagers' child, the dual role of child and parent can be difficult for the teen mother herself. In addition, both pregnancy and the demands of parenting can severely limit the teen's social contacts, possibly causing isolation and depression.

SmithBattle and Leonard (1998) suggest that for some adolescent women, the process of becoming a mother can be both "stressful and meaningful," creating "new understandings of the self and one's place in the world" (p. 36). Based on findings from qualitative studies, these authors believe that in disadvantaged communities where there are few educational, career or marriage opportunities, mothering can serve as a "rite of passage to adulthood." However, research over the past three decades has pointed to the negative effects of adolescent pregnancy on life outcomes such as educational attainment, economic status, marriage and family formation, and completed family size. The National Academy of Sciences report *Risking the Future* summarized the research through 1987 on the consequences of adolescent pregnancy (Hayes, 1987a; see chapter 5). This report states that considerable evidence shows that teen parenthood leads to "lower social and economic attainment of young mothers and their families and that it entails considerable health and developmental risks" (p. 123).

The lower socioeconomic status of young mothers and the families they head is linked to the truncated education that often accompanies pregnancy in adolescence (Card & Wise, 1978; Hofferth & Moore, 1979; Klepinger, Lundberg, & Plotnick, 1995; Mott & Marsiglio, 1985; Trussell, 1976). There is some evidence that while there are large differences in educational attainment in the years immediately following the birth of a child, adolescent mothers may "catch up" in the long run to those in their cohort who postpone childbearing (Furstenberg, Brooks-Gunn, & Morgan, 1987). Nonetheless, current research finds that, controlling for other environmental factors, adolescent childbearing results in a 50% reduction in the odds of completing high school; only 30% of mothers age 17 and younger will attain a high school diploma by age 30 (Maynard, 1996). Adolescent mothers are more likely to earn a high school equivalency diploma (GED) than women who delay childbearing until after the teen years, but a GED apparently does not make up the difference in earnings associated with high school graduation (Maynard, 1996).

In the United States, earning power is closely related to years of completed education. In decades past, the greatest difference was between high school graduates and nongraduates; in our increasingly technological society, it has become more necessary to complete education past the high school years. Adolescent mothers earn an average $5600 annually during the first 13 years of parenthood, less than half the poverty level (Maynard, 1996). Families headed by adolescent mothers more often live in poverty and receive public assistance (Moore & Burt, 1982); greater than 70% of these families receive welfare at some time, and 40% will be on welfare for five or more years following the first teen birth (Maynard, 1996).

There is also a link between the larger completed family size typical of women who begin their families as teens and economic status (Hayes, 1987b). A first birth during the teen years was reported years ago to be associated with a faster pace of childbearing (Card & Wise, 1978; Mott, 1986). Recent research indicates that adolescent mothers will have 24% more children than women who delay childbearing (Maynard, 1996). Larger families stretch the already tight budget of these teen-headed families; the costs of safe and reliable day care and transportation may impede young mothers' search for stable and well-paying employment (Hayes, 1987b). Coupled with lower educational levels, teen mothers are likely to have lower hourly wages and job status. Because adolescent mothers spend more time as single parents than do women who begin their families at age 20 or 21 (4 years vs. 10 months), these adolescent families do not generally have spouses upon whom to rely for financial assistance (Maynard, 1996). Fathers of babies born to adolescent mothers are likely to be poorly educated and of lower socioeconomic status themselves, increasing the chances of their children living in poverty, as well (Zabin & Hayward, 1993; Hardy & Zabin, 1991). In turn, some of the most measurable consequences of adolescent childbearing have been the well-documented negative effects later in life to children born to and raised by teen mothers, a subject beyond the scope of this chapter.

Recently, questions have been raised as to whether the effects of pregnancy in adolescence have been overstated (Hoffman, 1998). Studies in the 1990s have focused on the teen's environment—family and community—rather than the occurrence of childbearing itself as the major cause for the poor lifetime outcomes of teen mothers. Hoffman reviewed the findings of recent studies which use new methods of controlling for these environmental effects; although the methods are not perfect, he asserts that becoming a teen parent is not as catastrophic a life event as it has been characterized in the past. However, he finds that current improved research methods do not give evidence that "the independent causal effects of teenage parenting are positive, zero or even just marginally negative" (Hoffman, 1998, p. 239). He concludes that programs to reduce the incidence of early parenthood should continue until there are solid findings in either direction, as these programs can also ameliorate the effects of growing up in poverty.

Secondary Prevention Programs

Physical and emotional characteristics of adolescence along with environmental factors place the pregnant teen and her developing fetus at risk for complications and developmental problems. Adolescents have generally not completed their own physical growth; smaller stature and possibly the continued growth of the mother may put the fetus at risk for low birth weight (Zabin & Hayward, 1993; Hardy & Zabin, 1991). Although the exact etiology is unclear, it is the youngest pregnant teenagers (under age 15) who have higher rates of complications, prematurity, and/or low-birthweight babies than do older teens and adult women (Hayes, 1987b). This may be principally a function of size and maternal physical growth status, but socioeconomic factors are implicated as well.

Poor eating and other poor health habits are typical of adolescence, and the effects of these characteristics are compounded by the fact that nutritional needs are greater for teens than older women (Zabin & Hayward, 1993). Adolescents may also have a low awareness of their own health issues/needs (Hayes, 1987b) and may not be able to conceptualize the medical demands that are a part of pregnancy and childbirth. Access to and utilization of prenatal care and nutrition programs are more challenging for socially disadvantaged pregnant teens (Hardy & Zabin, 1991); secondary prevention programs have been designed to improve access to services to reduce the negative effects of pregnancy on the teen and her child.

Evidence seems clear that pregnancy outcomes can be just as good for teens as for older women if and only if the prenatal services provided to them are optimal—designed specifically to meet their needs. Given excellent prenatal care, most of the differentials in outcome disappear, but access to such care has a social as well as a medical component. Effective secondary prevention programs include prenatal care provided consistently by the same staff, with an increased number of visits by the teen over the course of the pregnancy. Other comprehensive services need to be provided, such as nutritional support and behavioral counseling that minimize the additional risks experienced by young mothers. The greatest levels of success in reducing risks to pregnant adolescents have been achieved using a team approach or case management system, where the services of varied providers can be coordinated in one place (Hardy & Zabin, 1991).

The Hopkins Adolescent Clinic (HAC) used this model, and teens receiving prenatal care in this clinic attended more prenatal visits, gained more weight, were less likely to experience anemia or toxemia; all of these results were significantly different from the control group results despite a similar level of medical care. Low- and very-low-birthweight babies were born nearly twice as frequently to mothers in the control as in the HAC group, and Apgar scores were significantly higher for HAC babies (Hardy & Zabin, 1991). Stevens-Simon and colleagues (1992) evaluated another comprehensive adolescent prenatal care program to determine whether the care and/or outcomes differed from those for adult women in a traditional prenatal clinic. They found that the adolescent women were more rapidly enrolled in a nutritional support and supplementation program, and more often referred to outside community agencies for nonobstetric assistance than were the adult women. At entry into prenatal care, the teens had lower hematocrits, poorer diets, and lower weight gain; later in gestation, these characteristics as well as birth outcomes were similar for the teen and adult groups (Stevens-Simon, Fullar, & McAnarney, 1992).

Home visitor programs have also been shown to improve pregnancy outcomes for adolescent women. One of the first studies of prenatal home visitation was carried out by Olds *et al.* (1986), who evaluated a program in which visiting nurses provided pregnant women with parent education, social support, and links to community services. Although not designed just for adolescents, one of the main program effects was a significant increase in the birth weight (nearly 400 g) of infants born to adolescents (Olds, Henderson, Tatelbaum, & Chamberlin, 1986). A more recent study of a paraprofessional home visitor program for pregnant adolescents (Rogers, Peoples-Sheps, & Suchindran, 1996) found the program associated with earlier entry into and increased use of prenatal care by teenagers, a variable highly correlated with successful outcomes. While there was no program effect on low birthweight, it was found that unmarried teens in the intervention group had a decreased risk of preterm birth, which is strongly related to infant mortality (Rogers *et al.*, 1996). The professional or paraprofessional home visitor program model appears promising as a means of affecting pregnancy and birth outcomes.

In a thorough review of the literature on prevention programs that focus on pregnant and parenting adolescents, Hoyer (1998) discusses the most effective programs by general type and identifies weaknesses in evaluation design and data analysis. She concludes that comprehensive programs appear the most effective in improving outcomes for teen mothers and their babies, but need to be implemented and well evaluated across the country in communities that differ ethnically, racially, and socioeconomically if that conclusion is to be supported.

Limitations of Programs and Research

As with primary prevention research, there are many limitations to secondary prevention programs and research. With respect to program design, secondary prevention programs are limited to providing health care and psychosocial supports; these programs cannot change the environment (community, family) in which the pregnant teenager lives and will parent her child. Many hospitals, health departments, and medical centers have basic teen program models, but few programs of this type have been evaluated, and even fewer results have been published in the literature. And secondary prevention programs need to be truly long-term and extend into the parenting years; evaluation needs to span many years to determine whether there is any effect on the adolescent and her child as they continue to develop.

Hoyer (1998) has pointed to numerous methodological issues regarding secondary prevention program evaluations. A major issue is the difficulty service providers find in randomly assigning teens to treatment or control groups. Although the lack of a true control group compromises the experimental design of research studies to determine program effectiveness, neither providers nor community members are comfortable denying services to teens. Also, because programs are often implemented as demonstration projects, selectivity can contaminate the results, and sample sizes are often too small to establish real differences between groups. These methodological issues must be surmounted so that strong program evaluations can be conducted to determine what works in preventing the secondary sequelae of adolescent pregnancy.

Summary

There are potential psychological, social, economic, and fertility effects for the adolescent and her child resulting from adolescent pregnancy and parenting; for maternal and child health outcomes to be optimized during this period of rapid development for both mother and child, pregnant teens need considerable psychosocial support along with amplified prenatal care. Given a strong level of support, results need not be significantly different from adult outcomes. Secondary prevention programs designed to improve the health of pregnant adolescents can ameliorate some of the consequences associated with adolescent pregnancy and childbearing; further evaluation and research regarding these programs will help to determine their most effective designs.

HEALTH POLICY IMPLICATIONS

It is clear from the consequences we have discussed above that there are economic and social consequences to adolescent childbearing in the United States on the individual level—to mother, family, and child. Economic consequences go well beyond the individual level, however, with serious consequences for the community and, indeed, the nation. The magnitude of these effects is difficult to describe because several economic and methodological assumptions have to be made to determine (1) the cause–effect relationships between poverty and early parenthood; (2) therefore, the degree to which subsequent economic hardship and its correlates should be included in measuring the effects of childbearing; and (3) the breadth of the effects that should be considered, as well as their temporal dimensions; that is, how far into the future should these effects be measured and attributed to the birth?

When measured by the direct costs of public assistance benefits and medical expenses, the annual cost of early childbearing (to girls 17 years of age and below) has been estimated at $3.7 billion (Maynard, 1996). Less direct costs (e.g., foster care, delinquency among children of adolescents, loss of tax revenue because of early childbearing's effects on work patterns) have been estimated at over $3 billion. Costs of a range of indirect social effects, even without the intergenerational costs implied, are estimated at close to $30 billion. Although studies produce alternative numbers, societal costs appear high whatever causal assumptions and statistical controls are employed. Many costs are reflected in federal, state, and local spending, which must also include the costs of preventive intervention, costs that are borne by the private as well as the public sector.

Savings attributable to intervention are equally difficult to estimate with the exception of those due to contraceptive services, whose costs can more easily be estimated than comprehensive intervention and whose effects are directly measured in terms of births and treatment of sexually transmitted infections averted. Studies have reported the magnitude of these savings (AGI, 1995, 1996), one with estimates specific to contraceptive method (Trussell, Koenig, Stewart, & Darroch, 1997) and one which reports savings of $3 to $4 for each $1 spent (Forrest & Samara, 1996).

CONCLUSIONS

As stated at the outset, the dimensions of the adolescent pregnancy and childbearing "problem" are societal as well as an individual. Individual interventions should not be expected, by themselves, to change emerging patterns of family formation or economic dependency, even if they appear successful in postponing sexual onset, pregnancy, or childbearing. Patterns of early childbearing vary in both their etiology and their nature; to address them effectively requires an understanding of a broad range of adolescent issues, an understanding that extends beyond reproductive health to the environment in which young people live. Although there is a critical role for individual intervention on both the health and social level, patterns of premarital conception and childbearing may ultimately change only if structural changes in their environment alter young people's picture of what a family might, realistically be, and how their current behavior relates to their long-term goals. An initiative must go well beyond medical service and sex education if it is to affect young people's opportunity structure—present and future, real and perceived.

Nonetheless, there is a critical role for the public health community, and the individual clinician, in the design and delivery of appropriate services (Zabin, 1990). From a child's earliest years, a clinician can begin to establish a confidential and supportive relationship with each young patient, such that, when entering the period of puberty, the clinic or medical office is seen as an appropriate place for supportive and confidential care. The health community can address the need for intervention at many points along the trajectory from sexual onset to childbearing and childrearing, with initiatives appropriate to the developmental stages of young boys and girls alike. Those interventions will have to address both the motivation to avoid childbearing and the motivation to use positive means to avoid it, and must include the medical and counseling services that support and legitimize both abstinence and contraception.

Support for effective intervention requires local data and local leadership; these will only emerge if the community understands the level and the nature of its problem. There, too, the medical and public health establishment have a critical role to play as providers, experts, and vocal advocates. Initiatives have to be powerful to overcome the normal instincts of young people in close, unsupervised proximity. But there is a normative structure on which to build: the vast majority of young people even in our highest risk communities do not want to bear children in their teen years (Zabin, Astone, & Emerson, 1993). It is in the interest of the health establishment—indeed, of the entire community—to support them with the services they require.

REFERENCES

Abma, J., Chandra, A., Mosher, W., Peterson, L., & Piccinino, L. (1997). Fertility, family planning, and women's health: New data from the 1995 National Survey of Family Growth. Series 23[no. 19]. 1997. National Center for Health Statistics. Vital and Health Statistics.

Abrahamse, A. F., Morrison, P. A., & Waite, L. J. (1988b). Beyond stereotypes: Who becomes a single teenage mother? (Rep. No. R-3489HHS/NICHD). Rand Corporation.

Abrahamse, A. F., Morrison, P. A., & Waite, L. J. (1988a). Teenagers willing to consider single parenthood: Who is at greatest risk? *Family Planning Perspectives, 20,* 13–18.

Ahn, N. (1994). Teenage childbearing and high school completion: Accounting for individual heterogeneity. *Family Planning Perspectives, 26,* 17–21.

Alan Guttmacher Institute (1994). *Sex and America's teenagers.* New York: The Alan Guttmacher Institute.

Alan Guttmacher Institute (1995). Issues in brief: Teenage pregnancy and the welfare reform debate. [On-line]. Available: http://www.agi-usa.org/pubs/ib5.html

Alan Guttmacher Institute (1996). Issues in brief: The impact of publicly funded family planning. [On-line]. Available: http://www.agi-usa.org/pubs/ib8.html

Alan Guttmacher Institute (1999a). Facts in brief: Teen sex and pregnancy, 1999. [On-line]. Available: http://www.agi-usa.org/pubs/fb_teen_sex.html

Alan Guttmacher Institute (1999b). Teenage pregnancy: Overall trends and state-by-state information. [On-line]. Available: http://www.agi-usa.org/pubs/teen_preg_stats.html

Astone, N. M., & Washington, M. (1994). The association between grandparental coresidence and adolescent childbearing. *Journal of Family Issues, 15*, 574–589.

Barth, R. P., Leland, N., Kirby, D., & Fetro, J. V. (1992). Enhancing social and cognitive skills. In B. C. Miller, J. J. Card, R. L. Paikoff, & J. Peterson (Eds.), *Preventing adolescent pregnancy* (pp. 53–82). Newbury Park, CA: Sage.

Billy, J. O. G., & Udry, J. R. (1985). The influence of male and female best friends on adolescent sexual behavior. *Adolescence, 20*, 21–32.

Brewster, K. L. (1994a). Neighborhood context and the transition to sexual activity among young black women. *Demography, 31*, 603–613.

Brewster, K. L. (1994b). Race differences in sexual activity among adolescent women: The role of neighborhood characteristics. *American Sociological Review, 59*, 408–424.

Bumpass, L., & McLanahan, S. (1989). Unmarried motherhood: Recent trends, composition, and black–white differences. *Demography, 26*, 279–286.

Burton, L. M. (1990). Teenage childbearing as an alternative lifecourse strategy in multigeneration black families. *Human Nature, 1*, 123–143.

Card, J. J., & Wise, L. L. (1978). Teenage mothers and teenage fathers: The impact of early childbearing on the parents' personal and professional lives. *Family Planning Perspectives, 10*, 199–205.

Coleman, J. S. (1961). *The adolescent society*. New York: The Free Press of Glencoe.

Coley, R. L., & Chase-Lansdale, P. L. (1998). Adolescent pregnancy and parenthood: Recent evidence and future directions. *American Psychologist, 53*, 152–166.

Cooksey, E. C. (1994). Factors in the resolution of adolescent premarital pregnancies. *Demography, 27*, 207–218.

Crane, J. (1991). The epidemic theory of ghettos and neighborhood effects on dropping out and teenage childbearing. *American Journal of Sociology, 96*, 1226–1259.

Dragastin, S. E., & Elder, G. H. (1975). *Adolescence in the life cycle*. Washington, DC: Hemisphere.

Dryfoos, J. G. (1990). *Adolescents at risk: Prevalence and prevention*. New York: Oxford University Press.

Duncan, G. L., & Hoffman, S. (1990). Welfare benefits, economic opportunities, and out-of-wedlock births among black teenage girls. *Demography, 27*, 519–535.

Eisen, M., & Zellman, G. L. (1992). A health beliefs field experiment: Teen Talk. In B. C. Miller, J. J. Card, R. L. Paikoff, & J. Peterson (Eds.), Preventing adolescent pregnancy (pp. 220-264). Newbury Park, CA: Sage.

Eisen, M., Zellman, G. L., & McAlister, A. L. (1990). Evaluating the impact of a theory-based sexuality and contraceptive education program. *Family Planning Perspectives, 22*, 261–271.

Elkind, D. (1975). Recent research on cognitive development in adolescence. In S. E. Dragastin & G. Elder (Eds.), *Adolescence in the life cycle*. New York: Wiley.

Elliott, D., & Morse, B. J. (1989). Delinquency and drug use as risk factors in teenage sexual activity. *Youth and Society, 21*, 32–60.

Ensminger, M. E. (1990). Sexual activity and problem behaviors among black, urban adolescents. *Child Development, 61*, 2032–2046.

Finer, L. B., & Zabin, L. S. (1998). Does the timing of the first family planning visit still matter? *Family Planning Perspectives, 30*, 30–33 & 42.

Forrest, J. D., & Samara, R. (1996). Impact of publicly funded contraceptive services on unintended pregnancies and implications for Medicaid expenditures. *Family Planning Perspectives, 28*, 188–195.

Forrest, J. D., & Singh, S. (1990). The sexual and reproductive behavior of American women, 1982–1988. *Family Planning Perspectives, 22*, 206–214.

Franklin, C., Grant, D., Corcoran, J., Miller, P. O., & Bultman, L. (1997). Effectiveness of prevention programs for adolescent pregnancy: A meta-analysis. *Journal of Marriage and the Family, 59*, 551–567.

Frost, J. J., & Forrest, J. D. (1995). Understanding the impact of effective teenage pregnancy prevention programs. *Family Planning Perspectives, 27*, 188–195.

Furstenberg, F. F., Brooks-Gunn, J., & Morgan, S. P. (1987). Adolescent mothers and their children in later life. *Family Planning Perspectives, 19*, 142–151.

Furstenberg, F. F., Levine, J. A., & Brooks-Gunn, J. (1990). The children of teenage mothers: Patterns of early childbearing in two generations. *Family Planning Perspectives, 22*, 54–61.

Hamburg, B. A. (1986). Subsets of adolescent mothers: Developmental, biomedical and psychosocial issues. In J. B. Lancaster & B. A. Hamburg (Eds.), *School-age pregnancy and parenthood*. New York: Aldine De Gruyter.

Hanson, S. L., Morrison, D. R., & Ginsburg, A. L. (1989). The antecedents of teenage fatherhood. *Demography, 26*, 579–596.

Hanson, S. L., Myers, D. E., & Ginsburg, A. L. (1987). The role of responsibility and knowledge in reducing out of wedlock childbearing. *Journal of Marriage and the Family, 49*, 241–256.

Hardy, J. B., & Zabin, L. S. (1991). *Adolescent pregnancy in an urban environment*. Baltimore, MD and Washington, DC: Urban and Schwarzenberg and The Urban Institute.

Hayes, C. D. (Ed.) (1987a). *Risking the future: Adolescent sexuality, pregnancy and childbearing*. Vol. 1. Washington, DC: National Academy Press.

Hayes, C. D. (Ed.) (1987b). Consequences of adolescent pregnancy. In *Risking the future: Adolescent sexuality, pregnancy and childbearing* (pp. 123–139). Washington, DC: National Academy Press.

Hayes, C. D. (Ed.) (1987c). Trends in adolescent sexuality and fertility. In *Risking the future: Adolescent sexuality, pregnancy and childbearing* (pp. 33–74). Washington, DC: National Academy Press.

Hayes, C. D. (Ed.) (1987d). Determinants of adolescent

sexual behavior and decision making. In *Risking the future: Adolescent sexuality, pregnancy and childbearing* (pp. 95–121). Washington, DC: National Academy Press.

Henshaw, S. K. (1998). Unintended pregnancy in the United States. *Family Planning Perspectives, 30,* 24–29 & 46.

Henshaw, S. K. (1999). U.S. teenage pregnancy statistics: With comparative statistics for women aged 20–24. [On-line]. Available: http://www.agi-usa.org/pubs/teen_preg_sr_0699.html

Hofferth, S. L., & Moore, K. A. (1979). Early childbearing and later economic well-being. *American Sociological Review, 44,* 784–815.

Hoffman, S. (1998). Teenage childbearing is not so bad after all...or is it? A review of the literature. *Family Planning Perspectives, 30,* 236–239, 243.

Hogan, D. P., Astone, N. M., & Kitagawa, E. M. (1985). Social and environmental factors influencing contraceptive use among black adolescents. *Family Planning Perspectives, 17,* 165–169.

Hogan, D. P., & Kitagawa, E. M. (1985). The impact of social status, family structure and neighborhood on the fertility of black adolescents. *American Journal of Sociology, 90,* 825–855.

Howard, M., & McCabe, J. B. (1990). Helping teenagers postpone sexual involvement. *Family Planning Perspectives, 22,* 21–26.

Howard, M., & McCabe, J. B. (1992). An information and skills approach for younger teens: Postponing sexual involvement. In B. C. Miller, J. J. Card, R. L. Paikoff, & J. Peterson (Eds.), *Preventing adolescent pregnancy* (pp. 83–109). Newbury Park, CA: Sage.

Hoyer, P. J. (1998). Prenatal and parenting programs for adolescent mothers. *Annual Review of Nursing Research, 16,* 221–249.

Jessor, R., & Jessor, S. L. (1977). *Problem behavior and adolescent development.* New York: Academic Press.

Kellam, S. G., Adams, R. G., Brown, C. H., & Ensminger, M. E. (1982). The long-term evolution of the family structure of teenage and older mothers. *Journal of Marriage and the Family,* 539–554.

Kellam, S. G., Ensminger, M. E., & Turner, R. J. (1977). Family structure and the mental health of children. *Archives of General Psychiatry, 34,* 1012–1022.

Kinsey, A. C., Pomeroy, W. B., & Martin, C. E. (1948). *Sexual behavior in the human male.* Philadelphia: W. B. Saunders.

Kinsey, A. C., Pomeroy, W. B., Martin, C. E., & Gebhard, P. (1953). *Sexual behavior in the human female.* Philadelphia: W. B. Saunders.

Kirby, D., Barth, R. P., Leland, N., & Fetro, J. V. (1991). Reducing the risk: Impact of a new curriculum on sexual risk-taking. *Family Planning Perspectives, 23,* 253–263.

Kirby, D., Short, L., Collins, J., Rugg, D., Kolbe, L., Howard, M., Miller, B. C., Sonenstein, F. L., & Zabin, L. S. (1994). School-based programs to reduce sexual risk behaviors: A review of effectiveness. *Vital Health Statistics, 109,* 339–360.

Klepinger, D. H., Lundberg, S., & Plotnick, R. D. (1995). Adolescent fertility and the educational attainment of young women. *Family Planning Perspectives, 27,* 23–28.

Koo, H. P., Dunteman, G. H., George, C., Green, Y., & Vincent, M. L. (1994). Reducing adolescent pregnancy through a school and community-based intervention: Denmark, South Carolina, revisited. *Family Planning Perspectives, 26,* 206–211, 217.

Lewis, C., & Ventura, S. (1990). Birth and fertility rates by education: United States 1980 and 1985. *Vital Health Statistics, 21.*

Marini, M. M. (1984). Women's educational attainment and the timing of entry into parenthood. *American Sociological Review, 49,* 491–511.

Marsiglio, W. (1987). Adolescent fathers in the United States: Their initial living arrangements, marital experience and educational outcomes. *Family Planning Perspectives, 19,* 240–251.

Martin, J. A., Smith, B. L., Mathews, T. J., & Ventura, S. J. (1999). Births and deaths: Preliminary data for 1998. [47 no. 25]. Hyattsville, MD, National Center for Health Statistics. National Vital Statistics Reports.

Maynard, R. A. (Ed.) (1996). *Kids having kids: A Robin Hood Foundation report on the costs of adolescent childbearing.* New York: Robin Hood Foundation.

McLanahan, S. (1983). Family structure and stress: A longitudinal comparison of two-parent and female-headed families. *Journal of Marriage and the Family,* May, 347–357.

McLanahan, S. (1985). Family structure and the reproduction of poverty. *American Journal of Sociology, 90,* 873–901.

McLanahan, S. S., & Bumpass, L. L. (1988). Intergenerational consequences of family disruption. *American Journal of Sociology, 94,* 130–152.

Miller, B. C. (1995). Risk factors for adolescent nonmarital childbearing. In *Report to Congress on out-of-wedlock childbearing* (pp. 217–227). Washington, DC: Dept. of Health and Human Services [DHHS Pub. No. (PHS) 95-1257].

Miller, B. C., & Moore, K. A. (1990). Adolescent sexual behavior, pregnancy, and parenting: Research through the 1980s. *Journal of Marriage and the Family, 52,* 1025–1039.

Moore, K. A., & Burt, M. R. (1982). The consequences of early childbearing. In *Private crisis, public cost: Policy perspectives on teenage childbearing* (pp. 17–32). Washington, DC: The Urban Institute Press.

Moore, K. A., Miller, B. C., Glei, D., & Morrison, D. R. (1995). *Adolescent sex, contraception, and childbearing: A review of recent research.* Washington, DC: Child Trends, Inc.

Moore, K. A., Simms, M. C., & Betsey, C. L. (1986). *Choice and circumstance: Racial differences in adolescent sexuality and fertility.* New Brunswick, NJ: Transaction Books.

Moore, K. A., Snyder, N. O., & Daly, M. (1991). *Facts at a glance*. Washington, DC: Child Trends, Inc.

Moore, K. A., Wenk, D., Hofferth, S. L., & Hayes, C. D. (1987). Statistical appendix (Table 3.1). In S. L. Hofferth & C. D. Hayes (Eds.), *Risking the future* (pp. 414–415). Washington, DC: National Academy Press.

Mosher, W. D., & McNally, J. W. (1991). Contraceptive use at first premarital intercourse: United States, 1965–1988. *Family Planning Perspectives, 23*, 108–116.

Mott, F. L. (1986). The pace of repeated childbearing among young American mothers. *Family Planning Perspectives, 18*, 5–12.

Mott, F. L. & Marsiglio, W. (1985). Early childbearing and completion of high school. *Family Planning Perspectives, 17*, 234–237.

Olds, D. L., Henderson, C. R., Tatelbaum, R., & Chamberlin, R. (1986). Improving the delivery of prenatal care and outcomes of pregnancy: A randomized trial of nurse home visitation. *Pediatrics, 77*, 16–28.

Philliber, S. (1996). Effective strategies to reduce teen pregnancy: An overview. In *Promising approaches to prevent adolescent pregnancy* (pp. 2–5). Washington, DC: Population Resource Center.

Philliber, S., & Namerow, P. (1995). *Trying to maximize the odds: Using what we know to prevent teen pregnancy*. Accord, NY: Philliber Research Associates.

Piccinino, L. J., & Mosher, W. D. (1998). Trends in contraceptive use in the United States: 1982–1995. *Family Planning Perspectives, 30*, 4–10 & 46.

Plotnick, R. D. (1992). The effects of attitudes on teenage premarital pregnancy and its resolution. *American Sociological Review, 57*, 800–811.

Rindfuss, R. R., Bumpass, L., & St. John, C. (1980). Education and fertility: Implications for the roles women occupy. *American Sociological Review, 45*, 431–447.

Robbins, C., Kaplan, H. B., & Martin, S. S. (1985). Antecedents of pregnancy among unmarried adolescents. *Journal of Marriage and the Family, 47*, 567–583.

Rodgers, J. L., Rowe, D. C., & Harris, D. F. (1992). Sibling differences in adolescent behavior: Inferring process models from family composition patterns. *Journal of Marriage and the Family, 54*, 142–152.

Rogers, M. M., Peoples-Sheps, M. D., & Suchindran, C. (1996). Impact of a social support program on teenage prenatal care use and pregnancy outcomes. *Journal of Adolescent Health, 19*, 132–140.

Rosenbaum, E., & Kandel, D. B. (1990). Early onset of adolescent sexual behavior and drug involvement. *Journal of Marriage and the Family, 52*, 783–798.

Rutter, M. (1990). Psychosocial resilience and protective mechanisms. In J. E. Rolf, A. S. Masten, D. Cicchetti, K. H. Nuechterlein, & S. Weintraub (Eds.), *Risk and protective factors in the development of psychopathology*. Cambridge: Cambridge University Press.

Schinke, S., Blythe, B., & Gilchrest, L. (1981). Cognitive-behavioral prevention of adolescent pregnancy. *Counseling Psychology, 28*, 451–454.

Singh, S., & Darroch, J. E. (1999). Trends in sexual activity among adolescent American women: 1982-1995. *Family Planning Perspectives, 31*, 212–219.

Smith, E. A. (1989). A biosocial model of adolescent sexual behavior. In G. R. Adams, T. Gullotta, & R. Montemayor (Eds.), *Biology of adolescent behavior and development* (pp. 143–167). Newbury Park, CA: Sage Publications.

Smith, E. A., Udry, J. R., & Morris, N. M. (1985). Pubertal development and friends: A biosocial explanation of adolescent sexual behavior. *Journal of Health and Social Behavior, 26*, 183–192.

SmithBattle, L., & Leonard, V. L. (1998). Adolescent mothers four years later: Narratives of the self and visions of the future. *ANS, Advances in Nursing Science, 20*, 36–49.

Stevens-Simon, C., Fullar, S., & McAnarney, E. R. (1992). Tangible difference between adolescent-oriented and adult-oriented prenatal care. *Journal of Adolescent Health, 13*, 298–302.

Trussell, T. J. (1976). Economic consequences of teenage childbearing. *Family Planning Perspectives, 8*, 184–190.

Trussell, T. J., Koenig, J., Stewart, F., & Darroch, J. E. (1997). Medical care cost savings from adolescent contraceptive use. *Family Planning Perspectives, 29*, 248–255, 295.

Udry, J. R. (1979). Age at menarche, at first intercourse, and at first pregnancy. *Journal of Biosocial Science, 11*, 433–441.

Udry, J. R., Billy, J. O. G., Morris, N. M., Groff, T. R., & Raj, M. H. (1985). Serum androgenic hormones motivate sexual behavior in adolescent boys. *Fertility and Sterility, 43*, 90–94.

Udry, J. R., & Cliquet, R. L. (1982). A cross-cultural examination of the relationship between ages at menarche, marriage, and first birth. *Demography, 19*, 52–63.

Udry, J. R., Talbert, L. M., & Morris, N. M. (1986). Biosocial foundations for adolescent female sexuality. *Demography, 23*, 217–230.

Upchurch, D. M., & McCarthy, J. (1990). The timing of a first birth and high school completion. *American Sociological Review, 55*, 224–234.

U.S. Census Bureau (1998). Resident population, by race, Hispanic origin, and single years of age: 1997 (Table No. 22). 9-29-1998. U.S. Census Bureau. Statistical Abstract of the United States: 1998.

Ventura, S. J., Mathews, T. J., & Curtin, S. C. (1999). Declines in teenage birth rates, 1991–1998: Update of National and state trends. [47, no. 26]. Hyattsville, MD, National Center for Health Statistics. National Vital Statistics Reports.

Ventura, S. J., Taffel, S. M., Mosher, W. D., Wilson, J. B., & Henshaw, S. K. (1995). Trends in pregnancies and pregnancy rates: Estimates for the United States, 1980–1992. [43, No. 11(S)]. Hyattsville, MD, National Center for Health Statistics. Monthly Vital Statistics Report.

Vincent, M. L., Clearie, A. F., & Schluchter, M. D. (1987). Reducing adolescent pregnancy through school and community-based education. *Journal of the American Medical Association*, *257*, 3382–3386.

Walter, H. J., & Vaughn, R. D. (1993). AIDS risk reduction among a multi-ethnic sample of urban high school students. *Journal of the American Medical Association*, *270*, 725–730.

Werner, E. E. (1985). Stress and protective factors in children's lives. In A. R. Nicol (Ed.), *Longitudinal studies in child psychology and psychiatry*. New York: Wiley.

Werner, E. E. (1986). A longitudinal study of perinatal risk. In D. C. Farran & J. D. McKinney (Eds.), *Risk in longitudinal development*. New York: Academic Press.

Wu, L. L., & Martinson, B. C. (1993). Family structure and risk of premarital birth. *American Sociological Review*, *58*, 210–232.

Zabin, L. S. (1990). Adolescent pregnancy: The clinician's role in intervention. *Journal of General Internal Medicine*, *5*, S81–S88.

Zabin, L. S. (1992). School-linked health services: The Johns Hopkins program. In B. C. Miller, J. J. Card, R. L. Paikoff, & J. Peterson (Eds.), *Preventing adolescent pregnancy* (pp. 156–184). Newbury Park, CA: Sage.

Zabin, L. S. (1994). Addressing adolescent sexual behavior and childbearing: Self esteem or social change? *Women's Health Issues*, *4*, 92–97.

Zabin, L. S., Astone, N. M., & Emerson, M. R. (1993). Do adolescents want babies? The relationship between attitudes and behavior. *Journal of Research on Adolescence*, *3*, 67–86.

Zabin, L. S., Hardy, J. B., Smith, E. A., & Hirsch, M. B. (1986). Substance use and its relation to sexual activity among inner-city adolescents. *Journal of Adolescent Health Care*, *7*, 77–87.

Zabin, L. S., & Hayward, S. C. (1993). *Adolescent sexual behavior and childbearing*. Vol. 26. Newbury Park, CA: Sage.

Zabin, L. S., Hirsch, M. B., & Emerson, M. R. (1989). When adolescents choose abortion: Effects on education, psychological status and subsequent pregnancy. *Family Planning Perspectives*, *21*, 248–255.

Zabin, L. S., Hirsch, M. B., Smith, E. A., & Hardy, J. B. (1986). Ages of physical maturation and first intercourse in black teenage males and females. *Demography*, *23*, 595–605.

Zabin, L. S., Hirsch, M. B., Streett, R., Emerson, M. R., Smith, M., Hardy, J. B., & King, T. M. (1988). The Baltimore pregnancy prevention program for urban teenagers: I. How did it work? *Family Planning Perspectives*, *20*, 182–187.

Zabin, L. S., Kantner, J. F., & Zelnik, M. (1979). The risk of adolescent pregnancy in the first months of intercourse. *Family Planning Perspectives*, *11*, 215–222.

Zabin, L. S., Wong, R., Weinick, R., & Emerson, M. R. (1992). Dependency in urban black families following the birth of an adolescent's child. *Journal of Marriage and the Family*, *54*, 496–507.

Zelnik, M., & Kantner, J. F. (1973). Sex and contraception among unmarried teenagers. In D. F. Westhoff (Ed.), *Toward the end of growth* (pp. 7–18). Englewood Cliffs, NJ: Prentice Hall.

Zelnik, M., & Kantner, J. F. (1977). Sexual and contraceptive experience of young unmarried women in the United States, 1976 and 1971. *Family Planning Perspectives*, *9*, 55–56, 58–63, 67–71.

Zelnik, M., & Kantner, J. F. (1980). Sexual activity, contraceptive use and pregnancy among metropolitan-area teenagers: 1971–1979. *Family Planning Perspectives*, *12*, 230–237.

14

Sexually Transmitted Infections

SEVGI O. ARAL and PAMINA M. GORBACH

INTRODUCTION

Sexually transmitted infections (STI) constitute a major burden of disease for women globally and include bacterial infections (syphilis, gonorrheal infection, chlamydial infection, and chancroid) and viral infections [herpes simplex virus (HSV), human papillomavirus (HPV), and hepatitis B virus (HBV)]. Rates of STIs in developing countries, especially those in Sub-Saharan Africa, far exceed those found in industrialized countries and STIs have been recognized as a major contributor to the global burden of disease (Gerbase *et al.*, 1998; Wasserheit, 1989; Brunham & Embree, 1992). In 1995 there were over 333 million cases of the four major curable STDs in adults between the ages of 15 and 49: 12 million cases of syphilis, 62 million cases of gonorrhea, 89 million cases of chlamydia, and 170 million cases of trichomoniasis, making STDs among the most common causes of illness in the world. Among industrialized countries, the United States has the highest rates of STI (Eng & Butler, 1997), including the easily curable infections like gonorrheal and chlamydial infections and syphilis. Women in all societies carry a greater burden of sexually transmitted infections, compared to men, for several reasons. First, STIs are more easily transmissible from men to women; second, greater proportions of women tend to be asymptomatic when infected with sexually transmitted pathogens, thus, women's infections are more likely to go undiagnosed and therefore untreated; third, women suffer severe sequelae of STI including infertility, pelvic inflammatory disease (PID), ectopic pregnancy, cervical cancer, fetal wastage, low birth weight, infant blindness, neonatal pneumonia, and mental retardation (Wasserheit & Holmes, 1992); fourth, universally, compared to men, women suffer more from the stigma attached to STI and their sequelae such as infertility. In many societies women's worth is defined in terms of her reproductive capacity and reproductive performance (Aral, 1992).

Perhaps the most important complication of STIs in general is the increased probability of acquisition and transmission of HIV in the presence of other STI (Fleming & Wasserheit, 1999). This becomes an even greater concern for women than men, because the best prevention methods (condoms and avoidance of risky sex) are those that require the cooperation, if not control of a man.

SEVGI O. ARAL • Division of STD Prevention, Centers for Disease Control and Prevention, Atlanta, Georgia 30333.   PAMINA M. GORBACH • Graduate School of Public Health, San Diego State University, San Diego, California 92182-4162.

Handbook of Women's Sexual and Reproductive Health, edited by Wingood and DiClemente. Kluwer Academic / Plenum Publishers, New York, 2002.

EPIDEMIOLOGY

This chapter focuses on the epidemiology of STIs in industrialized countries, where surveillance data are available. It is not possible to determine trends of STI over time in developing countries, because data have not been systematically collected and mostly come from sporadic studies of specific clinic or high-risk populations. In general, data on reported STIs from North America and many countries of Europe, as well as from Australia and New Zealand showed steady increases in the incidence of all STIs during the 1960s, with leveling off or decline of most of the bacterial STI but continual increases in viral STIs and genital chlamydial infections during the 1970s and 1980s. The incidence of gonorrhea and syphilis began to decline at different times, and declined at differing rates, in these industrialized countries. The sex ratio of males to females with bacterial STIs has declined for several decades. Gonorrhea and syphilis have continued to decline during the 1990s, and chlamydial infections have begun declining in Nordic countries, and in those areas of the United States and Canada and elsewhere where chlamydia control programs have been initiated. In the Southern Hemisphere, a few regions doing relatively well economically (e.g., Costa Rica, Thailand, and Harare, Zimbabwe) have experienced declining rates of bacterial STI during the 1990s. In contrast, some countries are experiencing explosive epidemics of bacterial STI [e.g., China (Michael *et al.*, 1998), Mongolia, (Purevdawa *et al.*, 1997), and Russia, and the Newly Independent States of the former USSR (Tichonova *et al.*, 1997)]. Also, many countries in Eastern Europe, Southern Africa, and Asia continue to experience epidemic increases in HIV infection.

BACTERIAL STI

Gonorrhea

The major bacterial STIs include gonorrhea, chlamydial infection, syphilis, and in many developing countries, chancroid. The male:female sex ratio for gonorrhea declined throughout much of this century; but increased, accelerating in the 1960s and 1970s, with use of selective culture media for isolation of *Neisseria gonorrhoeae* and with partner notification, both of which led to increasing detection of infected women during the 1960s and 1970s. This occurred simultaneously with the "sexual liberation" of women coinciding with the advent of oral contraception in the 1960s; and with decreasing rates of STI in homosexual men during the AIDS era (Aral & Holmes, 1999).

In the United States, the incidence of reported gonorrhea increased during World War II, peaked in 1946, then decreased until 1957, and subsequently increased again for nearly two decades, peaking at 473 per 100,000 in 1975. A rapid decline then continued at an accelerating pace to 124 in 1996, the lowest ever since the beginning of WWII (Division of STD Prevention, 1997). While there has been a recent surprising increase in gonorrhea of 8.9% between 1997 and 1998 from 122.0 cases to 132.9 cases per 100,000 persons, there has been a 72% decrease in the overall rate of gonorrhea from 1975 to 1998 (Centers for Disease Control, Division of Sexually Transmitted Diseases, 2000). It is too soon to tell if the increase in gonorrhea in the last few years is due to an increase in the accuracy of reporting or due to an actual resurgence of infection.

Comparisons of trends in the incidence of gonorrhea in industrialized countries are shown in Figure 1. Gonorrhea incidence per 100,000 population had fallen to 31.5 by 1994 in the United Kingdom; and to 18.6 in Canada by 1995. In summary, rates of reported gonorrhea in the United States in 1995 were 22.4 times those in Sweden, 7.8 times those in Canada, and 4.6 times those of the United Kingdom. This underestimates the true differences in rates, because smaller proportions (perhaps only about half of the cases of gonorrhea occurring in the United States) are reported.

STIs are differentially reported and treated in the United States with large differences be-

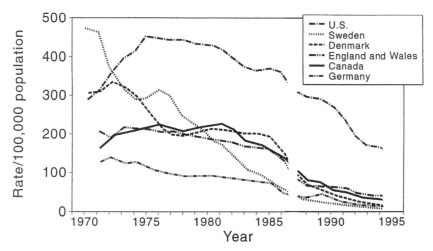

Figure 1. Gonorrhea trends: international comparisons.

tween the public and private sector persisting. In 1987, the number of cases reported from public STD clinics (526,000) was over twice as high as the number reported by private providers (255,000). While the proportion reported from STD clinics has been declining somewhat in recent years, with only 51.6% reported from STD clinics in 1996; for women nearly two thirds of gonorrhea cases were reported from non-STD clinic sources. The male: female ratio of reported incidence initially increased to over 3:1 by 1966, then declined rapidly to about 1.5:1 by 1973, and remained rather constant at that level through 1987 until it began to steadily decrease dropping to 1.1 by 1996 (Aral & Holmes, 1999).

Gonorrhea incidence among men who have sex with men (MSM), which had declined remarkably in response to the HIV epidemic, has started increasing in discrete local areas in the recent past. Between 1993 and 1996 the annual number of patients with urethral, pharyngeal, and/or rectal gonorrhea increased by 82% from 74 to 139, at a clinic serving MSM in Washington, D.C. At the same clinic the percent of gonorrhea patients tested for HIV who were HIV positive increased from 23% to 43% (Barrow et al., 1997). In addition, the GISP surveillance data show that urethral gonorrhea

among MSM has been increasing in several cities on the West Coast and in Denver (Centers for Disease Control and Prevention, 1997).

Syphilis

Syphilis may fluctuate in incidence more dramatically than gonorrhea as sexual behaviors change. Sweden provides an excellent example. A sharp rise occurred in the incidence of primary and secondary syphilis in both sexes in Sweden during World Wars I and II. Following WWI, the incidence of syphilis fell rapidly, coinciding with the increased availability of improved diagnostic tests and the arsenicals, rising during World War II, then falling again at the time of the introduction of penicillin. The incidence rose again during the sexual revolution of the early 1960s, and unlike gonorrhea, continued to increase after 1970, with epidemic spread among MSM until the recognition of AIDS in 1981. The incidence of syphilis per 100,000 population in Sweden then fell to 0.8 in 1995. The decline in the male:female ratio was less dramatic for syphilis than for gonorrhea. In the early 1900s it was about 2.5:1 and about 1.5:1 from the mid-forties to the mid-fifties. Thereafter, a dramatic reversal of this trend occurred, reaching a peak male:female ratio of 6.5:1 in 1982, then falling sharply again after recognition of the AIDS epidemic, and adoption of safer sex practices by MSM (Aral & Holmes, 1999).

In the United States, the incidence of primary and secondary syphilis rose during World War II, reaching a peak of 76 cases per 100,000 in 1947, then fell to a nadir of about 4 per 100,000 for 1955 to 1958 (Figure 2). In 1959 the trend reversed, and the incidence rose rapidly in men and women, to 12 per 100,000 in 1965, triple the level of a decade earlier. Factors considered responsible at the time included declining federal, state, and local appropriations for venereal disease control (federal dollar expenditures alone dropped from 17 to 3 million annually in 1955); a deemphasis on syphilis in medical teaching (e.g., in 1955, the phrase "and syphilology" was dropped from the *AMA Archives of Dermatology and Syphilology*); and a shift in management of syphilis from the public health clinic to the private office, with the availability of penicillin. From 1965 through 1980, the total incidence of primary and secondary syphilis changed very little, although the ratio of male:female cases increased steadily from about 1.5:1 up to about 3.5:1 in 1980.

Nationally, from 1982 through 1986, the reported national primary and secondary syphilis incidence in men had dropped steadily from 22.5 cases per 100,000 to 16.2 per 100,000, while rates in females remained unchanged. However, from 1985 to 1990, unlike the situation in Sweden, the incidence of primary and secondary syphilis increased sharply and unexpectedly in both men and women in the United States. A sharp rise in the number of reported cases of primary and secondary syphilis among Black men and women accounts for most of this increase. Sporadic, local syphilis outbreaks have contributed substantially to this national morbidity. Interestingly, these outbreaks have occurred in areas where earlier outbreaks of chancroid had occurred, and where heterosexual HIV seropositivity rates are highest, such as New York, Los Angeles, some areas in Texas, and in south Florida, all areas where crack-cocaine use and exchange of sex for drugs had become common (Aral & Holmes, 1999).

Since 1990 levels of primary and secondary syphilis morbidity per 100,000 in the United States have fallen dramatically, from 23.5 in men and 17.3 in women in 1990 to 3.6 among men and 2.9 among women in 1997. Even in the South, which has consistently reported greater morbidity than other regions, from

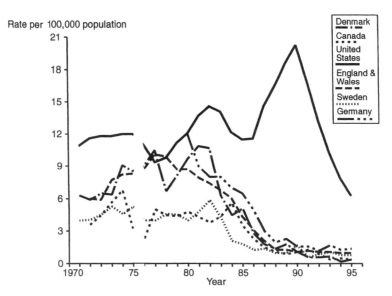

Figure 2. Syphilis trends: international comparisons.

1990 to 1995 the syphilis rate declined 64%, from 33.7 in 1990 to 12.1 in 1995. The male to female ratio of syphilis cases has been stable at 1.1 between 1990 and 1995 (Aral & Holmes, 1999). Data on sex preference, available on a national basis only through 1982, showed that the proportion of U.S. men with primary and secondary syphilis who named other men as sex partners (MSM) had increased from 23% in 1969 to 42% in 1982. From 1990 to 1998 the U.S. primary and secondary syphilis rate declined 87% (Centers for Disease Control, 2000) and is anticipated to continue to decrease. A concerted effort toward its elimination in the United States was launched in 1999 by the Centers for Disease Control.

Comparison of recent primary and secondary syphilis trends in selected industrialized countries since 1970 are interesting, with declining trends in all except the United States. As of 1995 primary and secondary syphilis rates per 100,000 population were 4.4 per 100,000 in the United States, 1.4 in Germany, 1.0 in England and Wales, 0.8 in Sweden, 0.4 in Denmark, and 0.4 in Canada (Figure 2).

Chlamydia Trachomatis Infections

Chlamydia trachomatis has become the most prevalent sexually transmitted bacterial infection in North America and Europe (Division of STD Prevention, 1997). The number of cases of chlamydial infection reported in Sweden based on diagnostic testing rose from 20,000 in 1983 to 38,000 in 1987, nearly equal to the number of cases of gonorrhea (40,000) reported in that country in 1970. Since 1988, the number of chlamydial infections has fallen steadily in Sweden, in association with implementation of routine screening for infection in women, and with strengthened partner notification.

In the United States, indirect estimates based on the incidence of syndromes associated with *C. trachomatis* as determined by visits to private physicians, or on the case ratio of *C. trachomatis* to *N. gonorrhoeae* infections, indicated over 4 million infections per year as of 1986 (Washington, 1986). Accurate national

time trends in incidence of proven *C. trachomatis* infections cannot yet be defined because of changes in reporting and increasing laboratory surveillance. Trends of nongonococcal urethritis (NGU) incidence in men provided a reasonable approximation, in the past, when the proportion of NGU cases attributable to *C. trachomatis* remained fairly consistent at about 40% between the early 1970s and the end of the 1980s (Cates, 1987; Judson, 1981). Based on the number of visits by men to private physicians' offices, NGU increased between the mid-1960s and the end of the 1980s in the United States as well as in the United Kingdom. In 1972 in the United States, the number of visits to private physicians' offices for NGU surpassed the number for gonococcal urethritis for the first time, and by 1987 NGU was more than twice as common as gonococcal urethritis. The increase in office visits for NGU relative to office visits for gonococcal urethritis was due mainly to a decline in gonorrhea after 1971, rather than an increase in NGU. However, in England, Wales, and other developed countries the reported number of cases of NGU continued to increase steadily, even as the reported number of cases of gonococcal urethritis declined. In recent years in the United States, a declining proportion of NGU has been attributable to chlamydial infection in some studies, making trends in NGU no longer a useful surrogate for trends in *C. trachomatis* infection (Aral & Holmes, 1999). Similarly, other indicators for the incidence of chlamydial infection, such as mucopurulent cervicitis, (Brunham *et al.*, 1984) or pelvic inflammatory disease (PID), do not provide useful surrogates for trends in genital chlamydial infections (Aral & Holmes, 1999).

Starting in the late 1980s efforts for early detection and treatment of chlamydial infections increased remarkably in the United States. The number of chlamydial infections per 100,000 population reported to the U.S. Centers for Disease Control increased steadily from 6.5 in 1984 to 207 in 1997; chlamydial infection now results in more disease notifications to state health departments and CDC than any other infectious disease.

During 1996, state-specific chlamydia positivity rates among 15- to 24-year-old women tested at selected family planning clinics ranged from 2.6% to 10.9%. Reported 1995 rates of chlamydia infection for women (290.3 per 100,000 population) were almost six times those for men (52.1 per 100,000 population), again reflecting testing bias. The prevalence of chlamydia test positivity dropped by almost two thirds during the first seven years of implementation of federally funded chlamydia screening in Pacific Northwest family planning clinics, after which rates have leveled off. Adolescents continue to have the highest rates of disease. More recently initiated chlamydia screening programs in other regions of the country are also showing declines in prevalence, demonstrating that serial monitoring of prevalence in family planning clinics, like serial monitoring in prenatal clinics, represents a useful approach to monitoring the impact of screening programs (Aral & Holmes, 1999).

Non-STD clinic-based surveys of chlamydial infection using urine-based DNA amplification testing in San Francisco (Klausner et al., 1997), Seattle (Marrazzo et al., 1997), San Diego (Gunn et al., 1998) and other parts of the world document high prevalence of infection among teenagers and young adults from the general population. High rates of urethral infection have also been found by screening young men, supporting extension of selective screening to young men as well (Marrazzo et al., 1997).

In summary, teenagers and young adults of both genders in the United States have high prevalence rates of chlamydial infection, particularly in high risk populations.

Chancroid

In the 1970s and 1980s most reported cases of chancroid in the United States occurred in sporadic outbreaks, in Los Angeles, Dallas, Boston, New York City, and several Florida cities, leading to an extraordinary increase from 850 cases in 1981 to 4986 cases of chancroid in the United States by 1987. Because chancroid may facilitate HIV transmission (Plummer et al., 1990; Hayes et al., 1995) and because recent

U.S. outbreaks of chancroid were in metropolitan areas and heterosexual populations of high HIV prevalence, this increased incidence was considered to be of great public health importance. Chancroid is recognized far more frequently among men than among women. For example, in the United States during 1987, the male:female sex ratio was 5.8:1 for reported cases of chancroid, compared with 0.94:1 for genital herpes. The link between lack of circumcision and STI is best established for chancroid (Moses et al., 1998), and cultural circumcision practices probably also have an important influence on the incidence of chancroid in different ethnic groups.

Patterns of commercial sex help to explain high male:female sex ratios, not only in recent U.S. outbreaks but in many developing countries of Africa, Asia, and Latin America where chancroid is endemic. For example, the prevalence of genital ulcers in sex workers in a poor neighborhood of Nairobi, Kenya, was an extraordinary 42% in the early 1980s (Kreiss et al., 1986), and the majority were culture-positive for Hemophilus ducreyi.

Since 1987, reported cases of chancroid have declined steadily in the United States (Division of STD Prevention, 1997), to 243 cases in 1997. However, the accuracy of the data early in the U.S. chancroid epidemic were questionable because of the lack of a readily available diagnostic test for H. ducreyi (DiCarlo et al., 1995; Morse et al., 1997). In Jackson, Mississippi in 1994–1995, use of a multiplex polymerase chain reaction assay for H. ducreyi identified chancroid as the major cause of genital ulcers (Morse et al., 1997). In two outbreaks, in New Orleans and Jackson, chancroid was associated with crack cocaine use, exchange of sex for drugs, and delayed health care seeking (DiCarlo et al., 1995; Morse et al., 1997).

Vaginal Trichomoniasis and Other Vaginal Infections

The National Therapeutic and Disease Index (NDTI) survey in the United States indicates a decline in initial visits to physicians offices for vaginal trichomoniasis from an estimated 579,000 in 1966 to 190,000 in 1988, with relatively unchanged rates since then (175,000 in 1997). During this same period, initial visits for other vaginal infections (etiology not defined) increased from an estimated 1,155,000 in 1966 to 4,474,000 in 1989, then declined irregularly to 3,100,000 in 1997 (Aral & Holmes, 1999). Estimates from the World Health Organization suggest that trichomoniasis accounts for nearly half of all curable infections in the world and based on their estimates for North America, 5 million new cases are extrapolated to occur annually in America (Cates, 1999).

Genital Herpes

Genital herpes simplex virus infection spread rapidly from the mid-1960s until the onset of the AIDS epidemic. The annual number of patient consultations with private physicians in office practice for newly diagnosed symptomatic genital herpes in the United States increased 12.5-fold, from 18,000 in 1966 to over 225,000 visits in 1990, then declined irregularly to 167,000 in 1997. People 20 to 29 years of age had more office visits than other age groups. Women outnumbered men in genital-herpes-related physician consultations, reflecting either true gender differentials in genital herpes incidence, or differences in health-care-seeking behavior (Aral & Holmes, 1999).

During the 1970s and 1980s media attention may have increased both physicians' and patients' awareness of the signs and symptoms of genital herpes, increasing the proportions of patients with genital herpes who sought physician consultations and received a correct diagnosis (Cates, 1987). However, based on the percentage of adults with serum antibody, the true annual incidence of new HSV-2 infections in the United States clearly exceeds the number of physician consultations for newly diagnosed symptomatic genital infections by several fold.

The most recent data on HSV-2 seroprevalence in the United States were collected in a stratified random sample of the U.S. population through the National Health and Nutrition Examination Survey (NHANES) III (1988–1994). According to these findings, in 1991 (midpoint of the survey), HSV-2 seroprevalence in persons 12 years of age and older was 21.9%, corresponding to 44.9 million infected persons. Seroprevalence was greater in women (25.6%) than in men (17.8%), and was greater in Blacks (45.9%) than in Whites (17.6%). Independent predictors of HSV-2 seropositivity included gender, race/ethnicity, age, education, poverty, cocaine use, and lifetime number of sex partners (Fleming et al., 1997). Only 9.2% of seropositive people reported a history of genital herpes. Between 1978 and 1991 age-adjusted HSV-2 seroprevalence increased 30%. The increase in seroprevalence was fivefold among 12- to 19-year-old Whites. Increases among Blacks and older Whites were smaller. Based on these figures, it has been estimated that there are up to one million new HSV-2 infections transmitted each year in the United States (Cates, 1999).

Genital Human Papillomavirus Infections

The associations between certain types of HPV and precancerous or invasive lesions of the cervix, vagina, vulva, anus, and penis have been clearly documented, (Koutsky & Kiviat, 1999) and as a result, interest in and physician awareness of genital HPV infections have increased. Presently, genital and anal HPV and HSV infections appear to be the most prevalent STIs in the United States (Aral & Holmes, 1999). As with genital HSV infections, HPV infections are far more often subclinical than they are associated with lesions recognized by the infected individual. By screening for HPV DNA every three months, using PCR amplification tests, the cumulative incidence of genital HPV infections in one study was 43% over a three-year period among sexually active female University students (Ho et al., 1998; Koutsky & Kiviat, 1999). Serologic tests for antibody to those types of HPV found in the genital tract are now helping to further define the epidemiology of genital HPV infection in the same way that serologic tests have elucidated the epidemiology of HSV-2 infection.

External genital warts are mostly caused by type 6 or 11 HPV, consequently, physician–patient consultations for this condition provide the best available indicator of trends in the incidence of genital infections by HPV types 6 or 11. Initial visits to physician's offices for genital warts increased from 55,695 in 1966 to over 351,370 in 1987; from 1987 to 1997, initial visits to physicians offices declined to around 145,000. The extent to which this rise and fall represents the natural history of the spread of the epidemic of HPV-6 and 11 through the United States population, rather than changes in health care seeking, diagnosis, or risk-taking behaviors, remains undefined.

Among sexually active women, the prevalence of cervical HPV DNA has been highest for teenagers and those in the early twenties, and lower for older women (Koutsky & Kiviat, 1999). The natural history of genital HPV infection in men remains largely undefined, although the short-term natural history of incident genital infection by various HPV types is being defined in women by serial cervicovaginal PCR testing, and cervical cytology, and by serologic studies. It appears that the median duration is for HPV-16 (about $1\frac{1}{2}$ years), and the shortest duration is for HPV-6 and 11 (about 5–6 months) (Ho *et al.*, 1998). Type-specific serum antibody detectable by current assays develops slowly over several months in the majority of infected women. The longer duration of HPV-16 shedding may help explain its relatively high incidence in the population.

Based upon these preliminary findings from cohort studies, and together with data from national surveys of sexual behavior, it is likely that the majority of adults in the United States—perhaps three quarters—have been infected with one or more types of genital HPV (Aral & Holmes, 1999). It has been estimated that there may be at least 5.5 million new HPV infections per year and a prevalence of productive HPV (persons with active shedding of HPV DNA) of 20 million (Cates, 1999).

STI COMPLICATIONS AND CONSEQUENCES

The major complications of sexually transmitted infections include AIDS; cancer (cervix, vagina, vulva, anus, penis, liver, Kaposi's sarcoma, and lymphoma T-cell leukemia); PID and related sequelae including infertility; complications of pregnancy and the puerperium; congenital, perinatal, and postnatal infections of the fetus/infant; various neurologic syndromes, and a variety of other diseases. Selected aspects of the epidemiology of these complications are discussed below.

Pelvic Inflammatory Disease

Trends in pelvic inflammatory disease reflect not only trends in incidence, but also changing diagnostic criteria, and changing management practices, which recently have involved decreasing rates of hospitalization. The U.S. National Survey of Family Growth (NSFG), performs repeated surveys of reproductive age women living in the United States, providing data on trends in PID (National Center for Health Statistics. Vital and health statistics, 1997). In 1995, 8% of women reported past treatment for PID, including 8% of Hispanic women, 7% of non-Hispanic White women, and 11% of Black women (National Center for Health Statistics. Vital and health statistics, 1997; Aral & Mosure, 1997; Aral & Wasserheit, 1998). PID was twice as common among women who reported vaginal douching regularly (12%) than among those who did not douche (6%). PID was also twice as common among those with 10 or more sex partners in their lifetimes (14%) as among women who had had two or three partners (7%). While the distribution of PID across population groups was similar in 1982, 1988, and 1995, the prevalence of PID apparently declined during this time from 14% in 1982 to 11% in 1988, and 8% in 1995 (National Center for Health Statistics. Vital and health statistics, 1997; Aral & Mosure, 1997; Aral & Wasserheit, 1998).

Infertility

There is growing evidence that STIs, specifically chlamydia and gonorrhea, are the primary cause of infertility problems in the world (Cates & Brunham, 1999). In the last few decades there has been an increase in infertility associated with an increase in the prevalence of STIs worldwide. Undiagnosed and untreated STIs often enter the upper reproductive tract of women where they cause inflammation and tubal occlusion due to scaring as a result of immune response. In industrialized countries it has been demonstrated that the first episode of PID results in 8–12% infertility, where a second episode can result in as much as 19–25% infertility and three or more episodes result in 40–50% infertility (Cates & Brunham, 1999; Sciarra, 1997). It has been reported that 20 to 40% of women infected with gonorrhea or chlamydia develop PID and about 20% of those cases result in infertility (Chandra & Stephen, 1998). Some of the variability in infertility resulting from PID has been attributed to the severity of the inflammation and the age at which a woman has PID. Generally more severe episodes of PID, which are more often associated with Chlamydia trachomatis infections, and PID at a younger age result in an increase in infertility (Cates & Brunham, 1999; Westrom & Eschenbach, 1999; Germain *et al.*, 1992). The World Health Organization estimated that 60–80 million couples are infertile throughout the world (Sciarra, 1997). However, information on the prevalence of infertility is difficult to obtain because infertility is generally only diagnosed in individuals seeking medical attention for impaired fecundity in developed countries. In developing countries, where health care is often unavailable, prevalence has primarily been estimated through epidemiological studies. In the United States, the annual incidence of STI-related infertility was estimated to be 125,000 cases per year. Other developed countries, such as England and Denmark report similar estimates of incidences of STI-related infertility. In Africa almost two thirds of infertility in women has been attributed to prior STI infection (Cates & Brunham, 1999). Sub-Saharan Africa has been estimated to have the highest reported rates of gonorrhea and chlamydia associated infertility (Sciarra 1997).

Ectopic Pregnancy

Ectopic pregnancy is the leading cause of pregnancy-related death during the first trimester, responsible for 9% of all pregnancy-related deaths in the United States in 1992. Women who have one ectopic pregnancy are at increased risk for another such pregnancy and for future infertility. In the United States, the reported number of hospitalizations for ectopic pregnancy increased from 17,800 in 1970 to 88,400 in 1989 (Centers for Disease Control and Prevention, 1995). Based on the National Hospital Discharge Survey (NHDS), the estimated number of hospitalizations for ectopic pregnancy was 64,400 in 1990, 55,600 in 1991, and 58,200 in 1992 (95% CI=48,600–67,700) for a rate of 10.6 per 1000 reported pregnancies (i.e., ectopic, legal abortions, and live births).

This analysis of the estimated number of ectopic pregnancies, based only on hospitalizations, indicates a decline since the late 1980s. However, in part this decline reflects the shift toward treating ectopic pregnancy in an outpatient setting. When data from NHDS are combined with data from the National Hospital Ambulatory Medical Care Survey (NHAMCS), the estimated total number of ectopic pregnancies in 1992 was 108,800 (Centers for Disease Control and Prevention, 1995), nearly double the estimated number of hospitalized cases. Thus, combining data for hospitalized an ambulatory cases suggests that the incidence of ectopic pregnancy, instead of declining in the late 1980s, may have increased steadily since 1970.

Surveillance data on ectopic pregnancy are not available for the period after 1992. However, estimates based on pregnancy outcome data collected in 1995 by the NSFG continue to indicate that ectopic pregnancies constituted

2% of all pregnancies during the 1987–1990 period and during the 1991–1994 period. The estimated yearly averages were 105,180 and 110,880 ectopic pregnancies for the two periods, respectively (Anjari Chandra, personal communication).

The increase in ectopic pregnancies over the past three decades was not confined to the United States. From the mid-1970s through the mid-1980s, the incidence of ectopic pregnancy more than doubled in many countries of the Western world, including Sweden, Norway, Ireland, Canada, and Finland, even as the incidence of gonorrhea was declining (Skjeldestad *et al.*, 1997). Suggested explanations include the effects of changes in the management of infertility, and ectopic pregnancy (leading to recurrent ectopic pregnancies), and an increasing incidence of silent or subclinical PID.

Adverse Outcomes of Pregnancy

While data are not available on trends of every type of AOP, recent studies provide estimates of the magnitude of the problem (Goldenberg *et al.*, 1997). Fetal or neonatal infections with five of the major sexually transmitted organisms—syphilis, herpes simplex virus, group B streptococcus, cytomegalovirus, and HIV—may have a devastating effect, including either death or long-term neurologic disability affecting between 1000 and 2500 infants per year in the United States. In contrast to these relatively rare outcomes, approximately 400,000 infants are born prematurely each year in the United States, and of these more than 20,000 die in the fetal or neonatal period and another 20,000 end up with long-term neurologic sequelae. As many as 100,000 of these preterm births and 5000 or more deaths, as well as a similar number of major disabilities, may be associated with maternal STIs. The greatest potential for achieving improvement in adverse outcomes of pregnancy associated with sexually transmitted diseases may lie in reducing the excess number of preterm births, many apparently associated with antenatal bacterial vaginosis.

Cervical Cancer

In the past, health care behavior has been less important in the epidemiology of incurable viral STIs than in the epidemiology of curable bacterial STI, as discussed below. One exception is cervical carcinoma, a complication of cervical HPV infection. Regular cervical cytologic screening allows early detection and treatment of cervical dysplasia, preventing progression to invasive cervical carcinoma. The incidence of cervical cancer is exceptionally high in developing countries which lack programs for preventing cervical cancer, and has been rising in some countries where the recommended frequency for cytology screening is relatively low. The higher incidence of cervical cancer in Blacks than in Whites in the United States could be attributable either to more frequent cervical HPV infection or to less frequent cytology screening or to both factors. Similarly, because early diagnosis and treatment of invasive cancer predicts better prognoses, the higher mortality rate for cervical cancer in Black women than in White women could also reflect differences in health care behavior.

SOCIAL AND DEMOGRAPHIC CORRELATES OF STI IN THE UNITED STATES

In the United States the prevalence, incidence and trends in incidence of all known STI vary by age, gender, racial ethnic background, socioeconomic status (SES), residence, and sexual preference. Comprehensive data on such correlates are available only to the extent that STI are reported and data on correlates are captured through the reporting system, including age, gender, and race ethnicity. Some of the available data are presented below, using gonorrhea and syphilis as examples.

The incidence and trends in incidence of reported gonorrhea cases in the United States differ by racial group. Between 1975 and 1984, the annual incidence of reported gonorrhea declined less among White women (8.9% decline) and White men (13.6%) than among men and women of other races (19.2% and 18.3%, respectively). Trends after 1984 reversed this picture; the race differential between Whites and Blacks grew between 1984 and 1987. In 1996, the incidence of reported gonorrhea per 100,000 was 826 among Black non-Hispanics, 106 among American Indian/Alaskan Natives, 69 among Hispanics, 26 among White non-Hispanics, and 18.6 among Asian/Pacific Islanders. Among 15- to 19-year-old African-American non-Hispanics, the 1996 reported gonorrhea incidence was 3791 per 100,000, the highest age, gender, and race-ethnicity-adjusted rates in the United States (Division of STD Prevention, 1997).

In the United States gonorrhea incidence has also been strongly associated with socioeconomic status (SES) and residence. For example, in 1986 and 1987 in Seattle, Washington, census tracts representing the lowest SES quartile accounted for 58% of reported gonorrhea (Rice et al., 1991). Data from the Gonococcal Isolate Surveillance Project (GISP) in the United States suggests a further concentration of morbidity among core transmitters as rates decline (Fox & Knapp, 1997). As rates of gonorrhea and pelvic inflammatory disease decline in many local areas, morbidity becomes concentrated in low SES core groups residing in low SES areas (Aral & Wasserheit, 1998). A recent analysis of gonorrhea morbidity in United States cities with >200,000 population showed that six factors accounted for 75% of the variation in gonorrhea morbidity in these cities: population density, percent households with female heads, city government general expenditure per capita, violent crime rate, percent of families below poverty level, and percent of births to mothers younger than 20 (Zaidi et al., 1997).

Nationally, an abrupt rise in primary and secondary syphilis in African-Americans began in 1986, coinciding with the crack cocaine epidemic, and continued through 1990, after which rates began to fall equally rapidly. During 1997, the incidence of primary and secondary syphilis per 100,000 in the United States was 22.0 among Blacks, 1.6 for Hispanics, 0.5 for Whites, and 0.6 for others. There are also clear geographic patterns associated with syphilis in the United States. In 1990, 58% of all U.S. counties reported no cases of primary or secondary syphilis. By 1997 this percentage was up to 7%, with 31 (1%) of 3115 counties reporting 50% of all primary and secondary syphilis cases! Highest rates occurred in the South where outbreaks of primary and secondary syphilis still occur.

A most interesting and concerning pattern in P & S syphilis morbidity is its overlap with seroprevalence of HIV among childbearing women, and with the incidence of gonorrhea particularly in southeastern United States. The most recent data available on prenatal HIV seroprevalence were for 1994, after which national antenatal HIV seroprevalence surveys were arbitrarily stopped by the U.S. Congress.

Finally, age is strongly associated with STIs, especially chlamydial infection and will be discussed in the following section. Many studies of adolescents have been conducted in STD and family planning clinics (Orr et al., 1996; Fortenberry et al., 1997; Martin et al., 1998; Burstein et al., 1998; Millstein & Moscicke, 1995) and in juvenile detention (DiClemente, 1991; Dyer et al., 1998). National data sources such as the CDC's Youth Risk Behavior Surveillance Survey (YRBSS), National Survey of Adolescent Males (NSAM), and the National Survey of Family Growth (NSFG) also provide important data on adolescents risk for STIs across the United States. Data from the 1997 YRBSS indicate that 48% of U.S. high school students have had sexual intercourse, with 16% having engaged in sexual intercourse with more than four partners. Over time, however, the trends seem to suggest a leveling off for sexual experience and increases for condom use in both the NASM and NSFG (Sonenstein et al., 1998). High rates of sexual activity among adolescents have been noted in other countries in surveys such as the Demographic Health Surveys but with great differences by region of the world. Among women, the proportion having first intercourse by age 17 in Mali (72%), Jamaica (53%), Ghana (52%), the United States (47%), and Tanzania (45%) is 7–10 times that in Thailand (7%) and the Philippines (6%). The proportion of men who have had intercourse before their seventeenth birthday in Jamaica (76%), the United States (64%) and Brazil (63%) is about 10 times the level reported in the Philippines (7%) (Singh *et al.*, 2000). While both male and females are initiating sex at a young age in many countries, there persists a difference in age among the partners in that many young females have older partners. For example, nearly two thirds (64%) of sexually active 15- to 17-year-old women have partners who are within 2 years of their age; 29% have sexual partners who are 3–5 years older, and 7% have partners who are 6 or more years older in the United States (Darroch *et al.*, 1999). Finally, relatively poor health care-seeking and access could be a factor in the high prevalence of STI in adolescent/young adult populations.

Other individual level factors correlated with STI are centered around the concept of self-efficacy. This includes the self-efficacy to use condoms and to choose partners (Catania *et al.*, 1989). Self-efficacy has been defined as an individual's belief that she has the skills to control her own behavior to achieve the desired outcome or goal (Bandura, 1987) and has been suggested as a critical factor in condom use (Bandura, 1987). Discrimination in sex partner choice and recruitment involves another facet of self-efficacy as individuals who do not assess the risks of their sexual partners and then decide whether or not to have sex with them and/or practice safe sex when doing so are at much greater risk of STI/HIV than individuals who are discriminating in partner choice (Aral *et al.*, 1991). However, individuals' ability to assess STD/HIV risk may be compromised by the other risks they have in their lives and weigh as less of a threat.

DETERMINANTS OF POPULATION TRANSMISSION DYNAMICS

Each of the three direct determinants of the rate of spread of STIs in a population—rate of exposure between infected and uninfected persons, efficiency of transmission per exposure, and duration of infectivity—are driven by a complex set of factors. Some of these factors are discussed below.

Determinants of Exposure: Trends and Patterns of Sexual Behavior

Our understanding of the relevant components of sexual behavior that influence risk of STI, including HIV infection, has changed considerably over the past few decades. A better understanding of the epidemiology of specific STIs, and the greater need for preventive interventions to change sexual behavior in the context of increasing viral STIs, initiated such changes in the early 1980s. The AIDS epidemic has been the single most important factor to both highlight the need for more systematic information on sexual behavior and facilitate an unprecedented increase in infection-related studies of sexual behavior.

The term "sexual behavior" involves many components: sexual experience and activity, age at sexual debut or "coitarche," current and lifetime number of sex partners, frequency of sexual intercourse, consistency of sexual activity, mode of recruitment of sexual partners, duration of sexual unions, and types of sexual practice (Aral & Cates, 1989). While the conjoint distribution of the component variables in the population determines aggregate exposure to the risk of STIs, the specific relationship between each of these variables and the risk of various STDs with differing natural histories, and the distribution of these variables across population subgroups, have by no means been fully defined.

The population at risk for STIs has been very simply defined in terms of age groups, often assuming those between ages 15 and 45 may engage in sexual intercourse with new partners. Further refinements of this concept have included in the population at risk only the sexually experienced, defined as persons who have ever had sexual intercourse (Bell & Holmes, 1984). However, current sexual activity, rather than sexual experience per se, is a more accurate measure of current exposure to the risk of STIs (Aral *et al.*, 1988).

One of the most frequently used risk markers in STI research is age at first sexual intercourse. This variable has often been employed to describe sexual activity levels of populations and to monitor the so-called sexual revolutions and evolutions. Age at sexual debut has two epidemiological functions: first as a true risk factor, causally related to disease outcome, and second as an indicator of other aspects of sexual activity. Etiologically, age at sexual debut has been independently associated with the development of cervical cancer in some studies, and in other studies with *C. trachomatis* antibody prevalence (Sanchez *et al.*, 1996) and with HIV infection, perhaps owing to the biological development of the female cervix during the teenage years. As a risk indicator, age at sexual debut is correlated with sociodemographic factors such as race and socioeconomic status, sexual behavior variables, number of sex partners, and specific STIs. Age at sexual debut together with age at first marriage has been the primary variable documenting the sexual revolution of the 1970s (Hofferth *et al.*, 1987).

Risk of exposure to an STI is directly associated not only with number of infected sex partners, but also with the prevalence of STI within one's pool of potential choice of sex partner(s). The number of sex partners within a specific time period, often one or three months, has been shown to be a risk factor for having gonorrhea (D'costa *et al.*, 1985), chlamydia (Handsfield *et al.*, 1986; Schacter *et al.*, 1983), genital herpes, and human papillomavirus infections (Syrjanen *et al.*, 1984). Lifetime number of sex partners is associated with the risk of cervical and other genital cancers, as well as with the prevalence of serum antibody reflecting past exposure to various STI (this is essentially true for all STI pathogens for which serologic tests are available). However, the relationship between number of sex partners and STI risk is not simple; it is of course influenced by the partner's sexual behavior, and the varying infectiousness of infected partners.

The most recent data on lifetime number of sex partners of reproductive age American women was collected in 1995 by the National Survey of Family Growth (National Center for Health Statistics: Vital and health statistics, 1997). The greatest percentage of women 15–44 years of age (24.6%) had had only one lifetime partner, but 12.7% reported 10 or more partners. The other recent source of data on sexual behavior in the United States, the National Health and Social Life Survey (NHSLS) found similar numbers and compared these numbers to data on sexual behavior from other industrialized countries. In the NHSLS 31.4% of women reported one lifetime sex partner, 36.4% reported two to four partners, and 29.6% reported five or more partners; in the United Kingdom 39.3% of women reported one lifetime partner, 35% reported two to four lifetime partners, 19.8% five or more; in France 46.1% of women reported one lifetime partner, 34.4% reported two to four lifetime partners, 13.7% five or more. For men, the pattern was similar. In the NHSLS 19.5% of men reported one lifetime sex partner, 20.9% reported two to four partners, and 56.2% reported five or more partners; in the United Kingdom 20.6% of men reported one lifetime partner, 29.0% reported two to four lifetime partners, 43.8% five or more; in France 21.4% of men reported one lifetime partner, 29.1% reported two to four lifetime partners, 45.0% reported five or more (Laumann *et al.*, 1994). Clearly, similar numbers of partners are reported in the United States, United Kingdom, and France although slightly more Americans report more partners.

Exposure to an STI transmitter depends upon how one chooses one's sex partners and on the prevalence of STI in the pool of available partners. Both in the general population and among STD clinic attendees, marked gender differentials exist in the recruitment of sex partners. Compared with men, women tend to report meeting their potential partners through less casual associations, and to know them better and for longer periods of time prior to becoming sexually involved with them (Sanchez *et al.*, 1996; Research and Forecasts, Inc., 1987;

Aral *et al.*, unpublished data). A nondiscriminating approach to sex partner recruitment increases the probability of sexual contact with members of high-risk core groups and thus of exposure to STI. Better understanding of patterns of partner recruitment in population subgroups will help explain some of the variability in STI risk.

Role of Sexual Mixing, Sexual Networks, and Partner Concurrency

Some of the most exciting developments in our understanding of the role of sexual behavior in determining the probability of exposure between infected and uninfected persons (and thus the rate of spread of STIs in the population), in the 1990s have been in the areas of patterns of partner mixing (Garnett & Anderson, 1993; Garnett *et al.*, 1996), sexual networks (Anderson *et al.*, 1990; Ghani *et al.*, 1997; Gupta *et al.*, 1989; Klovdahl, 1985), and partner concurrency (Morris & Kretzschmar, 1997). Deterministic mathematical modeling has been used to describe how patterns of sex partner mixing such as random, assortative (like with like), or disassortative, can influence the course of an HIV epidemic (Gupta *et al.*, 1989). Empirical data on patterns of mixing have been collected from surveys conducted in Uganda (Morris *et al.*, 1996), Thailand (Morris *et al.*, 1996a), Great Britain (Johnson *et al.*, 1992), France (AIDS and sexual behavior in France, 1992), and the United States (Laumann *et al.*, 1994) as well as a few smaller studies (Garnett & Anderson, 1993; Garnett *et al.*, 1996; Stoner *et al.*, in press; Aral *et al.*, 1999). Concurrent partnerships, (Laumann & Youm, 1999) existence of "bridge" persons, who have sex both with members of high risk groups and low risk groups (Gorbach *et al.*, 2000) or with groups specifically found to have high STI prevalence and with groups with low STI prevalence (Aral *et al.*, 1999); high density of sexual networks (i.e., a large number of sexual connections among all members of a group), variance in a population's distribution of number of sex partners (Anderson *et al.*, 1990), and the extent to which so called "core groups" are embedded in the general population are all, in theory, associated with faster spread of sexually transmitted infections in the population, and higher STI rates.

Determinants of Efficiency of Transmission per Exposure

Factors that influence the efficiency of transmission when infected and uninfected individuals are sexually exposed to each other include susceptibility of the uninfected host; cervical ectopy in women; circumcision status of men; use of contraceptives, barrier methods such as condoms and microbicides; sexual practices; inoculum size, which is a determinant of infectivity of the infected host; use of suppressive therapy; and inflammation and other reproductive tract infections (Aral & Holmes, 1999).

Condoms, used consistently and correctly, offer good protection against HIV and gonorrheal and chlamydial infections. However, male condoms may not completely prevent contact between the epithelium of the penis and the vulva and therefore may offer less protection against those STIs which commonly infect the squamous epithelium such as herpes simplex virus (HSV) and human papillomavirus (HPV) (Aral & Holmes, 1999). Studies which have explored the relationship between STI and condom use yield contradictory and unexpected findings due to a number of factors, including difficulty in accurately measuring consistent and correct condom use; the inherent biases of self-selection (where people who know they are at high risk tend to use condoms) in observational studies; and the confounding effects of prevalence of infection in sexual networks.

Determinants of Duration of Infectiousness

The primary determinant of duration of infectivity of specific STI is the natural history of that infection. Access to effective diagnostic and treatment services is an important factor which reduces duration of infection of bacterial STIs. In this context health-care-seeking behaviors of the population, behaviors of health care providers, and properties of the health care system all influence the duration of infectiousness (and infection) (Aral & Wasserheit, 1999).

Risk Markers and Risk Factors for STI

In STI epidemiology the terms risk factor, risk marker (or risk indicator), and risk determinant have been used interchangeably without much attention to the existence of a *causal* link between the relevant attribute or exposure and the disease or disease outcome. Similarly, little differentiation has been made between modifiable and nonmodifiable risk factors, an important distinction within the context of prevention.

Many of the traditional STI risk factors appear to be correlates of the probability of encountering an infected partner, whereas others may influence the probability of infection if exposed, or the probability of disease if infected. While the causal link between demographic variables and STIs can probably be explained in terms of coincidental differences in sexual behavior and/or disease prevalence, such variables may be most accurately referred to as risk markers or risk indicators. For example, single marital status and inner-city residence fall into this category.

Other variables, such as sexual behaviors and health care behaviors, are directly related to the probability of exposure to STIs, to infection following exposure, or to complications if infected, and can be referred to as true risk factors. Of the major sexual behavioral risk factors for STDs discussed earlier, all but specific sexual practices really represent attempts to measure the probability of exposure to an infected partner. Health care behaviors which can reduce the risk of acquiring STIs or prevent complications include use of condoms for prophylaxis, early consultation for diagnosis and treatment, compliance with therapy, and partner referral (Aral

& Wasserheit, 1999). Absence of such behaviors can be regarded as risk factors for STIs.

PREVENTION TRIALS FOR STI CONTROL

Prevention trials targeting particular risk factors for STI can help confirm the role of the risk factors, as well as guide preventive interventions that directly influence the epidemiology of STIs. The search for conclusive results in the evaluation of interventions to prevent STIs including HIV has resulted in increasing numbers of controlled prevention trials in the past decade. Such trials are generally classified either as behavioral or biomedical intervention trials, although in reality, even those based on a biomedical intervention require supportive behavioral intervention components (e.g., to motivate vaccine acceptance and compliance, and prevent relapse to riskier behaviors by those who might otherwise feel safe after vaccination); and, as discussed below, behavioral interventions benefit from biomedical outcome measures.

Behavioral Preventive Intervention Trials

In STI and HIV prevention several specific issues need to be considered. First, the behaviors targeted for change (e.g., sexual behaviors) are difficult to measure objectively. Dependence on self-reports of behavior creates additional problems in that interventions may change reports of behavior without changing the behavior itself (Aral & Peterman 1993). Second, individuals who change one risk behavior often change other risk behaviors in a countervailing direction, necessitating use of summary measures that reflect the net effects of these changes. Third, the transmission dynamics of STIs are influenced not only by sexual behavior but also by additional factors such as phase of the epidemic, population prevalence, transmission probability, duration of infectiousness, and specific characteristics of transmission networks, resulting in different trends in the incidence of various STIs in the same populations (Hamers *et al.*, 1995). Fourth, the nature of the relationship between sexual behavior and STI incidence varies across the phases of the epidemic (Wasserheit & Aral, 1996). At the individual level, the magnitude of risk associated with particular behaviors depends on the infectiousness of the infected partner. Finally, as eloquently stated recently, whereas adjustment for confounding factors may be feasible in epidemiologic studies of etiologic factors, bias in adoption of behavior change (or in intervention assignment) is inherently part of the practice of medicine and public health, and the idea that such bias can be simply adjusted away may be wishful thinking (Green, 1997). In the light of all these considerations, it is increasingly obvious that in evaluating behavioral interventions to prevent STIs, and HIV, data from randomized controlled trials are particularly important (Aral & Peterman, 1993), the choice of outcome measure is critical and the outcome measure of choice is the appropriate biomedical measure of the STI or STIs of interest.

Some remarkably important STI prevention trials have been completed recently. Among the most important of these, in terms of public health implications, is Project RESPECT. This project was designed to specifically evaluate the efficacy of individual HIV prevention counseling in changing high-risk behaviors and preventing new STIs. This study of high-risk heterosexuals is among the first randomized trials of HIV/STI prevention counseling (Kamb *et al.*, 1998). The study, conducted among HIV negative, heterosexual STD clinic patients enrolled from five U.S. inner-city STD clinics (Baltimore, Denver, Long Beach, Newark, San Francisco), compared (1) Enhanced Counseling, a four-session counseling intervention, each session of 1-hour duration, based on theories of behavioral science, social cognitive theory and the theory of reasoned action, and aimed at changing attitudes, self-efficacy, and perception of risk regarding consistent condom use with all sex partners; (2) Client-Centered HIV Prevention Counseling (two sessions of 20 minutes each), an intervention based on CDC's client-

centered counseling model recommended for use with HIV testing, and aimed at increasing clients' perceptions of personal risk, exploring barriers and facilitators around risk reduction, and negotiating an incremental risk reduction plan that emphasized consistent condom use with all sex partners; and (3) HIV Education (the control intervention which was purely informational, using two brief, didactic messages about HIV and STD prevention that encouraged consistent condom use with all sex partners, similar to the type of prevention messages given at most STD clinics). The Enhanced Counseling and Client-Centered Counseling interventions were significantly more effective than the HIV Education intervention at decreasing high-risk behaviors and preventing new STIs. These findings were consistent across study sites and gender. Most of the STI reduction occurred in the first six months. At 12 months there were no differences across intervention and control groups in condom use, but a 20% reduction in new STIs for counseling interventions remained significant (though the 12-month difference was attributable to the reductions achieved during the first six months). The amount and duration of the effect of counseling in Project RESPECT were modest, but from the population perspective even modest changes in behaviors of high risk STD clinic patients could have a substantial impact on STI and HIV transmission.

Another multisite randomized HIV prevention trial, coordinated by the National Institute of Mental Health, developed and evaluated a seven-session intervention targeting sexual behavior change among low income individuals at high risk for HIV infection (The NIMH multisite HIV prevention trial, 1998). Participants were largely recruited from STD clinics, with a smaller number from primary health care settings. The intervention group experienced significant reductions in reported unprotected sexual exposures and lower rates of gonococcal infection in men (based upon chart review), but urine LCR tests at 12 months showed no difference in prevalence of gonococcal or chlamydial infections. Taken together, Project RESPECT and the NIMH trial suggest an impact on behavior with transient reduction in bacterial STI incidence. The feasibility is low for wide-scale implementation in public health settings of the seven-session intervention employed in the NIMH trial. The impact of the two-session Project Respect trial was encouraging, but the need for "booster" counseling sessions to achieve more persistent effects requires more study.

A third randomized controlled study, a culture- and gender-specific risk-reduction intervention targeting African-American and Hispanic STD clinic patients in San Antonio, Texas, reduced reinfection rates with gonorrhea and chlamydia among high-risk minority women (Shain et al., 1997), and these effects apparently persisted for 12 months. The findings from this study suggest counseling can be effective in a small group as well as one on one.

In another effort researchers in the United Kingdom have conducted a four school randomized trial to assess the feasibility of a large randomized controlled trial of peer-led sex education in schools (Machekano et al., 1997). The findings suggest that evaluation of peer-led sex education through a randomized controlled trial is acceptable to schools, pupils, and parents. In general, pupils who received peer-led sex education responded more positively than those in control schools.

There are few examples of community-level randomized trials assessing STI/HIV behavior change. A recent study assessing the utility of HIV risk reduction workshops and community HIV prevention events among women living in 18 low-income housing developments in five U.S. cities demonstrated a significant reduction in recent risk behavior such as unprotected intercourse in the past two months from 50% to 37.6% and the percentage of protected acts of intercourse rose from 30.2% to 47.2%; significantly greater changes than noted in the control communities (Sikkema et al., 2000).

Biomedical Preventive Intervention Trials

A randomized controlled trial provided empirical evidence for the effectiveness of screening for cervical chlamydial infection followed by timely and appropriate treatment as the key strategy for the prevention of pelvic inflammatory disease (Scholes et al., 1996). Participants were unmarried female health maintenance organization enrollees 18 to 34 years of age with risk factors for chlamydial infection. They were randomized to receive chlamydia screening or routine care. In this study, cervical chlamydia screening led to a 56% reduction in the incidence of pelvic inflammatory disease during one year of follow-up.

Another intervention trial assessed the effect of nonoxynol-9 (N-9) film on the rates of gonococcal and chlamydial infections and HIV infection in a cohort of sex workers (Ryan, 1997). A two-year triple-masked multiclinic randomized controlled trial was conducted among 1292 HIV-negative, nonpregnant sex workers between the ages of 18–45 in Cameroon. Women who were randomized to use condoms and N-9 film or condoms and placebo film were counseled monthly to use both at every coital act and were examined monthly for a mean of 14 months. The study found no additional effect of N-9 over that of condoms on the rate of cervical infection or HIV infection in this population of sex workers. Although they reported high rates of condom use, the rate of new gonorrhea infections was 31.1 infections per 100 woman-years in the placebo group and 33.3 per 100 woman-years in the N-9 group (RR = 1.07, 95% C.I. 0.83–1.39). The rate of chlamydial infections was 22.2 per 100 woman-years for placebo users and 20.6 per 100 woman years for N-9 users (RR = 0.93, 95% C.I. 0.68–1.26).

A landmark HIV prevention trial randomized communities to biomedical intervention and control conditions to assess the effect of the community level intervention. This community randomized trial conducted in the Mwanza region of Tanzania was the first randomized trial to demonstrate an impact of a preventive intervention on HIV incidence in a general population. It showed that improved syndromic management of STI at the primary health care level reduced HIV incidence by about 40% (Grosskurth et al., 1995). HIV incidence was compared in six intervention communities and six pair-matched comparison communities. A random cohort of 1000 adults, 15–54 years of age, from each community was surveyed at baseline and at follow-up two years later. The intervention included establishment of a STD reference clinic, staff training in syndromic management, regular supervisory visits to health facilities, and provision of antimicrobials, and general population health education about STI and health care seeking for STI symptoms.

A subsequent HIV-prevention trial in the Rakai district of Uganda randomized clusters of villages to mass treatment of STI every 10 months versus antiparasitic treatment alone. Serologic screening and treatment for syphilis and syndromic management for STI were offered both to intervention and control villages. The study showed no effect on HIV incidence (Wawer, Gray, Sewankambo et al., 1999), but significant improvements in pregnancy outcomes (Grey et al., 1998). The differences in outcome of the Mwanza and Rakai studies are intriguing. The Mwanza study focused on treatment of symptomatic STI only, whereas the Rakai study provided antimicrobials to the entire population, some of whom had prevalent STI. The Rakai study offered serologic screening and treatment for syphilis, and syndromic management for STI both in the interventions and the control communities. Thus, absolute differences between intervention and control groups on prevalence of STI (other than trichomoniasis) at the point the Rakai study was terminated were small. The impact of systemic antimicrobial therapy on normal flora in uninfected individuals (e.g., suppression of potentially protective H_2O_2-producing lactobacilli or increasing vulvovaginal candidiasis; both potential risk factors for HIV acquisition) represent possible confounders of any beneficial impact on STI prevalence. Differences in the relative prevalence of STI and HIV in the Mwanza and Rakai districts (higher prevalence of HIV infection in Rakai) and basic differences in study design and in the nature of the interventions also may account for the differences in outcome (Aral & Holmes, 1999).

HEALTH POLICY INTERVENTIONS

Randomized controlled intervention trials at individual, group, or community levels, provide the best empirical evidence for the effectiveness of preventive measures. However, preventive measures with the greatest impact include so called structural interventions, often based upon policy changes. Use of randomized controlled trials to assess the effects of policy interventions is usually not feasible; more creative approaches are needed for this purpose.

One strategy is to combine information from many sources and check for consistency across data sets. This is the approach employed in assessing the effects of the policies adopted by the Thai HIV/AIDS Control Program, which required 100% condom use in commercial sex. Evaluation is based on reductions in STI cases in government clinics, and declines in HIV/STI observed through surveys of men and commercial sex workers. More recently, a comparison of two cohorts of military conscripts showed a decline in HIV incidence from 2.48 per 100 person-years between 1991 and 1993 to 0.55 per 100 person-years between 1993 and 1995. STI incidence declined even more, with an overall 10-fold decrease between 1991 and 1993 and 1993 to 1995 (Celentano et al., 1998). The most recent analysis of trends in prevalence of HIV infection among young men conscripted into the military during May or November each year show that the prevalence peaked in 1992 to 1993 and has been declining since, with possible leveling off in the most recent group of conscripts. Another approach has been used in demonstrating the effectiveness of alcohol taxation on reducing STI rates among youth (Chesson & Harrison, 1997). Between 1982 and 1994 there were 34 instances of a state beer tax increase in the United States. The investigators conducted a nonparametric quasi-experiment comparing the proportional changes in STI rates in states with and without a tax increase over the same period, and employed a time series econometric analysis, evaluating the effect of the level of beer taxation on the proportional changes in STI rates, controlling for legal minimum drinking age, per capita income, and state and year differences. The results showed that in 26 (77%) of the states with an increase in beer tax, there was a greater proportional decrease in gonorrhea rates among males in both the 15–19 and the 20–24 age groups as compared to the proportional change among the states without a tax increase. Similar patterns were observed for females. It was estimated that a $0.15 tax increase on a six-pack of beer would reduce gonorrhea incidence rates by roughly 10% among the 15- to 19-year age group. The feasibility, noninvasive nature, and relatively low cost of this study are remarkable, and of course its findings, not having been based on sample data, are completely generalizable to the study population. Nonobtrusive measures to assess the effectiveness of policy interventions to reduce STIs including HIV warrant further evaluation.

New Conceptual Framework: Ecological Risk

The epidemiological research listed above describes the characteristics of individuals at risk of STI. Such studies have been limited, however, to analyses of individual's risks without considering the social context in which the exposures occur. Empirical social science on sexuality, such as described in the NHSLS in the United States (Laumann et al., 1994), on the other hand, has generally had to infer public health implications because it has lacked the clinical data with which to define the sexual health status of its study participants. There is a need to integrate both empirical approaches in order to develop interventions aimed at the reduction of such risks and such interventions must be directed at not only individuals, the people most at risk, but at the larger social context in which individual behavior is determined.

While community level interventions have been recently initiated (described above) the focus, shifting from the individual to the community has skipped the critical levels of sexual dyad (or sexual partnership) and social

network (or peer group). A conceptual framework that identifies the factors affecting STI risk at multiple levels using an ecological approach may advance our understanding of such risks. An ecological perspective implies that behavior results from an interaction of both individual and environmental determinants (McLeroy et al., 1988). We propose an evolving ecological model that suggests a dependent variable and the independent variables that affect it at varying levels of directness. A call for such an approach throughout public health research that moves away from the "individualization" of risk that perpetuates the idea that risk is individually rather than socially determined has already been introduced (Diez-Roux, 1998). While some conceptualizations of reproductive risk to men and women and related interventions have addressed the role of peer groups on individual behavior (Janz et al., 1996) and addressed influential members of social groups, none have yet brought the partnership level into a holistic model. A new framework for conceptualizing risks to women and men of STI may be helpful. One such model introduced here postulates that STIs including HIV are affected through many levels (Figure 3). Specifically, it builds on the individual level by adding a sexual partnership level and separating social network influences from the broader community context. The overlapping spheres of this model represent the multiple levels in which sexual risk behavior occurs. New analytic tools for multilevel analysis have recently been developed and now make the analysis of such complexity technically feasible and able to be estimated statistically.

Levels of the Ecological Model: Individual, Partnership, Social Network, Community

Individual level risks were previously described in this chapter. New findings of risks for STIs at the partnership level have shown that certain patterns of partnerships discordant for age, race/ethnicity, and number of sexual partners represent risk factors for acquiring STI

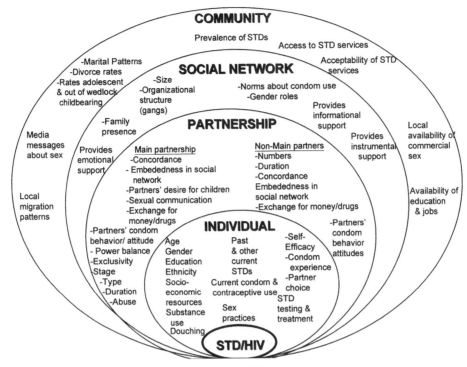

Figure 3. Ecological framework of STD risk for women and men.

(Aral *et al.*, 1999). New analyses of STI risk have tried to account for partner level risks as well as individual level risks. Using data from the 1995 NSFG, one such analysis found 27% of women of reproductive age to be at direct (through their own risk behavior) or indirect (through their partner's behavior) risk for STIs (Finer *et al.*, 1999).

Little research has been conducted on the types of sexual partnerships of people at risk, although there is considerable literature on the dyads of college students. Recent evidence suggests the sexual partnerships of the general U.S. population are predominantly made up of people of similar social characteristics, defined by Laumann *et al.* (1994) as "homophilous" or by Aral *et al.* (1999) as "concordant." Epidemiological research on STI, however, has revealed that people with STI are "heavy mixers" meaning they have sex with two or more partners outside of their own social strata (Catania *et al.*, 1995). This suggests such partnerships may be nonhomophilous or "discordant." "Discordant pairs" have been characterized as representing links across social networks and maybe responsible for the spread of STI between networks. In one study, partners of people with STI not only were nonmonogamous (inferred because either the index patient or partner, or both, had other partners), but were drawn from outside of the social network of the index patient and were likely to be involved in exchange of sex for drugs (Thomas *et al.*, 1995).

The social network level has been studied in terms of the norms generated regarding sexual behavior and condom use. Research on the roles of social norms has shown that consistency or inconsistency between social norms and behaviors that are preventative for STI is an important determinant of the type of social influence that networks and reference groups will exert on members regarding adoption of those behaviors (Catania *et al.*, 1989). Perception of social or peer norms concerning the acceptability of safer sex practices has been demonstrated to be an important determinant of HIV risk taking behavior (Kelly *et al.*, 1993). Specifically, if individuals believe that condom use or other safer sex behaviors are expected, supported, and likely to be reinforced within their peer network, they are more likely to conform to these perceived norms (Fisher & Misovich, 1990).

As described above, our understanding of the role of behaviors in determining individuals' risk of acquiring or transmitting infection and influencing the rate of spread of STI in the population is evolving rapidly. Improved understanding of how behaviors affect STI may be facilitated by multi-level ecological approaches, and may in turn help the development of more effective behavioral interventions aimed at prevention of STI.

REFERENCES

ACSF investigators (1992). AIDS and sexual behaviour in France. *Nature, 360*, 407–409.

Anderson, R. M., Gupta, S., & Ng, W. (1990). The significance of sexual partner contact networks for the transmission dynamics of HIV. *Journal of Acquired Immune Deficiency Syndromes, 3*, 417–429.

Aral, S. O. Unpublished data.

Aral S. O. (1992). Sexual behavior as a risk factor for sexually transmitted disease. In A. Germain, K. K. Holmes, P. Piot, & J. N. Wasserheit (Eds.), *Reproductive tract infections* (pp. 185–198). New York: Plenum Press.

Aral, S. O., Soskoline, V., Joesoef, R. M., & O'Reilly, K. R. (1991). Sex partner recruitment as risk factor for STD: Clustering of risky modes. *Sexually Transmitted Diseases, 18*, 10–17.

Aral, S. O., & Cates, W., Jr. (1989). The multiple dimensions of sexual behavior as risk factor for sexually transmitted disease: The sexually experienced are not necessarily sexually active. *Sexually Transmitted Diseases, 16*, 173–177.

Aral, S. O., & Holmes, K. K. (1999). Social and behavioral determinants of the epidemiology of STDs: Industrialized and developing countries. In K. K. Holmes, P. F. Sparling, P-A. Mårdh, S. M Lemon, W. E Stamm, P. Piot, & J. N. Wasserheit (Eds.), *Sexually transmitted diseases*, 3rd ed. (pp. 39–76). New York: McGraw-Hill.

Aral, S. O., & Mosure, D. (1997). Declining prevalence of pelvic inflammatory disease (PID) and vaginal douching among reproductive age US women: 1995. Abstract presented at the 12th Meeting of the International Society for STD Research. Seville, Spain.

Aral, S., & Peterman, T. (1993). Defining behavioral methods to prevent sexually transmitted diseases through intervention research. In M. S. Cohen, E. W. Hook III, & P. J. Hitchcock (Eds.), *Infectious disease clinics of North America: Sexually transmitted diseases in the AIDS era: Part I* (pp. 861–873). Philadelphia: W. B. Saunders.

Aral, S. O., & Wasserheit, J. N. (1999). STD-related health care seeking and health service delivery. In K. K. Holmes, P. F. Sparling, P-A. Mårdh, S. M Lemon, W. E Stamm, P. Piot, & J. N. Wasserheit (Eds.), *Sexually transmitted diseases*, 3rd ed. (pp. 1295–1305). New York: McGraw-Hill.

Aral, S. O., & Wasserheit, J. N. (1998). Social and behavioral correlates of pelvic inflammatory disease. *Sexually Transmitted Diseases, 25*, 378–385.

Aral, S. O., Hughes, J. P., Stoner, B., Whittington, W., Handsfield, H. H., Anderson, R. M., & Holmes, K. K. (1999). Sexual mixing patterns in the spread of gonococcal and chlamydial infections. *American Journal of Public Health, 89*, 825–833.

Aral, S. O., Schaffer, J. E., Mosher, W. D., & Cates, W., Jr. (1988). Gonorrhea rates: What denominator is most appropriate? *American Journal of Public Health, 78*, 702–703.

Bandura, A. (1987). Perceived self-efficacy in the exercise of control over AIDS infection. Paper presented at the National Institutes of Mental Health and Drug Abuse Research Conference on *Women and AIDS: Promoting Health Behaviors*, Bethesda, MD.

Barrow, R. Y., Hawley, P., Mertz, K., Litchfield, B., Knapp, J., Neal, S., Cohron, G., Levy, M., Health, J., & Levine, W. C. (1997). Increase in gonorrhea and HIV coinfection among men who have sex with men, Washington, DC. Abstract presented at the 12th Meeting of the International Society for STD Research. Seville, Spain, October 19–22.

Bell, T. A., & Holmes, K. K. (1984). Age-specific risks of syphilis, gonorrhea, and hospitalized pelvic inflammatory disease in sexually experienced United States women. *Sexually Transmitted Diseases, 22*, 291.

Brunham, R. C., & Embree J. E. (1992). Sexually transmitted diseases: Current and future dimensions of the problem in the third world. In A. Germain, K. K. Holmes, P. Piot, & J. N. Wasserheit (Eds.), *Reproductive tract infections: Global impact and priorities for women's reproductive health* (pp. 35–58). New York: Plenum Press.

Brunham, R. C., Paavonen, J., Stevens, C. E., Kiviat, N., Kuo, C.C., Critchlow, C. W., & Holmes, K. K. (1984). Mucopurulent cervicitis—the ignored counterpart in women of urethritis in men. *New England Journal of Medicine, 311*, 1–6.

Burstein, G. R., Caydos, C. A., Diener-West, M., Howell,

M. R., Zenilman, J. M., & Quinn, T. C. (1998). Incident chlamydia trachomatis infections among inner-city adolescent females. *Journal of American Medical Association*, 280, 521–526.

Catania, J. A., Binson, D., Dolcini, M. M., Stall, R., Choi, K. H., Pollack, L. M., Hudes, E. S., Canchola, J., Phillips, K., Moskowitz, J. T., & Coates, T. J. (1995). Risk factors for HIV and other sexually transmitted diseases and prevention practices among US heterosexual adults: Changes from 1990 to 1992. *American Journal of Public Health*, 85, 1492–1499.

Catania, J. A., Coates, T. J., & Greenblatt. (1989). Predictors of condom use and multiple partnered sex among sexually active adolescent women: Implications for AIDS related health interventions. Presented at The 5th International Conference on AIDS, Montreal, Canada.

Cates, W. Jr. (1999). Estimates of the incidence and prevalence of sexually transmitted diseases in the United States. American Social Health Association Panel. *Sexually Transmitted Diseases*, 26 (4 Suppl), S2-7.

Cates, W. Jr. (1987). Epidemiology and control of sexually transmitted diseases: Strategic evolution. *Infectious Disease Clinics of North America*, 1, 1–23.

Cates, W., & Brunham, R. C. (1999). Sexually transmitted diseases and infertility. In K. K. Holmes, P. F. Sparling, P. Mårdh, S. M. Lemon, W. E. Stamm, P. Piot, & J. N. Wasserheit (Eds.), *Sexually transmitted diseases*, 3rd ed. (pp. 1079–1087). New York: McGraw-Hill.

Celentano, D. D., Nelson, K. E., Lyles, C. M., Beyrer, C., Eiumtrakul, S., Go, V. F., Kuntolbutra, S., & Khamboonruang, C. (1998). Decreasing incidence of HIV and sexually transmitted diseases in young Thai men: Evidence for success of the HIV/AIDS control and prevention program. *AIDS*, 12, F29–F36.

Centers for Disease Control, Division of Sexually Transmitted Diseases (2000). 1998 Sexually Transmitted Disease Surveillance Report.

Centers for Disease Control and Prevention (1997). Gonorrhea among men who have sex with men—selected sexually transmitted diseases clinics, 1993–1996. *Morbidity and Mortality Weekly Report*, 46, 889–892.

Centers for Disease Control and Prevention (1995). Ectopic pregnancy—United States, 1990–1992. *Morbidity and Mortality Weekly Report*, 44, 46.

Chandra, A., & Stephen, E. H. (1998). Impaired fecundity in the United States: 1982–1995. *Family Planning Perspectives*, 30, 34–42.

Chesson, H., & Harrison, P. (1997). Alcohol and risky sex: The effect of beer taxes on sexually transmitted disease rates among youth. Abstract presented at the 12th Meeting of the International Society for STD Research. Seville, Spain, October 19–22, 1997 [Abstract no, O203].

Darroch, J. E., Landry, D. J., & Oslak, S. (1999). Age differences between sexual partners in the United States. *Family Planning Perspectives*, 31, 160–167.

D'Costa, L. J., Plummer, F. A., Bowmer, I., Fransen, L., Piot, P., Ronald, A. R., & Nsanze, H. (1985). Prostitutes are a major reservoir of sexually transmitted diseases in Nairobi, Kenya. *Sexually Transmitted Diseases*, 12, 64–67.

DiCarlo, R. P., Armentor, B. S., & Martin, D. H. (1995). Chancroid epidemiology in New Orleans men. *Journal of Infectious Diseases*, 172, 446–452.

DiClemente, R. (1991). Predictors of HIV-preventative sexual behavior in a high-risk adolescent population: The influence of perceived peer norms and sexual communication on incarcerated adolescents' consistent use of condoms. *Journal of Adolescent Health*, 12, 385–390.

Diez-Roux, A. V. (1998). Bringing context back into epidemiology: Variables and fallacies in multilevel analysis. *American Journal of Public Health*, 88, 216–222.

Division of STD Prevention (1997). *Sexually transmitted diseases surveillance, 1996.* U.S. Department of Health and Human Services, Public Health Service. Atlanta: Centers for Disease Control and Prevention.

Dyer, I. E., Miller, M. E., Richwald, G. A., Armbruster, J. E., Borenstein, L. A., Rotblatt, H., Morris, R. E., & Harvey, S. M. (1998). Chlamydia screening in juvenile custody facilities. In R. S. Stephens *et al.* (Eds.), *Chlamydial infections: Proceedings of the Ninth International Symposium on Human Chlamydial Infection.* Napa, CA, June 21–26.

Eng, T. R., & Butler, W. T. (1997). *The hidden epidemic: Confronting sexually transmitted diseases.* Washington, DC: National Academy Press. Institute of Medicine.

Finer, L. B., Darroch, J. E., & Singh, S. (1999). Sexual partnership patterns as a behavioral risk factor for sexually transmitted diseases. *Family Planning Perspectives*, 31, 228–236.

Fisher, J. D., & Misovich, S. J. (1990). Social influence and AIDS prevention behavior. In J. Edwards, R. S. Tindall, L. Health, & E. J. Posavac (Eds.), *Social influence process and prevention* (pp. 39–70). New York: Plenum Press.

Fleming, D. T., & Wasserheit, J. N. (1999). From epidemiological synergy to public health policy and practice: The contribution of other sexually transmitted diseases to sexual transmission of HIV infection. *Sexually Transmitted Infections*, 75, 3–17.

Fleming, D. T., McQuillan, G. M., Johnson, R. E., Nahmias, A. J., Aral, S. O., Lee, F. K., & St. Louis, M. E. (1997). Herpes simplex virus type 2 in the United States, 1976 to 1994. *New England Journal of Medicine*, 337, 1105–1111.

Fortenberry, J. D., Orr, D. P., Katz, B. P., Brizendine, E. J., & Blythe, M. J. (1997). Sex under the influence: A diary self-report study of substance use and sexual behavior among adolescent women. *Sexually Transmitted Diseases*, 24, 313–319.

Fox, K. K., & Knapp, J. S. (1997). Changing epidemiology of gonorrhea: Findings from a sentinel system. Abstract presented at the 12th Meeting of the International Society for STD Research. Seville, Spain, October 19–22.

Garnett, G. P., & Anderson, R. M. (1993). Contact tracing and the estimation of sexual mixing patterns: The epidemiology of gonococcal infections. *Sexually Transmitted Disease, 20*, 181–191.

Garnett, G. P., Hughes, J. P., Anderson, R. M., Stoner, B. P., Aral, S. O., Whittington, W. L., Handsfield, H. H., & Holmes, K. K. (1996). Sexual mixing patterns of patients attending sexually transmitted diseases clinics. *Sexually Transmitted Diseases, 23*, 248–257.

Gerbase, A. C., Rowley, J. T., Heymann, D. H., Berkley, S. F., & Piot, P. (1998). Global prevalence and incidence estimates of selected curable STDs. *Sexually Transmitted Infect, 74, Suppl 1*, S12–S16.

Germain, A., Holmes, K. K., Piot, P., & Wasserheit, J. N. (1992). *Reproductive tract infections: Global impact and priorities for women's reproductive health.* New York: Plenum Press.

Ghani, A. C., Swinton, J., & Garnett, G. P. (1997). The role of sexual partnership networks in the epidemiology of gonorrhea. *Sexually Transmitted Diseases, 24*, 45–56.

Goldenberg, R. L., Andrews, W. W., Yuan, A. C., MacKay, H. T., & St. Louis, M. E. (1997). Sexually transmitted diseases and adverse outcomes of pregnancy. *Clinics in Perinatology, 24*, 23–41.

Gorbach, P. M., Sopheab, H., Phalla, T., Leng, H. B., Mills, S., Bennett, A., & Holmes, K. K. Sexual bridging by Cambodian men: Potential importance for general population spread of STD/HIV epidemics. *Sexually Transmitted Diseases, 27*, 320–326.

Gorbach, P. M., Stoner, B. P., Aral, S. O., Whittington, W. L., Coronado, N., Connor, S., Handsfield, H. H., & Holmes, K. K. (1997). Sleeping around in Seattle: A qualitative assessment of sexual partnerships. Presented at The International Conference of Sexually Transmitted Disease Research, Seville Spain, October 19–21.

Green, S. B. (1997). The eating patterns study—the importance of practical randomized trials in communities. *American Journal of Public Health, 87*, 541–543.

Grey, R. H., Kingozi, G., Wabwira-Mangen, F., Serwadda, D. S., Li, C., Meehan, M., & Wawer, M. J. (1998). A randomized trial of STD control during pregnancy in Rakai, Uganda: Impact on maternal and infant health. 12th World AIDS Conference, Geneva, Switzerland, July 1998 [Abstract no 23276].

Grosskurth, H., Mosha, F., Todd, J., Mwijarubi, E., Klokke, A., Senkoro, K., Mayaud, P., Changalucha, J., Nicoll, A., & ka-Gina, G. (1995). Impact of improved treatment of sexually transmitted diseases on HIV infection in rural Tanzania: Randomised controlled trial. *Lancet, 346*, 530–536.

Gunn, R. A., Pdschun, G. D., Fitzgerald, S., Hovell, M. F., Farshy, C. E., Black, C. M., & Greenspan, J. R. (1998). Screening high-risk adolescent males for *Chlamydia trachomatis* infection. Obtaining urine specimens in the field. *Sexually Transmitted Diseases; 25*(1), 49–52.

Gupta, S., Anderson, R. M., & May, R. M. (1989). Networks of sexual contacts: Implications for the pattern of spread of HIV. *AIDS, 3*, 807–817.

Hamers, F. F., Peterman, T. A., Zaidi, A. A., Ransom, R. L., Wroten, J. E., & Witte, J. J. (1995). Syphilis and gonorrhea in Miami: Similar clustering, different trends. *American Journal of Public Health, 85*, 1104–1108.

Handsfield, H. H., Jasman, L. L., Roberts, P. L., Hanson, V. W., Kothenbeutel, R. L., & Stamm, W. E. (1986). Criteria for selective screening for *Chlamydia trachomatis* infection in women attending family planning clinics. *Journal of the American Medical Association, 255*, 1730–1734.

Hayes, R. J., Schulz, K. F., & Plummer, F. A. (1995). The cofactor effect of genital ulcers on the per-exposure risk of HIV transmission in sub-Saharan Africa. *Journal of Tropical Medicine & Hygiene, 98*, 1–8.

Ho, G. Y., Bierman, R., Beardsley, L., Chang, C. J., & Burk, R. D. (1998). Natural history of cervicovaginal papillomavirus infection in young women. *New England Journal of Medicine, 338*, 423–428.

Hofferth, S. L., Kahn, J. R., & Baldwin, W. (1987). Premarital sexual activity among U.S. teenage women over the past three decades. *Family Planning Perspectives, 19*, 46–53.

Janz, N. K., Zimmerman, M. A., Wren, P. A., Israel, B. A., Freudenburg, N., & Carter, R. J. (1996). Evaluation of 37 AIDS prevention projects: Successful approaches and barriers to program effectiveness. *Health Education Quarterly, 23*, 80–97.

Johnson, A. M., Wadsworth, J., Wellings, K., Bradshaw S., & Field, J. (1992). Sexual lifestyles and HIV risk. *Nature, 360*, 410–412.

Judson, F. N. (1981). Epidemiology of sexually transmitted hepatitis B infections in heterosexuals: A review. *Sexually Transmitted Diseases, 8(4 suppl)*, 336–343.

Kamb, M. L., Fishbein, M., Douglas, J. M. Jr., Rhodes, F., Rogers, J., Bolan, G., Zenilman, J., Hoxworth, T., Malotte, C. K., Iatesta, M., Kent, C., Lentz, A., Graziano, S., Byers, R. H., & Peterman, T. A. (1998). Efficacy of risk-reduction counseling to prevent human immunodeficiency virus and sexually transmitted diseases: A randomized controlled trial. Project RESPECT Study Group. *Journal of the American Medical Association, 280*, 1161–1167.

Kelly, J. A., Murphy, D. A., Sikkema, K. J., & Kalichman, S. C. (1993). Psychological interventions to prevent HIV infection are urgently needed: New priorities for behavioral research in the second decade of AIDS. *American Psychologist, 48*, 1023–1034.

Klausner, J. D., Delgado, V., Cahoon-Young, B., Morrow, S., McFarland, W., & Bolan, G. (1997). An update III. Knock-knock: Door-to-door population based survey of risk behavior and *Chlamydia trachomatis* prevalence in young women living in low income neighborhoods in the San Francisco Bay Area. 125th Meeting of the

American Public Health Association, November 9–13, Indianapolis, Indiana.

Klovdahl, A. S. (1985). Social networks and the spread of infectious diseases: The AIDS example. *Social Science & Medicine, 21*, 1203–1216.

Koutsky, L. A., & Kiviat, N. B. (1999). Genital human papillomarivurs. In K. K. Holmes, P. F. Sparling, P-A. Mårdh, S. M Lemon, W. E. Stamm, P. Piot, & J. N. Wasserheit (Eds.), *Sexually transmitted diseases*, 3rd ed. (pp. 347–359.). New York: McGraw-Hill.

Kreiss, J. K., Koech, D., Plummer, F. A., Holmes, K. K., Lightfoote, M., Piot, P., Ronald, A. R., Ndinya-Achola, J. O., D'Costa, L. J., & Roberts, P. (1986). AIDS virus infection in Nairobi prostitutes. Spread of the epidemic to East Africa. *New England Journal of Medicine, 314*, 414–418.

Laumann, E. O., & Youm, Y. (1999). Racial/ethnic group differences in the prevalence of STDs in the US: A network explanation. *Sexually Transmitted Diseases, 26*(5), 250–261.

Laumann, E. O., Gagnon, J. H., Michael, R. T., & Michaels, S. (1994). *The social organization of sexuality*. Chicago, University of Chicago Press.

Machekano, R., McFarland, W., Mzezewa, V., Ray S., Mbizvo, M., Bassett, M., Latif, A., Mason, P., Gwanzura, L., Moses, L., Ley, C., Brown, B., Parsonnet, J., & Katzenstein, D. (1997). A peer education intervention reduces HIV infection among factory workers in Zimbabwe. Abstract presented at the 5th Conference on Retroviruses and Opportunistic Infections, Chicago, Illinois, Feb. 1–5, 1997 [Abstract: Session 6, no. 15].

Marrazzo, J. M., White, C. L., Krekeler, B., Celum, C. L., Lafferty, W. E., Stamm, W. E., & Handsfield, H. H. (1997). Community-based urine screening for *Chlamydia trachomatis* with a ligase chain reaction assay. *Annals of Internal Medicine, 127*, 796–803.

Martin, D. H., Cohen, D., Farley, T. A., Kissinger, P., Nsuami, M., Rigol, J., Mroczkowski, T. (1998). Towards controlling *C. trachomatis* infections: Use of adolescent prevalence estimates for planning intervention strategies. In R. S. Stephens *et al.* (Eds.), Chlamydial infections: Proceedings of the Ninth International Symposium on Human Chlamydial Infection: Napa, CA, June 21–26.

McLeroy, K., Bibeau, D., Steckler, A., & Glanz, K. (1988). An ecological perspective on health promotion programs. *Health Education Quarterly, 15*, 351–377.

Michael, R. T., Wadsworth, J., Feinleib, J., Johnson, A. M., Laumann, E. O., & Wellings, K. (1998). Private sexual behavior, public opinion, and public health policy related to sexually transmitted diseases: A US-British comparison. *American Journal of Public Health, 88*, 749–754.

Millstein, S. G., & Moscicki, A. (1995). Sexually-transmitted disease in female adolescents: Effects of psychosocial factors and high risk behaviors. *Journal of Adolescent Health, 17*, 83–90.

Morris, M., & Kretzschmar, M. (1997). Concurrent partnerships and the spread of HIV. *AIDS, 11*, 641–648.

Morris, M., Podhisita, C., Wawer, M. J., & Handcock, M. S. (1996a). Bridge populations in the spread of HIV/AIDS in Thailand. *AIDS, 10*, 1265–1271.

Morris, M., Serwadda, D., Kretzschmar, M., Sewankambo, N., Wawer, M. (1996b). Concurrent partnerships and HIV transmission in Uganda. Abstract (#Tu.D.473) presented at the XI International Conference on AIDS, Vancouver, July 7–12, 1996.

Morse, S. A., Trees, D. L., Htun, Y., Radebe, F., Orle, K. A., Dangor, Y., Beck-Sague C. M., Schmid S., Fehler G., Weiss, J. B., & Ballard, R. C. (1997). Comparison of clinical diagnosis and standard laboratory and molecular methods for the diagnosis of genital ulcer disease in Lesotho: Association with human immunodeficiency virus infection. *Journal of Infectious Diseases, 175*, 583–589.

Moses, S., Bailey, R. C., & Ronald, A. R. (1998). Male circumcision: Assessment of health benefits and risks. *Sexually Transmitted Infections, 74*, 368–373.

National Center for Health Statistics (1997). *Vital and health statistics. Fertility, family planning, and women's health: New data from the 1995 national survey of family growth*. Series 23: data from the national survey of growth, no. 19. Hyattsville, MD.

NIMH Multisite HIV Prevention Trial: Reducing HIV sexual risk behavior (1998). The National Institute of Mental Health (NIMH) Multisite HIV Prevention Trial Group. *Science, 280*, 1889–1894.

NIMH Multisite HIV Prevention Trial (1997). *AIDS, 11*, Suppl 2, S1–63.

Orr, D. P., Langefeld, C. D., Katz, B. P., & Caine, V. A. (1996). Behavioral intervention to increase condom use among high-risk female adolescents. *Journal of Pediatrics, 128*, 288–295.

Plummer, F. A., Wainberg, M. A., Plourde, P., Jessamine, P., D'Costa, L. J., Wamola, I. A., & Ronald, A. R. (1990). Detection of human immunodeficiency virus type 1 (HIV-1) in genital ulcer exudate of HIV-1-infected men by culture and gene amplification. *Journal of Infectious Diseases, 161*, 810–811.

Purevdawa, E., Moon, T. D., Baigalmaa, C., Davaajav, K., Smith, M. L., & Vermund, S. H. (1997). Rise in sexually transmitted diseases during democratization and economic crisis in Mongolia. *International Journal of STD & AIDS, 8*, 398–401.

Research and Forecasts, Inc. (1987). *The Abbott report: STD's and sexual mores in the 1980's*. New York.

Rice, R. J., Roberts, P. L., Handsfield, H. H., & Holmes, K. K. (1991). Sociodemographic distribution of gonorrhea incidence: Implications for prevention and behavioral research. *American Journal of Public Health, 81*, 1252–1258.

Ryan, K. (1997). An RCT to measure the effect of nonoxynol-9 film use on cervical gonorrheal and chlamydial infections. Abstract presented at the 12th Meeting of the International Society for STD Research. Seville, Spain, October 19–22, 1997.

Sanchez, J., Gotuzzo, E., Escamilla, J., Carrillo, C., Phillips, I. A., Barrios, C., Stamm, W. E., Ashley, R. L., Kreiss, J. K., & Holmes, K. K. (1996). Gender differences in sexual practices and sexually transmitted infections among adults in Lima, Peru. *American Journal of Public Health*, 86, 1098–1107.

Schachter, J., Stoner, E., & Moncada, J. (1983). Screening for chlamydial infections in women attending family planning clinics. *Western Journal of Medicine*, 138, 375–379.

Scholes, D., Stergachis, A., Heidrich, F. E., Andrilla, H., Holmes K. K., & Stamm, W. E. (1996). Prevention of pelvic inflammatory disease by screening for cervical chlamydial infection. *New England Journal of Medicine*, 334, 1362–1366.

Sciarra, J. J. (1997). Sexually transmitted diseases: Global importance. *International Journal of Gynecology and Obstetrics*, 58, 107–119.

Shain, R. N., Piper, J. M., Newton, E. R., Perdue, S., Champion, J., Holden, A., Ramos, R., & Guerra, F. (1997). A controlled randomized trial of a risk-reduction intervention: Behaviors contributing to reduced rates at 12 months' follow-up. Abstract presented at the 12th Meeting of the International Society for STD Research. Seville, Spain, October 19–22, 1997.

Sikkema, K. J., Kelly, J. A., Winett, R. A., Solomon, L. J., Cargill, V. A., Roffman, R. A., McAuliffe, T. L., Heckman, T. G., Anderson, E. A., Wagstaff, D. A., Norman, A. D., Perry, M. J., Crumble, D. A., & Mercer, M. B. (2000). Outcomes of a randomized community-level HIV prevention intervention for women living in 18 low-income housing developments. *American Journal of Public Health*, 90, 57–63.

Singh, S., Wulf, D., Samara, R., & Cuca Y. P. (2000). Gender differences in the timing of first intercourse: Data from 14 countries. *International Family Planning Perspectives*, 26, 21–28 & 43.

Skjeldestad, F. E., Kendrick, J. S., Atrash, H. K. & Daltveit, A. K. (1997). Increasing incidence of ectopic pregnancy in one Norwegian county—a population based study, 1970–1993. *Acta Obstetrica et Gynecologica Scandinavica*, 76, 159–165.

Sonenstein, F. L., Ku, L., Lindberg, L. D., Turner, C. F., & Pleck, J. H. (1998). Changes in sexual behavior and condom use among teenaged males: 1988 to 1995. *American Journal of Public Health*, 88, 956–959.

Stoner, B. P., Whittington, W. L., Hughes, J. P., Aral, S. O., & Holmes, K. K. Comparative epidemiology of gonococcal and chlamydial network membership: Implications for transmission patterns (submitted)

Syrjanen, K., Vayrynen, M., Castren, O., Yliskoski, M., Mantyjarvi, R., Pyrhonen, S., & Saarikoski, S. (1984). Sexual behaviour of women with human papillomavirus (HPV) lesions of the uterine cervix. *British Journal of Venereal Diseases*, 60, 243–248.

Thomas, J. C., Kulik, A. L., & Schoenbach, V. J. (1995). Syphilis in the south: Rural rates surpass urban rates in North Carolina. *American Journal of Public Health*, 85, 1119–1121.

Tichonova, L., Borisenko, K., Ward, H., Meheus, A., Gromyko, A., & Renton, A. (1997). Epidemics of syphilis in the Russian Federation: Trends, origins, and priorities for control. *Lancet*, 350, 210–213.

Washington, A. E. (1986). In D. Oriel *et al.* (Eds.), *Incidence of* Chlamydia trachomatis *infections in the United States: Using reported* Neisseria gonorrhoeae *as surrogate, in Chlamydial infections* (p. 487). Cambridge, England: Cambridge University Press.

Wasserheit, J. N. (1989). The significance and scope of reproductive tract infections among Third World women. *International Journal of Gynecology and Obstetrics Suppl.* 3, 145–168.

Wasserheit, J. N., & Aral, S. O. (1996). The dynamic topology of sexually transmitted disease epidemics: Implications for prevention strategies. *Journal of Infectious Diseases*, 174, Suppl 2, S201–213.

Wasserheit, J. N., & Holmes, K. K. (1992). Reproductive tract infections: Challenges for international health policy, programs, and research. In A. Germain, K. K. Holmes, P. Piot, & J. N. Wasserheit (Eds.), *Reproductive tract infections* (pp. 7–33). New York: Plenum Press.

Wawer, M. J., Sewankambo, N. K., Serwadda, D., Quinn, T. C., Paxton, L. A., Kiwanuka, N., Wabwire-Mangen, F., Li, C., Lutalo, T., Nalugoda, F., Gaydos, C. A., Moulton, L. H., Meehan M. O., Ahmed, S., & Gray, R. H. (1999). Control of sexually transmitted diseases for AIDS prevention in Uganda: A randomised community trial. Rakai Project Study Group. *Lancet*, 353, 525–535.

Westrom, L., & Eschenbach, D. (1999). Pelvic inflammatory disease. In K. K. Holmes, P. F. Sparling, P-A. Mårdh, S. M Lemon, W. E Stamm, P. Piot, & J. N. Wasserheit (Eds.), *Sexually transmitted diseases*, 3rd ed. (pp. 801–802). New York: McGraw-Hill.

Zaidi, A. A., Roegner, R. L., Flock, M. L., & Levine, W. C. (1997). Socio-demographic factors associated with gonorrhea rates in the United States: An ecologic analysis. Abstract presented at the 12th Meeting of the International Society for STD Research. Seville, Spain, October 19–22.

15

HIV/AIDS

GINA M. WINGOOD and RALPH J. DICLEMENTE

INTRODUCTION

> Upon first meeting Janet, she just overflowed with energy. She had a smile that lit up a room and radiated warmth like the Summer sun. Her confidence was overwhelming. She was articulate, bright, and exuberant. She was proud to be the mother of three adolescent sons and a newborn. Janet spoke lovingly of her partner and showed everyone her new wedding band. At first glance, no one would know that Janet had been repeatedly abused as an adolescent, that she was a teen mother of twins, that she was a crack addict who was living with HIV, and that she had a son also living with HIV.
>
> Her sexual history revealed that she had never used condoms, even after she was diagnosed with HIV. Her recent marriage was preceded by a six-month courtship. Prior to this courtship Janet had sexual relations with many men. Janet mentioned that she had abstained from drugs during the past six months; however, she drank three to four times a week in quantities that would often result in intoxication. Emotionally, Janet was worn by the fact that her 18-year-old son had tried to kill someone and was sentenced to jail. Janet had also not disclosed her HIV serostatus to her partner.

While stories such as this are not atypical of women living with HIV, Janet's situation illustrates the need to examine HIV/AIDS among women not only as a biomedical phenomenon, but as important, to understand the social context of women's lives. Since the emergence of AIDS, one constant has been the disproportionate number of AIDS cases among disenfranchised women, including, those who are impoverished, drug-addicted, or are in relationships characterized by imbalances of power.

This chapter reviews the epidemiology of HIV among women, examine the psychosocial correlates of engaging in practices that increase women's vulnerability for HIV infection, and discuss interventions designed to reduce women's risk of HIV. Additionally, this chapter explores

GINA M. WINGOOD and RALPH J. DICLEMENTE • Department of Behavioral Sciences and Health Education, Rollins School of Public Health, Emory University, Atlanta, Georgia 30322.

Handbook of Women's Sexual and Reproductive Health, edited by Wingood and DiClemente. Kluwer Academic / Plenum Publishers, New York, 2002.

research examining secondary HIV prevention and health policy issues for women living with HIV.

EPIDEMIOLOGY

The acquired immunodeficiency syndrome (AIDS) was first described in 1981 among a cluster of gay and bisexual men in California (CDC, 1981a). Less well known is the fact that the first case of AIDS in a woman was also described later that year (CDC, 1981b). In the United States, AIDS, and its causal agent, human immunodeficiency virus (HIV), have occurred predominantly among gay men. However, in 1995, HIV/AIDS became the third leading cause of death among women 25 to 44 years of age, and the leading cause of death among African-American women, accounting for 22% of deaths in this age group (CDC, 1996). Further, time trend analysis suggests that nationally women have comprised an increasingly larger proportion of AIDS cases. For instance, women accounted for 7% of AIDS cases in 1986. Over time, however, women comprised a greater proportion of AIDS cases; 10% during 1988, 23.1% during 1995, and 24.2% in 2000 (CDC, 2000). While there has been a reported decrease in AIDS-related deaths by 23%, attributable in large part to the advent of more effective antiretroviral treatment (i.e., HAART) and a decrease in the incidence of AIDS cases for the first time in the United States since the beginning of the epidemic among men, AIDS cases have increased by 3% among women (CDC, 1997). As of June 2000, the CDC reported that nearly 124,911 women were living with AIDS and 36,814 women were living with HIV (CDC, 2000).

Unfortunately, this condition strikes many women during their young adult years. As of June 2000, 78% of women living with AIDS were 20–44 years of age (CDC, 2000). Given the long incubation time of HIV, a great number of new infections probably occur in women still in their teens or early twenties. Unfortunately, women tend to become infected with HIV at earlier ages than men. The percentage of cases attributed to heterosexual transmission for younger women was more than twice that for older women, and the greatest increases in AIDS incidence rates have been observed among very young women who were infected heterosexually (CDC, 2000).

Nationally, AIDS disproportionately affects ethnic minority women. As of June 2000, the proportion of women with AIDS who were African-American and Latina were 57.5% and 19.9%, respectively (CDC, 2000). Racial or ethnic disparity varies markedly by geographic area, and these rates largely reflect the disproportionate numbers of Black and Hispanic women with AIDS reported from the Northeast and Puerto Rico (CDC, 1998).

Among women diagnosed with AIDS in the United States, incidence rates are highest among African-American women, and those living in the Northeast and metropolitan areas. However, the group experiencing the greatest increase in incident AIDS cases between 1990 and 1995 occurred among women living in the South and in rural residences (Wortley & Fleming, 1997). High AIDS rates among ethnic minority women living in the South may be reflective of the fact that many of these women live in communities experiencing a confluence of situations that may enhance likelihood of exposure, including: extreme poverty, high rates of injection drug and crack cocaine use, high HIV seroprevalence rates among males, and nearly epidemic STD rates.

As of June 2000, the majority of AIDS cases among women, 39%, were attributed to heterosexual contact, whereas 27% were attributable to injection drug use (CDC, 2000). Heroin was once the injection drug of choice, but cocaine, amphetamines, and other drugs increasingly have been used intravenously and may be injected more frequently and involve more needle sharing than heroin (Chiasson et al., 1989). In 1994, heterosexual contact surpassed injection drug use as the predominant route of transmission to U.S. women with a diagnosis of AIDS (CDC, 1995b). When considering only women 20–24 years of age, 51%

of cases are attributed to heterosexual transmission, 12% were attributable to injection drug use, and 36% identified either no risk factor or a risk factor was not reported. Over the course of the epidemic, from 1983 to 1999, the proportion of AIDS cases among women attributed to heterosexual contact has increased substantially, from 15% to 40% (CDC, 2000). The findings suggest that AIDS cases attributable to heterosexual transmission are increasing faster than any other exposure category.

Rare modes of HIV transmission to women include female-to-female sexual transmission and artificial insemination. Most HIV infections among women who report sex with other women are related to other behavioral risk factors, such as injection drug use or having had sex with a man (Chu, Hammet, & Buehler, 1992). HIV infection by means of intravaginal insemination with donor sperm is rare (CDC, 1990). However, HIV screening of semen for artificial insemination is recommended but is not mandatory in the United States. While commercial sperm banks routinely screen semen for HIV, many physicians who perform inseminations do not require HIV testing for donors (CDC, 1994a).

BIOLOGICAL FACTORS INCREASING WOMEN'S SUSCEPTIBILITY TO HIV

Understanding the biological properties that increase women's susceptibility to HIV is pivotal. In their landmark study, Padian and colleagues discovered that as the receptive sexual partner in heterosexual intercourse women are at greater risk than men for HIV acquisition (Padian et al., 1987). The risk of acquiring HIV from a single act of intercourse is at least eight-fold greater from men to women than from women to men (Padian et al., 1987). Other female-specific biologic characteristics that may enhance the efficiency of heterosexual HIV transmission include having sex during menstruation, using oral contraceptives and having a cervical ectopy (Clementson, 1993). Further,

the type of sex that women have can increase their risk of HIV. Having unprotected anal receptive sex with an HIV-infected partner may be the most efficient way of acquiring infection sexually. In one study, women who had anal sex with their HIV-infected male partners were two to four times more likely to be infected than women reporting only vaginal sex (Peterman, Wasserheit, & Cates, 1992). Oral sex seems to be less risky than anal or vaginal sex, but few people report only oral sex (Downs & deVincenzi, 1996). Additionally, like HIV, many other STDs are more efficiently transmitted from men to women than from women to men. For example, the risk of a woman acquiring gonorrhea from a single act of intercourse may be as high as 60% to 90%; conversely, transmission from a woman to a man is markedly lower, about 20% to 30% (Judson, 1990). This is concerning as the presence of STDs further amplify the risk for transmission of HIV. While the factors influencing the efficiency of the sexual transmission of HIV have not been fully identified, it is clear that many biological cofactors increase women's susceptibility to HIV.

CORRELATES OF CONSISTENT CONDOM USE

The Significance of Consistent Condom Use

While epidemiological and biological data are informative with respect to quantifying the differential risk for STD/HIV infection, they provide less insight into the influence of pervasive cultural, gender-specific, and psychosocial factors that are the determinants of behavior (Wingood & DiClemente, 1992). Thus, reducing the risk of HIV infection among sexually active women requires the identification of factors associated with HIV-related sexual risk taking. A primary HIV prevention strategy for sexually active persons is to use condoms properly and consistently, that is during every episode of sexual intercourse.

Examining correlates of consistent condom use is important since findings from prospective studies indicate that condoms, when used consistently, can provide a 70% to 100% reduction in the risk of HIV transmission. In particular, findings from the European Study Group on Heterosexual Transmission of HIV observed no seroconversions among couples who used condom consistently while among inconsistent condom users the seroconversion rate was significantly higher, 4.8 per 100 person-years (deVincenzi, 1994). Moreover, predictions based on mathematical modeling suggest that, irrespective of the number of sexual partners and the prevalence of HIV among potential sex partners, consistent condom use can substantially reduce the risk of sexually transmitted HIV infection relative to never or half-time condom use (Fineberg, 1988). Thus, as empirical evidence supports the clinical and public health significance of consistent condom use for preventing HIV infection, future behavior change interventions should assess consistent condom use as a primary outcome measure for evaluating program efficacy. The next section will review studies that have examined correlates of consistent condom use among women.

Perceived Attitudes and Beliefs

One study conducted among a community-recruited sample of African-American women examined the correlates of consistent condom use over a three month period (Wingood & DiClemente, 1997). Compared to women who did not use condoms consistently, women who used condoms consistently were more than seven-and-a-half times more likely to perceive themselves as having high self-control over using condoms and more than six-and-a-half times more likely to perceive themselves as having greater control over their partner's use of condoms. Additionally, another study conducted among adolescent females recruited from a clinic noted that women who used condoms consistently were six-and-a-half times more likely to perceive that their partner preferred using condoms (Plichta et al., 1992).

Self-Efficacy

Self-efficacy is the level of confidence that individuals have in their ability to effect change in a specific practice (Bandura, 1994). Self-efficacy regarding sexual communication/negotiation is the confidence a women has in bargaining for safer sex in light of the social costs of such negotiations. While low sexual communication self-efficacy has been associated with HIV risk-taking (Catania et al., 1992), having high sexual communication self-efficacy has been associated with being a consistent condom user. A study conducted among young African-American women recruited from a community-based setting noted that compared to inconsistent condom users, consistent condom users were 13 times more likely to have high sexual assertiveness self-efficacy (Wingood & DiClemente, 1997). One may assume that communication self-efficacy may be a more important determinant for women than for men, because women must convince men to wear condoms. This assumption was supported in a recent study of STD clinic patients. In this study a significant self-efficacy by gender interaction was observed. Partialing the interaction indicated that self-efficacy was a significant predictor of condom use for women; however, it was not a significant predictor of condom use for men (LoConte, O'Leary, & Labouvie, 1997).

Partner-Related Factors

Partner characteristics and behavior patterns are essential in determining women's ability to protect themselves from HIV because male partners must agree to use condoms. Several partner-related variables appear to be associated with consistent condom use. Women who have older partners, who have partners that they perceive are less committed to the relationship (Wingood & DiClemente, 1997) and women who are in shorter relationships, less than 3 months in duration (Plichta et al., 1992), are more likely to use condoms consistently. This later study noted that having a briefer relationship is an important predictor of condom use even after when controlling for type of partner (main or casual), and the frequency of sexual intercourse. These findings suggest that women are more likely to use condoms early in a relationship with a new partner, but discontinue condom use when they perceive that their partners are committed to the relationship. Women may believe that requesting condom use during a committed relationship may be perceived by the partner as intimating that they are unfaithful and thus could threaten the stability of the relationship.

Pregnancy-Related Factors

The desire to become pregnant may be associated with not using condoms (Adler & Tschann, 1993). One study conducted among African-American women, for instance, observed that consistent condom users were eight-and-a-half times less likely to desire pregnancy (Wingood & DiClemente, 1997). This suggests that in HIV prevention programs for women, addressing the dual concepts of HIV prevention *and* pregnancy prevention may be an effective means of enhancing condom use. On the other hand, when a woman does decide to become pregnant, she must be counseled in ways to do so with relative safety, for example through joint HIV antibody testing with her partner.

CORRELATES OF HIV-RELATED SEXUAL RISK TAKING

Among women a high degree of individual compliance is necessary for condoms to be used consistently during sexual intercourse. For economically disadvantaged women, numerous behavioral, social, cultural, and gender-related factors may reduce their compliance with consistent condom use and, in doing so, elevate their risk of HIV exposure (Wingood & DiClemente, 1992). In addition to examining factors that protect women from acquiring HIV, such

as consistent condom use, it is also important to examine those factors that increase women's sexual risk of HIV. This means examining gender related factors that are strongly associated with HIV sexual risk taking such as noncondom use (never having used a condom) and having multiple sexual partners (having more than one sex partner). Understanding the social influences that shape sexual relationships for women is critical to the development and implementation of tailored and more efficacious programs designed to reinforce the adoption and maintenance of HIV preventive behaviors among women (Wingood & DiClemente, 1992). Next we will review the studies that have empirically examined the correlates of HIV-related sexual risk taking among women.

Sociodemographics

Socioeconomic status (SES) is an important correlate of behavior that affects health, access to health services, the risk of disease, the risk of an adverse outcome once disease occurs, and mortality (Adler & Tschann, 1993; Pappas et al., 1993). Socioeconomic factors exacerbating women's vulnerability to HIV are prevalent. Economic factors play an important role in enhancing women's risk of infection, as women having lower income levels (Peterson et al., 1992; Wingood & DiClemente, 1998) are less likely to use condoms. Additionally, African-American and Latina women are four- and three-and-a-half times less likely, respectively, to use condoms compared to White women (Catania et al., 1992). This may be a result of ethnic minority women having less access to optimal and quality preventive care, including STD clinics. Further, compared to White women disenfranchised ethnic minority women may have more immediate survival concerns, such as obtaining money for food and shelter, that may militate against the use of health-protective behaviors (Mays & Cochran, 1988).

A number of sociodemographic factors associated with having multiple sexual partners were reported in a nationally representative sample of 8450 women aged 15 to 44 (Seidman, Mosher & Aral, 1992). Women with multiple sex partners were almost seven times more likely to have experienced their initial intercourse when they were younger than 16 years of age, were nearly two-and-a-half times more likely to report living in an urban residence, and were twice as likely to report having no religious affiliation. Additionally, several studies have illustrated that marital status is associated with HIV risk taking, with unmarried women being more likely to have multiple sexual partners (Seidman, Mosher & Aral, 1992; Grinstead et al., 1993).

Perceived Beliefs and Attitudes

Beliefs associated with HIV-related sexual risk taking include believing that condoms have a negative impact on sexual enjoyment (Catania et al., 1992; Peterson et al., 1992), feeling that using condoms is embarrassing (Peterson et al., 1992), perceiving oneself to be at risk for HIV (Sikkema et al., 1995) (this result is probably due to the fact that using condoms lowers perceptions of risk), perceiving that your partner will think you are unfaithful if you ask them to use a condom (Wingood & DiClemente, 1998), and having a negative attitude toward sex (Harlow et al., 1993).

Low Self-Efficacy

As described above, partner characteristics and characteristics of a particular relationship figure prominently into women's efficacy judgments. A woman's decision to negotiate condom use is based on her perceptions of the costs and benefits to a particular relationship and the relationship's role in the woman's economic, social, and survival goals. Women's inability to negotiate condom use is one of the strongest correlates of never having used a condom (Wingood & DiClemente, 1998; Peterson et al., 1992; Catania et al., 1992; Harlow et al., 1993). A number of studies have reported that women with low levels of self-efficacy for using con-

doms (Peterson et al., 1992) and being able to avoid HIV (Harlow et al., 1993) are also more likely to engage in HIV related sexual risk taking.

Partners may be viewed in some cases as "barriers" to condom use, so that efficacy judgments are likely to vary depending on partner characteristics. For example, a woman might possess strong confidence in her ability to persuade her new, sensitive partner to use a condom, but lack confidence in her ability to do so with an abusive partner. This finding suggests that more accurate assessments of self-efficacy to negotiate and achieve condom use could be obtained by incorporating different levels of partner resistance (Forsyth & Carey, 1998).

Partner-Related Influences

At the core of partner-related influences exacerbating women's HIV risk are the power inequities that exist between the sexes. Power inequalities in heterosexual relationships are evident in social norms dictating monogamy for women and not for men, men having control over condom use, and violence directed toward women as well as the threats of such victimization. Several studies have demonstrated that monogamous women, women who have one sexual partner, and women who have a partner who is resistant toward using condoms (Wingood & DiClemente, 1998) are nearly four and three times, respectively, less likely to use condoms (Catania et al., 1992; Wingood & DiClemente, 1998). Another study found that women who were monogamous in their relationships perceived themselves to be at less risk, had lower intentions to use condoms, and used condoms less (St. Lawrence et al., 1998). Since most women who do become HIV-seropositive are infected by a primary partner this self-assessment of risk and its resulting behavior is, indeed, unfortunate (Carpenter et al., 1991; Marmor et al., 1990).

Other partner-related factors associated with HIV sexual risk taking include having a physically abusive partner (Wingood & DiClemente, 1997), having a sexually abusive partner (Kalichman *et al.*, 1998; Zierler & Krieger, 1997; Wingood & DiClemente, 1998) and fearing partner victimization (Harlow *et al.*, 1993; Kalichman *et al.*, 1998). Because condom requests from women may be attributed by some men to female infidelity, and in light of the fact that sexual jealousy is a well-documented trigger for violence, such fears may be realistic. A recent study of male inmates demonstrated that those with a history of severe domestic violence were likely to view hypothetical condom requests from a main partner more negatively than their nonviolent counterparts. This negative reaction was associated with lower likelihood of compliance with the request for condom use and greater likelihood of coercion (Neighbors, O'Leary, & Labouvie, 1999). The potential importance of this finding is underscored by the fact that in this sample, one highly relevant to HIV risk, 37% of respondents reported severe levels of violence on the Modified Conflict Tactics Scale.

Cultural Factors

Acculturation is the cultural learning and behavioral adaptation that takes place among individuals exposed to a new culture (Pavich, 1986). This concept has been repeatedly shown to modify the effect of many health factors among Latin populations (Marin, Gomez & Hearst, 1993). A telephone survey of 1592 Hispanic and 629 non-Hispanic White men and women aged 18–49 randomly selected from nine states in the northeastern and southwestern United States found that Hispanic women who were moderately or highly acculturated were more likely to have multiple sexual partners, 4.9 and 8.4 times, respectively, than were less acculturated women (Marin, Gomez & Hearst, 1993). Compared to less acculturated women, moderately or highly acculturated women, may be less likely to adhere to the traditional Latin culture that emphasizes the need for men to express their sexuality by having multiple sex partners and for women to

avoid such sexual expression (Pavich, 1986; Vasquez-Nuttal, Romero-Garcia, & DeLeon, 1987).

A cultural factor that has been shown to affect African-American women's risk of HIV is their perception of the sex-ratio imbalance. For African-American women who are considering marriage, there are fewer marriageable men, that is, males who are heterosexual, employed, and not incarcerated, than there are marriageable females. Given this sex-ratio imbalance, African-American women may be more likely to tolerate objectionable behavior whereas the male may feel less pressure to develop commitments and exert greater power within relationships (Gasch, Fullilove, & Fullilove, 1990; Wingood & DiClemente, 1995).

Alcohol and Crack Cocaine

There are several theories that attempt to explain the relationship between alcohol use and high-risk sexual behavior. One interpretation is that alcohol is a sexual disinhibitor that may place individuals at greater risk of becoming infected with STDs, including HIV, through unsafe sex. Another interpretation is that chronic alcohol use may serve as a marker for individuals who tend to practice a constellation of high-risk behaviors (Leigh & Stall, 1993). Both theories stress the effects of alcohol use as influencing high-risk sexual behaviors. One study reported that daily use of alcohol was associated with not using condoms (Wingood & DiClemente, 1998b), while moderate use of alcohol was associated with having multiple sexual partners (Wingood & DiClemente, 1998b; Sikkema, 1996).

Crack cocaine and the exchange of sex for drugs has emerged as major risk factors for HIV and HIV risk taking. Trading sex for drugs often involves having sex with multiple anonymous sex partners, thereby increasing a women's risk of HIV (DeHovitz *et al.*, 1994). Further, crack cocaine use is often associated with more frequent sex and less frequent condom use. Thus, the combination of more frequent sexual intercourse, low condom use, and more sex partners may enhance the risk of HIV infection.

Mental Health

Women, during the same years when they are at high risk of acquiring HIV infection, are also at high risk of being depressed. Prior research has demonstrated that among women, the period from 25 to 45 years of age is the time of the highest risk of depression (Weissman, 1987). One study reported that women between the age of 25 and 45 who reported depressive symptomatology as measured by the Center for Epidemiologic Studies–Depression scale, were more likely to engage in HIV risk taking (Orr et al., 1994).

Pregnancy-Related Factors

A study conducted among a clinic recruited sample of adolescent females noted that those who consistently used oral contraceptives were half as likely to use condoms compared with adolescents who did not consistently use oral contraceptives. This suggests that among this sample, condoms are being used as a method of birth control and not for disease prevention. In addition, another study noted that if one or both partners wished to conceive they were less likely to use condoms (Adler & Tschann, 1993). While it is important to stress the importance of condom use for both pregnancy and HIV prevention, the desire to become pregnant may undermine conscientious use of condoms.

Limited Access to Female Controlled Method

Unfortunately, the female condom represents the only female-controlled method that is effective against HIV. Although the first female condom was introduced in the 1920s, the female condom has only recently been approved for use in the United States and represents an important alternative to the male condom (CDC, 1993; IOM, 1996). The female condom

is an effective barrier to HIV (CDC, 1993). A multisite study observed a 2.5% unintended pregnancy rate and no STDs for U.S. women who used the female polyurethane condom consistently and correctly over a six-month period (Farr et al., 1994).

There are several major advantages of the female condom over the male condom. These advantages include: greater control by the woman, it can be inserted prior to sexual intercourse, it protects a greater area of the vagina, and the female condom is less likely to break compared to the male condom (Gollub, 1995). There are also several potential disadvantages to use of the female condom. These include its relative high cost (90 cents per condom), its appearance, and its initial acceptance by women (Gollub, 1995; Eldridge et al., 1995). Further, because it is detectable by the partner, negative attributions, such as female infidelity, are just as likely to occur as when use of a male condom is requested. The development of nondetectable methods of protection, such as topical microbicides, must remain a high research priority.

HIV PRIMARY PREVENTION PROGRAMS

There have been two published reports that have reviewed HIV risk-reduction interventions since the beginning of the AIDS epidemic for at-risk women. One study, published in 1997 by Exner et al., reviewed all interventions that were conducted in the United States, Canada and Puerto Rico (Exner, Seal & Ehrhardt, 1997). The other study, published in 1996 by Wingood & DiClemente, focused on randomized controlled HIV interventions that were conducted in the United States (Wingood & DiClemente, 1996). Both reviews suggest that the most efficacious HIV prevention programs for women were those that (a) are guided by social psychological theories; (b) only include women; (c) emphasize gender-related influences, such as, gender-based imbalances, and sexual assertiveness; (d) are peer led, and (e) require multiple sessions. Both reviews suggest that future research needs to address the environmental conditions impeding women's ability to protect themselves against HIV. Below we present several randomized controlled trials that have been effective at reducing women's risk of HIV. Several sexual risk reduction interventions for women are also described in the chapter by Drs. Aral and Gorbach on STDs.

Group-Based HIV Risk Reduction Interventions

A study conducted by Kelly and colleagues (1994) randomized inner-city women attending a primary care clinic to either a five-session intervention designed to enhance HIV awareness, condom use skills, sexual assertiveness skills, problem solving, risk-trigger management, and peer norms supportive of behavior change or an attention control focusing on other health promotion issues (Kelly *et al.*, 1994). Women were evaluated at baseline and at a three-month follow-up on risk behaviors. Results indicated that at three-months follow-up compared to the control condition, the HIV intervention was effective in significantly reducing the number of unprotected intercourse episodes (14.0 to 11.7, $p < .04$), increasing the percentage of occasions on which condoms were used (26% to 56%, $p < .001$), increasing postponement of sex until a condom was obtained (from 18.3% to 28.3%), and in refusing sex without a condom (21.2% to 26.6%). This study illustrates that women can respond effectively to intensive cognitive-behavioral skill-building interventions.

Another trial evaluated the efficacy of a community-based social skills HIV prevention intervention to enhance consistent condom use (DiClemente & Wingood, 1995). Women responded to recruitment materials and street outreach; those reporting the recent use of crack cocaine or injection drugs were excluded. Women were randomized to one of three conditions. Women randomized to the HIV education condition participated in a single session that provided HIV risk-reduction information. Women randomized to the delayed HIV education con-

trol condition received no HIV risk-reduction information until all follow-up interviews were completed. Women randomized to the peer-led social skills HIV intervention completed five 2-hour sessions that emphasized ethnic and gender pride, HIV risk-reduction information, sexual self-control, sexual assertiveness and communication skills, proper condom use skills, and developing partner norms supportive of consistent condom use. Women in the social skills intervention, compared to the delayed HIV education control condition, demonstrated increased consistent condom use (adjusted OR = 2.1, $p = .04$), greater sexual self-control (adjusted OR = 1.9, $p = .05$), greater sexual communication (adjusted OR = 4.1, $p = .002$), greater sexual assertiveness (adjusted OR = 1.8, $p = .05$), and increased partners' adoption of norms supporting consistent condom use (adjusted OR = 2.1, $p = .03$). No statistically significant differences in outcome variables were observed between the HIV education condition relative to the delayed HIV education control condition. This HIV prevention intervention was the first randomized trial to increase consistent condom use among women. This degree of intervention provides the greatest protection in preventing HIV transmission among sexually active individuals.

Eldridge, St. Lawrence, and colleagues conducted an HIV sexual risk-reduction study for women entering inpatient substance abuse treatment (Eldridge *et al.*, 1997). Known HIV-seropositive women were excluded from analysis. All patients in the facility received three hours of HIV education; this intervention comprised the control condition. Participants in the behavioral skills training (BST) condition received an additional four sessions that provided skill building for sexual negotiation and condom use. A randomized block design was used to avoid contamination between the treatment conditions. Self-administered questionnaires assessing risk behavior and a variety of possible intervention mediators were augmented by behavioral skills assessments at baseline, post-intervention and at a two-month follow-up. Retention at the follow-up assessment point was only 49%. However, among the remaining participants, women receiving BST exhibited significantly improved prevention attitudes and more positive expected partner reactions relative to control participants, evidenced as significant group-by-time interactions. In addition, BST participants exhibited improved skills for sexual communication and condom use. While there were no statistical differences between groups with respect to number of partners and number of drugs used, a significant treatment effect was obtained for proportion of intercourse acts during which a condom was used (increasing from 36% to 50%).

Carey and colleagues (1997) conducted a study targeting low-income women, but used a different intervention approach (Carey et al., 1997). This intervention provided, in addition to the types of skill building described in connection with many of the studies described above, a motivational enhancement component drawn from substance use intervention research. Women were randomized to receive this four-session intervention or to a wait-list control. Risk behavior and mediators were assessed at baseline, three weeks postintervention, and at a three-month follow-up. Results indicated that, compared with women in the control condition, those receiving the intervention reported increased risk sensitization, stronger intentions to practice safer sex, more communication with partners (at the three-week follow-up point only), and lower frequency of unprotected vaginal intercourse. This last effect was significant only at the three-week time point. The authors present effect size data, based on mediator as well as risk variables at the three-week assessment point, for their own study and for previous studies of women.

These data indicate the improved effectiveness of the intervention approach incorporating motivational enhancement. However, the efficacy of the intervention appears to be limited to a relatively brief follow-up period. As in many studies, there is the potential for treatment decay over time. Thus, one important area for further research is to develop and evaluate maintenance strategies designed to reduce long-term attenuation of treatment effects.

Couples HIV Interventions

Since transmission events are associated with sexual activity between individuals, targeting interventions tailored toward couples is an important option to reduce the couples' risk of HIV. Further, intervening with the couple forces us to examine the role that male partners can play in reducing women's risk of HIV infection. The limited research that has been conducted on the effectiveness of HIV primary prevention programs for heterosexual couples has observed substantial risk reduction as a result of counseling and testing programs involving serodiscordant couples, couples in which one partner is HIV-infected and the other is HIV-negative. Allen et al., counseled and followed 60 serodiscordant couples in Rwanda. All couples who participated in the intervention viewed an HIV/AIDS educational video, received free condoms and discussed the results of their HIV test results (Allen et al., 1992). HIV test results were distributed individually; however, the couples received their results together and discussed the implications of their test results with a counselor. At baseline 3% of couples reported using condoms and at 12-month follow-up 57% of couples reported using condoms. This study reported an HIV seroconversion rate of 4 per 100 man-years of follow-up and 9 per 100 women-years of follow-up. About 22 new infections would have occurred among serodiscordant couples based on rates among individuals who were not identified and not counseled as part of the study.

In another study, Padian et al. followed 144 serodiscordant couples in California (Padian et al., 1993). Of the index cases, 78% were men. Most male index cases were bisexuals, and most female index cases were infected through heterosexual intercourse with a previous sexual partner. The mean duration of the relationship for the couple at intake was 5.6 years. Couple counseling and risk assessments were conducted at average intervals of six months. Both condom use and sexual abstinence increased over time ($p < 0.001$ for both), and most behavior change occurred between intake and first follow-up visit. Among these couples, 32% reported being consistent condom users at entry into the study, and 75% reported being consistent condom users as much as nine years later. While this study had no control group, no new seroconversions were observed after 193 couple-years of follow-up. Couple counseling in combination with social support appears to be an effective means to promote and sustain behavior change among HIV-infected individuals and their heterosexual partners.

HIV Interventions Designed to Improve Access to STD Services

One example of an intervention designed to increase access to STD services and decrease HIV was conducted in the Mwanza region of Tanzania (Grosskurth et al., 1995). This landmark HIV prevention trial randomized communities to biomedical intervention and control conditions to assess the effect of the community level intervention. This intervention focused on (1) establishing an STD reference clinic, (2) training clinic staff in the diagnosis and treatment of STDs, (3) ensuring the continuous availability of medications to treat STDs, (4) conducting regularly scheduled visits to health facilities, and (5) providing health education about STD treatment. HIV incidence was compared in six intervention communities and six pair-matched comparison communities. A random cohort of 1000 adults, 15–54 years of age, from each community was surveyed at baseline and at follow-up two years later. This study observed a 42% reduction in HIV incidence as a result of the intervention. One of the largest impacts was seen in women aged 15–24. This study was the first randomized trial to demonstrate an impact of a preventive intervention on HIV incidence in a general population. The authors concluded that the availability of an aggressive STD screening and treatment intervention played an important part in reducing HIV transmission, particularly among women. While the findings are exciting, a subsequent trial was not able to demonstrate a significant reduction in HIV incidence (Wawer, Gray, Sewankambo, et al., 1998; Wawer, Sewankambo, Serwadda, et al., 1999). Thus, further research is needed to deter-

mine the implications of these disparate findings and the level of HIV prevention efficacy associated with aggressive community level STD case detection and treatment (Grosskurth, Gray, Hayes, Mabey, & Wawer, 2000).

SECONDARY SEQUELA IN WOMEN LIVING WITH HIV

Most of the research conducted on women has focused, to a large extent, on primary prevention of HIV. Fewer studies have addressed women living with HIV. Epidemiologic data indicate that women living with HIV are a growing population. However, women living with HIV remain an understudied and underserved population. The next few sections will discuss the lives of women who live with HIV.

As HIV infection is as much a social condition as it is a medical condition, living with HIV impacts a woman's physical, social, psychological and emotional aspects of living (Pergami et al., 1993). This may be particularly burdensome for those women whose lives are complicated by poverty, other chronic illnesses, discrimination, and unresponsive bureaucracies. These challenges are further compounded by the stigmatizing nature of HIV disease.

Stigma

Stigma is a mark or symbol perceived by segments of individuals within society, and connotes disgrace on those who bear the "mark." HIV seropositivity and AIDS represent markers for social stigma that invite prejudice and discrimination. Stigmatization in the case of AIDS is twofold, involving fears associated with the disease itself, and the disease's association with homosexuality and other similarly stigmatized and marginalized social groups (i.e., substance users) (Clatts & Mutchler, 1989).

The common perception of persons about people living with HIV evokes images of promiscuous and uncontrolled behavior. The disease is often defined in terms of political, religious, and moral boundaries that creates the backdrop for an "us" versus "them" mentality. One study reported that at least 20% of persons living with HIV and 43% of those with AIDS report direct experience with discrimination often resulting in feelings of social isolation and marginalization. Structural interventions are urgently needed to reduce stigmatization among individuals living with HIV (Bean *et al.*, 1989).

Women Living with HIV Are Exposed to Many Stressors

Several studies have examined the unique stressors that affect women living with HIV. Semple *et al.* (1993) identified the major stressors among Caucasian women living with HIV. The main HIV-related stressors were (1) being informed of their HIV serostatus (27.8%); (2) chronic financial strain (11.1%); (3) terminating an exclusive relationship as a result of learning their HIV serostatus (11.1%); (4) having a child develop behavioral problems subsequent to learning their serostatus (11.1%); (5) and death of a friend from AIDS (11.1%). Other studies report additional gender-specific stressors for women with HIV, such as (6) the caretaking responsibilities for an HIV-positive child; (7) the decision to continue or terminate a pregnancy; (8) the shame and stigma of having HIV; (9) the isolation of not knowing other women with HIV; (10) the lack of physicians' knowledgeable about the medical and gynecological conditions that are common among women with HIV; (11) and the lack of HIV support groups (Rehner, 1994; Selwyn *et al.*, 1989). These burdens are made worse by the absence of a supportive kin network to assist women in effectively coping with these stresses.

Women Living with HIV Residing in Rural Areas

While stressors are common among all women living with HIV, stressors such as stigma, secrecy and confidentiality may be more pronounced for women residing in non-urban areas (Roberts *et al.*, 1997; Mainous & Matheny, 1996). Prior to developing the WiLLOW program (discussed below) we conducted a series of qualitative interviews. One interview, typical of women's responses, was with a woman named Meg.

While the medical care provided by an urban HIV specialty clinic may be more comprehensive than the care provided in rural settings, it is not only the higher standard of care that motivates Meg's two hour journey to receive treatment at an urban center. Meg is fearful of the stigma associated with HIV—not only for herself but, more importantly, for her family; her children and grandchildren.

"They don't understand. No one would understand. They'd just condemn me and my family. One day we'd be part of the community, the next, we'd be social outcasts. It's not fair. But it's real."

Meg's assessment of the threat of stigmatization if local townspeople become aware of her condition probably is not much different from many other women with HIV living in rural areas. Meg's experiences as an HIV positive woman seeking medical care are consistent with the findings from a recent survey con-

---

Meg is a 40-year-old white widowed woman living with HIV residing in rural Alabama. Her HIV infection was diagnosed seven years ago following the death of her husband from AIDS. Meg has private medical insurance. While she and her children visit a family physician for their routine medical care in their hometown, the local physician is unaware of her HIV diagnosis. Once a month Meg drives two hours to see an infectious disease specialist in the urban medical center. She states, "I want to keep living there until my children are grown up." She further reports that she has no one with whom she can talk with about her disease. She is mildly depressed and nervous.

ducted among rural residents living with HIV in Kentucky (Roberts *et al.*, 1997). In this study, 74% of the residents went outside their county for HIV-related ambulatory care, with 64% of the respondents traveling to an urban area. The primary reasons for traveling to urban areas included concerns regarding confidentiality and beliefs that their physician was not knowledgeable about HIV.

Violence among Women Living with HIV

Women at highest risk for domestic violence are demographically similar to women living with HIV. Notably, the epidemiology of physical assault within personal relationships mirrors the epidemiology of HIV infection in women (Zierler & Krieger, 1997; Zierler, Witbeck, & Mayer, 1996). Overlapping risk factors include poverty, unemployment, drug dependency, childhood sexual and physical abuse, being younger than 30 years of age, and homelessness (Zierler & Krieger, 1997; Zierler, Witbeck, & Mayer, 1996; Brown, Melchior, & Huba, 1994; Fisher *et al.*, 1995). Violence and HIV also may be linked in other ways as well.

Partner notification, the practice of informing sex or needle-sharing partners that they have been exposed to HIV is recommended in many settings, whether done by HIV-infected persons themselves or by health care providers. Partner notification can give uninfected sexual partners an opportunity to reduce their exposure to HIV by practicing safer sex. However, the effectiveness of partner notification in preventing HIV infection is unknown. Further, several researchers have suggested that a diagnosis of HIV infection may trigger violence at the time of disclosure in significant relationships (North & Rothenberg, 1993; Rothenberg & Paskey, 1995). Zierler and colleagues examined the extent to which people in treatment for HIV infection experience their condition as a reason for violence within intimate relationships. In this study, 10.3% of the women reported that their HIV serostatus was a cause of harm, while 4.5% of men who had sex with men and 3.2% of heterosexual men reported that their HIV

serostatus was the cause of physical harm. These findings suggest that clinical settings providing HIV-related care may be an appropriate environment for routine assessment of violence. Programs to cross-train staff in antiviolence agencies and HIV clinical care facilities need to be developed for women and men living with HIV infection (Zierler *et al.*, 2000).

Limited Access to Clinical Trials

Historically, women have had less access to clinical trials than men (Cotton *et al.*, 1993). Several researchers have examined access to clinical trials among women living with HIV. These studies have shown that women living with HIV seem to be treated less aggressively than men living with HIV. Two studies have demonstrated that even after controlling for demographic factors, women living with HIV were less likely than men to be treated with zidovudine (Moore *et al.*, 1991; Stein *et al.*, 1991). Other studies have found that women, particularly ethnic minority women, are less likely than men to have received PCP prophylaxis (Moore *et al.*, 1994; Bastian *et al.*, 1993). Further, women living with HIV who are receiving services tend to receive fewer services than men living with HIV (Hellinger, 1993). These findings may be explained by several factors including women's ethnicity, exposure group and/or insurance status. These findings indicate a greater need to develop interventions that are designed to increase access to treatment and services for women living with HIV.

Pregnancy

Large longitudinal studies conducted among women living with HIV suggest that pregnancy is associated with some degree of immune compromise. Nevertheless, definitive conclusions about an association between pregnancy and HIV progression await further well-designed studies (DeHovitz, 1995).

While pregnancy may minimally affect the health of the HIV positive mother, pregnant women living with HIV can perinatally transmit the virus to their children. Many women first learn that they are HIV infected when they are tested during prenatal care (Wortley *et al.*, 1995). Unfortunately, women at greatest risk of HIV are those who receive limited or no prenatal care (Barbaccii *et al.*, 1990). Globally, rates of perinatal HIV transmission range from 14% to 40%, averaging about 29% in the United States. Factors that increase the risk of transmission include having a more advanced disease stage in the mother, higher levels of viral replication, and possibly having acquired primary HIV-1 infection during pregnancy (St. Louis *et al.*, 1993)

The Centers for Disease Control and Prevention recommends that given the safety and availability of current therapies for reducing perinatal transmission, clinicians should encourage all pregnant women to accept HIV counseling and testing (CDC, 1995a). These recommendations stem from the findings of a landmark study, the ACTG 076 study (CDC, 1994c). This phase III, randomized, double-blind, and placebo-controlled clinical trial was designed to evaluate the safety and efficacy of zidovudine (also known as AZT) administered to HIV-infected pregnant women and their infants in reducing the rate of mother-to-infant HIV transmission. Enrollment in this study was halted after interim analyses of 364 infants demonstrated a significant reduction in HIV infection in the group receiving AZT as compared with the placebo control group (8.3% vs. 25.5%, $p = .00006$). Further, no congenial anomalies were believed to be related to AZT administration (CDC, 1994b). Research in the area of perinatal transmission is now examining if ZDV or other therapies administered during labor and delivery can also reduce perinatal HIV transmission.

SECONDARY PREVENTION OF HIV

There are several compelling clinical and public health reasons to design a secondary prevention program for women living with HIV

aimed at building supportive social networks, increasing coping skills and reducing stress, risky sexual behaviors, and sexually transmitted diseases (STDs). First, an effective program could reduce the risk of disease progression among women living with HIV that may result from women's exposure to other strains of HIV or sexually transmitted diseases during unprotected sex. Second, an effective program could promote the quality of life among women living with HIV that may result from reducing stressors, enhancing coping skills and building stronger social networks. Third, an effective program could reduce risk of HIV transmission to seronegative sexual partners. Finally, an effective program could reduce risk of HIV transmission to their unborn children. Presently, there are very few psychosocial interventions designed to increase the quality of life or enhance coping for women living with HIV. In this section, we present a program entitled, *WiLLOW*, an acronym that stands for Women involved in Life Learning from Other Women (Wingood & DiClemente, 2000a).

WiLLOW is a randomized behavioral trial that has two primary aims (1) to enhance the quality of life and (2) to increase safer sex practices among women living with HIV. *WiLLOW* is grounded in a Social Support Networks framework as well as the Transactional Model of Stress and Coping. In the *WiLLOW* program, women participate in four 4-hour group sessions, administered on consecutive weeks, led by a health educator and HIV-positive peers.

In the first session, after providing an overview of the *WiLLOW* program, women engage in activities that are designed to foster women's gender pride, sense of self-worth, and self-esteem. This session also focuses on enhancing women's social support network, increasing the amount of practical, emotional, and information support needed, and preventing "burnout" among those individuals that currently provide support.

The second session emphasizes emotion-focused and problem-focused coping. Women are taught to use emotion-focused coping strategies to reduce stressor that are unchangeable or difficult to change. Emotion-focused strategies include stress management, relaxation techniques, releasing emotional tension through use of humor or participating in spiritual and religious activities, engaging in positive self-talk, and exercising. Women are also taught to use problem-focused coping strategies to reduce stressors that are modifiable. Problem-focused coping strategies include decision making, problem solving, and assertiveness training.

The third session focuses on sexual risk-reduction education. During this session, the health educator presents information to increase participants' knowledge of STD prevention strategies, educates women about the effect of STDs on a compromised immune system and the potential for perinatal transmission of STDs and HIV. Peer educators model proper condom use and provide corrective feedback to women role playing condom use demonstrations.

The fourth session addresses how sexuality occurs within the context of a larger social relationship. In this session women engage in an activity where they identify healthy and unhealthy characteristics of relationships. Unhealthy relationships are characterized as relationships in which many of these qualities are lacking. Subsequently, the health educator defines emotional abuse, physical and sexual abuse. Then participants discuss how being in an abusive relationship can make it difficult to receive support and practice safer sex. At the end of this session women again recite the poem *Phenomenal women* by Maya Angelou and receive Certificates of Empowerment for completing the program. This is a very powerful and moving session. Women exchange hugs, reinforce the need to stay in touch with one another, and begin solidifying their relationships with one another. Indeed, clinical staff have commented that they see marked changes in participant's attitudes, their sense of self, and their willingness to interact with each other. As one Nurse commented, "…before they would come into the waiting room and sit quietly in a corner. They wouldn't talk to anyone. They'd just sit there. Not reading anything, just sitting and mostly staring blankly into space. After they go

through *WiLLOW*, you can see them starting to talk with other women, carrying their head up high, asking questions about where to get one service or another and they are participating on advisory councils. It's as though they had come out of a cocoon."

In essence, *WiLLOW* fosters the development of friendships and social support networks among the group members and enhances pride in oneself. Of the 800 group sessions that could have been completed by these women (200 women attending four sessions) only seven sessions have been missed, yielding a participation rate of 99%.

The *WiLLOW* program has as its overarching goal the improvement in women's ability to build supportive social networks that may increase their coping skills and reduce risky sexual practices and, as a consequence, their risk for STDs. Building supportive social networks is viewed as creating a "family" for women living with HIV. Unfortunately, there are few secondary prevention programs for women living with HIV. Given the potential adverse health consequences associated with unprotected sexual intercourse among women living with HIV, both for the woman and her sex partner, such interventions could make a significant impact in reducing the spread of HIV as well as promoting the mental and social health of women living with HIV. Moreover, the integration of social support and sexual risk-reduction program efforts with clinical services may strengthen the social networks of women living with HIV.

HEALTH POLICY

Cost-of-illness measures provide a sense of the magnitude of the impact of an illness, as well as a point of reference for the consideration of program budgets and intervention priorities (Siegel, 1999). Estimates of the economic cost of illness have been developed for many of the major causes of morbidity and mortality in the United States (NIH, 1995). However, although the health burden imposed by HIV among women is considerable, little research has been devoted to quantifying the economic impact of this condition in the United States. This section discusses the economic burden of HIV among women nationally.

The economic burden of HIV is measured in terms of direct and indirect costs (Siegel, 1999). Direct costs refer to the expenditures for health care and represent the value of goods and services (i.e., physicians, health educators, transportation), the costs of laboratory services and pharmaceuticals, and the costs of hospitalization for HIV. Indirect costs refers to the loss of productivity, lost wages due to being unable to work, lost wages due to premature death, and the value of output forgone by individuals with HIV and HIV-related disability. In 1994, the annual cost of sexually transmitted HIV-related illness was estimated to be $6.7 billion, with slightly over $5 billion being direct costs (IOM, 1997).

The studies assessing indirect cost use gender-specific average wages to place a value on income lost attributable to HIV morbidity. Because HIV disproportionately affects people earning lower wages (ethnic minorities, younger people and the impoverished), it could be argued that a lower wage could be used to estimate lost income. However, it can also be argued that use of gender specific wages for women undervalues the economic burden created by HIV among women (Curran, 1980).

While the cost to women, their families and society, in general, is considerable, there are efforts underway to determine the cost effectiveness of prevention interventions for women. One researcher who has been in the forefront of examining cost-effectiveness of HIV prevention interventions for women is Dr. David Holtgrave. Holtgrave et al. conducted a retrospective economic evaluation (Holtgrave & Kelly, 1996) of a recent randomized controlled HIV risk reduction trial conducted by Sikkema and colleagues which was shown to increase women's condom use behaviors (Sikkema et al., 1996). The aim of the economic evaluation was to determine the intervention's cost per client, the cost per quality-adjusted life-year (QALY)

saved, and whether the intervention was cost effective (Holtgrave, 1996).

To determine the cost of providing the intervention on a per-client basis Holtgrave et al. identified the categories of resources consumed by the intervention (i.e., an hour of group facilitation time; an hour of transportation time for a client, materials cost per client per session). For each resource category, the team then estimated the number of units of the resource consumed and the dollar value of each unit of each resource category. This information provided the basic data with which to estimate the cost per client for the intervention. The total societal cost of the intervention was $269 per client for participating in the entire intervention or $26,914 for all study participants receiving the intervention.

Next the authors used the observed behavioral results from the randomized trial as input into a mathematical model of HIV transmission. The model that was used posited that the cumulative probability of HIV infection over a given time period is a function of six factors, including (1) the client's number of sexual partners, (2) number of sexual acts per partner, (3) the infectivity of each sexual act, (4) the level of condom use, (5) the effectiveness of condom use at reducing infectivity and (6) the HIV seroprevalence level among the network of one's sexual partners. This study also determined that the number of HIV infections averted by participating in the intervention was 0.38.

Finally, the authors estimated the cost per quality-adjusted life years (QALY) saved by participating in the intervention. The intervention cost was $2054 for each quality-adjusted life-year saved; this is favorable compared with other life-saving programs. Moreover, under most scenarios, this HIV prevention intervention was cost effective.

Local policy makers can benefit from economic evaluation of HIV prevention interventions. The economic evaluation of this program suggests that effective HIV prevention programs for women is a wise investment. However, a remaining question is how to fine-tune allocation of these resources across different female populations so as to maximize their prevention potential.

SUMMARY AND CONCLUSIONS

Perhaps the interventions with the greatest potential for HIV prevention are those aimed at changing the social and environmental processes that facilitate HIV transmission (Wingood & DiClemente, 2000b). Interventions at the superstructural level attempt to identify and change deep rooted and pervasive attitudes and structures in society that facilitate HIV transmission. Example of structures and attitudes at the societal level that increase women's risk include sexism and the lower value often attached to women and women's work (du Guerny & Sjoberg, 1993). Change strategies at the superstructural level include focusing on women's educational and vocational training to enhance women's economic independence, reducing stereotyped sexist images of women in the media, and promoting the development of more effective women-controlled barrier methods. Unfortunately, changing these societal level structures will not be radical nor swift. Nevertheless, without a comprehensive and coordinated national program that addresses the broader societal factors that support and reinforce women's risk exposures and behaviors, efforts to reduce women's HIV risk may not achieve their full potential.

REFERENCES

Adler, N. E., & Tschann, J. M. (1993). Conscious and preconscious motivation for pregnancy among female adolescents. In A. Lawson & D. L. Rhode (Eds.), *The politics of pregnancy: Adolescent sexuality and public policy* (pp. 144–158). New Haven, CT: Yale University Press.

Allen, S., Serufilira, A., Bogaerts, J., Varr de Perre, P., Nsengumuremyi, F., Lindan, C., Carael, M., Wolf, W., Coate, T., & Hulley, S. (1992). Confidential HIV testing and condom promotion in Africa: Impact on HIV and gonorrhea rates. *Journal of American Medical Association, 268*(23), 3338–3343.

Bandura, A. (1997). *Self-efficacy: The exercise of control.* New York: W. H. Freeman.

Bandura, A. (1994). Social cognitive theory and exercise of control over HIV infection. In R. J. DiClemente & J. Peterson (Eds.), *Preventing AIDS. Theories and methods of behavioral interventions* (pp. 25–59). New York: Plenum.

Barbacci, M. B., Dalabetta, G. A., Repke, J. T., Talbot, B. L., Charache, P., Polk, B. F., & Chaisson, R. E. (1990). Human immunodeficiency virus infection in women attending an inner-city prenatal clinic: Ineffectiveness of targeted screening. *Sexually Transmitted Diseases, 17,* 122–126.

Bastian, L., Bennett, C. L., Adams, J., Waskin, H., Divine, G., & Edlin, B. R. (1993). Differences between men and women with HIV-related *Pneumocystis carinii* pneumonia. *Journal of the Acquired Immune Deficiency Syndrome, 6,* 617–623.

Bean, J., Keller, L., Newbury, C., & Brown, M. (1989). Methods for the reduction of AIDS social anxiety and social stigma. *AIDS Education and Prevention, 1,* 194–221.

Brown, V. B., Melchior, C. R., & Huba, G. J. (1994). Mandatory partner notification of HIV test results: Psychological and social issues for women. *AIDS Public Policy Journal, 9,* 86–92.

Carey, M. P., Maisto, S. A., Kalichman, S. C., Forsyth, A. D., Wright, E. M., & Johnson, B. T. (1997). Enhancing motivation to reduce the risk of HIV infection for economically disadvantaged urban women. *Journal of Consulting and Clinical Psychology, 65,* 531–541.

Carpenter, C. J., Mayer, K. H., Stein, M. D., Leibman, B. D., Fisher, A., & Fiore, T. (1991). Human immunodeficiency virus infection in North American women: Experience with 200 cases and a review of the literature. *Medicine, 70,* 307–325.

Catania, J. A., Coates, T. J., Kegeles, S., Fullilove, M. T., Peterson, J., Marin, B., Siegel, D., & Hulley, S. (1992). Condom use in multi-ethnic neighborhoods of San Francisco: The population-based AMEN (AIDS in multi-ethnic neighborhoods) study. *American Journal of Public Health, 82,* 284–287.

Centers for Disease Control and Prevention (1981a). Pneumocystis pneumonia—Los Angeles. *Morbidity and Mortality Weekly Report, 30,* 250–252.

Centers for Disease Control and Prevention (1981b). Follow-up on Kaposi's sarcoma and pneumocystis pneumonia. *Morbidity and Mortality Weekly Report, 30,* 409–410.

Centers for Disease Control and Prevention (1990). HIV-infection and artificial insemination with processed semen. *Morbidity and Mortality Weekly Report, 39,* 249–256.

Centers for Disease Control and Prevention (1993). Barrier protection against HIV infection and other sexually transmitted diseases. *Morbidity and Mortality Weekly Report, 42,* 589–591, 597.

Centers for Disease Control and Prevention (1994a). Guidelines for preventing transmission of human immunodeficiency virus through transplantation of human tissue and organs. *Morbidity and Mortality Weekly Report*, *43*, 1–17.

Centers for Disease Control and Prevention (1994b). Birth outcomes following zidovudine therapy in pregnant women. *Morbidity and Mortality Weekly Report*, *43*, 409–416.

Centers for Disease Control and Prevention (1994c). Zidovudine for the prevention of HIV transmission from mother to infant. *Morbidity and Mortality Weekly Report*, *43*, 285–287.

Centers for Disease Control and Prevention (1995a). U.S. Public Health Service recommendations for human immunodeficiency virus counseling and voluntary testing for pregnant women. *Morbidity and Mortality Weekly Report*, *44*(RR-7), 1–12.

Centers for Disease Control and Prevention (1995b). Update: AIDS among women—United States, 1994. *Morbidity and Mortality Weekly Report*, *44*, 81–84.

Centers for Disease Control and Prevention (1996). Update: Mortality attributable to HIV infection among persons aged 25–44 years—United States, 1994. *Morbidity and Mortality Weekly Report*, *45*, 121–125.

Centers for Disease Control and Prevention (1997). Update: Trends in AIDS incidence, deaths, and prevalence— United States, 1996. *Morbidity and Mortality Weekly Report*, *46*, 165–173.

Centers for Disease Control and Prevention (1998). Midyear edition. *HIV/AIDS Surveillance Report*, *10*, 1–40.

Centers for Disease Control and Prevention (2000). Midyear-end edition. *HIV/AIDS Surveillance Report*, *12*, 1–40.

Chiasson, R. E., Bacchetti, P., Osmond, D., Brodie, B., Sande, M. A., Moss, A. R. (1989). Cocaine use and HIV infection intravenous drug users in San Francisco. *Journal of the American Medical Association*, *261*, 561–565.

Chu, S. Y., Hammet, T. A., & Buehler, J. W. (1992). Update: Epidemiology of reported cases of AIDS in women who report sex only with other women, United States, 1980–1991 (letter). *AIDS*, *6*, 518–519.

Clatts, M., & Mutchler, K. (1989). AIDS and the dangerous other: Metaphors of sex and deviance in the representation of disease. *Medical Anthropology*, *10*, 105–114.

Clemetson, D. B., Moss, G. B., Willerford, D. M., Hensel, M., Emonyi, W., Holmes, K. K., Plummer, F., Ndinya-Achola, J., Roberts, P. L., & Hillier, S. (1993). Detection of HIV DNA in cervical and vaginal secretions: Prevalence and correlates among women in Nairobi, Kenya. *Journal of the American Medical Association*, *269*, 2860–2864.

Cotton, D. J., Finkelstein, D. M., He, W., & Feinberg, J. (1993). Determinants of accrual of women to a large, multicenter clinical trials program of human immunodeficiency virus infection. *Journal of Acquired Immune Deficiency Syndrome*, *6*, 1322–1328.

Curran, J. W. (1980). Economic Consequences of pelvic inflammatory disease in the United States. *American Journal of Obstetrics and Gynecology*, *138*, 848–851.

DeHovitz, J. A. (1995). Natural history of HIV infection in women. In H. Minkoff, J. A. DeHovitz, & A. Duerr (Eds.), *HIV infection in women* (pp. 57–71). New York: Raven Press.

DeHovitz, J. A., Kelly, P., Feldman, J., Sierra, M., Clarke, L., Bromberg, J., Wan, J. Y., Vermund, S. H., & Landesman, S. (1994). Sexually transmitted diseases, sexual behavior, and cocaine use in inner-city women. *American Journal of Epidemiology*, *140*(12), 1125–1134.

deVincenzi, I. (1994). A longitudinal study of human immunodeficiency virus transmission by heterosexual partners. European Study Group on Heterosexual Transmission of HIV. *New England Journal of Medicine*, *331*, 341–346.

DiClemente, R. J., & Wingood, G. M. (1995). A randomized controlled trial of an HIV sexual risk reduction intervention for young adult African-American women. *Journal of the American Medical Association*, *274*, 1271–1276.

Downs, A. M., & deVincenzi, I. (1996). Probability of heterosexual transmission of HIV. *Journal of Acquired Immune Deficiency Syndrome and Human Retrovirology*, *11*, 388–395.

du Guerny, J., & Sjoberg, G. (1993). Inter-relationship between gender relations and the HIV/AIDS epidemic: Some possible considerations for policies and programmes. *AIDS*, *7*, 1027–1034.

Eldridge, G. D., St. Lawrence, J. S., Little, C. E., Shelby, M. C., Brasfield, T. L., Service, J. W., & Sly, K. (1997). Evaluation of an HIV risk reduction intervention for women entering inpatient substance abuse treatment. *AIDS Education and Prevention*, *9*(1 Suppl.), 62–76.

Elford, J. (1987). Moral and social aspects of AIDS: A medical students' project. *Social Science & Medicine*, *24*, 543–549.

Exner, T. M., Seal, D. W., & Ehrhardt, A. A. (1997). A review of HIV interventions for at-risk women. *AIDS and Behavior*, *1*, 93–124.

Farr, G., Gabelnick, H., Sturgen, K., & Dorflinger, L. (1994). Contraceptive efficacy and acceptability of the female condom. *American Journal of Public Health*, *84*, 1960–1964.

Fineberg, H. V. (1988). Education to prevent AIDS: Prospects and obstacles. *Science*, *239*, 592–596.

Fisher, B., Hovell, M., Hofstetter, C. R., & Hough, R. (1995). Risks associated with long-term homelessness among women: Battery, rape, and HIV infection. *International Journal of Health Services*, *25*, 351–369.

Forsyth, A. D., & Carey, M. P. (1998). Measuring self-efficacy in the context of HIV risk-reduction: Research challenges and recommendations. *Health Psychology*, *17*, 559–568.

Gasch, H., Fullilove, M. T., & Fullilove, R. E. (1990) "Can do" thinking may enable safer sex. *Multicultural Inquiry & Research on AIDS Quarterly Newsletter*, *4*, 5–6.

Gollub, E. L. (1995). Women-centered prevention techniques and technologies. In A. O'Leary & L. S. Jemmott (Eds.), *Women at risk: Issues in the primary prevention of AIDS* (pp. 43–82). New York: Plenum.

Grinstead, O. A., Faigeles, B., Binson, D., & Eversley, R. (1993). Sexual risk for human immunodeficiency virus infection among women in high-risk cities. *Family Planning Perspectives, 25,* 252–256.

Grosskurth, H., Mosha, F., Todd, J., Mwijarubi, E., Klokke, A., Senkoro, K., Mayaud, P., Changalucha, J., Nicoll, A., & ka-Gina, G. (1995). Impact of improved treatment of sexually transmitted diseases on HIV infection in rural Tanzania: Randomized controlled trial. *Lancet, 346,* 530–536.

Grosskurth, H., Gray, R., Hayes, R., Mabey, D., & Wawer, M. (2000). Control of sexually transmitted diseases for HIV-1 prevention: Understanding the implications of the Mwanza and Rakai trials. *Lancet, 355,* 1981–1987.

Harlow, L. L., Quina, K., Morokoff, P. J., Rose, J. S., & Grimley, D. M. (1993). HIV risk in women: A multi-faceted model. *Journal of Applied Biobehavioral Research, 1,* 3–38.

Hellinger, F. J. (1993). The use of health services by women with HIV infection. *Health Services Research, 28,* 544–561.

Holtgrave, D. R., & Kelly, J. A. (1996). Preventing HIV/AIDS among high-risk urban women: The cost-effectiveness of a behavioral group intervention. *American Journal of Public Health, 11,* 347–357.

IOM (Institute of Medicine) (1997). *The hidden epidemic: Confronting sexually transmitted diseases,* T. R. Eng *et al.* (Eds.). Washington DC: National Academy Press.

IOM (1996). *Contraceptive research and development: Looking to the future.* In P. F. Harrison, & A. Rosenfield (Eds.). Washington, DC: National Academy Press.

Judson, F. N. (1990). Gonorrhea. *Medical Clinics of North America, 74,* 1353–1367.

Kalichman, S. C., Williams, E. A., Cherry, C., Belcher, L., & Nachimson, D. (1998). Sexual coercion, domestic violence, and negotiating condom use among low-income African American women. *Journal of Women's Health, 7,* 371–378.

Kelly, J. A., Murphy, D. A., Washington, C. D., Wilson, T. S., Koob, J. J., Davis, D. R., Ledezma, G., & Davantes, B. (1994). The effects of HIV/AIDS intervention groups for high-risk women in urban clinics. *American Journal of Public Health, 84,* 1918–1922.

Leigh, B. C., & Stall, R. (1993). Substance use and risky sexual behavior for exposure to HIV: Issues in methodology, interpretation, and prevention. *American Psychologist, 48,* 1035–1045.

LoConte, J., O'Leary, A., & Labouvie, E. (1997). Psychosocial correlates of HIV-related sexual behavior in an inner-city STD clinic. *Psychology and Health, 12,* 589–601.

Mainous, A. G. III, & Matheny, S. C. (1996). Rural human immunodeficiency virus health service provision. Indications of rural-urban travel for care. *Archives of Family Medicine, 5,* 469–473.

Marin, B., Gomez, C. A., & Hearst, N. (1993). Multiple heterosexual partners and condom use among Hispanics and non-Hispanic Whites. *Family Planning Perspectives, 25,* 170–174.

Marmor, M., Krasinski, K., Sanchez, M., Cohen, H., Dubin, N., Weiss, L., Manning, A., Bebenroth, D., Saphier, N., & Harrison, C. (1990). Sex, drugs, and HIV infection in a New York City hospital outpatient population. *Journal of Acquired Immunodeficiency Syndromes, 3,* 307–318.

Mays, V. M., & Cochran, S. D. (1988). Issues in the perception of AIDS risk and risk reduction activities by Black and Hispanic/Latino women. *American Psychologist, 43,* 949–957.

Moore, R. D., Stanton, D., Gopalan, R., & Chaisson, R. E. (1994). Racial differences in the use of drug therapy for HIV disease in a urban community. *New England Journal of Medicine, 330,* 763–768.

Moore, R. D., Hidalgo, J., Sugland, B. W., & Chaisson R E. (1991). Zidovudine and the natural history of the acquired immunodeficiency syndrome. *New England Journal of Medicine, 324,* 1412–1416.

Neighbors, C. J., O'Leary, A., & Labouvie, E. (1999). Domestically violent and non-violent male inmates' evaluations and responses to their partner's requests for condom use: Testing a social-information processing model. *Health Psychology, 18,* 427–431.

NIH (National Institutes of Health) (1995). Public Health Service: Disease specific estimates of direct and indirect costs of illness and NIH support. November.

North, R. L., & Rothenberg, K. H. (1993). Partner notification and the threat of domestic violence against women with HIV infection. *New England Journal of Medicine, 329,* 1194–1196.

Orr, S. T., Celentano, D. D., Santelli, J., & Burwell, L. (1994). Depressive symptoms and risk factors for HIV acquisition among black women attending urban health centers in Baltimore. *AIDS Education and Prevention, 6,* 230–236.

Padian, N., Marquis, L., Francis, D. P., Anderson, A. E., Rutherford, G. W., O'Malley, P. M., & Winkelstein, W. Jr. (1987). Male-to-female transmission of human immunodeficiency virus. *Journal of the American Medical Association, 258,* 788–790.

Padian, N., O'Brien, T., Chang, Y., Glass, S., & Francis, D. (1993). Prevention of heterosexual transmission of human immunodeficiency virus through couple counseling. *Journal of Acquired Immune Deficiency Syndromes, 6,* 1043–1048.

Pappas, G., Queen, S., Hadden, W., & Fisher, G. (1993). The increasing disparity in mortality rates between socioeconomic groups in the United States, 1960 and 1986. *New England Journal of Medicine, 329,* 103–109.

Pavich, E. G. (1986). A Chicano perspective on Mexican culture and sexuality. *Journal of Social Work and Human Sexuality, 4,* 47–65.

Pergami, A., Gala, C., Burgess A., Durbano, F., Zanello, D.,

Riccio, M., Invernizzi, G., & Catalan, J. (1993). The psychosocial impact of HIV infection in women. *Journal of Psychosomatic Research, 37*, 687–696.

Peterman, T. A., Wasserheit, J. N., & Cates, W. (1992). Prevention of the sexual transmission of HIV. In V. T. DeVita, S. Hellman, & S. A. Rosenberg (Eds.), *AIDS etiology, diagnosis, treatment and prevention* (pp. 443–450). Philadelphia: Lippincott.

Peterson, J. L., Grinstead, O. A., Golden, E., Catania, J. A., Kegeles, S., & Coates, T. J. (1992). Correlates of HIV risk behaviors in Black and White San Francisco heterosexuals: The population-based AIDS in Multiethnic Neighborhoods (AMEN) study. *Ethnicity & Disease, 2*, 361–370.

Plichta, S. B., Weisman, C. S., Nathanson, C. A., Ensminger, M. E., & Robinson, J. C. (1992). Partner-specific condom use among adolescent women clients of a family planning clinic. *Journal of Adolescent Health, 13*, 506–511.

Rehner, T. A. (1994). Depression in Alabama women with HIV. Doctoral Dissertation at the School of Social Work in the Graduate School of the University of Alabama.

Roberts, N. E., Collmer, J. E., Wispelwey, B., & Farr, B. M. (1997). Urbs in rure redux: Changing risk factors for rural HIV infection. *American Journal of Medical Science, 314*, 3–10.

Rothenberg, K., & Paskey, S. J. (1995). The risk of domestic violence and women with HIV infection: Implications for partner notification, public policy, and the law. *American Journal of Public Health, 85*, 1569–1576.

Seidman, S., Mosher, W., & Aral, S. (1992). Women with multiple sexual partners: United States, 1988. *American Journal of Public Health, 82*, 1388–1394.

Selwyn, P. A., Carter, R. J., Schoenbaum E. E., Robertson, V. J., Klein, R. S., & Rogers, M. F. (1989). Knowledge of HIV antibody status and decisions to continue or terminate pregnancy among intravenous drug users. *Journal of the American Medical Association, 261*, 3567–3571.

Semple, S. J., Patterson, T. L., Temoshok, L. R., McCutchan, J. A., Straits-Troster, K. A., Chandler, J. L., & Grant, I. (1993). Identification of psychobiological stressors among HIV-positive women. *Women & Health, 20*, 15–36.

Siegel, J. B. (1999). The economic burden of sexually transmitted diseases in the United States. In K. K. Holmes, P. A. Mardha, S. M. Lemon, W. E. Stamm, P. Piot, & J. Wasserheit (Eds.), *Sexually transmitted diseases* (pp. 1367–1380). New York: McGraw-Hill.

Sikkema, K. J., Heckman, T. G., Kelly, J. A., Anderson, E. S., Winett, R. A., Solomon, L. J., Wagstaff, D. A., Roffman, R. A., Perry, M. J., Cargill, V., Crumble, D. A., Fuqua, R. W., Norman, A. D., & Mercer, M. B. (1996). HIV risk behaviors among women living in low-income, inner-city housing developments. *American Journal of Public Health, 86*, 1123–1128.

St. Lawrence, J. S., Eldridge, G. D., Reitman, D., Little, C. E., Shelby, M. C., & Brasfield, T. L. (1998). Factors influencing condom use among African American women: Implications for risk reduction interventions. *American Journal of Community Psychology, 26*, 7–28.

St. Louis, M. E., Kamenga, M., Brown, C., Nelson, A. M., Manzila, T., Batter, V., Behets, F., Kabagabo, U., Ryder, R. W., & Oxtoby, M. (1993). Risk for perinatal HIV-1 transmission according to maternal immunologic, virologic, and placental factors. *Journal of the American Medical Association, 269*, 2853–2859.

Stein, M. D., Piette, J., Mor, V., Wachtel, T. J., Fleishman, J., Mayer, K. H., & Carpenter, C. C. (1991). Difference in access to zidovudine (AZT) among symptomatic HIV-infected persons. *Journal of General Internal Medicine, 6*, 635–640.

Vasquez-Nuttal, E., Romero-Garcia, I., & DeLeon, B. (1987). Sex roles and perceptions of femininity and masculinity of Hispanic women. *Psychology of Women Quarterly, 11*, 409–425.

Wawer, M., Gray, R. H., Sewankambo, N. K., *et al.* (1998). A randomized community-based trial of intense sexually transmitted disease control for AIDS prevention, Rakai, Uganda. *AIDS, 12*, 1211–1225.

Wawer, M., Sewankambo, N. K., Serwadda, D., *et al.* (1999). Control of sexually transmitted diseases for AIDS prevention in Uganda: A randomized community trial. *Lancet, 353*, 525–535.

Weissman M. (1987). Advances in psychiatric epidemiology: Rates and risks for major depression. *American Journal of Public Health, 77*, 445–451.

Wingood, G. M., & DiClemente, R. J. (1997). Gender-related correlates and predictors of consistent condom use among African-American women: A prospective analysis. *International Journal of STD & AIDS, 8*, 1–7.

Wingood, G. M., & DiClemente, R. J. (1998b). The influence of psychosocial factors, alcohol, drug use on African-American women's high risk sexual behavior. *American Journal of Preventive Medicine, 15*, 54–60.

Wingood, G. M., & DiClemente, R. J. (1998). Partner influences and gender-related factors associated with noncondom use among young adult African-American women. *American Journal of Community Psychology, 26*, 29–53.

Wingood, G. M., & DiClemente, R. J. (1996). HIV sexual risk reduction interventions for women: A review. *American Journal of Preventive Medicine, 12*(3), 209–217.

Wingood, G. M., & DiClemente, R. J. (1995). Understanding the role of gender relations in HIV prevention research. *American Journal of Public Health, 85*, 592.

Wingood, G. M., & DiClemente, R. J. (2000a). The WiLLOW Project: Mobilizing social networks of women living with HIV to enhance coping and reduce sexual risk behavior. In W. Pequegnat, & J. Szapocznik (Eds.), *Working with Families in the Era of HIV/AIDS* (pp. 281–298). Newbury Park, CA: Sage.

Wingood, G. M., & DiClemente, R. J. (2000b). Applying a

theoretical framework of gender and power to understand the exposures and risk factors for HIV among women. *Health Education & Behavior, 27*, 539–565.

Wingood, G. M., & DiClemente, R. J. (1992). Cultural, gender and psychosocial influences on HIV-related behavior of African-American female adolescents: Implications for the development of tailored prevention programs. *Ethnicity and Disease, 2*, 381–388.

Wortley, P. M., & Fleming, P. L. (1997). AIDS in women in the United States. *Journal of the American Medical Association, 278*, 911–916.

Wortley, P. M., Chy, S. Y., Diaz, T., Ward, J. W., Doyle, B., Davidson, A. J., Checko, P. .J., Herr, M., Conti, L., & Fann, S. A. (1995). HIV testing patterns: Where, why, and when were persons with AIDS tested for HIV? *AIDS, 9*, 487–492.

Zierler, S., & Krieger, N. (1997). Reframing women's risk: Social inequalities and HIV infection. *Annual Review of Public Health, 18*, 401–436.

Zierler, S., Cunningham, W. E., Andersen, R., Shapiro, M. F., Bozzette, S. A., Nakazono, T., Morton, S., Crystal, S., Stein M., Turner, B., & St. Clair, P. (2000). Violence victimization after HIV infection in a US probability sample of adult patients in primary care. *American Journal of Public Health, 90*, 208–216.

Zierler, S., Witbeck, B., & Mayer, K. (1996). Sexual violence, women and HIV infection. *American Journal of Preventive Medicine, 12*, 304–310.

16

Sexual Dysfunction

NINA WILLIAMS and SANDRA L. LEIBLUM

INTRODUCTION

The end of the twentieth century bombards us with explicit sexuality as part of daily discourse. Art, journalism, the Internet, and movies routinely reveal the erotic exploits of both famous and infamous individuals. Cultural historians in the next century may be surprised to discover that actual comfort with sex and effortless performance tended to be rather rare, regardless, and perhaps because, of the public spectacle.

Both genders make ubiquitous sexual complaints, but women experience twice as many sexual problems as men. According to the most recent nationally based population survey of sexual habits, the National Health and Social Life Survey (Michael, Gagnon, Laumann, & Kalata, 1994), 43% of American women complained of some type of sexual problem. One out of every three women said they were uninterested in sex (compared to one out of six men), and 20% reported that sex provided little pleasure (compared to 10% of men). While this finding that so many women do not enjoy sex seems obviously troublesome, it is our first lesson into the cultural embeddedness of sexual

NINA WILLIAMS • Highland Park, NJ 08904. SANDRA L. LEIBLUM • Department of Psychiatry, Robert Wood Johnson University of Medicine and Dentistry, Piscataway, New Jersey 08855.

Handbook of Women's Sexual and Reproductive Health, edited by Wingood and DiClemente. Kluwer Academic / Plenum Publishers, New York, 2002.

"pathology." A century ago, spontaneous female sexual desire was considered a psychiatric disease.

In fact, defining sexual health and dysfunction in women is no easy matter. The process is so shaped by cultural values, political and religious agenda, and economic forces that the outcome is always temporary. Richgels (1992) argues "sexuality is as much a cultural product as diet, etiquette, or the means of production" (p. 125).

The rates of sexual dysfunction cited above are not unusual; similar figures are routinely obtained in surveys all over the world (Dunn, Croft, & Hackett, 1998). Nor is the gender difference easy to explain. The architecture of genitalia favor women. Compared to men's exposed apparatus, women's genitals are better protected and far more resilient. For most of a woman's life (the game changes after menopause), there are very few physiological sources of sexual trouble. Why is it, then, that so many women have difficulty expressing and enjoying their sexuality? Guilt and inhibition are certainly primary suspects. Female socialization presents many double binds about sex that women must disentangle. As the baby-boom generation enters middle age, the biological, medical and psychological risk factors associated with aging gain wider attention. Finally, women's sexuality appears powerfully influenced by the emotional state of the sexual bond. It is not easy to determine which came first, the bad sex or the bad relationship.

It is beyond the scope of this chapter to fully explore all of the factors underpinning our definitions and treatments of sexual dysfunctions in women. Our goal is to describe the state of our knowledge of this topic—so central to women's sense of health and well-being—at the end of the century. We begin by defining the terms currently used to describe sexual functioning and to review the scope of the problem. A review of cultural, psychological, behavioral, and medical factors related to sexual dysfunction and some case examples will be provided. The rapidly changing state of treatment for sexual disorders will be reviewed, as well as the status of research on this topic.

EPIDEMIOLOGY

Societal definitions of "normalcy," shifts in clinical practice, and relevant research combine to create and recreate a diagnostic classification system. As new expectations bloom and old beliefs fade away, old concepts (such as nymphomania) are discarded and new disorders are "identified." How deep these changes go is not always clear. Some authors argue that the "rhetoric of liberation" displayed in such public documents as sex manuals and videos conceals the unchanged imposition of external standards on women rather than granting them permission to explore their own sexuality (Altman, 1984). With the realization that the language used to describe disorders carries significant symbolic weight, the clinical nomenclature evolves but the underlying concepts may not. For instance, "frigidity" was the term commonly used for decades to describe a woman with diminished or absent sexual drive. Now the term has been rejected not only for lacking precise information but for being pejorative and disrespectful. Only recently, however, has the diagnosis of hypoactive sexual desire (the new term) required that the *woman* report considerable personal dissatisfaction with the state of her libido (rather than her partner's discontent alone).

The most recent edition of the *Diagnostic and Statistical Manual of Mental Disorders* (DSM-IV; American Psychiatric Association, 1994)

conceptualizes sexual disorders as "disturbances (rather than inhibitions) in the processes that characterize the sexual response cycle or by pain associated with sexual intercourse" (p. 493). The sexual disorders listed are (a) sexual desire disorders, namely hypoactive sexual desire or sexual aversion disorder; (b) sexual arousal disorders; (c) orgasmic disorders; and (d) sexual pain disorders. All disorders are further classified according to whether they are lifelong or acquired, generalized or situational, and due to psychological factors or combined factors. In DSM-IV, attention has been paid to the role of psychological distress and interpersonal difficulty in the definition of sexual dysfunction, although most of the criteria for diagnosis continue to be somewhat subjective and relatively arbitrary (Leiblum, 1998).

The Sexual Response Cycle

The model of sexual functioning used as the basis for the classification system of the DSM-IV is the triphasic process described by Kaplan (1974). Kaplan's model begins with the desire phase, by which is meant "the experience of specific sensations that motivate the individual to initiate or become responsive to sexual stimulation" (Rosen & Beck, 1988, p. 42). Desire is conceptualized as under central neurophysiological control. The second phase, arousal, refers to the vasocongestion of the genitals, leading to erection in men and to lubrication and swelling of the vaginal walls in women. In the final phase, orgasm, the pelvis produces pleasurable reflex muscle contractions. Sipski and Alexander (1998) note that Kaplan's model is criticized for several reasons; desire does not always precede arousal and orgasm, and the latter phases are described in simplistic terms, as if arousal and orgasm were merely reflex mechanisms. As the following variety of arousal and orgasmic dysfunctions show, this is not the case.

Hypoactive Sexual Desire Disorder (HSD)

Hypoactive sexual desire is the most common female sexual complaint. One large-scale recent study reported an incidence rate of 65%

(Rosen, Taylor, Leiblum, & Bachmann, 1993). Prevalence estimates range from 17% to 60% (Spector & Carey, 1990). The National Health and Social Life Survey (Michael, Gagnon, Laumann, & Kolata, 1994), completed by over 3400 men and women, reported that one out of three women complained of sexual disinterest during the previous year, compared to one out of six men. Women and men with HSD report significantly lower levels of sexual fantasy and lower frequency of intercourse.

Approximately 40% of women with primary HSD diagnosis also receive secondary diagnoses of arousal or orgasm disorders (Beck, 1995). Depression, dependency, anxiety, generalized symptom distress, and poor dyadic adjustment are common in individuals with HSD. Because the studies producing these findings have been correlational, however, no conclusions can be drawn about the direction of the effect.

Despite their frequency, desire disorders are difficult to diagnose and study. There are no reliable physical "markers" of sexual desire in women (a difficulty encountered repeatedly in this area of women's health). Researchers have attempted to define hypoactive desire operationally as the lower-than-average frequency of intercourse, but this is not a valid correlation. Women often engage in sexual encounters despite a lack of internal desire and fail to initiate sexual interactions when they do experience desire (Garde & Lunde, 1980). In 1998, an interdisciplinary conference was convened by the Sexual Health Council of the American Foundation of Urological Diseases to evaluate and revise the existing definition and classification of female sexual dysfunction based on available scientific information and current research and clinical data (Consensus Conference on Female Sexuality, 1998). The Consensus Conference noted that while the DSM-IV definition of HSD focuses on internal markers of desires (e.g., sexual fantasies and thoughts), as well as physical sensations, for women even the mental experience of desire may be reflected and reactive rather than spontaneous or initiatory. Finally, both men and women may decide to be asexual without receiving a diagnosis of HSD.

Sexual Aversion Disorder (SAD)

Sexual aversion disorder is defined in the DSM-IV as persistent and recurrent extreme aversion and avoidance of all or almost all genital contact with a partner. Sexual aversion disorder is distinguished from hypoactive desire disorder because the women who have SAD not only avoid sexual situations but respond to them with physical reactions of anxiety and/or disgust. One recent clinical example involved a woman who participated in intercourse, but vomited immediately after sex. Beyond specific avoidance of genital contact, there may be variations in what other behaviors may be avoided. Some women avert any genital contact, tolerating other types of sexual touch, while other women seem to generalize their genital aversion to behaviors that others might regard as only vaguely sexual (Anderson & Cyranowski, 1995). Several authors have argued that sexual aversion is a variant of panic disorder (Crenshaw, 1985; Kaplan, 1988).

Female Sexual Arousal Disorder (FSAD)

FSAD is the pervasive or recurrent inability to respond to sexual stimulation or to maintain an adequate lubrication-swelling response, coupled with marked distress or interpersonal difficulty. The disorder is not diagnosed if it is due exclusively to the direct physiological effects of a substance or medical condition (although as discussed later in this chapter such effects are increasingly common).

Michael et al. (1994) found that 19% of women aged 18–59 complained of recurrent lubrication difficulties. Lack of physical arousal was noted by approximately 14% of women in an outpatient gynecological clinic and the incidence of persistent or recurrent lubrication problems increased to 44% in postmenopausal women (Rosen, Taylor, Leiblum, & Bachmann, 1993).

Thus, complaints of difficulty becoming aroused sexually are common in women, although they are rarely diagnosed in isolation from hypoactive sexual desire or orgasmic disorder (DeAmicis, Goldberg, LoPiccolo, Friedman, & Davis, 1985). In practice, it is often difficult to distinguish sexual arousal disorders from sexual desire disorders. Women who do not become sexually excited and avoid sex altogether are likely to be diagnosed with hypoactive sexual desire. Women who do not become aroused and fail to reach orgasm are likely to receive the diagnosis of female orgasmic disorder (Leiblum, 1998).

Segraves and Segraves (1991) note that FSAD is rarely diagnosed in women who do not also have a desire or orgasmic dysfunction. These authors have suggested that FSAD may not in fact be a separate clinical entity. Determining the answer to this question is difficult. Despite the prevalence and potential impact of FSAD on other aspects of sexual function in women, few studies have been done of the pathophysiology or treatment of the disorder. While the definition of FSAD emphasizes physiological arousal, many women report arousal problems despite adequate physiological markers of arousal. Despite evidence that sexually functional women are easily able to gauge their level of genital arousal (and use it to gauge their level of desire), many women with arousal problems may be unaware of whether or not they are lubricating adequately (Beck, 1995). Unlike male arousal disorder, when the absence of an erection despite adequate stimulation is easily recognized by observers, a valid and reliable physical indicator of arousal in women has yet to be identified. Thus, despite the classification system's emphasis on physical signs, the woman's subjective identification of lack of arousal is crucial in making the diagnosis.

Female Orgasmic Disorder (FOD)

Anorgasmia is defined as the inability to achieve orgasm under some or all conditions of sexual stimulation. Michael et al. (1994) reported that about 30% of women reached orgasm only sometimes or less frequently and only 25% always achieved an orgasm during sex with their primary partner.

The type and intensity of stimulation needed to trigger orgasm in women varies widely. Consequently, the clinician must base the diagnosis on her or his judgment that the woman has had "adequate" stimulation, opening the diagnosis to varying expectations of what is reasonable for a particular woman given her age and sexual experience. The complaint must also cause marked distress or interpersonal difficulty.

Historically, high rates of orgasmic disorder have been reported in clinical and nonclinical samples. In recent years, many women have benefited from increased sexual permission and education regarding effective techniques for sexual self-arousal as well as encouragement to be more assertive when interacting with a partner (Hurlbert, Apt, & Rabehl, 1993).

Orgasmic dysfunction is either primary, secondary, or situational. A woman with primary orgasmic dysfunction has never been able to achieve orgasm under any conditions or stimulation, while a woman with secondary orgasmic dysfunction has been orgasmic in the past but is not now. Situational orgasmic dysfunction describes women who are able to have orgasms under some circumstances (e.g., during masturbation or with a particular partner) but unable to have orgasms under other circumstances. The most common instance of situational orgasmic disorder is when the woman is unable to experience orgasm during heterosexual intercourse.

With the lessening of cultural emphasis on the "vaginal orgasm" (that is, the orgasms experienced during intercourse), many women have found themselves quite easily orgasmic with manual, oral, or self-stimulation. There seems little doubt that women are readily orgasmic if not restricted by a negative sexual upbringing and unrealistic social expectations. Yet anywhere from 20–30% of women continue to have difficulty achieving orgasm, especially during intercourse, which has led many researchers and clinicians to wonder why situational anorgasmia warrant diagnosis as a sexual dysfunction at all (Hurlbert et al., 1993).

Although female orgasmic dysfunction does have an operational definition (the presence or absence of orgasm), the sources and varieties of female orgasm are not simple to classify. Whipple and Komisaruk (1999) describe many instances of women who "do not fit into the stereotypical pattern of sexual response described in the literature" (p. 34). These authors and others have described women who are able to climax in response to erotic imagery in the absence of any physical stimulation, who have complete spinal cord injury or complete excision of the clitoris in ritual female circumcision yet experience orgasm, and who achieve orgasm from vaginal stimulation alone. Hurlbert *et al.* (1993) argue that individual and relationship variables are better predictors of female sexual satisfaction than such variables as number of orgasms experienced. Their study indicated that what women enjoy most in an erotic exchange is foreplay, orgasm, sex, and afterplay; what women want more of, however, is foreplay, afterplay, sex, and orgasm.

Sexual Pain Disorders

Dyspareunia, or recurrent or persistent genital pain associated with sexual intercourse, is quite common in women, with incidence figures of between 10 and 15% (Leiblum, 1996a; Laumann, Paik, & Rosen, 1999). Vaginismus, the recurrent or persistent involuntary spasm of the musculature of the outer third part of the vagina, which interferes with sexual intercourse, is reported by 12–17% of women who present to sex therapy clinics (Rosen & Leiblum, 1995). These conditions often coexist; both cause anxiety, sexual avoidance, complaints of pain upon penetration, and lack of lubrication. Dyspareunia and vaginismus are particularly frequent sexual complaints among perimenopausal and postmenopausal women. The Female Consensus Conference (1998) proposed a new diagnostic category—noncoital sexual pain disorder—defined as recurrent or persistent genital pain induced by noncoital sexual stimulation. The incidence of this complaint remains unknown.

As in so many female sexual dysfunctions, the patient's subjective complaints of pain and the physician's physical findings do not always correspond. Medical conditions or organic factors may be present, although not easily diagnosed. Conditioned anxiety, involuntary muscle contractions, problems with sexual excitement, vaginal lubrication, and lack of desire can all contribute to muscular tightness and reports of pain. Both dyspareunia and vaginismus can be specifically conditioned to the sexual situation involving a specific partner and not be apparent during a physical examination. Thus, while medical evaluation is an important part of the standard diagnostic practice of sexual dysfunction, the absence of medical findings does not invalidate the clinical diagnosis.

Binik and his colleagues have argued that dyspareunia should be viewed as a pain disorder rather than a sexual dysfunction. Reissing, Binik, & Khalife (1999) note that most clinicians regard dyspareunia as ascribable either to a particular physical pathology or, if a discernible physical cause is undetectable, as a reflection of psychosexual conflict. They suggest that this model is both inaccurate and disrespectful to the patient. They suggest dyspareunia should be assessed and treated like any other pain disorder (e.g., lower-back pain). The important issue is the central phenomenon of the problem, namely the pain rather than its location. Using a pain model, one would carefully evaluate the pain complaint and assess the degree of interference with everyday life, including sexual relations. One would also anticipate that a single intervention, whether medical or psychological, would be unlikely to resolve the problem (Leiblum, 1999).

Limitations of the Current Classification System

The classification of sexual disorders in the DSM-IV presents several significant problems. First, there is an attempt, following Masters and Johnson's (1970) depiction of human sexual inadequacy, to create parallels between male and female sexual disorders. While this works for some disorders, it is untenable for others. For example, as mentioned above, male erectile disorder is fairly obvious to diagnose while the corresponding disorder, female arousal difficulty, is much more difficult to confirm, not only by the woman, but often by her partners as well. Second, the lack of objective, explicit operational criteria for diagnosing several disorders and the significant level of comorbidity among sexual dysfunctions lead to poor reliability and validity of the various diagnostic categories. The DSM-IV diagnostic system describes a smooth linear progression of sexual behavior, from desire to arousal to orgasm. While this is occasionally the case, often it is not.

Finally, deriving accurate epidemiological statistics is extremely difficult when researching human sexual activities. Despite the wide availability of more information about sexuality than ever before, women vary enormously in their openness to recognizing, reporting, and seeking treatment for these problems.

While maintaining the current DSM-IV classification schema based on the sexual response cycle, The Consensus Conference recommended several significant changes (1998), Among them was the decision to make the woman's *personal* distress an integral aspect of diagnosis, rather than relying only on physiological response or interpersonal distress.

Even with the proposed revised classification, however, problems remain. First, the unwarranted assumption remains that the sexual response cycle unfolds in linear, independent phases and that each may be diagnosed independently of the others. As noted, there is a high degree of overlap between disorders; most disorders tend to co-occur and to occur on a continuum of severity (Leiblum, 1998). The assumption of processes in women parallel to those observed in men has not been challenged. Objective, operational definitions of female sexual disorders do not exist and diagnosis will tend to be rather imprecise and global until research specific to women's sexuality (rather than generalization from male research to women) establishes a more useful body of knowledge about feminine desire, arousal, and orgasm (Leiblum, 1999).

The recognition and legitimization of personal distress as an essential ingredient of diagnosis is very important because it acknowledges and validates the subjective nature of sexual problems. However, there is no agreement about the degree of distress needed to warrant a diagnosis or even what constitutes a sexual complaint and what constitutes a dysfunction. Nonetheless, there is little doubt that both male and female sexual difficulties detract from emotional and relationship satisfaction and diminish quality of life (Laumann *et al.*, 1999).

Finally, although hypoactive sexual desire disorder and female orgasmic disorder are the most common diagnoses given, the major complaints clinicians hear from women about their sexual lives center on their dissatisfaction with such nongenital behaviors as affection, communication, and nongenital touching as well as issues of attraction and passion. These factors should be assessed as well as genital response for greater validity in evaluating female sexual disorders in both research and clinical practice.

PSYCHOSOCIAL AND BEHAVIORAL CORRELATES RELATED TO FEMALE SEXUAL DYSFUNCTION

Sexual behavior is a function of both biological and psychosocial influences and risk factors from both of these domains are implicated in the etiology and maintenance of sexual problems. Sexual disorders in most women are caused or maintained by psychological rather than physical factors. The exceptions—postmenopausal, elder, and chronically medical ill women—are discussed at length in the section following on biomedical factors. Yet, however, a disorder begins, sexual problems ultimately affect the body, the behavior, the individual psychology, and the interpersonal dynamics of a relationship for every woman who is affected. Even a woman in her sixties with hormonally based lubrication problems discovers that her sense of her body's health and integrity is altered, which can lead to depression, avoidance of sexual encounters, and misunderstanding with her lover. The psychosocial and behavioral factors that most commonly affect sexual functioning are discussed below.

Developmental Factors

Most women are reared in families and cultures that have, at best, ambivalent feelings about female sexual expression. The contradiction between the beliefs that men are more interested in sex than women and that women's sexuality is so volatile that it must be carefully controlled by men has not been reconciled. Thus, women are often taught to regard their genitals as shameful, their sexual feelings as sinful, their exploration of their bodies as dirty, and their premarital sexual activity as damaging their worth and reputation. Religious and cultural taboos on masturbation, dating, or sex education leave many women ignorant about even the most basic facts of female anatomy. Such factors are often implicated in the etiology of hypoactive sexual desire, sexual aversion, and vaginismus.

Traumatic Events

Abundant research documents that sexual abuse is a significant risk factor for desire and arousal disorders in women, especially when the abuse occurs before puberty (Sarwer & Durlak, 1996; Kinzl, Traweger, & Biebl, 1995). A history of abuse often contributes to dyspareunia and vaginismus but this history is by no means universally present. Sexual aversion is generally associated with a past history of sexual or gynecological trauma. Trauma includes not only childhood sexual abuse, but physical abuse, violent defloration, rape, and sexual assault (Golding, Wilsnack, & Learman, 1998). Women who have experienced medical, particularly gynecological, trauma may also report intrusive thoughts, sensations, and emotions during sexual encounters. For example, a client who was subjected to repeated bladder catheterizations during early childhood experienced panic attacks and vaginismus during routine gynecological exams because the sounds and sights of a doctor's office triggered flashbacks.

Emotional Problems and Stress

Both men and women who experience emotional or stress-related problems are more likely to be found in all categories of sexual dysfunction (Laumann et al., 1999). For example, a drop in household income of greater than 20% is associated with a reduction in both desire and arousal.

Depression has long been known to diminish sexual desire. In one of the earliest studies looking at the influence of hormones on sexual desires, Schreiner-Engel and Schiavi (1986) found that an early history of depression was associated with hypoactive sexual desire, especially in women. More recently, Beck (1995) reported that anger and anxiety both reduced desire in women, with anger showing a more marked effect. Eating disorders also diminish sexual interest and pleasure, particularly in anorexic women (de Silva, 1993). Many clinicians believe sexual aversion disorder might best be viewed as a phobia and removed from the sexual desire category. Moreover, the effect of many psychiatric medications on desire and orgasmic delay has been well documented (Segraves, 1988).

Relationship Status

Interestingly, the association between being married and having orgasms during sex with a partner is very strong; married women reported always or usually having orgasms more often than women who were never married and not cohabiting at the time of the interview (Michael et al., 1994). That orgasmic consistency is so strongly related to being in a committed relationship is particularly striking because it exceeds the influences of such factors as education, religion, or ethnicity (Michael et al., 1994; Heiman & Grafton-Becker, 1989).

When a relationship is conflicted, however, the ways in which the conflict can affect the sexual partnership are endless: resentment and antagonism toward one's sexual partner, sexual clumsiness and inconsideration, inadequate foreplay and time for arousal, personal upsets and anxieties that prevent concentration on sensual exchange, struggles for power and control, and "negative fantasies" that focus on the unattractive aspects of one's partner are a few of the most common (Leiblum & Rosen, 1989; Pietropinto, 1988). A study showing that women became less interested in sex when they were angry concluded that this was a gender difference; women were more likely than men to want to terminate the encounter under these conditions (Beck, 1995). Another gender difference of note is that while in men, performance anxiety has been implicated in arousal difficulties, anxiety not only does not inhibit arousal in women but may even increase it in comparison with a neutral alternative (Beggs, Calhoun, & Wolchik, 1987).

Ease with Sexuality

Trudel, Ravart, and Matte (1993) found that, compared to people with HSDD, those who reported a satisfactory level of desire wanted, initiated, and had partnered sex more often, masturbated more frequently, and felt more positive emotions and greater satisfaction during sex. Another author suggested that "sexually functional clients appear to have little difficulty describing their sexual desire," relying on the frequency of genital arousal, sexual daydreams, and partnered sex to gauge their level of desire (Beck, 1995, p. 191).

Clearly, sexual desire includes emotional, cognitive and motivational factors; just as clearly, the woman who is at ease in noticing her body's responses and accepting sexual feelings will be better able to function sexually. Because women with HSDD typically have sexual problems in arousal and orgasm as well, and female sexual assertiveness and pleasure in sexual thoughts are powerful indicators of sexual satisfaction, the most powerful aphrodisiac for women may be giving them permission to understand and explore their desire (Trudel *et al.*, 1993; Hurlbert *et al.*, 1993). Researchers attempting to identify the component parts of sexual aversion noted that sexual fears and sexual self-consciousness and self-criticism appear

to be the most relevant cognitive factors (Katz, Gipson, Kearl, & Kriskivich, 1989; Katz, Gipson, & Turner, 1992). Correlational analyses indicated higher self-reported levels of sex drive are linked with more frequent sexual fantasies, particularly in women (Anderson & Cyranowski, 1995).

Social Constructions of Female Sexuality

Feminist theorists note that women's freedom to experience their sexuality freely remains constrained by the meanings such behavior has in our culture. Richgels (1992) writes that "women gain access to class through their sexual behavior and breaking the sexual rules of a culture can at once declass them.... Because one of the most important functions of sexual behavior for women has been to maintain their class status and economic survival, the desire for sexual expression in a freely chosen union has been a luxury many women still cannot afford" (p. 130). Even well-educated, financially secure, heterosexual women must listen to high school students refer to classmates as "sluts" or "frigid;" read about a powerful public figure devalued for using her sexuality to succeed or for being cold or unattractive if she has not, or witness the oppression of lesbian and bisexual women. No woman experiences this without feeling psychologically restrained in the expression of her own body's and heart's wishes.

Thus, free sexual expression for women symbolizes not only the positive expressions of pleasure, desire, love, and play but her placement within a valued or devalued class, her shameful urges, and her physical vulnerability. This paradox is a critical difference in how sexuality is experienced by men and women (Richgels, 1992).

Freed of the assumption that women's definitions of sexual normalcy are a corollary of men's definitions, how does one's perspective on sexual dysfunction begin to shift? Might desire flee its expectation of consistency and instead ebb and flow with the menstrual cycle, pregnancy, lactation, and menopause? Would women continue to regard their heterosexual partner's achievement of erection as essential to a successful sexual encounter? More than one elder woman, her husband newly rejuvenated by sildenafil citrate (Viagra), has complained that she misses the slower, gentler pace of sex based on kisses and caresses. Would coital orgasms remain the elusive golden ring of "great" sex or would sexual exploration extend to the clitoris and other erotically charged parts of the body? Both feminist and more empirical researchers agree that in a woman-centered sexuality, the quality of relatedness between lovers would become integrated with their bond in other aspects of their lives, not split off as if it could develop in a separate domain.

BIOMEDICAL FACTORS RELATED TO FEMALE SEXUAL DYSFUNCTION

Gender and Age

Because women have nearly twice as many sexual problems as men, gender seems to be a risk factor for sexual dysfunction. Although gender is a biological fact, its relation to sexual dysfunction is not clear. As we have seen, gender does seem to be a culturally mediated variable, and its connection to sexual dysfunction may be related to differences in how men and women are socialized. Research into this question has not yet been done (Eisenberg, 1999). Age is a risk factor in that most sexual difficulties are progressive and because hormonal changes after menopause reduce vaginal elasticity and lubrication, and thin vaginal tissue. Aging is particularly related to sexual arousal and sexual pain disorders in women (Warnock, Bundren, & Morris, 1997). Other factors related to reduced sexual functioning as women age include increased occurrence of physical illness and pain, the use of medications that affect libido, and the loss of their male partners to death (Renshaw, 1996).

A recent survey into the sexual habits of older Americans found that half the women aged 45–59 had intercourse at least once a week. In the 60–74 age range, the figure dropped to 24%, and among women 75 and older to 7% (although more than one fourth of the women over 75 who still had a partner reported having intercourse once a week). Nonetheless, two thirds of those over 45 were satisfied with their sex lives, and both genders endorsed having a good relationship as more important to their quality of life than having a satisfying sexual relationship (Toner, 1999).

Endocrine Function

Circulating levels of androgens affect sexual function in both genders. A relationship exists between sexual behaviors and the menstrual cycle but the nature of the relationship to sexual desire and the specific hormonal events underlying changes in behavior is unclear.

For women, it is primarily at menopause, when there is a marked drop in estrogen production that complaints of dyspareunia appear. While some women are not affected by changes in genital tissues and reduced lubrication, particularly if they have maintained a regular pattern of sexual exchange, many peri- and postmenopausal women report increased sexual discomfort, leading to avoidance or aversion.

Whether a woman proceeds through a natural menopause or through one induced by a hysterectomy (a surgery one out of three women has had by the age of 60), the lost production of androgens may affect sexual desire as well; one study found that 36% of women over 75 "would be quite happy never having sex again" in contrast to 5% of men in that age group (Toner, 1999).

While the loss of estrogen is clearly implicated in vaginal atrophy and lubrication inadequacy, it is testosterone that is primarily responsible for libido in both men and women. Androgen replacement increases the level of sexual activity in hypogonadal men and there is increasing evidence that testosterone therapy increases both libido and erotic sensitivity in women as well (Sherwin & Gelfand, 1985). Testosterone deficiency in women is associated with a variety of complaints, including diminished or absent sexual interest; reduced clitoral, vaginal, and nipple sensitivity; milder orgasms; and diminished vitality and energy (Rako, 1999).

These authors argue that a woman's libido may be compromised when she goes on a regimen of estrogen replacement since estrogen has the effect of stimulating the production of SHBG (sex hormone binding globulin), which binds up whatever available testosterone a woman may be producing in her ovaries and adrenal glands. This is more of a problem for hysterectomized women than for naturally menopausal women, although it can contribute to reduced sexual interest and sensation for both groups of women. Some studies have found that postmenopausal women treated with estradiol (synthetic estrogen) and testosterone implants showed greater improvements in sexuality than women who received estradiol alone (Sherwin & Gelfand, 1985; Warnock, Bundren, & Morris, 1997).

Wallen and Lovejoy (1993) emphasize that even hormonal effects on sexual behavior—seemingly the most biological of influences—respond strongly to social context and are not strict regulators of sexual behavior. Thus, under some social circumstances hormone levels will predict accurately the occurrence of sexual behavior; in others, the same hormonal conditions will be unrelated to the occurrence of sexual activity. In fact, endocrine researchers argued 60 years ago that what distinguished human adaptation from that of other primates was the ability to engage in sexual activity *without* hormonal influence, allowing sexual activity to be used in other than reproductive contexts.

A number of researchers have found in studies comparing age-matched women with and without HSDD that there are no notable differences in any endocrine function, including levels of testosterone, estradiol, progesterone, and prolactin. This finding suggests that while physical aspects of sexual function, such as vaginal lubrication, are affected by hormones given to peri- and postmenopausal women, the exact relationship between sexual desire and hormones is unclear (Beck, 1995; Wallen &

Lovejoy, 1993; Galyer, Conaglen, Hare, & Conaglen, 1999).

Harding (1998) writes that "scientific" explanations for sexual desire in women are not static but have changed over the centuries, oddly in step with the social values of a given time. In the eighteenth century, for instance, the idea that men and women were structurally different was used to prove that the pattern of male–female social relations was natural and inevitable. At the dawn of industrialization in the nineteenth century, these biological differences were used to devalue women's supposedly closer connection to nature and to glorify men's connection to civilization. In the late twentieth century, hormones are used to justify a perception that women lack control over their bodies and emotions.

General Health

Whether acute or chronic, illness creates a number of physical and emotional effects that reduce interest in, capacity for, and pleasure from sexual exchange and account for the significant increase in sexual pain among chronically ill women. One reason is the experience of illness itself, with pain, anxiety, physical restriction, alterations in appearance, mood changes, fatigue, and uncertainty all playing a part. Treatments for the illness can be physically frightening, painful, or intrusive and require medication, surgeries, and hospitalizations. Women report that life events such as threats to employment or money worries, and the responses of spouse, children, and extended family had major impact on their sexual feelings during illnesses. When an illness becomes chronic or the outcome of treatment is not clear, both physical and psychological effects can become overwhelming.

Some illnesses have specific impact on sexual functioning because of the features of the disease or condition itself. A history of urinary tract symptoms increases the odds ratio of experiencing both arousal and sexual pain disorders by sevenfold (Laumann *et al.*, 1999). A past history of a sexually transmitted disease also increases the chances of low desire in women (although interestingly it does not appear to increase the risk of sexual dysfunction in men). Goldstein and Berman (1998) suggest that difficulties with vaginal engorgement due to abnormal circulation in the vagina or clitoris during sexual stimulation may be due to atherosclerotic vascular disease. While the terms used by researchers into this hypothesis ("vaginal engorgement insufficiency" and "clitoral erectile insufficiency") may be off-putting in their attempt to create a parallel female version of male erectile disorder, it is reasonable to consider the impact of vascular factors as a contributing element in the etiology of FSAD and FOD.

Recently, focal vulvitis or vulvar vestibulitis has received much attention as a cause of female dyspareunia. In fact, unlike most of the female sexual disorders, there are a host of physical conditions that are prevalent in the genesis of dyspareunia and must be carefully ruled out before a psychogenic diagnosis is made (Park *et al.*, 1997). Physically significant etiological factors include hymeneal scarring, pelvic inflammatory disease, and various vulvar conditions (Rosen & Leiblum, 1995). Dyspareunia is often secondary to vaginismus or chronic lack of lubrication (Steege & Ling, 1993). Although the DSM-IV criteria for dyspareunia specifies that the disturbance not be caused exclusively by vaginismus or lack of lubrication, Meana and Binik (1994) challenge that position, arguing that deficiency in lubrication is usually associated with such psychological concomitants as fear.

The impact of gynecological surgery on female sexuality has been reported to result in outcomes ranging from positive, through no change, to negative. Few studies have specified which aspects of the sexual response cycle were investigated. A recent study compared women who had hysterectomies and those who had other abdominal surgery for changes in sexual desire (Galyer *et al.*, 1999). While sickness and fatigue were reported as affecting sexual desire, no respondent indicated that her hysterectomy or other surgery had altered her desire. Interestingly, no significant differences in androgen

levels were found, in contrast to previous studies.

Chronic nongynecological disorders that affect sexual functioning include spinal cord injury (psychogenic lubrication absent, orgasm inhibited in about half the women affected). Half of the women with multiple sclerosis experience sexual dysfunction at some point in their disease; because the emotional and physical effects of MS are intertwined and can affect sexuality alone or in concert, the etiology of these effects is not clear. Victims of a stroke report decreased libido, arousal, and orgasm. Women with breast, ovarian, and cervical cancer report higher rates of dyspareunia. The effects of traumatic brain injury, neuromuscular disorders, diabetes, cardiac and pulmonary disease are well known in men but have not yet been studied in women (Sipski & Alexander, 1998). Table 1 summarizes medication conditions that affect sexual functioning.

Medication

A wide variety of medications are associated with sexual dysfunction. A partial list of these medications and their effects is shown in Table 2. Prescription medications for hypertension, psychiatric illness, cancer, glaucoma, and birth control and over-the-counter medications for such symptoms as hay fever, pain, and indigestion can affect sexual functioning.

The largest medication-related impact on sexual functioning in recent years has been the antidepressants known as selective serotonin retook inhibitors; some researchers report that 70% of people who take SSRIs may develop sexual dysfunction (McGahuey, Delgado, & Gelenberg, 1999). One reason this high figure has emerged now, nearly a decade after the first SSRIs were released, is that physicians were not asking patients about sexual effects of these medications and patients, used to lowered libido because of their depressions, did not recognize this as a medication-related side effect. The most common effect of SSRIs is absent or delayed orgasm, although desire and arousal difficulties have also been reported. The effects are

TABLE 1. Medical Conditions Affecting Women's Sexual Functioning

Medical condition	Effect
Diabetes	Lowered desire, dyspareunia from vaginal dryness and irritation, decreased genital sensitivity
Heart and lung diseases	Anxiety about the possibility of exacerbating condition can interfere with desire, arousal and orgasm (also true when partner is patient)
Autoimmune diseases	(75–90% affect women)
Lupus	Diminished desire, diminished lubrication, dyspareunia, depression
Arthritis	Painful intercourse
Scleroderma	Scarring of genitals leads to dyspareunia
Sjogrens	Dyspareunia, lack of lubrication
Thyroid disease	Can lead to androgen inadequacy, lowered desire
Multiple sclerosis	Blocks genital enervation, diminished arousal and orgasm
Epilepsy	Arousal problems, dyspareunia, vaginismus
Spinal cord injuries	Desire remains intact, women with total SCI as high as T7 can experience orgasm through fantasy and sexual contact
Pelvic prolapse	Dyspareunia
Sexually transmitted diseases	Fear of contracting can cause loss of desire; STDs can cause dyspareunia
Chemotherapy	Deprivation of estrogen inhibits arousal and can lead to dyspareunia
Radiation therapy	Deprivation of testosterone inhibits desire, fantasy, arousal, and orgasm
Oopherectomy	Deprevation of estrogen and testosterone
Hysterectomy	Nerve damage, possibility of shortened vagina but studies differ; loss of desire may be psychological or pain related
Breast surgery	Effects limited to chemo- or radiation therapy
Vulvodynia	Dyspareunia
Yeast infection	Dyspareunia
Endometriosis	Dyspareunia
Pelvic adhesions	Dyspareunia
Uterine fibroids	Dyspareunia
Ovarian cysts	Dyspareunia
Retroverted (tipped) uterus	Dyspareunia

Note: Reichman (1998); Sipski & Alexander (1998).

related to the dosage and develop gradually (Rosen, Lane, & Menza, 1999a; Labbate, Grimes, Hines, Oleshansky, & Ariana, 1998).

Pregnancy and Breast-Feeding

The advent of oral contraceptives ushered in a period of great sexual expectations among both men and women. The fear of unwanted pregnancy tends to dampen desire, and efforts to prevent conception through such "natural" means as the rhythm method or withdrawal divorced sexual opportunities from sexual interest, or interrupted the building of sexual pleasure for many. Although couples who are actively seeking to conceive a child often report the endeavor provides a boost in desire, arousal, and orgasm, the situation tends to change during pregnancy. Between 60% and 85% of women report nausea during the first trimester, and a third of these women miss work because of its severity (Gawande, 1999). Fatigue, a common feature of pregnancy in the first and third trimesters, may reduce sexual desire. During the second trimester, as the nausea and the exhaustion recede, couples often enjoy a renaissance of pleasure. Interestingly, perhaps because the vascular supply to the pelvis is dramatically increased during pregnancy, some women report increased arousal and orgasmic capacity. During the third trimester, interest may wane as the woman's body becomes unwieldy (and

TABLE 2. Medications Affecting Women's Sexual Functioning

Medication	Effect
Monophasic birth control pills	Lowered desire
Depo-Provera	Lowered desire
Hormone replacement therapy	Lowered desire
Antihormones	
Lupron	Lowered desire
Synarel	Lowered desire
Danazol	Raised/lowered desire
Antidepressants	Lowered desire, arousal, delayed, or inhibited orgasm
All except Remeron, Welbutrin, Serzone	
Antipsychotics	Lowered desire, inhibited arousal, and orgasm
Tranquilizers	Lowered desire, inhibited arousal, and orgasm
Especially Clonazepam	
Mood stabilizers	
Lithium	Possibly lowered desire and arousal
Tegretol	Possibly lowered desire
Blood pressure medications	
Diuretics	Diminished arousal
Spironolactone	Lowered desire and arousal
Inderal, Lopressor, and Tenormin	Inhibited arousal
Digoxin	Lowered desire and arousal
Clonidin, Methyldopa, Quanthedine, and Reserpine	Lowered desire
Antacids	All shown to be capable of causing lowered desired, arousal
Antibiotics	problems, inhibited orgasm, or diminished genital sen-
Anticholesterol	sation
Antiepileptics	
Antifungals	
Antihistamines	
Anti-inflammatories	
Cancer chemotherapy	
Drugs to treat glaucoma	

Note: Physicians' Desk Reference (2001), Bancroft (1980), Gitlin (1994), Medical Letter on Drugs & Therapeutics (1992), Reichman (1998).

may be seen by the woman or her partner as less desirable), fatigue mounts, and the couple (or their physician) worries about precipitating early labor through female orgasm.

The postpartum period is the time of greatest risk for mood disorder in women, perhaps because of the tumultuous shift in hormonal balance following childbirth. Depression and anxiety have global effects on sexual functioning. Sexual pain may occur on resumption of intercourse, particularly if the woman has received an episiotomy. Strikingly, childbirth does not cure vaginismus; vaginismic women who have had vaginal births are not likely to see a remission in their symptoms when they attempt to resume intercourse.

Some breast-feeding women report a loss in sexual desire and arousal. This may be due to the transformation of the breast from a primarily sexual organ to the nourisher of a baby, which leads some women to refrain from including breast stimulation during sexual activity while lactating. Regardless of feeding method, however, mothers of small children are less likely to have the time, energy, or privacy needed to pursue a fully satisfying sexual relationship.

Infertility and Its Treatment

Sex for procreation can become mechanical and unpleasurable when a couple experiences infertility. When months of unsuccessful attempts become years of frustration and disappointment, it is not surprising that couples begin to lose sexual desire and avoid physical intimacy. Couple intimacy suffers if interventions are not taken to correct the situation.

In some respects, infertility is similar in its effects on sexual health to other chronic medical disorders, such as multiple sclerosis or autoimmune diseases, that disturb a sense of well-being. Feelings of depression, inadequacy, anxiety, and low self-esteem are common concomitants of infertility. Although not life-threatening in any way, infertility challenges a sense of bodily integrity, self-concept, emotional stability, future plans, and the fulfillment of social roles (Daniluk, 1998; Leiblum, 1996). However, unlike other medical stressors, infertility is often associated with feelings of shame and guilt, which add to its burden. Moreover, infertility typically occurs in the context of a couple relationship and, consequently, both partners are usually profoundly affected by the diagnosis, treatment, and interventions associated with the infertility experience.

Although infertility is indisputably stressful for both genders, the reasons for the stress appear to differ for men and women (Andrews, Abbey, & Halman, 1992). For men, the dynamics of feelings about infertility appear similar to stress reactions associated with other life problems, such as financial or vocational problems. For women, however, fertility problems appear to constitute a unique stressor in that there are stronger and more deleterious effects on sexual self-esteem, sexual dissatisfaction, and a sense of self-efficacy. In couples in which one partner is fertile and the other is not, shame, self-blame, and guilt may be so great that the individual diagnosed with infertility feels unworthy of his partner's love and commitment. Some couples urge their mates to seek other relationships or believe their union should be dissolved.

The fertile partner may feel angry, antagonistic, or resentful, and these feelings may be expressed either directly, by way of furious accusation, or indirectly, by emotional or physical withdrawal. While it may seem obvious that the infertility workup and the extended nature of infertility treatment might reduce sexual satisfaction and function, the research evidence is somewhat contradictory. Most investigations do not focus on sexual adjustment explicitly and often only one or two questions about sexual functioning are included in infertility research studies. While many studies find evidence of sexual disruptions, others do not (Daniluk, 1988; Fagan, Schmidt, & Rock, 1986; Freeman, Boxer, Rickels, Tureck, & Mastroianni, 1985; Freeman, Garcia, & Rockels, 1983; Leiblum, Kemmann, & Lane, 1987; Platt & Leiblum, 1994).

Nevertheless, there are many ways in which the sexual relationship changes during the years of infertility evaluations and treatment. For example, time devoted to sensual foreplay may be abbreviated as well as efforts to increase arousal. While male ejaculation is clearly necessary for conception, female orgasm is not, and, therefore, efforts devoted to stimulating female orgasm are sometimes abandoned.

When ovulation induction injections have been used, the pressure to have sexual intercourse during the fertile period is considerable. Reliable and prompt ejaculation becomes the goal of sexual relations and sexual intimacy at nonfertile times of the month often is abandoned. For couples whose sexual adjustment was tenuous to begin with, infertility treatment can damage sexual response and pleasure. Men with unreliable erections may experience erectile failure and sexual apathy or avoidance. Women with a history of inhibited sexual desire may become sexually avoidant at times other than ovulation.

While infertility can cause sexual problems, sexual problems also can be responsible for lack of success in conception. The woman with vaginismus often comes for treatment only when she wants to get pregnant (Leiblum, 1995). Typically, vaginismic couples have colluded in avoiding resolution of their sexual problems. Often, these couples have conflicted marriages, in which the husband is angry and disappointed about the lack of intercourse, but is fearful or reluctant to force the issue.

Sexual problems other than vaginismus can lead to infertility. The man with erectile failure or ejaculatory delay or inability may be unable to deposit semen in close enough proximity to the vagina that conception occurs. The couple who engage in infrequent sex may miss the window of opportunity for conception. It is important to take a complete sexual history when dealing with couples who are experiencing infertility. While sexual problems are rarely the primary or single cause of reproductive failure, they may contribute to a reduced probability of conception. Further, when sexual problems do occur, they are magnified if the couple feels thwarted in their quest for a biological child.

Finally, the sexual competency of both partners should be assessed before assuming one or the other is responsible for the infertility problems. For example, a vaginismic woman was referred by her gynecologist for sex therapy. The physician assumed she was responsible for the failure to conceive. However, upon evaluation the husband was found to have significant difficulty getting and maintaining erections. His erectile problems were so humiliating that he avoided sexual contact. Only after his wife announced she was leaving the marriage if he did not become physically engaged with her did the husband consent to treatment (Leiblum, 1996b).

PSYCHOLOGICAL SEQUELAE AND SECONDARY PREVENTION

Psychological Sequelae

Throughout this chapter, we have attempted to point out the effect of sexual problems on women's sense of well-being. Sexual success has become a sign of adult power so potent that 8- and 10-year-old girls are already dieting to produce the body media displays as sexually appealing. The problem is that this body—and the sexuality it suggests—are impossible goals for virtually all girls and women to achieve. An eating disordered woman on the verge of change in treatment often describes her regret at giving up the quest to achieve and maintain an unattainable standard of female beauty, her self-control manifest as she conquers the body's inconvenient appetites (including sexual pleasure). It is only as this truce with physical desire is negotiated that sexual interest reemerges (Williams *et al.*, 1999).

Similarly, the woman with sexual problems who compares herself to the social paradox of chaste, controlled sexually responsiveness (so like the impossibly buxom and trim body of the supermodel), encounters such mixed messages that disconnection from one's messily contradictory emotions and withdrawal from the erotic enterprise has a real appeal. Women who participated in a group the authors led to treat hypoactive sexual desire found common ground in their belief that their lives would be simpler and more pleasant if they did not have to think about sex, much less participate in it. Each felt threatened and shamed by her partner's sexual demands, yet also superior to these appetites. Each voiced her inner conflict between feeling like a defective child, excluded from adult womanhood, and her contempt for women who were naturally responsive.

The ways in which any sexual problem will affect a woman vary enormously, despite these commonalities. The specifics of a woman's history, psychology, culture, support, and relationships each mitigate or exacerbate the psychological sequelae of sexual dysfunction. The following case vignette illustrates the range of emotional consequences.

As this example shows, a sexual dysfunction can not only create problems in achieving pleasure or an intimate connection with a lover, but impose a sense of defect and alienation on a woman. The ostensible public permission now given to women to be sexually desirous and orgasmic makes some women feel even more defective for failing to approximate the ideal. B, used to professional competition and success, was depressed by her "failure" in this arena. The suggestion that she consider an antidepressant only increased her sense that she was abnormal. In the following section, B's treatment will be described.

Vignette

B, a 39-year-old professional woman, presented with primary orgasmic dysfunction and a situational lack of desire. Her reason for seeking help was that she was feeling sexually attracted to a male colleague and was feeling it might be possible to have an orgasm; she reported no desire for her husband.

B's memories of early childhood centered on her father, who seemed to prefer his sons' accomplishments to B's. B's mother was described as critical and competitive; B feared being like her. Despite the regular arrival of younger siblings, B received no sex education except prohibitions against masturbation and spending time alone with boys.

When she was 11, a male relative fondled B's genitals while she slept. As she slowly woke, she flooded with pleasant sensations, then became fearful and guilty when she realized what was happening and turned away. She never told anyone about this molestation. In adolescence, B's relationship with her body was adversarial; she hated her physical transformation and concealed the onset of menstruation for several months. She reported no sexual play or attraction to either gender in high school or college. B lost her virginity to a friend in her early twenties because she felt it was time for her to do so. She enjoyed arousing her lover but reported no physical sensation during the experience.

Subsequent lovers were initially challenged, but eventually contemptuous of her inability to reach orgasm, rejecting her as "frigid" or a "freak of nature." B married a man who was not especially interested in sex; eventually he complained about her lack of enthusiasm and she made two efforts at resolving her problem in therapy. B reported feeling somewhat baffled about why her lack of interest and pleasure in sex mattered so much to others but she was also mortified by the failure of these treatments, both of which had recommended masturbation. The marriage settled into a companionable detachment.

In her late thirties, B became attracted to a coworker's ribald sense of humor and lack of inhibition. Their interest in each other grew over months of long, searching conversations about their marriages and sexual fantasies. B's guilt and anxiety about the flirtation conflicted with her realization that she was becoming sexually aroused for the first time in her adult life. Her attraction seemed to have opened a door, B said, but she could not bring herself to cross the threshold.

EFFECTIVENESS OF SEX THERAPY

Most female sexual dysfunctions have a good prognosis. Individual, couples, and group therapy have all demonstrated success, and approaches combining these modalities are also quite effective. Pharmacological interventions may be important as well in reducing generalized anxiety or depression associated with the sexual or relationship problem. The difficulty is in obtaining reliable data on outcome. There

are fewer studies of the efficacy of psychological treatments in the past few years. Recent outcome funding has been placed on studying the effects of medical treatments, and none of the medical studies have compared these outcomes to those obtained by psychological techniques.

Desire Disorders

Desire disorders are difficult to treat. The causes are so intertwined, leading to or following other sexual dysfunctions. Patient and thorough assessment is needed to separate the relevant biological, psychological, and interpersonal variables, and treatment generally requires an even more laborious sorting through of these variables as various issues are resolved and others emerge. In couples for whom the problem appears to be one of desire discrepancy rather than inhibited desire in one partner (one person wants sex twice a week, the other four times), treatment will work to guide the couple to a compromise. If fatigue, boredom, or a limited sexual repertoire contribute, script modification has been useful. But it is not always the case that removing the more desirous partner's pressure or resolving concrete obstacles to desire results in active sexual interest. Extensive, insight-oriented treatment is then needed to explore individual conflicts about sexual feelings or interpersonal intimacy.

An approach called "orgasm consistency training" has been described as equally effective for women with low sexual desire and those who have infrequent orgasms (Hurlbert et al., 1993). The authors suggest that female interest and satisfaction in partnered heterosexual sex increases when the woman achieves orgasm before the man does. The program teaches directed masturbation for the woman, couples sensate focus exercises, and techniques to improve voluntary male control over the timing of ejaculation. With respect to the latter, the motto "ladies come first" is thought to increase female sexual interest as well as increasing communication, affection, and sexual awareness between partners. An integral part of their approach is the use of the coital alignment technique, described below in the section on orgasmic disorders.

Another, less structured strategy begins with the observation that when desire problems emerge from relational conflicts, the nature of these conflicts will differ depending on the development stage of the relationship. A couple having desire problems early in a marriage may be struggling around issues of merging two approaches to life, while a couple whose desire discrepancy emerges after many years may be so

melded together that they lack the emotional differentiation from which erotic attraction seems to emerge (Lobitz & Lobitz, 1996). The treatment approach is to identify the couple's developmental stage and to remove the emotional obstacles to further sexual intimacy.

Sexual aversion is relatively resistant to conventional forms of sex therapy (Crenshaw, 1985). Some success has been reported with the combined use of antianxiety medication and sex therapy that was modified to accommodate the special needs of these patients, who avoid any touching or communication that might lead to sexual involvement (Crenshaw, 1985; Kaplan, Fyer & Novick, 1982).

Female Arousal Disorder

There are few specific treatments for FAD, which is instead addressed obliquely through interventions for hypoactive sexual desire or orgasmic disorder. In the 1970s biofeedback was tried to enhance sexual arousal but success was modest (Rosen & Beck, 1988). Women may experience some symptomatic relief by using the artificial lubricants available at pharmacies, although these treatments do not increase vasocongestion to the pelvis. Moreover, lubricant use can mask an arousal disorder, as if the goal were simply to facilitate penetration rather than to address obstacles to the woman's biological and emotional responsivity to sexual contact.

Recent efforts to delineate the relationship of general autonomic arousal on sexual response in women have found significant increases in both physiological and subject measure of sexual arousal after general autonomic arousal. The combined effects of the general arousal and false feedback to the women that they were becoming aroused combined to produce arousal in women with FSAD comparable to that observed in sexually functional women (Palace & Gorzalka, 1992). These findings converge with research indicating that general physical exercise increases arousal (Eisenberg, 1999).

Since vasoactive drugs such as sildenafil citrate (Viagra) have been so effective in men with erectile disorder, Goldstein and Berman

(1998) are investigating their use in women to facilitate smooth muscle relaxation and increase blood flow to the genitals. The results of these efforts are too preliminary to judge, although the section below on pharmacological treatments points out the enthusiasm with which these approaches are being greeted in the medical community (and the pharmaceutical industry).

Orgasmic Disorders

The basic components of sex therapy for primary orgasmic disorder include some form of directed masturbation training, sex education and permission, enhancement of coital orgasm frequency through the bridge technique or concurrent clitoral stimulation, and the use of women's sexual enhancement groups (Barbach, 1975; Heiman & Grafton-Becker, 1989; Schoever & Leiblum, 1994; Williams & Leiblum, 1997). Clinically directed masturbation is the most clearly beneficial intervention for the woman with primary orgasmic dysfunction. Recent studies indicate that orgasmic success is associated with sexual assertiveness (Hurlbert, 1991) and comfort with masturbation (Kelly, Strassberg, & Kircher, 1990).

Treatment of secondary anorgasmia must be individualized, although couples treatment is usually a critical component of treatment.

Without involving the partner, interpersonal resentment, distrust, or anxiety can thwart the motivation for being intimate or the safety to abandon oneself to pleasure that is so necessary for orgasmic release. Sensate focus assignments and coaching the couple on giving and receiving sexual feedback are particularly helpful.

In cases of situational orgasmic dysfunction, the success in the transfer of orgasm to coitus is often low whatever treatment is used. The technique of coital alignment has been suggested as a means of enhancing and increasing female coital orgasms and mutual orgasms (Eichel, Eichel, & Kule, 1988). Basically, coital alignment is the "riding high" variation of the missionary position with genitally focused pressure–counterpressure during intercourse; a follow-up study found that although women enjoyed the technique, it did not result in coital orgasm for most of them (Kaplan, 1992b). Thus, the question of whether striving for coital orgasm is either realistic or necessary must be challenged. A large number of women are unable to reliably achieve this goal; are coital orgasms a legitimate focus of treatment in the absence of other sexual complaints? To aid a woman in her pursuit of what seems like a socially designated achievement seems less helpful than reducing the couple's anxiety about relinquishing this definition of a sexual pinnacle.

Case Example

In the case of B, described earlier in this chapter, a behavioral approach to B's anorgasmia had foundered because B resisted suggestions that she look at her body, touch her genitals, or masturbate with a vibrator. B had also seen an interpersonal therapist and felt that simply discussing her marriage and her sexual history would take too long; she wanted to have an orgasm the next time she and the lover met. As her aversion to self-stimulation was discussed, B described her persistent belief that masturbation was sinful and her humiliation when previous efforts to masturbate had not stirred the slightest sensation. The turning point came when B realized that the arousal she felt while being fondled in childhood meant she was physiologically capable of sexual sensations. B began to look at herself as capable of achieving her goal. She had once concluded that she was simply defective, "not truly feminine"; now she wondered if she had "numbed out" her genitals.

B began to practice deep muscle relaxation and to pay more careful attention to a variety of bodily sensations. As B then began to weave an erotic fantasy, she found this was a way of bypassing her disturbing sense of badness, which seemed only stirred when she touched herself. With reassurance that it was normal and productive to explore any sexual image or impulse, B found she could increase her sensation by altering her position during the fantasy (for instance, lying on her stomach and pressing her pelvis into a pillow). B reported that her muscles were tightening, her nipples becoming erect, and her vagina lubricating. She admitted her fear that if she climaxed she would lose control of her body and her mind. She connected her panic to her feelings during the molestation and even further back to a moment when she felt her father had rejected her because she was too needy. B realized she was asking the female therapist to reassure her about her body's normalcy as she wished she'd been able to ask her mother. At the next session, B announced she had had an orgasm, using fantasy and body position to arouse her. This success did not immediately generalize to coital orgasm, however. B found her concentration on her pleasure was diluted when she had too many external stimuli (like a partner). Couples therapy was not possible because of her reluctance to disclose the source of her new sexual awareness to her husband. Satisfied with her new found ability to enjoy orgasm during oral sex and digital penetration, B's focus in therapy gradually shifted to an ongoing exploration of the dangers she perceived in intimacy.

Sexual Pain Disorders

The general psychological strategy for treating vaginismus and dyspareunia involves a combination of sexual education; systematic desensitization, in fantasy and in practice; couples therapy; exercises to increase voluntary control over the pubbococcygeal muscles; and vaginal self-dilation (Lazarus, 1989; Leiblum, Pervin, & Campbell, 1989; Meana & Binik, 1994). Usually good success is achieved with well-motivated patients and supportive partners. Partner involvement is critical.

In dyspareunia, treatment must also include assessment and correction of any physiological contributors to sexual pain. The existence of such factors should not lead to dismissing psychological and relationship factors, however. Although one study found surgery to be successful with women who had dyspareunia from vulvar vestibulitis, the authors found that all the patients needed an additional course of sex therapy to fully resolve their sexual pain (Fordney, 1978; Meana & Binik, 1994).

In cases of dyspareunia, therefore, it is important that assessment include a multi-disciplinary team working together to consider the different aspects of the pain—the possible neurological, muscular, affective, and interpersonal contributors—and treatment should be similarly coordinated. Understanding the parameters (location, intensity, quality, elicitors, time course) of the pain and the circumstances of its occurrence is crucial since it legitimatizes the pain complaint and helps guide intervention. Gynecologists should be involved in the assessment process along with clinicians. Determining which subtype of dyspareunia (e.g., vulvar vestibulitis, vaginal atrophy, mixed pain disorder) the woman is experiencing is important as well (Leiblum, 1999).

Binik and his collaborators believe that all reports of dyspareunia include both psychogenic and organogenic elements and that both must be taken seriously. Interestingly, these researchers have found that women who attribute their pain to psychosocial causes tend to report higher pain scores, higher levels of distress, lower marital adjustment, and more sexual problems than those women ascribing their pain to physical causes (Meana, Binik, Khalife, & Cohen, 1999). In addition to determining the exact site of the pain, the therapist should ask about when the pain began, the severity of the discomfort, and whether there were any precipitating factors that occurred before the onset of the symptom. For example, nonspecific pain that occurs subsequent to date rape would be treated differently from dyspareunia occurring during the postpartum period following episiotomy. One especially puzzling aspect of dyspareunia is the observation that some women are able to function sexually despite the report of great pain and others cannot. Similarly, the rated intensity of pain does not usually correlate with physical findings. Behavioral disruption cannot be reliably predicted from a gynecological exam or even a past history.

PHARMACOLOGICAL TREATMENTS

Bartlik, Kaplan, Kaminetsky, Roentsch, & Goldberg (1999a) reviewed emerging data about medications with the potential to enhance sexual responsivity in women. Although these findings are quite preliminary, based on clinical anecdotes or studies of small groups of women, recent research in sex therapy is increasingly focused on medical therapies. It seems likely that such medications will become the object of great interest by physicians and consumers in pursuit of rapid solutions to sexual complaints.

Desire Disorders

Testosterone, progesterone, and estrogen are all being evaluated for their effect on sexual response. Testosterone levels are positively correlated with frequency of masturbation and arousal (Bancroft & Wu, 1983; Schreiner-Engel, Schiavi, Smith, & White, 1991). Postmenopausal women treated with testosterone and estrogen (versus estrogen alone) reported improved sexual desire (Studd, Collins, Chakravarti, Newton, Oram, & Parsons, 1977). Estrogen can facilitate arousal, and because restoring estrogen levels postmenopause feminizes breast, skin and genitals, estrogen is thought to improve self-esteem and indirectly desire. But estrogen may also have a negative effect on sexual desire and arousal by indirectly reducing free testosterone. Raloxifene hydrochloride, a selective estrogen agonist used to prevent osteoporosis in menopausal women, reportedly increased libido in both peri- and postmenopausal women, probably due to increased testosterone levels. Some sources report that progesterone stimulates libido, whereas other indicate the reverse (Lee, 1997; Kaplan, 1974). The increase in libido that some women experience during late pregnancy and premenstrually has been attributed to elevated levels of progesterone, but synthetic derivatives of progesterone are used to reduce sexual drive in sex offenders.

Sexual Arousal

The prevailing medical tactic for increasing female sexual arousal is based on the assumption that vasodilation, the process by which the penis becomes erect, will similarly result in increased blood flow and arousal in the female pelvis. This may prove to be less successful than sildenafil citrate in men in part because blood circulates in and out of the clitoris, not remaining inside as it does in an erect penis. However, researchers are already experimenting with drugs such as sildenafil, phentolamine meslylate, and phentolamine (oral medications for erectile disorders), and aprostadil, a topical vasodilator, on women. One writer cited the example of a male patient's wife who co-opted his use of the vasoactive cream. Although the husband had no reaction, the wife reported heightened arousal, lubrication, vaginal engorgement, and better orgasms when she applied it to her vulva (Bartlik et al., 1999a).

Following the findings that general autonomic arousal increases sexual arousal, investigators speculate that medications like ephedrine, which augments peripheral sympathetic activity, seem to enhance sexual excitement. The herb ma huang contains ephedrine and has long been believed to increase sexual excitement. It is not clear that the improvements these drugs provide are worth the common side effect of anxiety or the potential for abuse.

Apomorphine, a direct dopamine receptor agonist has shown both vasodilation effect on the genitals and central action on parts of the brain inducing sexual response. Mixtures of sildenafil with dopaminergic agents like apomorphine and/or testosterone may eventually be used to treat severe female sexual dysfunction (Bartlik et al., 1999a). Rosen et al. (1999b) cautions that even "if … vasodilator drugs are effective in increasing vaginal engorgement, the clinical benefits in terms of sexual performance or satisfaction will need to be independently assessed" (p. 143).

Orgasmic Disorders

A number of strategies have been proposed to treat delayed or absent orgasm due to antidepressants, including reducing dosage, taking drug holidays, and changing medication or adding other medications to counteract the effects. The main problem of these approaches is the loss of the antidepressant effect in reduced dosage and drug holidays and the potential for side effects, drug interactions, and added costs.

A number of researchers have pointed out that several antidepressants (bupropion, nefazadone, and mirtrzapine) do not appear to decrease orgasm (Bartlik et al., 1999a; Rosen et al., 1999a). Bupropion was originally tested as a treatment for low desire in undepressed patients. Statistically significant improvement was found in more than 60% of the treated patients (vs. 10% of controls). Nefazadone may be a superior antidepressant for postmenopausal women, particularly those with diminished sexual responsivity secondary to declining levels of endogenous testosterone.

Sildenafil citrate (Viagra) is being tried on women who want to achieve multiple orgasms or are learning to gain control over their orgasmic ability. As yet, no empirical evidence supports this usage. Methylphenidate and dextroamphetamine are also helpful in alleviating delayed or inhibited orgasm secondary to SSRI use. Psychostimulants appear to improve all

sexual arenas, with women responding more vigorously than men, but the abuse potential of these medications is high. Herbal medications such as ginkgo biloba, ginseng, and ma huang have also been reported to reverse SSRI-caused sexual dysfunction, but no published controlled studies have been done and all three have potentially dangerous side effects (ginseng can enhance the growth of hormonally responsive tumors, ginkgo has a blood-thinning action, and ma huang can increase anxiety).

HEALTH POLICY IMPLICATIONS

For a number of financial, political, and social reasons, research into sexual dysfunction has primarily focused on male erectile disorder. Even now, as researchers investigate the possibility of vascular insufficiency in FAD, the interest has been sparked by the enormous success of medications in treating erectile disorders in men. Part of this inequity may be related to the greater variability in female sexual functioning, with its sources in medical, intrapsychic, historical, and relational substrates. For example, given the wide variability across women in the ease and potency of sexual arousal, it is difficult to identify what is normal and what is inadequate for any individual woman. Further, what may be satisfying at one stage of a woman's reproductive life may not be satisfying at another, due to changes in the hormonal ecology, demands of efforts to conceive, carry, and nurture children, and relationship satisfaction.

Three recent shifts in the climate around women's health research have potentially positive effects on our understanding of women's sexual dysfunction. The first, a growing interest in gender-based biology among researchers, promises a more complex appreciation of how women's sexual functioning is not "based on" or "derived from" male models. The Society for Women's Health Research (1998) has identified gender differences in virtually every system of the human body. "The findings from gender-based biology have the potential to revolutionize the way we understand health and disease for both men and women. These differences extend beyond the obvious areas like reproductive differences to areas such as reactions to specific drugs and how men and women respond to the same disease or treatment" (Greenberger, 1999, p. 1).

Estrogen may underlie gender-based biological differences that both directly and indirectly affect sexual dysfunction. Currently, research is exploring estrogen's effect on serotonin levels in the brain, which is correlated with depression, a leading medical cause of desire disorders. Other promising areas include investigations of differences in metabolism, distribution and side effects of drugs in men and women; there is currently considerably more information about the effects of medication on sexual functioning in men than in women. The NIMH spent $81.2 million on research on women's mental health in 1997, including research into the psychosocial and biological factors underlying eating disorders (which often lead to loss of desire); study of the finding that serious mental disorders among women often have their onset during childbearing, particularly the postpartum period; and clinical efforts to prevent depression in infertile women and to treat posttraumatic stress, which is correlated with desire, arousal, and sexual pain disorders (Parron, 1999).

The second cultural shift that may bode well for research into women's sexual health is the aging of the baby-boomer generation, which means that the first generation of American women who were encouraged to accept and explore their sexual pleasure is now entering menopause. Because age is a risk factor for all sexual dysfunction, a growing percentage of Americans may encounter sexual difficulties in the twenty-first century. The Association of Reproductive Health Professionals and the Society for Women's Health research have undertaken a three-year educational initiative that will address the issues of sexuality and reproductive health among adults over 50 (Mature Sexuality, 1999). Specific health issues to be addressed include vaginal dryness, erectile dysfunction, overactive bladder, diabetes, depression, osteo-

porosis, and Alzheimer's disease. A woman's sexual health can be adversely affected by the decline in a male partner's erectile functioning, particularly if the couple is rigid or conservative in its sexual script, emphasizing intercourse as the only "real" sexual encounter. This public health initiative, Mature Sexuality, will feature patient and provider education campaigns; conferences and continuing education of professionals; an extensive survey of sexual behavior among older adults; and an Internet resource center. The ARHP is also collaborating with the National Institutes of Health on research and public health initiatives on the benefits and risk of sex steroids for women during the perimenopause (Mature Sexuality, 1999).

Finally, producing economically viable solutions to women's sexual problems has become increasingly attractive to commercial enterprises since the overwhelming success of sildenafil citrate (Viagra). *The New York Times* wrote "a host of pharmaceutical companies are working to do for women what Viagra does for men. To do this effectively, they need far more scientific data on female sexual response than is presently available" (Eisenberg, 1999, p. F7). Researchers describe being deluged by offers of funding in dramatic contrast to the difficulty they have had in recent years obtaining research funds to study psychological causes of sexual problems. This is particularly striking because none of the recent outcome research has compared the effectiveness of sex therapies with medical therapies. The rush of funding may lead to such fundamental science as mapping the innervation of the female genitalia or identifying surgical approaches to hysterectomy that reduce nerve damage, work that needs to be done. Vivian Pinn, director of the Office of Research on Women's Health at the NIH, stated: "Because there is so little scientific data, interventions to treat women's sexual problems have lagged behind those developed for men. We've brought breast cancer and menopause out of the closet. It's time to address the issues of sound research initiatives to better define women's sexual functions and dysfunctions" (Eisenberg, 1999, p. F7).

CONCLUSIONS

We have, after all, long given up any expectation of a neat parallelism between male and female sexual development (Freud, Standard Edition 1931, 21:226). Over and over, our look into women's sexual problems confronts us with false dichotomies, the first being the idea that function and dysfunction can be neatly categorized (Wincze & Carey, 1991). Women's sexuality is not a version of male sexuality but neither, as long as men and women are lovers, is it so divorced from male sexuality that comparisons can be ignored. Most sexual problems are not a function of social expectations alone, but neither can they be truly understood nor lasting solutions devised without acknowledgment of their context. Sex is neither solely individual or social, psychological or medical, political or natural, empirical or deconstructed. What female sexuality is, finally, is contentious: a battleground in a very old struggle to delineate, to pin down exactly what women want and need.

There is a great deal to rejoice over in the state of research and practice with women who have sexual problems. The strict divisions that once existed between models of psychological treatment have gradually given way to more integrated approaches, including behavioral, systemic, and dynamic models of change. As biological treatments become more widely available, it seems likely that they, too, will become part of an increasingly sophisticated repertoire of interventions. All of this could provide distressed women a greater range of choices in how to resolve their sexual problems. As one woman put it recently, miffed by her lover's popping a pill to enhance his erection: "Why should he get the certainty of arousal while I still have to work at it?" Yet, the rapid expansion of technological solutions exposes even more fundamental questions. Those missing answers may ultimately be more constructive than any number of problem-based solutions. What do we mean when we refer to the sexual self in women? These meanings are relative, not fixed (Daniluk, 1998). Consider, as one example of this unexplored complexity, the im-

pact of changes in a woman's social role on her sexuality over the life span. We know that sexual problems increase for women as they age, but many women over 40 attribute this not to perimenopausal hormonal changes but to the realization that, as their bodies change, they lose a potent source of power in the culture. No longer is service as eager or rules as easily bent as they were when one was 20; instead, one feels virtually penniless in the sexual economy. Younger women are stunned by their new sexual power; infertile women suffer the loss of sexual privacy and eroticism in the drive to conceive; women with careers and small children struggle over satisfying the emotional and physical demands of job, children, and spouse; elder women face the deaths of spouses and the daunting reality of years alone. What might happen if researchers and clinicians of women's sexuality studied these questions?

REFERENCES

Altman, M. (1984). Everything they always wanted you to know: The ideology of popular sex literature. In C. S. Vance (Ed.), *Pleasure and danger: Exploring female sexuality* (pp. 115–130). Boston: Routledge & Kegan Paul.

American Psychiatric Association (1994). *Diagnostic and statistical manual of mental disorders*, 4th ed. Washington, DC: American Psychiatric Association.

Andersen, B. L., & Cyranowski, J. M. (1995). Women's sexuality: Behaviors, responses, and individual differences. *Journal of Consulting and Clinical Psychology*, 63(6), 891–906.

Andrews, F., Abbey, A., & Halman, L. (1992). Is fertility-problem stress different? The dynamics of stress in fertile and infertile couples. *Fertility and Sterility*, 57, 1247–1253.

Bancroft, J. (1980). Androgens and sexual behavior in women using oral contraceptives. *Clinical Endocrinology*, 12, 327–340.

Bancroft, J., & Wu, F. C. W. (1983). Changes in erectile responsiveness during androgen replacement therapy. *Archives of Sexual Behavior*, 12, 59–68.

Barbach, L. (1975). *For yourself: The fulfillment of female sexuality*. New York: Doubleday.

Bartlik, B., Kaplan, P., Kaminetsky, J., Roentsch, G., & Goldberg, J. (1999a). Medications with the potential to enhance sexual responsivity in women. *Psychiatric Annals*, 29(1), 46–52.

Bartlik, B., Legere, R., & Andersson, L. (1999b). The combined use of sex therapy and testosterone replacement therapy for women. *Psychiatric Annals, 29*(10), 27–33.

Beck, J. G. (1995). Hypoactive sexual desire disorder: An overview. *Journal of Clinical and Consulting Psychology, 63*(6), 919–927.

Beggs, V. E., Calhoun, K. S. & Wolchik, S. A. (1987). Sexual anxiety and female sexual arousal: A comparison of arousal during sexual anxiety stimuli and sexual pleasure stimuli. *Archives of Sexual Behavior, 16*, 311–319.

Consensus panel conference report on female sexual dysfunction: Definitions, classification & outcomes (1998, October). Sexual Health Council, American Foundation of Urology.

Crenshaw, T. L. (1985). The sexual aversion syndrome. *Journal of Sex & Marital Therapy, 11*(4), 285–292.

Daniluk, J. C. (1998). *Women's sexuality across the life span: Challenging myths, creating meanings.* New York: Guilford Press.

DeAmicis, L., Goldberg, D. C., LoPiccolo, J., Friedman, J., & Davies, L. (1985). Clinical follow-up on couples treated for sexual dysfunction. *Archives of Sexual Behavior, 150*, 197–200.

de Silva, P. (1993). Sexual problems in women with eating disorders. In J. Ussher & C. Barker (Eds.), *Psychological perspectives on sexual problems* (pp. 79–109). London: Routledge.

Drugs that cause sexual dysfunction: An update. (1992). *The Medical Letter on Drugs & Therapeutics, 34*(Aug. 7, 876), 73–78.

Dunn, K. M., Croft, P. R., & Hackett, G. I. (1998). Sexual problems: A study of the prevalence and need for health care in the general population. *Family Practice, 15*(6), 519–524.

Eichel, E., Eichel, J., & Kule, S. (1988). The technique of coital alignment and its relation to female orgasmic response and simultaneous orgasm. *Journal of Sex & Marital Therapy, 14*(2), 129.

Eisenberg, A. (1999). A boost to research of women's sexuality. *The New York Times,* 7/13/99, F7.

Fagan, P., Schmidt, C., & Rock, J. (1986). Sexual functioning and psychological evaluation of in vitro fertilization transfer. *Fertility and Sterility, 46*, 668–672.

Fordney, D. S. (1978). Dyspareunia and vaginismus. *Clinical Obstetrics and Gynecology, 21*, 205–221.

Freeman, E., Boxer, A., Rickels, K., Tureck, R., & Mastroianni, L. (1985). Psychological evaluation and support in a program of in vitro fertilization and embryo transfer. *Fertility and Sterility, 46*, 668–672.

Freeman, E., Garcia, C., & Rickels, K. (1983). Behavioral and emotional factors: Comparisons of anovulatory infertile women with fertile and other infertile women. *Fertility and Sterility, 40*, 195–201.

Freud, S. (1931). Female sexuality. *Standard Edition, 22*, 226.

Galyer, K. T., Conaglen, H. M., Hare, A., & Conaglen, J. V. (1999). The effect of gynecological surgery on sexual desire. *Journal of Sexual & Marital Health, 25*, 81–88.

Garde, K., & Lunde, I. (1980). Female sexual behavior: A study in a random sample of 40 year old women. *Maturitas, 2*, 225–240.

Gawande, Atul, (1999, July). A queasy feeling. *The New Yorker,* 7/5/99, 34–41.

Gitlin, M. (1994). Psychotropic medications and their effects on sexual function: Diagnosis, biology and treatment approaches. *Journal of Clinical Psychiatry, 55*(9), 406–413.

Golding, J. M., Wilsnack, S. C., & Learman, L. A. (1998). Prevalence of sexual assault history among women with common gynecological symptoms. *American Journal of Obstetrics and Gynecology, 179*(4), 1013–1019.

Goldstein, I., & Berman, J. R. (1998). Vasculogenic female sexual dysfunction: Vaginal engorgement and clitoral erectile insufficiency syndrome. *International Journal of Impotence Research, 10*, S84–90.

Greenberger, P. (1999). Annual update on women's health research, discoveries and implications. Address given at The Society for Women's Health Research's eighth annual scientific advisory meeting, Washington DC: November 2, 1998. Quoted in SWHR's website: information@womens-health.org.

Harding, J. (1998). *Sex acts: Practices of femininity and masculinity.* London: Sage.

Heiman, J. R., & Grafton-Becker, V. (1989) Orgasmic disorders in women. In S. R. Leiblum, & R. C. Rosen (Eds.), *Principles and practice of sex therapy; Update for the 90s* (pp. 51–88). New York: Guilford Press.

Hurlbert, D. F., Apt, C., & Rabehl, S. M. (1993). Key variables to understanding female sexual satisfaction: An examination of women in nondistressed marriages. *Journal of Sex & Marital Therapy, 19*(2), 154–165.

Hurlbert, D. F. (1991). The role of assertiveness in female sexuality. A comparative study between sexually assertive and sexually nonassertive women. *Journal of Sex & Marital Therapy, 17*, 183–190.

Kaplan, H. S. (1974). *The new sex therapy.* New York: Brunner-Mazel.

Kaplan, H. S. (1977). Hypoactive sexual desire. *Journal of Sex & Marital Therapy, 3*, 3–9.

Kaplan, H. S. (1988). Intimacy disorders and sexual panic states. *Journal of Sex & Marital Therapy, 14*(10), 3–12.

Kaplan, H. S. (1992a). A neglected issue: The sexual side effects of current treatments for breast cancer. *Journal of Sex & Marital Therapy, 18*, 3–9.

Kaplan, H. S. (1992b). Does the CAT technique enhance female orgasm? *Journal of Sex & Marital Therapy, 18*(4), 285–302.

Kaplan, H. S., Fyer, A. J., & Novick, A. (1982). The treatment of sexual phobias: The combined use of antipanic medications and sex therapy. *Journal of Sex & Marital Therapy, 8*(1), 3–28.

Katz, R. C., Gipson, M. T., Kearl, A., & Kriskovich, M. (1989). Assessing sexual aversion in college students: The Sexual Aversion Scale. *Journal of Sex & Marital Therapy, 15*, 135–140.

Katz, R. C., Gipson, M. T., & Turner, S. (1992). Brief report: Recent findings on the Sexual Aversion Scale. *Journal of Sex & Marital Therapy, 18*, 141–145.

Kelly, M. P., Strassberg, D. S., & Kircher, J. R. (1990). Attitudinal and experiential correlates of anorgasmia. *Archives of Sexual Behavior, 19*, 165–172.

Kinzel, J. F., Traweger, C., & Biebl, W. (1995). Sexual dysfunctions: Relationship to childhood sexual abuse and early family experiences in a nonclinical sample. *Child Abuse & Neglect, 19*(7), 785–792.

Labbate, L. A., Grimes, J., Hines, A., Olehansky, M. A., & Arana, G. W. (1998). Sexual dysfunction induced by selective serotonin reuptake antidepressants. *Journal of Sexual & Marital Therapy, 24*, 3–12.

Laumann, E., Paik, A., & Rosen, R. (1999). Sexual dysfunction in the United States: Prevalence, predictors, and outcomes. *Journal of the American Medical Association, 281*(6), 537–544.

Lazarus, A. (1989). Dyspareunia: A multimodal psychotherapeutic perspective. In S. Leiblum, & R. Rosen. (Eds.), *Principles and practice of sex therapy: An update for the 1990s* (pp. 92–111). New York: Guilford Press.

Lee, J. R. (1997). *Natural progesterone: The multiple roles of a remarkable hormone.* Sebastopol, CA: BLL Publishing.

Leiblum, S. R. (1999). Critical overview of new consensus-based definitions and classification system. Paper presented at Female Sexual Dysfunction Conference, Boston, October.

Leiblum, S. (1998). Definition and classification of female sexual disorders. *International Journal of Impotence Research: Basic & Clinical Studies, 10*, S104–106.

Leiblum, S. R. (1996a). Sexual pain disorders. *Treatment of psychiatric disorders: The DSM*, 4th ed. Washington, DC: American Psychiatric Press.

Leiblum, S. R. (1996b). Love, sex, and infertility: The impact of infertility on couples. In S. R. Leiblum (Ed.), *Infertility: Psychological issues and counseling strategies.* New York: Wiley.

Leiblum, S. R. (1995). Relinquishing virginity: The treatment of a complex case of vaginismus. In R. Rosen, & S. Leiblum (Eds.), *Case studies in sex therapy* (pp. 250–263). New York: Guilford Press.

Leiblum, S. R., Pervin, L. A., & Campbell, E. H. (1989). The treatment of vaginismus: Success and failure. In S. Leiblum, & R. Rosen (Eds.), *Principles and practice of sex therapy: Update for the 90s.* New York: Guilford Press.

Leiblum, S. R., Kemmann, E., & Lane, M. (1987). The psychological concomitants of in vitro fertilization. *Journal of Psychosomatic Obstetrics and Gynecology, 6*, 166–178.

Lobitz, W. C., & Lobitz, G. K. (1996). Resolving the sexual intimacy paradox: A developmental model for treating sexual desire disorders. *Journal of Sex & Marital Therapy, 22*(2), 71–84.

Masters, W. H., & Johnson, V. E. (1970). *Human sexual inadequacy.* Boston: Little, Brown.

Mature sexuality: A new provider and consumer education initia-

tive on sexuality and mid-life to older adulthood (1999). Press release from the Association of Reproductive Health Professionals in conjunction with the Society for Women's Health Research. *SWHR website*: information @womens-health.org

McGahuey, C. A., Delgado, P. L., & Gelenberg, A. J. (1999). Assessment of sexual dysfunction using the Arizona Sexual Experiences Scale (ASEX) and implications for the treatment of depression. *Psychiatric Annals, 29*(1), 39–45.

Meana, M., & Binik, Y. (1994). Painful coitus: A review of female dyspareunia. *The Journal of Nervous and Mental Disease, 182*(5), 264–272.

Meana, M., Binik, Y. M., Khalife, S., & Cohen, D. (1999). Psychosocial correlates of pain attributions in women with dyspareunia. *Psychosomatics, 40*(6), 497–502.

Michael, R. T., Gagnon, J. H., Laumann. E., & Kolata, G. (1994). *Sex in America: A definitive survey.* Boston: Little Brown.

Palace, E. M., & Gorzalka, B. B. (1992). Differential patterns of arousal and sexually functional and dysfunctional women. *Journal of Abnormal Psychology, 99*, 403–411.

Park, K., Goldstein, I., Andry, C., Siroky, M. B., Krane, R. J., & Azadzoi, K. M. (1997). Vasculogenic female sexual dysfunction: The hemodynamic basis for vaginal engorgement insufficiency and clitoral erectile insufficiency. *International Journal of Impotence Research, 9*, 27–37.

Parron, D. L. (1999). National Institute of Mental Health annual update on women's health research: Discoveries and implications. *SWHR website*: information@ womens-health.org

Pietropinto, A. (1988). Male contributions to female sexual dysfunction. *Medical Aspects of Human Sexuality, 20* (12), 84–91.

Physicians' Desk Reference (2001). Montvale, NJ: Medical Economics.

Platt, L., & Leiblum, S. R. (1994). Infertile men and infertile women. A psychosocial comparison. Poster presented at the meeting of the American Society of Psychosomatic Obstetrics and Gynecology, Washington DC, November.

Rako, S. (1999). Testosterone deficiency and supplementation for women: Matters of sexuality and health. *Psychiatric Annals, 29*(1), 23–26.

Reichman, J. (1998). *I'm not in the mood: What every woman should know about improving her libido.* New York: William Morrow.

Renshaw, D. C. (1996). Sexuality. In J. Sadavoy, & L. W. Lazarus (Eds.), *Comprehensive review of geriatric psychotherapy* (pp. 419–432). Washington, DC: American Psychiatric Press.

Reissing, E. D., Binik, Y. M., & Khalife, S. (1999). Does vaginismus exist? A critical review of the literature. *Journal of Nervous and Mental Disease, 187*(5), 261–274.

Richgels, P. B. (1992). Hypoactive sexual desire in heterosexual women: A feminist analysis. *Women & Therapy*, *12*(1/2), 123–135.

Rosen, R. C., Lane, R. L., & Menza, M. (1999a). Effects of SSRIs on sexual function: A critical review. *Journal of Clinical Psychopharmacology*, *19*(1), 67–85.

Rosen, R. C., & Leiblum, S. R. (1995). Treatment of sexual disorders in the 1990s: An integrated approach. *Journal of Consulting and Clinical Psychology*, *63*(6), 877–890.

Rosen, R. C., Taylor, J., Leiblum, S., & Bachmann, G. (1993). Prevalence of sexual dysfunction in women. Results of a survey study of 329 women in an outpatient gynecological clinic. *Journal of Sex & Marital Therapy*, *19*(3), 171–188.

Rosen R. C., & Beck J. G. (1988). *Patterns of sexual arousal: Psychophysiological processes and clinical applications*. New York: Guilford Press.

Sarwer, D. B., & Durlak, J. A. (1996). Childhood sexual abuse as a predictor of adult female sexual dysfunction. *Child Abuse & Neglect*, *20*(10), 963–972.

Schreiner-Engel, P., & Schiavi, R. (1986). Lifetime psychopathology in individuals with low sexual desire. *Journal of Nervous and Mental Disorders*, *174*, 646–651.

Schreiner-Engel, P., Schiavi, R. C., Smith, H., & White, D. (1991). The relationship between pituitary-gonadal function and sexual behavior in healthy aging men. *Psychosomatic Medicine*, *53*(4), 363–374.

Schoever, L. R., & Leiblum, S. R. (1994). The stagnation of sex therapy. *Journal of Psychology and Human Sexuality*, *6*, 5–10.

Segraves, R. T. (1988). Psychiatric drugs and inhibited female orgasm. *Journal of Sex & Marital Therapy*, *14*, 202–207.

Segraves, R. T., & Segraves, K. B. (1991). Diagnosis of female arousal disorder. *Journal of Sex & Marital Therapy*, *6*, 9–13.

Sherwin, B. B., & Gelfand, M. M. (1985). Sex steroids and affect in the surgical menopause: A double-blind, cross-over study. *Psychoneuroendocrinology*, *10*, 325.

Sipski, M. L., & Alexander, C. (1998) Sexuality and disability. In J. DeLisa, & B. Gans (Eds.), *Rehabilitation medicine: Principles and practice*, 3rd ed. (pp. 1197–1229). Philadelphia: Lippincott-Raven.

Spector, I. P., & Carey, M. P. (1990). Incidence and prevalence of the sexual dysfunctions: A critical review of the empirical literature. *Archives of Sexual Behavior*, *19*(4), 389–408.

Steege, J., & Ling, F. W. (1993). Dyspareunia: A special type of chronic pelvic pain. *Obstetrics and Gynecology Clinics of North American*, *20*, 779–793.

Studd, J. W. W., Collins, W. P., Chakravarti, S., Newton, J. R., Oram, D., & Parsons, A. (1977). Oestradiol and testosterone implants in the treatment of psychosexual problems in postmenopausal women. *British Journal of Obstetrics and Gynaecology*, *84*, 314–315.

Toner, R. (1999). A majority over 45 say sex lives are just fine. *The New York Times*, 8/4/99, A17.

Trudel, G., Ravart, M., & Matte, B. (1993). The use of the multiaxial diagnostic systems for sexual dysfunctions in the assessment of hypoactive sexual desire. *Journal of Sex & Marital Therapy*, *19*(2), 123–130.

Wallen, K., & Lovejoy, J. (1993). Sexual behavior: Endocrine function and therapy. In J. Schulkin (Ed.), *Hormonally induced changes in mind and brain* (pp. 71–97). San Diego: Academic Press.

Warnock, J. K., Bundren, J. C., & Morris, D. W. (1997). Female hypoactive sexual desire disorder due to androgen deficiency: Clinical and psychometric issues. *Psychopharmacology Bulletin*, *33*(4), 761–765.

Whipple, B., & Komisaruk, B. R. (1999). Beyond the G spot: Recent research of female sexuality. *Psychiatric Annals*, *29*(1), 34–37.

Williams, N., & Leiblum, S. R. (1997). Treatment of orgasmic dysfunction in women. In J. J. Sciarra (Ed.), *Gynecology and obstetrics*, rev. ed. Philadelphia: Lippincott-Raven.

Williams, N., Loeb, K., Boudette, R., Cortese, K., Logue, N., McEneaney, A., & Nolet, W. (1999). The body has two appetites: Eating disorders and sexual dysfunction. Presentation at The Human Sexuality Program, Robert Wood Johnson Medical School, Piscataway, NJ, January.

Wincze, J. P., & Carey, M. P. (1991). *Sexual dysfunction: A guide for assessment and treatment*. New York: Guilford Press.

17

Cervical Cancer

COLLEEN M. MCBRIDE and DELIA SCHOLES

INTRODUCTION

It is estimated that by the end of 1999 in the United States, 12,800 new cases of invasive cervical cancer will be diagnosed and that 4800 women will die. Worldwide, cervical cancer is the second most common cancer among women and the leading cause of death in many non-industrialized nations (Parkin, 1998). As is true generally for cancer, the burden of cervical cancer morbidity and mortality falls disproportionately on minority women and those who have inadequate access to health care. These statistics are disheartening, given the widely held view that cervical cancer is the most preventable of the major cancers (Ponten et al., 1995; Sigurdsson, 1999).

In this chapter we provide an overview of the cervical cancer problem in the United States. We begin by providing definitions and rates of cervical cancer and its precursor conditions, and review associated social and behavioral risk factors. In the second section, we summarize the primary and secondary intervention approaches that have been brought to bear

on the problem and the personal experiences of women who are coping with cervical cancer. Also considered is the cost-effectiveness of alternative intervention approaches and the implications for health policy. We conclude with recommendations for promising new directions in cervical cancer prevention.

DEFINITIONS AND EPIDEMIOLOGY

Definitions

The term "cervical neoplasia" currently encompasses a variety of cellular abnormalities of the cervix including invasive cervical cancer (ICC), localized malignancies (cervical carcinoma in situ, CIS), and various other noninvasive or premalignant conditions. The majority (80%) of invasive cervical cancers are squamous cell carcinomas that nearly always arise from cellular changes occurring at the squamocolumnar junction, that is, where the squamous cell epithelium of the outer cervix intersects with the columnar epithelium of the cervical canal leading to the uterine cavity (Kiviat, Koutsky, & Paavonen, 1999). Adenocarcinomas of the cervix originate in glandular tissue and comprise most of the remaining invasive tumors (another 10%) (Kiviat et al., 1999).

The identification of a variety of premalignant lesions has formed the basis for most of the

COLLEEN M. MCBRIDE • Duke University Comprehensive Cancer Center, Durham, North Carolina 27710. DELIA SCHOLES • Group Health Cooperative of Puget Sound Center for Health Studies, Seattle, Washington 98101-1448.

Handbook of Women's Sexual and Reproductive Health, edited by Wingood and DiClemente. Kluwer Academic / Plenum Publishers, New York, 2002.

cervical cancer prevention efforts to date. As these more common noninvasive cellular abnormalities were identified, the terms "dysplasia" and later "cervical intraepithelial neoplasia" (CIN) were introduced to order and classify them. These changes were categorized into a presumed continuum, CIN I, II, and III (mild, moderate, severe dysplasia/CIS), based on the amount of the epithelium occupied by abnormal cells. However, in recent years, evidence of an orderly progression of lower-grade cervical lesions toward malignancy has been called into question. The emergence of human papillomavirus (HPV) as a likely causal agent for most squamous cell cervical neoplasias has introduced new complexities and led to modifications of the existing classification system.

Incidence and Prevalence

Cervical cancer incidence rates (based on age-adjusted data) vary widely, from well below 10/100,000 women in North America, Europe, and China, to rates in excess of 50/100,000 women in some parts of Africa and Latin America (Parkin, 1998; Schoell, Janicek, & Mirhashemi, 1999). Approximately 80% of all cases of cervical cancer occur in developing nations, where cervical cancer mortality also continues to be high (Parkin, 1998; Sigurdsson, 1999).

In the United States, there have been notable declines in both incidence and mortality in recent decades. The nearly 80% drop in incidence between 1950 and 1991, as well as accompanying drops in mortality are attributed largely to the introduction of widespread cytologic screening programs during the 1950's (Kiviat et al., 1999; Schoell et al., 1999).

While the overall age-adjusted incidence of cervical cancer for U.S. women is approximately 9/100,000, incidence rates vary by age, race or ethnicity, and socioeconomic status. The incidence of invasive cervical cancer increases with age. However, the median age at diagnosis is 48 years, relatively young when compared to many other cancers (Schoell et al., 1999). Rates for cervical carcinoma *in situ* (CIS) are notably

higher and have quite the reverse pattern. Incidence rates increase through the teens, climbing steeply until the mid-twenties, and declining rapidly thereafter (Kiviat et al., 1999). Beginning with virtually no cases before age 15, incidence climbs steeply throughout the reproductive years to around 15/100,000 by the mid-thirties. Rates continue at this level through mid-life years and well into old age (Kiviat et al., 1999).

The occurrence of premalignant conditions is not reliably captured since there is no mandatory reporting requirement for these conditions. However, studies assessing the prevalence of CIN have reported rates as high as 13.7% in sexually transmitted disease (STD) clinic populations and as low as 1% in family planning clinics (Kiviat et al., 1999). Data from the National Breast and Cervical Cancer Early Detection Program indicate that around 10–11% of cervical specimens have low-grade cellular abnormalities (Mitchell et al., 1996).

Comparison by race and ethnic status has shown that the incidence of cervical cancer is about two times higher for African-American women than for White women (13/100,000 versus 7/100,000, respectively) (Schoell et al., 1999). Rates are slightly higher for Alaskan Native and Hispanic women (around 16/100,000) (Parker, Davis, Wingo, Ries, & Heath, 1998). Encouragingly, some of the steepest declines in incidence also have been among African-American women (Schoell et al., 1999). Racial-ethnic differences are also evident in mortality statistics: five-year survival is approximately 72% for White women, and 59% for African-American women (Parker et al., 1998). This is likely to be due, in part, to diagnoses occurring at later stages (Kiviat et al., 1999).

Women with lower incomes or educational levels experience higher rates of cervical cancer after adjusting for race. Differences in these statistics may be due to increased risk; higher STD rates and differences in sexual/ contraceptive behaviors also have been reported for different SES and ethnic groups. Insurance status and access to preventive services are also likely contributors. The recent Commonwealth

Fund survey "Women's Health: Current Trends and Issues" noted considerable disparity in the proportion of women receiving Pap tests: 57% of low-income women versus 77% of high income women (Commonwealth Fund, 1999). This report also noted that, despite positive economic trends, the proportion of women under age 65 who were uninsured is at its highest level ever (approximately 25% of the women surveyed).

Behavioral and Social Correlates

The observation in the last century of markedly lower occurrence of uterine cancer among nuns when compared to married women prompted consideration of an array of behavioral and sociodemographic risk factors for cervical cancer. Numerous factors related to sexual activity (lifetime number of sexual partners in the woman, woman's male partner, and early sexual debut), as well as contraceptive exposures (oral contraceptives, barrier methods), smoking, ethnicity and SES, and the intake of certain nutrients have been found to be associated with invasive cervical cancer and lower-grade abnormalities (Kiviat et al., 1999; Schiffman & Brinton, 1995; Schoell et al., 1999). A variety of sexually transmitted pathogens also have been examined; it is here that the most notable recent findings have occurred. A number of epidemiological and clinical studies employing various methodologies and conducted in a variety of populations have shown consistently strong associations between HPV infection and cervical cancer (relative risks of 10 and above), that are biologically plausible in terms of viral actions on host cells, are stronger with increasing viral load and temporally precede cervical neoplasia (Kiviat et al., 1999; Koutsky, 1997; Schiffman & Brinton, 1995). To date over 80 types of HPV have been identified, with evidence that around 20 types have a greater capacity to induce abnormal cellular changes in the cervical epithelium. The most consistent and frequent associations have been with HPV types 16, 18, 45, and 56 (Koutsky, 1997).

At present HPV is estimated to be the most prevalent sexually transmitted infection in the U.S. population (American Social Health Association and Kaiser Family Foundation, 1998); an estimated 15% of all sexually active adults in the United States are infected (Koutsky, 1997). The association between HPV and cervical cancer suggests that successful STD prevention strategies could also help prevent cervical cancer. The identification of selected high risk types also has spurred interest in development of HPV vaccines and screening modalities (Koutsky, 1997; Lowy & Schiller, 1999).

Given HPV's etiologic importance, studies with the greatest validity are those that have evaluated exposures as cofactors or as independent risk factors after accounting for HPV status. A number of case-control studies have documented increased risk associated with behaviors after controlling for HPV status. A study by Daling et al., for example, stratified women with cervical tumors into those with evidence of HPV infection and those without. When compared to controls, risk estimates for current smokers were elevated in both case groups (Daling et al., 1996). A clinic-based study of documented high-grade CIN by Becker et al. (1994) also found current smoking to be an independent predictor of disease after accounting for HPV infection.

Some studies of contraceptive practices among U.S. women, particularly use of oral contraceptives (OC), also have adjusted for HPV (Negrini et al., 1990). Negrini et al. examined women with a range of cervical abnormalities ranging from atypia to high-grade squamous cell intraepithelial lesions (HSIL), noting elevations in the risk of HSIL in OC users that increased with duration of use (Negrini et al., 1990). After adjusting for HPV status, Daling noted an increased risk of cervical cancer among women who had used OCs at an early age (Daling et al., 1996). Becker, however, noted an independent protective effect of ever-use of OCs (Becker et al., 1994).

Sexual history variables found to increase risk after controlling for HPV include a greater number of lifetime partners and having a history of STDs (herpes) (Becker et al., 1994; Daling *et al.*, 1996). Low educational attainment and a greater number of pregnancies also have been associated with increased risk of cervical cancer (Becker *et al.*, 1994; Schiffman & Brinton, 1995).

Screening for Cervical Cancer

In 1943, Papanicolau reported that epithelial cells scraped from the squamo-columnar junction of the uterine cervix could identify minor cellular changes and lesions, thus allowing for early detection of a malignancy that at the time was frequently fatal. The Pap test rapidly gained currency in many European countries and in the United States and led to the implementation of mass screening programs during the next few decades. The detection of cervical neoplasias through screening along with appropriate follow-up and treatment is still the foundation of cervical cancer control.

Although the efficacy of Pap testing has never been evaluated experimentally, compelling evidence has come from examination of the notable declines in incidence and mortality where widespread screening has been initiated (Sigurdsson, 1999). Despite notable successes in previous decades, the proportion of U.S. women who report having received a recent Pap test (approximately 67%) has not improved since 1993 (Commonwealth Fund, 1999); this proportion is considerably lower for low-income and some minority women.

The Pap test long has been considered to be an accurate screening tool. However, in the mid-1980s there began to be widespread concern about the potential for a high false negative rate (Kiviat *et al.*, 1999; Linder, 1997). The accuracy of screening results was found to vary substantially, due to specimen adequacy, varying interpretation of results, and, later, the need to note signs of HPV infection (Linder, 1997; Cannistra & Niloff, 1996). This has led to exploration of new screening technologies and quality assurance procedures (Kiviat *et al.*, 1999; Linder, 1997; Mitchell *et al.*, 1996).

These concerns prompted a re-evaluation of the classification of cervical specimens. A new classification schema called the Bethesda system was introduced in 1988 (Nguyen & Nordqvist, 1999) with the objectives to standardize Pap test reporting and make classification and reporting of cervical samples simpler, more complete, and better reflect biological processes. In this schema, the term "squamous intraepithelial lesion" is used to denote premalignant epithelial changes; these are further classified as low-grade squamous intraepithelial lesions (LSIL) (previously CIN 1, and abnormalities with evidence of HPV); and high-grade squamous intraepithelial lesions (HSIL) (previously classified as CIN II and III). In addition, a new category of lower-grade lesions was created, atypical squamous cells of undetermined significance (ASCUS). A similar category, atypical glandular changes of undetermined significance (AGCUS) was created for glandular cell abnormalities. These latter categories have become controversial in the intervening years, as the proportion of samples receiving this classification has soared. Understanding of the significance of these lesions and clear guidance on how to manage them are lacking.

In sum, there have been notable declines in cervical cancer incidence and mortality in the United States over the past several decades. An important etiologic agent has been identified, as well as several other potentially modifiable behavioral risk factors. Screening for cervical cancer is also undergoing improvement. Nonetheless, the incidence and mortality rates in the United States continue to belie the prevention potential of this malignancy.

PRIMARY PREVENTION

Primary prevention has not been a predominant intervention approach, despite consistent evidence that some modifiable risk factors, as well as a sexually transmitted pathogen increase women's risk for cervical cancer. Interventions to promote delayed sexual debut, use of barrier contraceptives, limiting sexual partners and smoking cessation have proliferated over the past decades, but few have linked these behaviors to cervical cancer prevention.

The few interventions that have emphasized primary prevention of cervical cancer have been in the area of smoking cessation. One such intervention provided written self-help guides and telephone counseling to women smokers who were seeking cervical cancer screening in a large managed care organization (McBride, Scholes, Grothaus, Curry, Ludman, & Albright, 1999). Rates of cessation were compared for women who received this minimal intervention approach and those who were randomized to receive usual care. The written intervention materials informed women smokers that nicotine metabolites could be found in cervical mucus and that these constituents were likely factors underlying the occurrence of abnormal pap smears. Results at 3- and 12-month follow-ups indicated no difference between usual care and intervention groups. However, interviews suggested that women were not convinced of the link between cervical cancer and smoking because they had not heard about this association from their providers. This skepticism may have been reinforced by how few providers discussed smoking cessation during routine health visits (only 58% as reported by this sample) (McBride, Scholes, Grothaus, Curry, & Albright, 1998). In a similar intervention, Rimer and colleagues provided feedback of the level of cotinine in cervical mucus to motivate women smokers to consider cessation. Unfortunately, the logistical difficulties inherent in giving timely feedback of test results compromised delivery of the intervention. Future interventions may do well to enlist providers to give messages about the role of cigarette smoking in the development of cervical cancer. Biomarker feedback or other methods to increase women's awareness of cervical exposure to carcinogens resulting from cigarette smoking also might increase the efficacy of these interventions (Audrain, Gritz, Rimer, Emmons, Lerman, & Orleans, 1994).

SECONDARY PREVENTION

Secondary prevention in the form of screening for premalignant cervical abnormalities using the Pap test has been the dominant cervical cancer prevention strategy. Intervention approaches have had two primary foci: (1) encouraging screening among underscreened groups (some minority groups, older, rural, and low-income women), and (2) promoting adherence to follow-up recommendations for cervical abnormalities/lesions. These approaches have focused on health care system "in reach" strategies and on proactive outreach strategies to encourage women to seek screening at recommended intervals and to encourage requisite follow-up of abnormal results. In both instances, these approaches have been developed primarily to address the psychological and system barriers that impede compliance.

This section will summarize the problems of underscreening and nonadherence to recommended follow-up, as well as the related psychological and system barriers. The section will conclude with an overview of the intervention approaches that have been evaluated to promote screening and follow-up and the personal stories of two women diagnosed with cervical cancer.

Barriers to Screening

As noted earlier, about one third of women have not had a Pap test in the recommended one-to-three year interval (Commonwealth Fund, 1999). Older women, those with low income, the uninsured, and some minority groups (e.g., Hispanic and Southeast Asian) have the lowest annual screening rates and go for longer intervals without screening. Reported barriers to cervical cancer screening have been consistent across a broad array of studies and populations. These include having inadequate access to health care, lack of awareness of the importance of screening, aversion to the discomforts of screening, fear of finding cancer, and logistical barriers such as having to take time off work for screening (Lantz, Stencil, Lippert, Beversdorf, Jaros, & Remington, 1995; Mamon, Shediac, Crosby, Sanders, Matanoski, & Celentano, 1990; Paskett, White, Carter, & Chu, 1990).

Other system factors also may be related to screening participation. Women who report relying on provider recommendation for Pap screening are more likely to be underscreened than women who know how often and why Pap testing should be done. Moreover, the low screening rates among older women who have been seen by their providers suggest that there also may be provider bias in referral for and in opportunistic conduct of screening (Mamon *et al.*, 1990).

Barriers to Follow-up of Abnormal Results

Prompt treatment of cervical lesions is a critical component of secondary prevention. Unfortunately, up to half of women fail to return for care (Marcus *et al.*, 1992; Stewart, Buchegger, Lickrish, & Sierra, 1994). Treatment of low-grade abnormalities usually entails outpatient procedures including repeat Pap smear, colposcopy, cervical biopsy, endocervical curettage, and/or cryosurgery. Later stage disease requires more invasive treatments such as conization of the cervix, hysterectomy, chemotherapy, and/or radiation therapy.

A number of barriers have been associated with nonadherence. Inadequate access to health care has been shown to decrease the likelihood that women will seek follow-up (Paskett *et al.*, 1990). Structural features of the health care system in which follow-up examinations and treatment occur in locations other than the primary care facility may further increase the logistical challenges of seeking follow-up (Kaplan, Bastani, Marcus, Breslow, Nasseri, & Chen, 1995). Moreover, psychological reactions including fear or worry about finding cervical cancer and treatment effects, discomfort or embarrassment, related sleep and mood disturbances, all have been associated with the notification of abnormal results, and may decrease willingness to seek follow-up (Lerman, Miller, Scarborough, Hanjani, Nolte, & Smith, 1991; Paskett *et al.*, 1990). Other knowledge-related factors including a lack of understanding of the meaning of abnormal results and the purpose of follow-up increased nonadherence in one study (Paskett *et al.*, 1990). Similarly, in another

study, 50% of patients indicated that they did not understand the purpose of the follow-up visit (Lerman *et al.*, 1992), and in some cases women mistakenly thought that the abnormal result meant that they already had cervical cancer (Paskett *et al.*, 1990). Some studies have suggested that these reactions may be associated with women's attentional style (Miller, Roussi, Altman, Helm, & Steinberg, 1994). Women who display a high degree of vigilance toward threatening cues (called "monitors") may experience stronger reactions than women who avoid or distract themselves from threatening cues ("blunters"). Evidence suggests that social support may buffer concerns and increase adherence particularly among women who have strong emotional reactions to abnormal test results and among African-American women (Crane, 1996).

INTERVENTION APPROACHES TO PROMOTE SCREENING

"In Reach" Health System Approaches

Health care system "in reach" approaches have focused primarily on (1) reminder systems or other prompts to women patients who are due for screening and/or their providers; and (2) systems to encourage providers to conduct opportunistic screening during unrelated visits.

Reminder systems that encourage patients to schedule Pap screening visits or prompt providers to recommend screening for their patients have had limited success (Burack *et al.*, 1998; Shea, DuMouchel, & Bahamonde, 1996). A meta-analysis of 16 randomized controlled trials showed that, in contrast to breast and colorectal cancer screening, computerized reminder systems resulted in no improvement in cervical cancer screening rates (odds ratio (OR) = 1.15, 95% confidence intervals (CI) = .89–1.49) (Shea *et al.*, 1996). Similarly, while Lantz and colleagues reported a significant increase in the proportion of women who received all needed cancer screening tests (i.e., both mammography and cervical screening) there was no individual impact on women who were in need of cervical screening alone (Lantz *et al.*, 1995). Endorsement by women's personal provider has been shown to increase the effectiveness of reminders (Bowman, Sanson-Fisher, Boyle, Pope, & Redman, 1995). Women who had not received a Pap test in the prior three years and who were randomized to receive a letter from their general practitioner were almost twice as likely to seek screening as women who received usual care, a general invitation or a pamphlet that described the importance of screening.

The limited success of reminder systems may be because these approaches do not help women overcome system-related barriers or their fears and other concerns about screening. Personalizing these approaches may increase them. Outreach telephone calls to offer barrier specific counseling and assistance with appointment scheduling increased the effectiveness of a reminder system (Lantz *et al.*, 1995). The mailed reminder and follow-up telephone call was seven times more effective in getting women to receive needed Pap screening than usual care. Innovative tailored reminder systems including birthday cards and newsletters (Rimer *et al.*, in press) to encourage compliance are also promising.

More comprehensive and linked systems also may increase rates of screening. Ansell and colleagues evaluated a conceptually based screening program set up to address both personal and system barriers to breast and cervical cancer screening (Ansell, Lacey, Whitman, Chen, & Phillips, 1994). Their program included computer tracking, free screening, follow-up care, active recruitment, and 20-minute informational sessions to increase knowledge about the importance of screening that was administered by culturally aware nurses. Screening history was recorded in a computerized management system that stored dates of tests and appointments. At follow-up, women reported significant increases in knowledge, 86% of women who were prompted by letter received an exam within two months, and 70% of those in need of follow-up for an abnormal result received appropriate care. National programs such as the National Breast and Cervical Cancer Early De-

tection Program have instituted similar comprehensive screening programs in 35 states and 9 American Indian tribes (Henson, Wyatt, & Lee, 1996). This program has addressed many of the barriers to low-income and underscreened women by underwriting costs, providing referrals for medical treatment of abnormalities, and disseminating public information and education. Participation rates resulting from these programs look promising—particularly for minority women—but rigorous evaluation of these activities has not been undertaken.

Approaches such as opportunistic screening as patients come into contact with the health care system have increased screening rates. Ward and colleagues (Ward, Boyle, Redman, & Sanson-Fisher, 1991) evaluated a minimal and a maximal intervention aimed at providers and patients. In both conditions, providers advised women of the need for Pap screening and offered to perform it during the current visit. Those who consented were screened immediately. In the minimal condition, providers suggested that women who declined screening should schedule an appointment within one week. In the maximal condition, providers attempted to persuade women who declined of the importance of Pap screening, and explore women's personal barriers. While both interventions were equally effective, providers were significantly less likely to use the maximal than the minimal approach, even though the maximal intervention on average required only 91 seconds. Older women were most likely to accept opportunistic screening. Similarly, in another study, older African-American women were approached in the waiting room and offered cervical cancer screening. Of the women approached, 71% agreed to participate, of whom 92% chose to be screened immediately (Mandelblatt *et al.*, 1993). However, one-third of the women who were subsequently referred for abnormal results did not return for follow-up care.

In summary, invitation or prompting systems by themselves are not effective in encouraging women with significant barriers to seek screening. Intervention components that allow for personalization and that address women's barriers have the greatest chance to be effective. Comprehensive health-system-based approaches may have the greatest impact on screening. However, as has been acknowledged for other screening behaviors, conceptually based interventions that consider the complex interplay of individual and system factors are needed (Curry, & Emmons, 1994).

Finally, a significant limitation to these "in reach" approaches is that they do not reach uninsured women. Larger societal actions and targeted outreach will be required to include this important target group.

Outreach Approaches

Intervention strategies to increase screening also have been conducted outside of health care settings. The majority of these interventions have relied on lay health advisors who reach out to women in a defined community to provide information and assistance in overcoming cultural and logistical barriers to screening. Lay health advisor interventions have been developed for diverse populations, that include Middle Eastern and East African (McAvoy & Raza, 1991), Southeast Asian (Bird, McPhee, Ha, Le, Davis, & Jenkins, 1998), Native American (Dignan et al., 1996; Hodge, Fredericks, & Rodriguez, 1996), Hispanic (Navarro, Senn, McNicholas, Kaplan, Roppe, & Campo, 1998), inner-city African-American (Sung, Blumenthal, Coates, Williams, Alema-Mensah, & Liff, 1997), and White (Margolis, Lurie, McGovern, Tyrrell, & Slater, 1998) women. Health advisors have included community peers (Navarro et al., 1998; Sung et al., 1997), traditional healers (Hodge et al., 1996), and mainstream health professionals (McAvoy & Raza, 1991). Health advisors generally visit women individually in their own homes (McAvoy & Raza, 1991) or in group meetings at homes and in neighborhood centers (Hodge et al., 1996; Navarro et al., 1998). The majority of these interventions consist of a single visit that typically includes an educational presentation, written pamphlets, and/ or videos depicting Pap screening procedures,

all conveyed in the native language of the community. However, at least one intervention included three visits by a lay health worker (Sung et al., 1997) and others have included health fairs and financial incentives (Bird et al., 1998).

Outreach interventions have had the greatest success in increasing Pap screening rates among white women with low income (Margolis et al., 1998), Hispanic, Asian, and Native American women (Dignan et al., 1996), with notably less success among African-American women (Margolis et al., 1998; Sung, et al., 1997). The cost of these interventions and the feasibility of permanently incorporating lay advisors into communities has yet to be evaluated. Other widely used outreach approaches such as telephone counseling that have shown great promise in other areas of behavior change (McBride & Rimer, 1999) have been used less often to promote cervical cancer screening.

Media-based strategies to promote cervical cancer screening also have not been used widely. However, the few studies conducted indicate that culturally sensitive radio announcements can reach important target groups and promote screening (Mitchell, Hirst, Mitchell, Staples, & Torcello, 1997; Yancey & Walden, 1994). One encouraging example is an Australian study (Mitchell et al., 1997) that developed and evaluated the impact of ethnically tailored radio announcements to encourage yearly Pap smears. The announcements made in 11 languages gave a telephone number of an interpreter for women who needed further information. Results indicated that women who were living in the target neighborhoods were significantly more likely to seek screening than women in the comparison group. Another small case study (Yancey & Walden, 1994) following the use of a video to promote screening among Hispanic women also showed promising results. After the video was shown at a community meeting of 27 Hispanic women, word-of-mouth dissemination resulted in over 100 requests for Pap tests over the next three weeks (Yancey & Walden, 1994). Thus, media-based interventions may have the potential to quickly and efficiently reach specific target groups, and, in turn, increase the likelihood that these women will seek needed screening.

INTERVENTIONS TO PROMOTE ADHERENCE TO FOLLOW-UP

"In Reach" Approaches

Interventions developed to increase adherence to follow-up for abnormal results have been focused primarily on "in reach" approaches directed to (1) all women with abnormal results to prevent nonadherence (Miller, Siejak, Schroeder, Lerman, Hernandez, & Helm, 1997; Paskett et al., 1990; Tomaino-Brunner, Freda, & Runowicz, 1996); or (2) women who have failed to schedule appointments in a recommended time frame or missed appointments (Lerman et al., 1992) (Marcus et al., 1998). These approaches primarily have focused on the evaluation of written educational materials to reassure women about follow-up and on personalized counseling to address individual barriers.

In one study (Tomaino-Brunner, Freda, Damus, & Runowicz, 1998), a one-page handout was sent to minority women patients who were scheduled for colposcopy. The handout mailed, one week prior to the appointment, detailed the reason for the visit and their referral for colposcopy, as well as a description of the procedure and why it was essential. Women receiving this intervention increased their related knowledge but showed no decrease in anxiety levels compared to a control group. A similar approach by Paskett and colleagues (1990) resulted in an increase in rates of follow-up compared to a control condition (OR = 1.7; 95% CI .91–3.20). The effectiveness of similar written interventions has not been increased by framing techniques that differentially emphasize the gains or losses of seeking follow-up treatment (Lauver & Rubin, 1990).

Alternatively, mail and telephone contacts, have been delivered in a triage model. In this approach, initial written reminders and informational brochures are followed by single or serialized telephone counseling contacts for women who fail to make or keep follow-up appointments (Miller et al., 1997). Telephone counseling was associated with a significant increase in adherence to colposcopy when compared to usual care (68% versus 50%) (Miller et al., 1997). Barriers counseling significantly improved adherence rates when compared to simple appointment confirmation (76% versus 68%). Similarly, Lerman and colleagues (1992) found that women who received telephone barriers counseling were almost three times more likely to seek follow-up care than women who received no intervention. A significant increase also was observed in women scheduling a subsequent Pap visit.

Generally, approaches to increase adherence have been more successful than usual care and most successful with women who were married, had high-grade abnormalities, and were nonsmokers (Marcus et al., 1998; Miller et al., 1997; Paskett et al., 1990). Addition of incentives such as travel vouchers have not increased adherence suggesting that other barriers to follow-up may outweigh specific logistical impediments (Marcus et al., 1998).

Appointment reminders, educational brochures and telephone counseling are all relatively low in cost and thus may be feasibly incorporated into existing delivery systems and practice settings. However, evaluating their "real world" sustainability is still lacking.

Underscreening for cervical cancer and nonadherence to follow-up recommendations of abnormal screening results continue to be significant problems for women in the United States. Interventions to promote screening and follow-up, in particular those that have taken a comprehensive multilevel approach by targeting both women's personal barriers and system barriers, and that have tracked compliance, have shown the most promising results. These interventions are consistent with conceptual models of program planning such as the Precede Proceed model (Green & Kreuter, 1991) and Social Cognitive Theory (Baranowski, Perry, & Parcel, 1997) that recommend substantial involvement of the target group and that seek to address multiple levels of influence.

COPING WITH CERVICAL CANCER

Patients with gynecologic cancers and their families experience a high degree of psychological distress in the initial months following the diagnosis that for some, can continue long term (Auchincloss & McCartney, 1998). Cervical cancer and its related treatment have enormous implications for quality of life, fertility, and for broader family and social roles. Evaluation of support services to enhance coping with cancer sequelae is in its infancy. Results from the few services that have been evaluated suggest that they can reduce distress and enhance coping (Nezu, Nezu, & Houts, 1999). More recently, computer-based resources are expanding the reach of support services and helping women overcome access barriers (Gustafson et al., 1993). A number of web sites are currently available (e.g., OncoLink and Center for Cervical Health) that offer information about the disease, link women to other relevant web sites, and provide testimonials from women living with cervical cancer, as well as chat rooms and email options for online support.

The personal stories of two women and their experiences after their diagnosis of cervical cancer can best highlight the personal toll of cervical cancer that will affect over 12,000 women this year.*

These stories emphasize the needed development and evaluation of a broad array of services for women who are coping with the immediate impact of cervical cancer and its long term consequences.

HEALTH POLICY IMPLICATIONS

The current state-of-the-science in the epidemiology of cervical cancer and related interventions have a number of implications for health policy. Primary prevention interventions

---

*The personal profiles are provided courtesy of the OncoLink and Center for Cervical Health web sites—www.oncolink.org and www.cervicalhealth.org.

are not as yet a major focus for cervical cancer prevention, and should receive more emphasis within health care systems, particularly those serving younger and high-risk populations (e.g., Medicaid, high-prevalence communities).

Cervical cancer screening efforts to date have had an enormous public health benefit in the United States. Emphasis on further broadening the availability and use of screening should continue to be a major priority. Morbidity and mortality from cervical cancer continues to be higher in the United States than in countries that have nationally organized health care systems, national screening programs, and centralized registries. Estimates based on a 30-year screening period and 80% participation rate indicate that potential years of life lost due to cervical cancer could be reduced by half and up to 63% (Segnan, 1994). The number of life years gained per 1000 individuals has been estimated at up to 68 years among women in the Netherlands (Segnan, 1994).

The greatest public health challenge and potential for benefit is to increase screening rates among those who have never been screened, who have long intervals between screenings, or who feel they no longer need screening. To this end, public health resources and interventions must continue to be directed to women who are older, have low income, belong to minority groups (in particular newly immigrant women), and those who lack access to health services or have significant barriers to receiving care.

Very few estimates of the cost-effectiveness of different intervention approaches to improve screening rates are available. The few evaluations suggest that appointment-reminder interventions, while more successful in recruiting women to attend screening, may be less marginally cost-effective due to additional staff costs than opportunistic approaches and chart identification (Hyndman, Straton, Pritchard, & Le Sueur, 1996).

While the Pap smear is a relatively inexpensive test, costs to the patient vary widely from $25 to $160 per test (Helms & Melnikow, 1999). This variability is not accounted for by duration of visit, location of practice or spe-

Vignette 1

Margaret, a 45-year-old mother of three young children, was in the midst of an acrimonious divorce when her cancer was diagnosed. At the time, the cancer appeared to be localized. However, because the tumor was fairly large, she received radiation implant treatment prior to surgery to shrink the tumor. Two weeks after the implant, Margaret returned to the hospital for a radical hysterectomy. Surgery showed that the cancer had spread to her lymph nodes. Throughout her two years of treatment and eventual hysterectomy, Margaret wondered whether she was being perceived as someone who was now facing the consequences of her prior sexual behaviors. She coped with this and her fears about the future by relying on the support of her family, coworkers, and the Internet which enabled her to connect with other cancer patients and their families. Margaret, now one-year cancer free, finds herself wondering whether she will have any future intimate relationships.

cialty (Helms & Melnikow, 1999). Public and commercial laboratory costs as well as reimbursement from public and private insurance also vary considerably. Treatment costs differ from setting to setting: the cost of colposcopy can range from $50 to $450 and costs of cryotherapy range from $30 to $280. However, regardless of the estimate, treatment costs for cervical cancer are consistently higher than costs related to prevention.

Recent changes in the classification system for cellular and tissue specimens, while an improvement in many ways, have had important cost implications, as well. The costs of treating low-grade abnormalities (ASCUS and AGCUS) have escalated in recent years with debatable cancer prevention benefit (Kurman, Henson, Herbst, Noller, & Schiffman, 1994). Fully 50 million Pap tests are performed annually in the United States, resulting in an estimated 2.5 million low-grade cervical lesions (Kurman *et al.*, 1994). The estimated cost of clinical management of these low-grade lesions is $6 billion annually (Walsh, 1998). Improved classification and the addition of HPV testing as part of cervical cancer screening have the potential to improve screening accuracy and could result in significant cost savings. Also promising is progress in the development of prophylactic and therapeutic HPV vaccines.

Vignette 2

Elizabeth, a married mother of a young daughter, was diagnosed with advanced cervical cancer in her late thirties. Elizabeth had the standard treatment including a complete hysterectomy followed by radiation and chemotherapy. A major concern for Elizabeth was recovering the health benefits that she lost when she was no longer able to keep her job during her course of treatment and recovery. As a married woman, she has been distressed by changes in the quality of her sex life following the surgery and treatment. She also continues to cope with symptoms that resulted from intensive abdominal radiation including lack of bladder and bowel control and the limits these conditions place on her freedom. She currently is in remission and participating in a clinical trial to evaluate new treatments to prevent the recurrence of her cervical cancer.

340   COLLEEN M. MCBRIDE and DELIA SCHOLES

CONCLUSIONS

Cervical cancer continues to be a significant public health concern in the United States, more so than is observed in other developed countries. This is unfortunate given the availability of a low cost, increasingly reliable screening test that can detect premalignant cellular changes. Current knowledge of the epidemiology of this condition and of the current and emerging detection and treatment modalities allow the possibility of eradicating cervical cancer, currently achievable for few cancers. However, significant challenges remain:

- Promoting screening among under-screened women and adherence to follow-up of abnormal findings through the use of efficacious interventions must be an important public health priority. The needs of under- and uninsured women pose the greatest challenges.
- Primary prevention opportunities are currently underutilized. The relationship between cervical cancer and a highly prevalent sexually transmitted pathogen (HPV) has not been fully exploited by public health interventions. Primary prevention interventions addressing sexual and other modifiable behaviors (smoking, contraception) offer promise for reducing women's risk for other cancers and reproductive health problems as well. These interventions could have particular benefit when targeted to young women who are at greatest risk of contracting HPV. However, raised awareness of the HPV/cervical cancer linkage must be developed with sensitivity to the potential for increasing the stigma of cervical cancer.
- This suggests that one-size-fits-all screening and follow-up interventions do not work. Rather, the system-based or outreach interventions likely to be most effective will involve personal contact, be comprehensive in scope, and involve multiple levels of influence and be based on respected conceptual models. Strategies that show particular promise include lay health counselors, written information and outreach reminder calls to increase understanding of the purpose of screening and follow-up, efforts to reduce a woman's personal barriers to care seeking and

"opportunistic" screening. Recent advances in computer technology and graphical programs offer exciting opportunities to individually customize these interventions.
- Additional evaluation of efforts to sustainably incorporate efficacious intervention approaches into communities or clinical practice settings are needed.
- Further study of optimal follow-up and treatment of the burgeoning numbers of low-grade cervical abnormalities also is needed. These abnormalities not only present considerable cost for health care systems, but substantial psychological costs to women resulting from their uncertain significance.
- Lastly, evaluation of support and other follow-up services for cervical cancer patients are needed. The internet offers exciting opportunities to link women to support networks and provide information and services in the short and long term that have substantial potential benefit to these women and their families.

REFERENCES

American Social Health Association and Kaiser Family Foundation (1998). American Social Health Association.

Ansell, D., Lacey, L., Whitman, S., Chen, E., & Phillips, C. (1994). A nurse-delivered intervention to reduce barriers to breast and cervical cancer screening in Chicago inner city clinics. *Public Health Reports, 109*, 104–111.

Auchincloss, S. S., & McCartney, C. F. (1998). Gynecologic cancer. In J. C. Holland & W. Breitbart (Eds.), *Psycho-oncology*. New York: Oxford University Press.

Audrain, J., Gritz, E., Rimer, B., Emmons, K., Lerman, C., & Orleans, T. (1994). Biomarkers in smoking cessation treatment. *Annals of Behavioral Medicine, 16*, 39.

Baranowski, T., Perry, C. L., & Parcel, G. S. (1997). How individuals, environments, and health behavior interact: Social cognitive theory. In K. Glanz, F. M. Lewis, & B. K. Rimer (Eds.), *Health behavior and health education* (pp. 153–178). San Francisco: Jossey-Bass.

Becker, T. M., Wheeler, C. M., McGough, N. S., Parmenter, C. A., Jordan, S. W., Stidley, C. A., McPherson, R. S., & Dorin, M. H. (1994). Sexually transmitted diseases and other risk factors for cervical dysplasia among southwestern Hispanic and non-Hispanic white women. *Journal of the American Medical Association, 271*, 1181–1188.

Bird, J. A., McPhee, S. J., Ha, N. T., Le, B., Davis, T., & Jenkins, C. N. (1998). Opening pathways to cancer screening for Vietnamese-American women: Lay health workers hold a key. *Preventive Medicine*, *27*, 821–829.

Bowman, J., Sanson-Fisher, R., Boyle, C., Pope, S., & Redman, S. (1995). A randomised controlled trial of strategies to prompt attendance for a Pap smear. *Journal of Medical Screening*, *2*, 211–218.

Burack, R. C., Gimotty, P. A., George, J., McBride, S., Moncrease, A., Simon, M. S., Dews, P., & Coombs, J. (1998). How reminders given to patients and physicians affected pap smear use in a health maintenance organization: Results of a randomized controlled trial. *Cancer*, *82*, 2391–2400.

Cannistra, S. A., & Niloff, J. M. (1996). Cancer of the uterine cervix. *New England Journal of Medicine*, *334*, 1030–1038.

Commonwealth Fund (1999). *Health concerns across a woman's lifespan: The Commonwealth Fund 1998 survey of women's health*.

Crane, L. A. (1996). Social support and adherence behavior among women with abnormal Pap smears. *Journal of Cancer Education*, *11*, 164–173.

Curry, S. J., & Emmons, K. M. (1994). Theoretical models for predicting and improving compliance with cancer screening. *Annals of Behavioral Medicine*, *16*, 302–316.

Daling, J. R., Madeleine, M. M., McKnight, B., Carter, J. J., Wipf, G. C., Ashley, R., Schwartz, S. M., Beckmann, A. M., Hagensee, M. E., Mandelson, M. T., & Galloway, D. A. (1996). The relationship of human papillomavirus-related cervical tumors to cigarette smoking, oral contraceptive use, and prior herpes simplex virus type 2 infection. *Cancer Epidemiology, Biomarkers & Prevention*, *5*, 541–548.

Dignan, M., Michielutte, R., Blinson, K., Wells, H. B., Case, L. D., Sharp, P., Davis, S., Konen, J., & McQuellon, R. P. (1996). Effectiveness of health education to increase screening for cervical cancer among eastern-band Cherokee Indian women in North Carolina. *Journal of the National Cancer Institute*, *88*, 1670–1676.

Green, L. W., & Kreuter, M. W. (1991). *Health promotion planning: An educational and environmental approach*. Mountain View: Mayfield.

Gustafson, D., Wise, M., McTavish, F., Taylor, J., Smalley, R., Wolberg, W., & Stewart, J. (1993). Development and pilot evaluation of a computer based support system for women with breast cancer. *Journal of Psychosocial Oncology*, *11*, 69–93.

Helms, L. J., & Melnikow, J. (1999). Determining costs of health care services for cost-effectiveness analyses: The case of cervical cancer prevention and treatment. *Medical Care*, *37*, 652–661.

Henson, R. M., Wyatt, S. W., & Lee, N. C. (1996). The National Breast and Cervical Cancer Early Detection Program: A comprehensive public health response to two major health issues for women. *Journal of Public Health Management Practice*, *2*, 36–47.

Hodge, F. S., Fredericks, L., & Rodriguez, B. (1996). American Indian women's talking circle. A cervical cancer screening and prevention project. *Cancer*, *78*, 1592–1597.

Hyndman, J. C. G., Straton, J. A. Y., Pritchard, D. A., & Le Sueur, H. (1996). Cost-effectiveness of interventions to promote cervical screening in general practice. *Australian and New Zealand Journal of Public Health*, *20*, 272–277.

Kaplan, C. P., Bastani, R., Marcus, A., Breslow, L., Nasseri, K., & Chen, L. (1995). Low-income women with cervical abnormalities: Individual and system factors affecting follow-up. *Journal of Women's Health*, *4*, 179–188.

Kiviat, N., Koutsky, L. A., & Paavonen, J. (1999). Cervical neoplasia and other STD-related genital tract neoplasias. In K. K. Holmes, P.-A. Mardh, P. F. Sparling, S. M. Lemon, W. E. Stamm, P. Piot, & J. N. Wasserheit (Eds.), *Sexually transmitted diseases* (pp. 811–832) New York: McGraw-Hill.

Koutsky, L. (1997). Epidemiology of genital human papillomavirus infection. *American Journal of Medicine*, *102*, 3–8.

Kurman, R. J., Henson, D. E., Herbst, A. L., Noller, K. L., & Schiffman, M. H. (1994). Interim guidelines for management of abnormal cervical cytology. The 1992 National Cancer Institute Workshop. *Journal of the American Medical Association*, *271*, 1866–1869.

Lantz, P. M., Stencil, D., Lippert, M. T., Beversdorf, S., Jaros, L., & Remington, P. L. (1995). Breast and cervical cancer screening in a low-income managed care sample: The efficacy of physician letters and phone calls. *American Journal of Public Health*, *85*, 834–836.

Lauver, D., & Rubin, M. (1990). Message framing, dispositional optimism, and follow-up for abnormal Papanicolaou tests. *Research in Nursing & Health*, *13*, 199–207.

Lerman, C., Hanjani, P., Caputo, C., Miller, S., Delmoor, E., Nolte, S., & Engstrom, P. (1992). Telephone counseling improves adherence to colposcopy among lower-income minority women. *Journal of Clinical Oncology*, *10*, 330–333.

Lerman, C., Miller, S. M., Scarborough, R., Hanjani, P., Nolte, S., & Smith, D. (1991). Adverse psychologic consequences of positive cytologic cervical screening. *American Journal of Obstetrics & Gynecology*, *165*, 658–662.

Linder, J. (1997). A decade has passed.... The Pap smear and cervical cancer. *American Journal of Clinical Pathology*, *108*, 492–498.

Lowy, D. R., & Schiller, J. T. (1999). Papillomaviruses: Prophylactic vaccine prospects. *Biochimica et Biophysica Acta*, *1423*, M1–8.

Mamon, J. A., Shediac, M. C., Crosby, C. B., Sanders, B., Matanoski, G. M., & Celentano, D. D. (1990). Innercity women at risk for cervical cancer: Behavioral and utilization factors related to inadequate screening. *Preventive Medicine*, *19*, 363–376.

Mandelblatt, J., Traxler, M., Lakin, P., Kanetsky, P., Thomas, L., Chauhan, P., Matseoane, S., & Ramsey, E. (1993). Breast and cervical cancer screening of poor, elderly, black women: Clinical results and implications. Harlem Study Team. *American Journal of Preventive Medicine, 9*, 133–138.

Marcus, A. C., Crane, L. A., Kaplan, C. P., Reading, A. E., Savage, E., Gunning, J., Bernstein, G., & Berek, J. S. (1992). Improving adherence to screening follow-up among women with abnormal Pap smears: Results from a large clinic-based trial of three intervention strategies. *Medical Care, 30*, 216–230.

Marcus, A. C., Kaplan, C. P., Crane, L. A., Berek, J. S., Bernstein, G., Gunning, J. E., & McClatchey, M. W. (1998). Reducing loss-to-follow-up among women with abnormal Pap smears. Results from a randomized trial testing an intensive follow-up protocol and economic incentives. *Medical Care, 36*, 397–410.

Margolis, K. L., Lurie, N., McGovern, P. G., Tyrrell, M., & Slater, J. S. (1998). Increasing breast and cervical cancer screening in low-income women. *Journal of General Internal Medicine, 13*, 515–521.

McAvoy, B. R., & Raza, R. (1991). Can health education increase uptake of cervical smear testing among Asian women? *British Medical Journal, 302*, 833–836.

McBride, C. M., & Rimer, B. K. (1999). Using the telephone to improve health behavior and health service delivery. *Patient Education and Counseling, 37*, 3–18.

McBride, C. M., Scholes, D., Grothaus, L., Curry, S. J., & Albright, J. (1998). Promoting smoking cessation among women who seek cervical cancer screening. *Obstetrics & Gynecology, 91*, 719–724.

McBride, C. M., Scholes, D., Grothaus, L. C., Curry, S. J., Ludman, E., & Albright, J. (1999). Evaluation of a minimal self-help smoking cessation intervention following cervical cancer screening. *Preventive Medicine, 29*, 133–138.

Miller, S. M., Roussi, P., Altman, D., Helm, W., & Steinberg, A. (1994). Effects of coping style on psychological reactions of low-income, minority women to colposcopy. *Journal of Reproductive Medicine, 39*, 711–718.

Miller, S. M., Siejak, K. K., Schroeder, C. M., Lerman, C., Hernandez, E., & Helm, C. W. (1997). Enhancing adherence following abnormal Pap smears among low-income minority women: A preventive telephone counseling strategy. *Journal of the National Cancer Institute, 89*, 703–708.

Mitchell, H., Hirst, S., Mitchell, J. A., Staples, M., & Torcello, N. (1997). Effect of ethnic media on cervical cancer screening rates. *Australian & New Zealand Journal of Public Health, 21*, 265–267.

Mitchell, M. F., Tortolero-Luna, G., Wright, T., Sarkar, A., Richards-Kortum, R., Hong, W. K., & Schottenfeld, D. (1996). Cervical human papillomavirus infection and intraepithelial neoplasia: A review. *Journal of the National Cancer Institute, Monographs*, 17–25.

Navarro, A. M., Senn, K. L., McNicholas, L. J., Kaplan, R.

M., Roppe, B., & Campo, M. C. (1998). Por La Vida model intervention enhances use of cancer screening tests among Latinas. *American Journal of Preventive Medicine, 15*, 32–41.

Negrini, B. P., Schiffman, M. H., Kurman, R. J., Barnes, W., Lannom, L., Malley, K., Brinton, L. A., Delgado, G., Jones, S., & Tchabo, J. G. (1990). Oral contraceptive use, human papillomavirus infection, and risk of early cytological abnormalities of the cervix. *Cancer Research, 50*, 4670–4675.

Nezu, C. M., Nezu, C. M., & Houts, P. S. (1999). Relevance of problem-solving therapy to psychosocial oncology. *Journal of Psychosocial Oncology, 16*, 5–26.

Nguyen, H. N., & Nordqvist, S. R. (1999). The Bethesda system and evaluation of abnormal pap smears. *Seminars in Surgical Oncology, 16*, 217–221.

Parker, S. L., Davis, K. J., Wingo, P. A., Ries, L. A., & Heath, C. W., Jr. (1998). Cancer statistics by race and ethnicity. *CA: A Cancer Journal for Clinicians, 48*, 31–48.

Parkin, D. M. (1998). Epidemiology of cancer: Global patterns and trends. *Toxicology Letters, 102–103*, 227–234.

Paskett, E. D., White, E., Carter, W. B., & Chu, J. (1990). Improving follow-up after an abnormal Pap smear: A randomized controlled trial. *Preventive Medicine, 19*, 630–641.

Ponten, J., Adami, H. O., Bergstrom, R., Dillner, J., Friberg, L. G., Gustafsson, L., Miller, A. B., Parkin, D. M., Sparen, P., & Trichopoulos, D. (1995). Strategies for global control of cervical cancer. *International Journal of Cancer, 60*, 1–26.

Rimer, B. K., Conaway, M., Lyna, P., Glassman, B., Yarnall, K., Lipkus, I. M., & Barber, T. (in press). The impact of tailored interventions on a community health center population. *Patient Education and Counseling*.

Schiffman, M. H., & Brinton, L. A. (1995). The epidemiology of cervical carcinogenesis. *Cancer, 76*, 1888–1901.

Schoell, W. M., Janicek, M. F., & Mirhashemi, R. (1999). Epidemiology and biology of cervical cancer. *Seminars in Surgical Oncology, 16*, 203–211.

Segnan, N. (1994). Cervical cancer screening. Human benefits and human costs in the evaluation of screening programmes. *European Journal of Cancer, 30A*, 873–875.

Shea, S., DuMouchel, W., & Bahamonde, L. (1996). A meta-analysis of 16 randomized controlled trials to evaluate computer-based clinical reminder systems for preventive the ambulatory setting. *Journal of the American Medical Informatics Association, 3*, 399–409.

Sigurdsson, K. (1999). Cervical cancer, Pap smear and HPV testing: An update of the role of organized Pap smear screening and HPV testing. *Acta Obstetrica et Gynecologica Scandinavica, 78*, 467–477.

Stewart, D. E., Buchegger, P. M., Lickrish, G. M., & Sierra, S. (1994). The effect of educational brochures on follow-up compliance in women with abnormal Papanicolaou smears. *Obstetrics & Gynecology, 83*, 583–585.

Sung, J. F., Blumenthal, D. S., Coates, R. J., Williams, J.

E., Alema-Mensah, E., & Liff, J. M. (1997). Effect of a cancer screening intervention conducted by lay health workers among inner-city women. *American Journal of Preventive Medicine, 13*, 51–57.

Tomaino-Brunner, C., Freda, M. C., Damus, K., & Runowicz, C. D. (1998). Can precolposcopy education increase knowledge and decrease anxiety? *Journal of Obstetric, Gynecologic, & Neonatal Nursing, 27*, 636–645.

Tomaino-Brunner, C., Freda, M. C., & Runowicz, C. D. (1996). "I hope I don't have cancer:" Colposcopy and minority women. *Oncology Nursing Forum, 23*, 39–44.

Walsh, J. M. (1998). Cervical cancer: Developments in screening and evaluation of the abnormal Pap smear. *Western Journal of Medicine, 169*, 304–310.

Ward, J. E., Boyle, K., Redman, S., & Sanson-Fisher, R. W. (1991). Increasing women's compliance with opportunistic cervical cancer screening: A randomized trial. *American Journal of Preventive Medicine, 7*, 285–291.

Yancey, A. K., & Walden, L. (1994). Stimulating cancer screening among Latinas and African-American women. A community case study. *Journal of Cancer Education, 9*, 46–52.

18

Breast Cancer

ROBERT A. SMITH and DEBBIE SASLOW

INTRODUCTION

Although incidence and mortality rates vary greatly in the world's regions, breast cancer is the most common cancer diagnosed among women in the world, representing 21% of all newly diagnosed cases in 1990. Among women, breast cancer also is the most common cause of death from cancer (Parkin & P. Pisani, 1999). With few exceptions, the highest age-standardized incidence rates in the world are found in developed countries, and the lowest rates are in less developed countries (see Table 1). Although age-standardized incidence rates have been relatively stable in the United States in recent years (Ries *et al.*, 2000a), rates in most other countries have been increasing, and this is especially true in developing nations. According to a recent report, the world incidence of breast cancer is projected to be 1.45 million new cases in 2010, an 82% increase over 1990 incidence estimates (Parkin & P. Pisani, 1999). Breast cancer also occurs in men, but is very rare by comparison. In the United States, annual incidence among men is less than one percent of the incidence among women (Greenlee, Murray, Bolden, & Wingo, 2000).

ROBERT A. SMITH and DEBBIE SASLOW • American Cancer Society, Atlanta, Georgia 30329

Handbook of Women's Sexual and Reproductive Health, edited by Wingood and DiClemente. Kluwer Academic / Plenum Publishers, New York, 2002.

Because the incidence of breast cancer begins to increase relatively early in adult life, and because of social and cultural considerations, it is among women's greatest health concerns. However, in the last two decades there has been considerable progress in breast cancer control. Today we have a better understanding about factors associated with the etiology of breast cancer (Henderson, Pike, Bernstein, & Ross, 1996), and there have been advances in estimating lifetime risk according to various breast cancer risk profiles (National Cancer Institute, 1999a; Rockhill, Weinberg, & Newman, 1998). There has been progress in our understanding of the role of family history as a risk factor for breast cancer, which based on the age at diagnosis and number of first degree relatives may contribute little excess risk, or a lifetime risk greater than 50% if a woman has inherited a mutation in a breast cancer susceptibility gene. For women with a family history suggestive of heritable breast cancer, guidelines for counseling and testing have been developed and are widely endorsed by leading medical organizations (American Society of Clinical Oncology, 1996). Several decades of intensive research has shown convincingly that early detection of breast cancer with mammography is associated with a significantly improved prognosis (Shapiro *et al.*, 1998; Tabar, Dean, Duffy, & Chen, 2000; Tabar *et al.*, 1985). The availability and utilization of mammography in the United States is high, and outside the United States the

TABLE 1. Incidence of Breast
Cancer in Females by World Region

Country	Rate per 100,000
North America	86.30
Australia/New Zealand	71.69
Northern Europe	68.31
Southern Europe	49.51
Eastern Europe	35.95
Southern Africa	31.46
Japan	28.61
Southeastern Asia	22.51
Western Africa	19.02
Other Eastern Asia	17.85
China	11.77

Source. Parkin, Pisani, & Ferlay (1999). Global cancer statistics. *CA Cancer Journal for Clinicians, 49,* 33–64.
Note. Age standardized incidence rates are calculated using the weights of the world standard population.

number of countries offering organized screening programs is increasing. Over time there also has been progress in treatment, including evolution in surgical approaches from the disfiguring radical mastectomy to breast conserving therapy, and continual evolution in the use of radiation, adjuvant therapy, and chemotherapy (Morrow & Harris, 2000). Progress in treatment and trends toward a more favorable stage at diagnosis means that women now have more treatment options, and decisions about treatment also may be influenced by progress in breast reconstruction for women who choose a mastectomy (Fine, Mustoe, & Fenner, 2000). Finally, there is better understanding today that the needs of breast cancer patients go beyond the initial course of clinical therapy and should include attention to women's psychosocial needs. It is in this area that our understanding of the challenges and needs of breast cancer patients has not been paralleled by either an availability or an appreciation for the importance of access to supportive care services (Ganz, 1995; Lee, 1997).

This chapter will focus on the descriptive epidemiology of breast cancer, and psychosocial aspects of breast cancer among women with and without the disease. Unless noted, all subsequent material pertains to female breast cancer in the United States.

DESCRIPTIVE EPIDEMIOLOGY

Breast cancer constitutes a heterogeneous group of disease subtypes that arise in the mammary gland. Breast cancer arises within breast tissue, which consists of 15 to 20 lobes. Each lobe is made up of lobules, which in turn consist of grape-like clusters of milk-secreting glands called alveoli. A branching system of ducts serves to drain milk from the milk-producing alveoli to the nipple. The breast parenchyma is interspersed and surrounded by fat and connective tissues. Most breast cancer is referred to as infiltrating ductal breast cancer because the malignancy arises within the branching ductal system and becomes invasive when it spreads from the ducts to the surrounding structures. The utilization of mammography also has led to the detection of ductal carcinoma *in situ* (DCIS), which is uncommonly palpable and therefore is usually detected when an abnormal sign suggestive of breast cancer is identified on a mammogram. DCIS is regarded as an uncertain, but potential precursor to invasive disease. DCIS usually is treated in a manner similar to minimal breast cancer (Page & Jensen, 1996).

Estimates of Disease Burden

According to current incidence and mortality estimates, in a hypothetical cohort of U.S. women approximately 1 in 8 will be diagnosed with breast cancer in her lifetime, and 1 in 30 will die from this disease (Ries *et al.*, 2000a). Excluding cancers of the skin, invasive breast cancer is the most frequently diagnosed malignancy among U.S women, accounting for nearly one in three new diagnoses of cancer. According to estimates from the American Cancer Society, 182,800 women would be diagnosed with invasive breast cancer, an additional 42,600 women would be diagnosed with DCIS, and 40,800 women would die from breast cancer in 2000 (Greenlee *et al.*, 2000).

Trends in Incidence and Mortality

When evaluating long-term trends, or comparing rates between different populations, cancer rates are commonly age-adjusted to remove the potential influence that differing age distributions within or between populations. Since the U.S. population is aging, long-term trends in crude rates can be expected to increase on that basis alone. Thus, in order to evaluate the underlying epidemiology of breast cancer, aggregate rates are generally age-adjusted. The long-term trend in the age-adjusted incidence of breast cancer is distinguished by two markedly different periods. Incidence data from Connecticut (available since 1935), five geographic regions (from 1950 to 1985), and data from 1973 to 1980 from the NCI's Surveillance, Epidemiology, and End Results Program (SEER) show a gradual annual increase between the mid-1930s and the early 1980s in the age-adjusted incidence rate of invasive breast cancer of about 1% per year (Devesa *et al.*, 1987). However, between 1980 and 1987, the age-adjusted incidence rate of breast cancer increased from 85.0 to 112.3 new cases per 100,000 women, a relative increase over the period of 32%, or an average increase of approximately 4% per year (Figure 1). Since 1987, when age-adjusted incidence rates peaked, the incidence rate has remained relatively stable and ranged between 106.6 new cases (1989) to 115.8 new cases (1997) per 100,000 women.

The incidence of breast cancer increases with age (Figure 2). The diagnosis of breast cancer is rare before age 30, accounting for only an estimated 700 cases in 2000, which is about 0.4% of the total estimated cases for that year (American Cancer Society Surveillance Program, 2000). After age 30, the proportionate increase in incidence rates is rapid. Between age 30 and 44, the incidence rate of breast cancer approximately doubles in each successive five-year age group. Between age 44 and 54, the rate of increase declines and the age-incidence curve becomes less steep. After age 55, age-specific rates continue to increase at a steady, but less dramatic rate, and peak at age 75 (Ries *et al.*, 2000a).

During the past two decades, a growing appreciation for the prognostic benefit of early breast cancer detection and a growing awareness of the capability of mammography to detect occult breast cancer has resulted in a significant increase in the proportion of women who have ever had a mammogram (MMWR, 1996). Earlier age-specific trends (also shown in Figure 2 for the period 1978–1981) show the pattern of age-specific incidence before the widespread use of mammography. Prior to the most recent period, the age-specific incidence rate was higher with each successive age group. The most recent distribution of age-specific incidence rates (1993–1997) shows a peak in rates for women at ages 75–79, after which rates fall off to approximately the level for women ages 65–69, a pat-

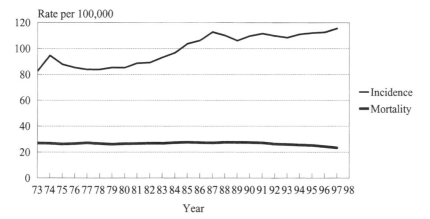

FIGURE 1. Breast cancer incidence and mortality rates, U.S. females, 1973–1997. (Ries *et al.*, 2000a). Rates are per 100,000 females, age-adjusted to the 1970 U.S. standard population.

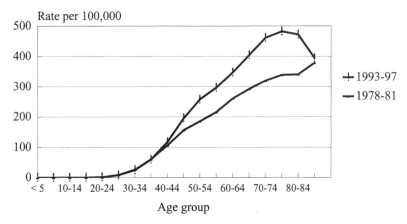

FIGURE 2. Average age-specific breast cancer incidence rates, U.S. females, 1978–1981 and 1993–1997. (Ries *et al.*, 2000a). Rates are per 100,000 females within the specified age category.

tern that is similar for both White and Black women (Ries *et al.*, 2000a). This shift in the pattern of age-specific rates was first observed in 1984 and has been evident since that time. A shift to lower age-specific rates in older women during this time period is probably best explained by a combination of two factors; specifically, the correlation of lead time with age, and declining screening rates after age 65 (Kessler, 1992; Smith, 1995).

In the United States, until 1987 breast cancer was the leading cause of cancer death among women, whereas it is now the second leading cause of death from cancer. The mortality rate from breast cancer has been remarkably stable over the previous 50 years, ranging from an average of 26.0 per 100,000 for the period 1956–1958 to 27.1 per 100,000 for the period 1986–1990 (see Figure 1 for the trend since 1973). However, in early 1995, it was announced that mortality data from 1989 to 1992 had revealed a decline in the breast cancer mortality rate for White women of approximately 6%, the largest decline ever observed (Smigel, 1995). No overall decline in deaths was observed for Black women. Since this announcement, overall mortality rates have continued to decline among white women, and the most recent data suggests that overall rates have begun to decline in Black women (Ries *et al.*,

2000b). Declines in mortality rates are seen in white women under and over age 50, whereas the recent mortality trend shows only a small decline in mortality rates among black women aged 50 years and younger. However, among Black women aged 50 years and older, the average annual increase in the mortality rate has only recently reversed. Similar mortality declines such as those observed in white women aged 50+ may become evident.

Breast cancer survival is strongly influenced by stage at diagnosis. When breast cancer is diagnosed while still localized to the breast, five-year survival as measured by the most recent survival data is 96.5% (Ries *et al.*, 2000a). When the disease has spread to the lymph nodes, the prognosis is poorer and five-year survival is 77%, and if it has spread to distant organs, five-year survival is only 21%.

Ethnicity and Breast Cancer

White women have higher age-adjusted incidence rates compared with Black women (118.4 vs. 103.0 per 100,000), and notable differences are evident in trends over time (Ries *et al.*, 2000a). Between 1973 and 1997 age-adjusted rates increased 28.3% among White women, and 33.0% among Black women. Among women under age 50 years of age, incidence rates are higher in Black women compared with White women (33.2 vs. 31.8), and the 1973–1997 trend reveals that rates for Black women under age 50 increased 19.0% compared with only 2.4% for Whites. Conversely, among women ages 50 years and older, incidence rates are higher among White women compared with Black women (385.1 vs. 322.1), although as with younger women, Black women show a higher percentage change in rates over the 25-year period (38% vs. 34%).

Trends in Incidence and Mortality: Some Conclusions

The recent increase in the incidence trend did occur in parallel with structural trends that supported greater utilization of mammography: increasing availability of mammography, increasing provider and public acceptance, increased promotion of mammography by public health agencies, and insurance coverage for the exam. Recent analyses have also concluded that the entirety of the recent increase is not due solely to the influence of increasing the rate of detection of occult disease (Liff, Sung, Chow, Greenberg, & Flanders, 1991; White, Lee, & Kristal, 1990). This conclusion is expected since it would be unlikely that a trend observed since the mid-1930s would suddenly be replaced entirely by another. Holford, Roush, and McKay (1991) have shown higher age-specific incidence for successive cohorts of women born since 1870, providing evidence that there has been a true underlying increase in disease continuing to contribute, at least in part, to the recent increase in incidence rates. White, Lee, and Kristal (1990) have concluded that an increase in screening accounts for the increase in incidence in women between the ages of 55–64 years, but does not completely account for the increase in rates among women under age 55, or older than age 65. Likewise, Liff, Sung, Chow, Greenberg, and Flanders (1991) concluded that an increase in the utilization of mammography and a true increase in the rate of disease explain the recent trend.

The recent decline in breast cancer mortal-ity is undoubtedly a function of improved stage at diagnosis and improved treatment, including both surgical technique and adjuvant therapy with tamoxifen. Recent surveys conducted in nearly all U.S. states show that the majority of women age 40 years and older have ever had a mammogram at some time, and a majority report mammography in the past two years (American Cancer Society, 1999). Since utilization of mammography began to increase, there has been steady improvement in the stage at diagnosis among incident breast cancer cases, improvements in near-term survival, and a decline in the breast cancer mortality rate.

RISK FACTORS

Breast Cancer Etiology

It is generally accepted that higher levels of endogenous hormones, in particular estrogens, are an important factor in the etiology of breast cancer, although the basic etiology underlying the association between known risk factors and breast cancer is not well understood (Henderson *et al.*, 1996; Pike, 1987; Pike, Krailo, Henderson, Casagrande, & Hoel, 1983). Presently, a model of breast cancer pathogenesis proposed by Pike and colleagues provides a consistent exemplar for the age-incidence curve, as well as observations of associations between incidence, age, and various reproductive risk factors (Pike, 1987; Pike *et al.*, 1983). Steroid hormones, in particular estradiol, influence proliferation of breast cells, and greater rates of cell division in turn increase the likelihood of genetic damage and thus the risk of tumorigenesis. Since greater rates of cell division will accumulate among women with earlier menarche, later menopause, shorter menstrual cycles, and late first full-term pregnancy, higher risks of breast cancer in these women are compatible with this model. Thus, according to the model, it is not the calendar age, per se, that influences breast cancer risk, but the "age" of breast tissue as determined by greater exposure to ovarian hormones, greater rates of cell division, and therefore greater risk of genetic damage. Other factors associated with higher circulating levels of endogenous hormones are also consistent with this theory, such as dietary influences on estrogen levels, the effects of exercise on age at menarche and menstrual cycle length, or the use of postmenopausal hormone replacement therapy (Kelsey, 1993).

Breast Cancer Risk Factors

Numerous factors associated with higher and lower levels of endogenous and exogenous estrogens, as well as other risk factors, have been associated with breast cancer risk. These include early age at menarche, late age at menopause, nulliparity and late age at first live birth, and postmenopausal obesity (Kelsey, 1993). High-dose exposure to radiation, not breast-feeding, history of some types of benign breast disease (i.e., proliferative disease with atypical hyperplasia, sclerosing adenosis, etc.), history of lobular carcinoma in situ, history of breast cancer, and family history of breast cancer in one or more first degree relatives have also been associated with breast cancer risk (Bernstein, Henderson, Hanisch, Sullivan-Halley, & Ross, 1994; Colditz et al., 1995; Colditz, Rosner, & Speizer, 1996; Huang et al., 1997). Lifestyle factors (i.e., a diet high in animal fats and alcohol consumption) remain important areas for investigation, as does the influence of regular physical activity.

Most of the observed risk factors for breast cancer are not particularly strong, and have limited value for counseling women about individual risk (Rockhill, Kawachi, & Colditz, 2000). Further, few of these risk factors are modifiable, and while they influence absolute risk over time, the magnitude of risk differences among the majority of women would not justify any difference in general screening recommendations nor be relevant for more far-reaching decisions related to prevention that will be discussed below (Smith, 1999). For most women, the most important risk factor is age, since breast cancer risk increases with increasing age. However, risk factors that can distinguish a woman at higher risk are her personal history of biopsy-confirmed benign breast disease or breast cancer, and her family history (Smith, 1999).

Family History

It has been recognized for some time that risk varies with the pattern of incidence in the family, especially with respect to the age and number of affected first degree relatives. For this reason, a careful and detailed assessment of the patient's family history is important in both assessing and communicating risk (American Society of Human Genetics, 1994). Among all women with a family history of breast cancer, risk is highest in women with families characterized by early age of onset of breast cancer, bilateral or multifocal disease, and two or more first-degree relatives with breast and/or ovarian cancer. This pattern of family history suggests a high probability of having a mutation in a dominantly inherited breast cancer susceptibility gene with high penetrance. Heritable breast cancer is estimated to account for 5–10% of all newly diagnosed cases, and 25% of cases diagnosed with breast cancer before age 30 (Newman, Millikan, & King, 1997). Lifetime risk of breast cancer among carriers of an alteration on BRCA1 or BRCA2 is similar, exceeding 50%, and risk of early onset disease is also high (Offit, 1998; Struewing et al., 1995, 1997). Previously, lifetime risk of breast cancer among mutation carriers was estimated to exceed 85%, but it appears these earlier estimates were influenced by investigations in very-high-risk families.

Risk Estimation

There is an inherent interest in knowing and quantifying risk among some women and clinicians, and tools are available that can calculate risk over successive decades and for a lifetime (to age 90) based on a woman's individual profile (National Cancer Institute, 1999a). Since breast cancer screening is not without individual costs as measured by the chance of an abnormal interpretation, diagnostic procedures, anxiety, etc., some have argued that these tools can help women and their providers make informed decisions about screening (Gail & Rimer, 1998). One can conjecture that some women will prefer to know their risk, and some will not, and that some that have learned their risk may, in hindsight, find that learning their personal risk may have increased, rather than alleviated, anxiety (Gerrard, Gibbons, & Reis-Bergen, 1999).

Furthermore, for average-risk women, small differences in lifetime risk may be magnified beyond their significance, especially since these models have greater precision for estimating aggregate risk compared with individual risk (Rockhill & Colditz, 1999). For these reasons, individuals trained in risk estimation and communication should do assessments of individual risk. However, for counseling purposes, risk factors that have greatest relevance to decisionmaking are a woman's age, her personal history of biopsy-confirmed benign breast disease or breast cancer, and her family history (Smith, 1999).

PRIMARY PREVENTION: CAN BREAST CANCER BE PREVENTED?

Until recently, the potential to prevent breast cancer was hardly discussed beyond the occasional reminder that prevention would be preferable to early detection if only there were an obvious and practical strategy. For the most part, breast cancer risk factors have been regarded as essentially (family history) or practically (reproductive decisions) nonmodifiable. Although there are clear indications of reproductive decisions a woman might make to reduce her risk of breast cancer, such as the timing of childbirth, birth spacing, or prophylactic oophorectomy, these decisions are neither as straightforward as it might seem, nor without significant individual harms, or costs to career opportunities. Further, and perhaps more important, none are by any means a *certain* route to

individual prevention. However, more recent research has identified behaviors that are associated with lower breast cancer risk and that fall into the category of individual choices that are not as drastic or life defining as those listed above.

The evidence remains inconclusive that engaging in physical activity or consuming a diet low in fat and/or high in fruits, vegetables, soy, or fiber has a substantial effect on breast cancer risk. However, there is sufficient emerging evidence to support lifestyle changes related to diet and physical activity because of their proven value for cardiovascular health, other health conditions, quality of life, and the possibility that they may reduce the risk of breast cancer. For example, alcohol consumption has been shown to be a risk factor for breast cancer. Among women who have ever consumed alcoholic beverages compared with women who never drink, risk of breast cancer was 40% greater, and consumption of an average of 5 or more grams per day was associated with a higher risk compared with less than 5 grams (Bowlin et al., 1997). Although data on the association between diet and breast cancer (particularly dietary fat) has been mixed, recent evidence suggests that among premenopausal women the consumption of five or more servings of fresh fruits and vegetables (compared with less than two servings per day) was associated with a lower risk of premenopausal breast cancer (Zhang et al., 1999). Also, this association was stronger among women with a family history (Zhang et al., 1999). Weight gain is positively associated with breast cancer risk after menopause compared with women whose weight has not changed (Huang et al., 1997). This association was observed only among women who had never taken postmenopausal hormones, suggesting that avoiding weight gain after menopause could significantly reduce breast cancer risk. Indeed, the role of diet and physical activity in breast cancer risk may be mediated, in part, though the combined effect on energy expenditure and maintaining a healthy body mass index. Although postmenopausal hormones have been shown to have beneficial effects on reducing menopausal symptoms, risk of cardiovascular mortality, and bone loss due to osteoporosis, long-term use has also been associated with an increased risk of breast cancer (Colditz, 1999). The accumulation of evidence suggests that women would benefit from careful assessment of the comparative benefits and risks associated with hormone replacement therapy, since breast cancer risk may be increased without comparable decreases in risk of other chronic conditions, particularly if they are at low risk for cardiovascular disease and osteoporosis.

In addition to possible mechanisms to reduce breast cancer risk described above, there is a growing emphasis on chemoprevention as a potential route to breast cancer risk reduction. The observation that adjuvant treatment with tamoxifen not only reduced the risk of breast cancer recurrence, but also risk of breast cancer in the contralateral breast (Fisher et al., 1989), led investigators to explore the potential for chemoprevention in women at higher than average risk (Nayfield, Karp, Ford, Dorr, & Kramer, 1991). To test the hypothesis that tamoxifen might prevent breast cancer, the National Surgical Adjuvant Breast and Bowel Project (NSABP) Breast Cancer Prevention Trial enrolled 13,388 women at higher than average breast cancer risk (Fisher et al., 1998). Participants were randomized to receive a placebo or tamoxifen at 20 mg/day for five years. After 47.7 months of follow-up, a 47% reduction in the risk of invasive breast cancer was observed in the experimental group. Similar results have been observed with raloxifene, in which the serendipitous observation of a 54% reduction in breast cancer incidence in the experimental group in a study of the drug's effect on reducing risk of osteoporosis (Jordan, 1998). However, the early findings of protective effects associated with selective estrogen receptor modulators (SERMS) such as tamoxifen and raloxifene raise many questions for which the absence of answers limits our ability to conjecture about the role SERMS may eventually play in breast cancer incidence reduction. For example, experts disagree about whether observed incidence re-

ductions will endure: does tamoxifen prevent breast cancer, postpone breast cancer, or both? More remains to be learned about the dose and duration of therapy and whether it may vary by age, underlying risk, and other factors. For some women, the expected benefits of tamoxifen must be balanced by observed risks (endometrial cancer, blood clots, stroke, and pulmonary embolism). Among some older women the balance of risks and benefits may be so unfavorable that they eliminate from eligibility those whose use of tamoxifen has the greatest potential to contribute to reduction in breast cancer incidence. A recent report in the Journal of the National Cancer Institute concluded that tamoxifen was most likely to benefit younger women at higher risk of breast cancer because their higher breast cancer risk outweighed the lower potential for adverse effects (Gail et al., 1999). Finally, some women taking tamoxifen have experienced significant quality of life side effects (vasomotor, gynecological, and sexual functioning) (Day et al., 1999). These side effects may cause some eligible women to choose not to take tamoxifen, and may affect duration of use among women who have initiated chemoprevention. There is reason to be optimistic about the potential for chemoprevention of breast cancer, and additional designer estrogens are being studied, and even more with more favorable benefit/risk characteristics are likely to emerge. However, until these drugs are tested in clinical trials, the uncertainty about their effectiveness and acceptability to patients and providers essentially prevents any realistic projections at this time for the role these drugs may play in preventing breast cancer.

SECONDARY PREVENTION: THE LOGIC FOR EARLY DETECTION

The single most effective tool for the early detection of breast cancer is mammography. Guidelines for early breast cancer detection emphasize a combination of breast self-examination (BSE), clinical breast examination (CBE), and mammography as a complete program of surveillance. After age 40, the principle role of BSE and CBE are to identify masses that were not detected on mammography due to test limitations, rapid tumor growth, or human error.

Breast Self-Examination

The American Cancer Society recommends that BSE should begin at age 20 and be performed monthly. There are various techniques for BSE, but all are focused on a systematic palpation of breast and axillary tissue and a visual inspection of the breasts. Any one technique may be chosen on the basis of personal preference since the overriding goal of BSE is for a woman to become familiar with what is normal breast composition for her. Because some premenopausal women experience breast discomfort near the time of menstruation, they may find BSE is more comfortable 8–10 days after the beginning of their period.

Clinical Breast Examination

CBE involves physical palpation of the breast by a trained clinician. Today, its role in early breast cancer detection is defined primarily by a woman's age. Between the ages of 20–40, CBE is the clinical compliment to BSE and is recommended every three years. Beginning at age 40, CBE should be done annually, and ideally, near and prior to the time of the annual mammogram. Technique is important and should be systematic. A competent physical examination includes palpation in small segments, from the nipple to the periphery of the breast including the axilla (Donegan, 1995).

Mammography

Screening mammography is an x-ray examination of the breasts to detect abnormalities that may be breast cancer. Mammography has evolved from the use of general purpose x-ray equipment to today's dedicated imaging equipment, and during the past decade significant progress has been made to improve the image quality of mammograms and to lower radiographic dose (Hendrick, 1992). Image quality and interpretive skills also have been improved through the American College of Radiology's Mammography Accreditation Program and the Mammography Quality Standards Act of 1992, which requires a facility to meet a broad range of technical and personnel standards in order to be certified by the Food and Drug Administration (FDA) to be a provider of mammography services (Food and Drug Administration (CDRH), 1999; Hendrick, 1989).

A screening mammogram includes two views of each breast: one of which is a craniocaudal view (CC), which is taken from the top of the breast, and the other is a mediolateral oblique view (MLO), which is taken from the side. Prior to taking the x-ray, the radiologic technologist positions a woman's breast in a compression device, which evens the thickness of the breast, separates breast tissues that may obscure a lesion, and improves the overall quality of the image. Compression involves some discomfort, but is essential to insure accuracy. After the examination, a radiologist examines the film for abnormalities. Abnormalities that cannot be resolved with additional imaging generally will proceed to biopsy with fine-needle aspiration, ultrasound or radiographic-directed core needle biopsy, or surgical excision.

At this time, no other imaging modality is recommended for primary screening for breast cancer. Ultrasound may be used to resolve abnormalities that are palpable, but not seen on a mammogram; to differentiate cystic from solid masses; and in some rare instances to screen for nonpalpable masses when the breast is comprised of such dense parenchyma that screen-film mammography is not useful (Jackson, 1993). Other imaging modalities that will likely have a role in breast imaging in the future are digital mammography and magnetic resonance imaging (MRI) (Li, Qian, & Clarke, 1997; Orel et al., 1997). Light scanning (diaphanography and transillumination), thermography, and xeromammography are not recommended for breast cancer screening (Bassett, Hendrick, Bassford, et al., 1994).

PSYCHOSOCIAL ISSUES RELATED TO BREAST CANCER

Whether a woman is getting a mammogram, facing a diagnosis of breast cancer, or living as a long-term survivor, she is likely to experience some of the psychosocial sequelae associated with breast cancer. Among all common risks to women's health, breast cancer is among women's greatest health concerns. Prior to the availability of screening and the emerging trend in broad-based, multichannel efforts to educate women about breast cancer, breast cancer was less commonly visible in the public domain. However, breast cancer is a major focus of public health programs, and probably has a greater presence in the mass media and the day-to-day domain than any other health issue. For example, October has been designated as breast cancer awareness month, and throughout the month there is more intensive media attention as well as a broad range of events focused on raising awareness about breast cancer at the national and community level. Throughout the year in communities across the country various groups organize running events and other activities dedicated to raising funds for breast cancer research. Corporations have entered into partnerships with advocacy groups to contribute funds for research through cause-related marketing, wherein a company pledges a percentage of profits from sales to support breast cancer research or other breast-cancer-related public health initiatives. The media and popular press not only regularly report new research findings about all aspects of breast cancer, but articles covering a variety of generalized topics seem to be present on a newsstand at all times.

Anxiety about Breast Cancer: Risk and Perceived Risk

The ubiquitous presence of breast cancer in the public domain has both benefits and costs. Clearly benefits arise from increasing awareness, both generalized awareness as well as awareness about individual risk, recommendations about screening, and reports of new developments in preventive and clinical care. However, so much attention has also given rise to confusion, to awareness that news and messages are often contradictory (or appear contradictory), and to a higher than expected level of anxiety about breast cancer that researchers worry has become pervasive, especially among young women (Black, Nease, & Tosteson, 1995). Various polls have found that younger women tend to overestimate their risk, whereas older women tend to underestimate their risk. This leads to increased fear among younger women and underutilization of mammography screening by older women.

A high risk or perceived high risk of breast cancer often creates anxiety. For some, the fear is so great as to result in avoidance of screening. However, for the most part, perceived risk of breast cancer has been correlated with an increased likelihood of breast cancer screening. Women with a positive family history, women who have had a suspicious mammogram, and women who believe they are more vulnerable to breast cancer are more likely to have had a recent mammogram and to intend to continue regular screening (McCaul, Branstetter, Schroeder, & Glasgow, 1996). Women whose abnormal mammogram leads to a surgical biopsy are more likely to intend to obtain screening mammograms in the future, although they are also more likely to believe they are at increased risk for breast cancer (Pisano, Earp, Schell, Vokaty, & Denham, 1998).

Women who face the highest risk of breast cancer are those who carry a genetic mutation in one of the breast cancer susceptibility genes (e.g., BRCA1/2). Although many women who carry a BRCA mutation are highly motivated to participate in early detection screening, others exhibit extreme fear that manifests in avoidance of mammograms and breast exams (Watson *et al.*, 1999). This is particularly true for individuals with high levels of cancer-related stress or fear of getting cancer (Lynch *et al.*, 1997). Such women may require psychological or psychiatric counseling to overcome their anxiety. Some women from high-risk families who receive a negative result for the BRCA1/2 genetic test may have a false sense of security regarding their risk of developing breast cancer and disregard the need for annual mammograms and clinical breast examinations. These women need to be counseled that they are still at some risk of getting breast cancer, i.e., the same risk as women who do not have a family history, and that it is important for them to follow standard screening guidelines.

Psychosocial Issues Associated with Breast Cancer Screening

Breast cancer screening causes a certain amount of stress for the woman being screened, particularly before the exam and while awaiting the results. Most women who receive a normal result following mammography screening do not experience psychological distress, and may exhibit relief and/or decreased levels of concern about breast cancer (Lowe, Balanda, Del Mar, & Hawes, 1999; Scaf-Klomp, Sanderman, van de Wiel, Otter, & van den Heuvel, 1997). Anxiety is the primary psychological effect associated with mammography screening, and is most common in women who receive an abnormal result (Steggles, Lightfoot, & Sellick, 1998). Upon reviewing a two-view screening mammogram, a radiologist may determine that additional images are needed due to what appears to be an abnormality, or due to technical reasons. Thus, it is not uncommon for women undergoing screening to be told they have an abnormal result, when in fact they do not have cancer, and there is a high probability that the initial area of concern will shortly be determined to be normal. However, it is also the case that women generally are unaware that abnormal findings on the initial screening mammogram are common and generally resolved toward a final determination that the exam is normal (Fine, Rimer, & Watts, 1993; Lerman,

Trock, Rimer, Jepson, et al., 1991; Sutton, Saidi, Bickler, & Hunter, 1995). Women who receive a suspicious result often experience anxiety and worries about breast cancer that may affect their moods and daily functioning, even if follow up tests confirm they do not have cancer (Lerman, Trock, Rimer, Boyce, et al., 1991). Lowe et al. showed that the increased concern about breast cancer was sustained for at least one month, whereas increased levels of anxiety, insomnia, physical well-being, and social functioning returned to baseline levels within one month of receiving the negative result (Lowe et al., 1999). Fine, Rimer, and Watts reported that women whose physicians had informed them about what to expect during screening had approximately half the rate of anxiety that was observed in women whose physicians had not discussed the screening procedure in advance (Fine et al., 1993). Thus, it appears that screening-related anxiety can be significantly reduced with some advance counseling by a woman's health care provider.

Other studies have shown that women who received a false positive result reported no adverse psychological effects 5 or 8–10 weeks after screening (Gilbert et al., 1998; Scaf-Klomp et al., 1997). One survey found that 99% of women who participated in a mammography screening program indicated that they had a positive attitude toward mammography regardless of whether they received a false positive result (Gram & Slenker, 1992). More recent findings also suggest that in spite of the anxiety associated with screening results suggestive of breast cancer, women accept false positive results as an inevitable part of the process of early detection. A report by Schwartz and colleagues revealed that women were highly tolerant of false-positive results, and this high level of tolerance was evident regardless of whether or not a woman had previously received a false-positive result (Schwartz, Woloshin, Sox, Fischhoff, & Welch, 2000). Since nearly two thirds of women felt that 500 false-positive exams per life saved was reasonable, and 39% would tolerate more than 10,000 false-positive exams per life saved, it appears that the value women place on the potential of mammography to save lives far exceeds concerns about harms.

Although the medical community should strive to minimize the number of false positives from mammography screening, inevitably there is a point where attempts to minimize the false positive rate results in missed cancers. Thus, women should be informed that false positive results are common, necessary, and some will inevitably require resolution with a biopsy. Women can lower their odds of a false-positive result by using the same mammography facility each year so that their provider is able to have ready access to films from previous exams for comparison.

Psychosocial Issues and the Breast Cancer Patient

According to Rowland and Massie (2000), Meyerowitz's 1980 delineation of the psychosocial impact of a diagnosis of breast cancer remains useful today (Meyerowitz, 1980). Meyerowitz described three broad areas in which women diagnosed with breast cancer were affected: psychological discomfort (fear, anxiety, depression, and anger); changes in life patterns (due to fatigue, physical discomfort, activity level, and changes in marital or sexual relationships); and fears and concerns (loss of the breast, hair loss due to treatment, fear about lymphedema, recurrence, and premature death). According to Rowland and Massie (2000), other key factors affecting the psychosocial impact of breast cancer include age, stage in the lifecycle, personality and coping style, and interpersonal support from family and friends.

A breast cancer diagnosis is often associated with high levels of anxiety, uncertainty, and difficulty making decisions (Northouse, 1992). Some breast cancer patients are more affected than others, and researchers have begun to identify specific characteristics that may predict which women are more likely to suffer from depression, anxiety, and other psychologi-cal symptoms. Such traits include pessimism (Carver et al., 1994; Epping-Jordan et al., 1999), cognitive avoidance coping (McCaul et al., 1999; Stanton & Snider, 1993), younger age (Epping-Jordan et al., 1999), intrusive thoughts, (Epping-Jordan et al., 1999), and self-blame (Glinder & Compas, 1999). Higher levels of distress were associated with insomnia, fatigue, and loss of concentration, particularly in women younger than age 55 (Cimprich, 1999; Epping-Jordan et al., 1999). However, it is interesting to note that women who had been diagnosed recently with breast or gynecologic cancer exhibited significantly less distress, including depression and anxiety, than women recently diagnosed with other types of cancer as well as other common medical conditions, and even identified many positive aspects from the cancer experience (Ganz, 1996).

Anxiety and depression tend to decrease significantly in the year following diagnosis and surgery, with no difference in psychological effects between women undergoing mastectomy versus lumpectomy or breast conservation (Goldberg et al., 1992). Age, education, and marital status were found to have little or no association with long-term distress levels (Maunsell, Brisson, & Deschenes, 1992), and although younger age is associated with higher distress levels at the time of diagnosis, this association is no longer evident several months later (Compas et al., 1999). However, the level of psychological distress is often associated with the degree of functional impairment, physical symptoms, and side effects, with fatigue being the most common and difficult problem (Bower et al., 2000; Budin, 1998; Longman, Braden, & Mishel, 1999; Pasacreta, 1997). Fatigue, depression, and anxiety all have been observed to have a negative impact on patient quality of life (Longman et al., 1999). Physical symptoms can lead to disruption in other areas, with significant psychosocial consequences. Schover (1997) has noted that even among couples with a satisfying sex life and perceived good sexual communication, physical symptoms can be so disruptive that they overwhelm the couple's sexual rapport and bond.

"… Eva had been warned that her chemotherapy would make her menopausal, and she was already experiencing annoying hot flashes. To minimize vaginal dryness, she used a gel lubricant the first time she and her husband tried sex. To her shock, however, Eva had great difficulty getting aroused. When her husband caressed her breasts, her only thought was about breast cancer. When he brushed his hand over her belly, she felt the soreness of her scar from breast reconstruction. She wanted the light off so that he would not see her without pubic hair and with only one nipple. After a long time of caressing, she signaled him to go ahead and try penetration. Even with the lubricant, Eva's vagina felt dry and tight. Thrusting hurt. She tried to hide her feelings, but tears dripped out of her eyes and her husband stopped. He held her while she sobbed. 'I don't think I'll ever be normal again,' she gasped. 'What are we going to do?' He tried to reassure her that he loved her and would live without sex until she felt more ready." (Schover, 1997)

Schover (1997) describes a common outcome of couple's communication breakdowns on issues of sexuality, a kind of prolonged impasse due to an ability to talk, communicate thoughts, questions, and fears, and a deep desire to avoid hurting each other's feelings.

Long-term Effects

The majority of long-term survivors of breast cancer who are free from disease do not experience prolonged depression and anxiety (Dorval, Maunsell, Deschenes, Brisson, & Masse, 1998; Ellman & Thomas, 1995). However a significant minority of breast cancer patients continue to experience psychological distress for years following diagnosis and treatment (Spiegel, 1997). A high level of distress for up to 18 months after surgery was associated with a prior history of depression, prior history of stressful life events, and with disease stage (regional versus localized) (Maunsell *et al.*, 1992).

Long-term effects that may affect the quality of life for survivors of breast cancer include numbness, arm problems and swelling (lymphedema), continued thoughts about recurrence and nervousness associated with follow up, concerns regarding health insurance coverage, body image, sexual interest and function, and problems with dating for those who are single (Dorval *et al.*, 1998; Ganz *et al.*, 1996; Polinsky, 1994). In *Breast cancer: The complete guide*, Hirshaut and Pressman (2000) included a patient's description of the period leading up to her five-year check-up after a mastectomy.

Recurrence

Women who have been diagnosed with breast cancer are at greater risk for a second primary tumor in the contralateral breast, or recurrence of breast cancer in the same breast. Risk of recurrence is influenced by the age at diagnosis, disease-related characteristics (tumor

"After that night, Eva's husband did not bring up the topic of sex.… He wanted to wait to try sex again until she felt ready. He was horrified at the idea of hurting her physically. Because he did not communicate these thoughts to Eva, however, she feared that he was no longer attracted to her. Even as she felt better, she was reluctant to initiate sex. What if her husband just went along because he felt sorry for her?" (Schover, 1997)

"... I didn't have a man in my life at the time and I thought to myself, okay, kid you better fill up your life with other things because romance is out from now on. Well, then I met Michael and I have to tell you I was shaking like a leaf the first time he even stood close to me because I was afraid he'd feel how my breast was gone and be really repelled. But that's not the way it turned out at all. In fact, when I told him, I think it opened him up to a lot of tenderness that was good for both of us and that's stayed on in our relationship" (Hirshaut & Pressman, 2000).

size, histology, etc.), and treatment characteristics (Morrow & Harris, 2000). The diagnosis of recurrent breast cancer may have greater psychosocial impact on a woman than her original diagnosis (Jenkins, May, & Hughes, 1991), although for many women the opposite is true which, as Bull has noted (Bull *et al.*, 1999), is testament to the strength and resilience of many breast cancer survivors. Upon diagnosis, psychological issues that were present during the original diagnosis and treatment tend to resurface. Additional psychosocial effects associated with recurrence include grief, fear, injustice, anger, and difficulty communicating with a significant other about the recurrence (Chekryn, 1984). Both the fear of recurrence and recurrence itself may induce a sense of loss of control over one's life and may increase health worries (Northouse, 1981), panic and anxiety (Maher, 1982), and major depressive illness (Jenkins *et al.*, 1991). Some association has been reported between psychological adjustment to metastatic or recurrent breast cancer and expressing emotion and having a "fighting spirit" (Classen, Koopman, Angell, & Spiegel, 1996). Although quality of life does improve in the months following the recurrence diagnosis, most areas of quality of life remain lower than they were prior to the diagnosis (Bull *et al.*, 1999).

Psychosocial Support

Overall, there is good evidence that psychosocial interventions focused on reducing stress, increasing knowledge, and improving coping skills are beneficial to breast cancer pa-

tients (Rowland & Massie, 2000). Improvements following these interventions include reduced stress, greater sense of control, improved body image and sexual function, and greater adherence to the prescribed course of therapy (Rowland & Massie, 2000). In addition, recent studies have shown that women participating in a support group focused on reducing stress in areas of daily life affected by breast cancer treatment showed improved immune function (Andersen *et al.*, 1998), suggesting that psychosocial interventions may influence not only psychological well-being but also improve survival. Additional support for this hypothesis was Spiegel *et al.*'s demonstration that women with advanced breast cancer randomized into a weekly group therapy session survived an average of 18 months longer than women in the control group that did not receive therapy demonstrates improved outcomes for women who receive psychosocial support (Spiegel, Bloom, Kraemer, & Gottheil, 1989). Karen Stabiner (Stabiner, 1997) described the sentiments of the women in such a support group:

They wondered if they ever would get to be old—and since there was no way to tell, they wondered how to live in the meantime. Should they do all the things they had never done—take off to Europe, quit that dead-end job? Or should they behave like everyone else, go to work in the morning, save money for the future? Healthy people deceived themselves, but the women in this room had irrefutable proof that the body could betray you at any moment without warning.

So they debated and marked time. The five-year cure statistic might not hold up, but there was one thing that was true—each year the chance of recurrence declined. Sixty percent of all recurrences happened in the first three years. If they got past that marker, the odds would shift in their favor. Maybe by then there would be a new treatment. That was what survival was really all about—hanging on long enough to find something that worked (Stabiner, 1997).

Psychosocial interventions can take numerous forms based on whether counseling is one-on-one or in a group, of short, longer, or open-ended duration. Some studies have found that group therapy can help reduce distress among recently diagnosed patients (Spiegel *et al.*, 1999), others have found that support groups had no effect on distress levels and that distress decreased over time regardless of participation in a cancer support group (Samarel, Fawcett, & Tulman, 1997). As Rowland and Massie (2000) have observed, overall the evidence points to a benefit from psychosocial interventions, and while some women may have experienced the same degree of improvement on their own without the experience of a structured intervention, no study has ever shown that women who received an intervention did worse than their peers in a control group.

HEALTH POLICY

Based on the estimated average annual incidence, in the United States every 15 minutes six women are diagnosed with invasive breast cancer or DCIS, and one woman dies of this disease. Deaths from breast cancer are the second most common cause of cancer mortality among U.S. women, accounting for nearly one in five deaths from cancer, and are a leading cause of premature mortality from cancer. On average a woman dying of breast cancer has lost 19.4 years of life she might have had if she had not died of this disease (Ries *et al.*, 2000a). The National Cancer Institute estimates that in 1999 there were 2.04 million women with a prior diagnosis of invasive breast cancer in the United States (National Cancer Institute, 1999b).

In the past 20 years, there has been a growing emphasis on the various elements of health policy that contribute to the control of breast cancer, including reimbursement for

screening, regulation of screening technology, programs for low-income women, and increased research funding. In 1981, Illinois was the first state to pass legislation requiring reimbursement for mammography. Between 1987 and 1992, 43 states passed similar reimbursement laws, and by 2000, 49 states and the District of Columbia had passed insurance reimbursement legislation (CDC, 2000a). In 1986, with funding from the American Cancer Society, the American College of Radiology (ACR) established the Mammography Accreditation Program (MAP), which was a voluntary program of oversight and professional peer review of a facility's mammography quality. By 1992, the Mammography Quality Standards Act had been passed, requiring all facilities in the United States offering mammography to be accredited by a private accrediting group and certified by the Food and Drug Administration (Hendrick, Smith, & Wilcox, 1993). The MQSA made a matter of law key provisions of the ACR's MAP, including standards for quality control and professional standards for radiologists, technologists, and medical physicists.

In 1990, Congress passed the Breast and Cervical Cancer Mortality Prevention Act, leading to the creation of the Centers for Disease Control's National Breast and Cervical Cancer Early Detection Program. By September 1999, more than 1.1 million mammograms had been provided to low-income women, with approximately 7300 breast cancers detected through the program (CDC, 2000b). In 1992 Congress passed the Breast Cancer Research Program, which allocated $300 million to breast cancer research to be administered by the Department of Defense. By late 1999, allocations had exceeded 1 billion dollars (National Breast Cancer Coalition, 2000).

Cost-Effectiveness

Cost-effectiveness studies in medicine are focused on the net cost of achieving a particular health-related outcome (Eisenberg, 1989). Thus, the estimate of the cost-effectiveness of breast cancer screening is an estimate of the marginal cost per year of life saved (MCYLS). The MCYLS is the fraction of the marginal costs of screening divided by the marginal effectiveness. In this case, the marginal costs of screening are the costs incurred by implementing a screening program minus the costs of observation without screening. The marginal effectiveness is the years of life gained in the screened group minus the years of life expected in the group not undergoing screening.

In general, breast cancer screening meets conventional criteria for cost-effectiveness insofar as the MCYLS generally is less than $40,000. Rosenquist and Lindfors (1998) updated an earlier cost-effectiveness analysis with data available at the 1997 National Institute's of Health Consensus Development Conference on Breast Cancer Screening in Women Ages 40–49 (National Institutes of Health Consensus Development Panel, 1997) and also in accordance with new recommendations from the United States Preventive Services Panel on Cost Effectiveness in Health and Medicine (Weinstein, Siegel, Gold, Kamlet, & Russell, 1996). Their model followed the methodology of their earlier effort (Lindfors & Rosenquist, 1995), i.e., program cost-effectiveness was evaluated for women ages 40–79 under different assumptions of potential mortality reductions and different age-specific screening intervals. Applying a discount rate of 3%, they estimated the MCYLS to be $18,800 with annual screening offered to women ages 40–79. In this case, a mortality reduction of 36% was assumed for annual screening of women aged 40–49, and between 44–46% for women aged 50–79.

CONCLUSION

For the foreseeable future, breast cancer will remain a major health problem for women Compared with other cancers affecting women, incidence begins to rise at an earlier age. This means not only that preventive health measures become a part of a woman's routine care at an earlier age, but also that women experience breast cancer in family and friends among the generation that came before them, but also their own generation, and the generation that followed their own.

The decision to screen women for breast cancer is based on the importance of the disease as a public health problem, and the ability of screening tests to save lives. While there has been great progress in the implementation of breast cancer screening in many countries, the full potential of early detection as a disease control strategy remains unfulfilled. While a majority of women age 40 and older have had a mammogram, most women are not screened at recommended intervals, and access to screening still is a problem for a significant percentage of medically underserved women.

The diagnosis of breast cancer often is overwhelming, and in the past decade a growing range of treatment options and considerations have increased the complexity of decision making at a time when anxiety is high. With cancer treatment often comes significant side effects, both psychosocial and physical, with the latter often having secondary psychosocial effects. The end of treatment is usually met with mixed emotions: joy and relief combined with fear and uncertainty as patients suddenly end their watchful regimen and frequent contact with providers. As women enter a posttreatment period, they face the challenge of recovery and a return to normal life, but a risk of reoccurrence and, in many cases, long-term risks of late onset complications such as lymphedema are an ever-present concern. In a high proportion of women diagnosed with breast cancer these concerns may be lifelong because, overall, survival from breast cancer is favorable compared with other cancers. Nevertheless, long-term survival is very poor for women with distant metastases, and for these women, clinicians, patients, and families face unique and great challenges related to end-of-life issues.

In conclusion, progress in breast cancer control has been stimulated by a unique partnership between the scientific and clinical community, and women. In the United States mortality has declined since 1990, and greater gains can be expected from improvements in early detection programs and progress in treatment. Yet, there still is a need for progress in implementing what we have learned from research, as well as addressing unmet and new clinical and psychosocial research challenges.

REFERENCES

American Cancer Society (1999). *Cancer risk report: Prevention and control, 1999.* Atlanta: American Cancer Society.

American Cancer Society Surveillance Program (2000). Estimated new cancer cases by sex and age. Atlanta: American Cancer Society.

American Society of Clinical Oncology (1996). Statement of the American Society of Clinical Oncology: Genetic testing for cancer susceptibility, Adopted on February 20, 1996. *J Clin Oncol, 14*(5), 1730–1736; discussion 1737–1740.

American Society of Human Genetics (1994). Statement of the American Society of Human Genetics on genetic testing for breast and ovarian cancer predisposition. *A J Hum Genet, 55*, i–iv.

Andersen, B. L., Farrar, W. B., Golden-Kreutz, D., Kutz, L. A., MacCallum, R., Courtney, M. E., & Glaser, R. (1998). Stress and immune responses after surgical treatment for regional breast cancer. *J Natl Cancer Inst, 90*(1), 30–36.

Bassett, L., Hendrick, R., Bassford, T. *et al.* (1994). *Quality determinants of mammography. Clinical practice guideline No. 13* (AHCPR Publication No. 95-0632). Rockville, MD: Agency for Health Care Policy and Research, Public Health Service, U.S. Department of Health and Human Services.

Bernstein, L., Henderson, B. E., Hanisch, R., Sullivan-Halley, J., & Ross, R. K. (1994). Physical exercise and reduced risk of breast cancer in young. *J Natl Cancer Inst, 86*(18), 1403–1408.

Black, W. C., Nease, R. F., Jr., & Tosteson, A. N. (1995). Perceptions of breast cancer risk and screening effectiveness in women younger than 50 years of age. *J Natl Cancer Inst, 87*(10), 720–731.

Bower, J. E., Ganz, P. A., Desmond, K. A., Rowland, J. H., Meyerowitz, B. E., & Belin, T. R. (2000). Fatigue in breast cancer survivors: Occurrence, correlates, and impact on quality of life. *J Clin Oncol, 18*(4), 743–753.

Bowlin, S. J., Leske, M. C., Varma, A., Nasca, P., Weinstein, A., & Caplan, L. (1997). Breast cancer risk and alcohol consumption: Results from a large case-control study. *Int J Epidemiol, 26*(5), 915–923.

Budin, W. C. (1998). Psychosocial adjustment to breast cancer in unmarried women. *Res Nurs Health, 21*(2), 155–166.

Bull, A. A., Meyerowitz, B. E., Hart, S., Mosconi, P., Apolone, G., & Liberati, A. (1999). Quality of life in women with recurrent breast cancer. *Breast Cancer Res Treat, 54*(1), 47–57.

Carver, C. S., Pozo-Kaderman, C., Harris, S. D., Noriega, V., Scheier, M. F., Robinson, D. S., Ketcham, A. S., Moffat, F. L., Jr., & Clark, K. C. (1994). Optimism versus pessimism predicts the quality of women's adjustment to early stage breast cancer. *Cancer, 73*(4), 1213–1220.

CDC (2000a). *State laws relating to breast cancer.* Atlanta: Centers for Disease Control Office, Program and Policy Information.

CDC (2000b). *Ten years of progress: The National Breast and Cervical Cancer Early Detection Program.* CDC. Available: *http://www.cdc.gov/cancer/nbccedp/anniversary.htm.*

Chekryn, J. (1984). Cancer recurrence: Personal meaning, communication, and marital adjustment. *Cancer Nurs, 7*(6), 491–498.

Cimprich, B. (1999). Pretreatment symptom distress in women newly diagnosed with breast cancer. *Cancer Nurs, 22*(3), 185–194; quiz 195.

Classen, C., Koopman, C., Angell, K., & Spiegel, D. (1996). Coping styles associated with psychological adjustment to advanced breast cancer. *Health Psychol, 15*(6), 434–437.

Colditz, G. A. (1999). Hormones and breast cancer: Evidence and implications for consideration of risks and benefits of hormone replacement therapy. *J Women's Health, 8*(3), 347–357.

Colditz, G. A., Hankinson, S. E., Hunter, D. J., Willett, W. C., Manson, J. E., Stampfer, M. J., Hennekens, C., Rosner, B., & Speizer, F. E. (1995). The use of estrogens and progestins and the risk of breast cancer in postmenopausal women. *N Engl J Med, 332*(24), 1589–1593.

Colditz, G. A., Rosner, B. A., & Speizer, F. E. (1996). Risk factors for breast cancer according to family history of breast cancer. For the Nurses' Health Study Research Group. *J Natl Cancer Inst, 88*(6), 365–371.

Compas, B. E., Stoll, M. F., Thomsen, A. H., Oppedisano, G., Epping-Jordan, J. E., & Krag, D. N. (1999). Adjustment to breast cancer: Age-related differences in coping and emotional distress. *Breast Cancer Res Treat, 54*(3), 195–203.

Day, R., Ganz, P. A., Costantino, J. P., Cronin, W. M., Wickerham, D. L., & Fisher, B. (1999). Health-related quality of life and tamoxifen in breast cancer prevention: A report from the National Surgical Adjuvant Breast and Bowel Project P-1 Study. *J Clin Oncol, 17*(9), 2659–2669.

Devesa, S. S., Silverman, D. T., Young, J. L., Jr., Pollack, E. S., Brown, C. C., Horm, J. W., Percy, C. L., Myers, M. H., McKay, F. W., & Fraumeni, J. F., Jr. (1987). Cancer incidence and mortality trends among whites in the United States, 1947–84. *J Natl Cancer Inst, 79*(4), 701–770.

Donegan, W. L. (1995). Diagnosis. In W. L. Donegan and J. S. Sprah (Eds.), *Cancer of the breast,* 4th ed. (pp. 157–205). Philadelphia: W. B. Saunders.

Dorval, M., Maunsell, E., Deschenes, L., Brisson, J., & Masse, B. (1998). Long-term quality of life after breast cancer: Comparison of 8-year survivors with population controls. *J Clin Oncol, 16*(2), 487–494.

Eisenberg, J. M. (1989). Clinical economics. A guide to the economic analysis of clinical practices. *JAMA, 262* (20), 2879–2886.

Ellman, R., & Thomas, B. A. (1995). Is psychological well-being impaired in long-term survivors of breast cancer? *J Med Screen, 2*(1), 5–9.

Epping-Jordan, J. E., Compas, B. E., Osowiecki, D. M., Oppedisano, G., Gerhardt, C., Primo, K., & Krag, D. N. (1999). Psychological adjustment in breast cancer: Processes of emotional distress. *Health Psychol, 18*(4), 315–326.

Fine, M. K., Rimer, B. K., & Watts, P. (1993). Women's responses to the mammography experience. *J Am Board Fam Pract, 6*(6), 546–555.

Fine, N. A., Musto, T. A., & Fenner, G. (2000). Breast reconstruction. In J. R. Harris, M. E. Lippman, M. Morrow, & C. K. Osborne (Eds.), *Diseases of the breast,* 2nd ed. (pp. 561–576). Philadelphia: Lippincott Williams & Wilkins.

Fisher, B., Costantino, J., Redmond, C., Poisson, R., Bowman, D., Couture, J., Dimitrov, N. V., Wolmark, N., Wickerham, D. L., Fisher, E. R., *et al.* (1989). A randomized clinical trial evaluating tamoxifen in the treatment of patients with node-negative breast cancer who have estrogen receptor-positive tumors. *N Engl J Med, 320*(8), 479–484.

Fisher, B., Costantino, J. P., Wickerham, D. L., Redmond, C. K., Kavanah, M., Cronin, W. M., Vogel, V., Robidoux, A., Dimitrov, N., Atkins, J., Daly, M., Wieand, S., Tan-Chiu, E., Ford, L., & Wolmark, N. (1998). Tamoxifen for prevention of breast cancer: Report of the National Surgical Adjuvant Breast and Bowel Project P-1 Study. *J Natl Cancer Inst, 90*(18), 1371–1388.

Food and Drug Administration (CDRH) (1999). *Compliance guidance: The mammography quality standards act final regulations.* Washington, D.C.: U.S. Department of Health and Human Services.

Gail, M., & Rimer, B. (1998). Risk-based recommendations for mammographic screening for women in their forties. *J Clin Oncol, 16*(9), 3105–3114.

Gail, M. H., Costantino, J. P., Bryant, J., Croyle, R., Freedman, L., Helzlsouer, K., & Vogel, V. (1999). Weighing the risks and benefits of tamoxifen treatment for preventing breast cancer [published erratum appears in *J Natl Cancer Inst* 2000 Feb 2;92(3):275]. *J Natl Cancer Inst, 91*(21), 1829–1846.

Ganz, P. A. (1995). Advocating for the woman with breast cancer. *CA Cancer J Clin, 45*(2), 114–126.

Ganz, P. A., Coscarelli, A., Fred, C., Kahn, B., Polinsky, M. L., & Petersen, L. (1996). Breast cancer survivors: Psychosocial concerns and quality of life. *Breast Cancer Res Treat, 38*(2), 183–199.

Gerrard, M., Gibbons, F. X., & Reis-Bergen, M. (1999). The effect of risk communication on risk perceptions: The significance of individual differences. *JNCI Monographs, 25,* 94–100.

Gilbert, F. J., Cordiner, C. M., Affleck, I. R., Hood, D. B., Mathieson, D., & Walker, L. G. (1998). Breast screening: The psychological sequelae of false-positive recall in women with and without a family history of breast cancer. *Eur J Cancer, 34*(13), 2010–2014.

Glinder, J. G., & Compas, B. E. (1999). Self-blame attributions in women with newly diagnosed breast cancer: A prospective study of psychological adjustment. *Health Psychol, 18*(5), 475–481.

Goldberg, J. A., Scott, R. N., Davidson, P. M., Murray, G. D., Stallard, S., George, W. D., & Maguire, G. P. (1992). Psychological morbidity in the first year after breast surgery. *Eur J Surg Oncol, 18*(4), 327–331.

Gram, I. T., & Slenker, S. E. (1992). Cancer anxiety and attitudes toward mammography among screening attenders, nonattenders, and women never invited. *Am J Public Health, 82*(2), 249–251.

Greenlee, R. T., Murray, T., Bolden, S., & Wingo, P. A. (2000). Cancer statistics, 2000. *CA Cancer J Clin, 50*(1), 7–33.

Henderson, B., Pike, M., Bernstein, L., & Ross, R. (1996). Breast cancer. In D. Schottenfeld & J. Fraumeni (Eds.), *Cancer epidemiology and prevention.* New York: Oxford University Press.

Hendrick, R. E. (1989). Quality control in mammography: The American College of Radiology's Mammography Screening Accreditation Program. *Curr Opin Radiol, 1*(2), 203–211.

Hendrick, R. E. (1992). Quality assurance in mammography. Accreditation, legislation, and compliance with quality assurance standards. *Radiol Clin North Am, 30*(1), 243–255.

Hendrick, R. E., Smith, R. A., & Wilcox, P. A. (Eds.) (1993). *ACR accreditation and legislative issues in mammography.* Chicago: RSNA.

Hirshaut, Y., & Pressman, P. I. (2000). *Breast cancer: The complete guide,* 3rd ed. New York: Bantam Books.

Holford, T. R., Roush, G. C., & McKay, L. A. (1991). Trends in female breast cancer in Connecticut and the United States. *J Clin Epidemiol, 44*(1), 29–39.

Huang, Z., Hankinson, S. E., Colditz, G. A., Stampfer, M. J., Hunter, D. J., Manson, J. E., Hennekens, C. H., Rosner, B., Speizer, F. E., & Willett, W. C. (1997). Dual effects of weight and weight gain on breast cancer risk. *JAMA, 278*(17), 1407–1411.

Jackson, V. P., Hendrick, R. E. Kepans, D. B. (1993). Imaging the dense breast. *Radiology, 188*(2), 297–301.

Jenkins, P. L., May, V. E., & Hughes, L. E. (1991). Psychological morbidity associated with local recurrence of breast cancer. *Int J Psychiatry Med, 21*(2), 149–155.

Jordan, V. C. (1998). Antiestrogenic action of raloxifene and tamoxifen: Today and tomorrow. *J Natl Cancer Inst, 90*(13), 967–971.

Kelsey, J. L. (1993). Breast cancer epidemiology: Summary and future directions. *Epidemiol Rev*, 15(1), 256–263.

Kessler, L. G. (1992). The relationship between age and incidence of breast cancer. Population and screening program data. *Cancer*, 69(7 Suppl), 1896–1903.

Lee, C. O. (1997). Quality of life and breast cancer survivors. Psychosocial and treatment issues. *Cancer Pract*, 5(5), 309–316.

Lerman, C., Trock, B., Rimer, B. K., Boyce, A., Jepson, C., & Engstrom, P. F. (1991). Psychological and behavioral implications of abnormal mammograms. *Ann Intern Med*, 114(8), 657–661.

Lerman, C., Trock, B., Rimer, B. K., Jepson, C., Brody, D., & Boyce, A. (1991). Psychological side effects of breast cancer screening. *Health Psychol*, 10(4), 259–267.

Li, L., Qian, W., & Clarke, L. P. (1997). Digital mammography: Computer-assisted diagnosis method for mass detection with multiorientation and multiresolution wavelet transforms. *Acad Radiol*, 4(11), 724–731.

Liff, J. M., Sung, J. F., Chow, W. H., Greenberg, R. S., & Flanders, W. D. (1991). Does increased detection account for the rising incidence of breast cancer? *Am J Public Health*, 81(4), 462–465.

Lindfors, K. K., & Rosenquist, C. J. (1995). The cost-effectiveness of mammographic screening strategies [published erratum appears in *JAMA* 1996 Jan 10; 275(2):112]. *JAMA*, 274(11), 881–884.

Longman, A. J., Braden, C. J., & Mishel, M. H. (1999). Side-effects burden, psychological adjustment, and life quality in women with breast cancer: Pattern of association over time. *Oncol Nurs Forum*, 26(5), 909–915.

Lowe, J. B., Balanda, K. P., Del Mar, C., & Hawes, E. (1999). Psychologic distress in women with abnormal findings in mass mammography screening. *Cancer*, 85(5), 1114–1118.

Lynch, H. T., Lemon, S. J., Durham, C., Tinley, S. T., Connolly, C., Lynch, J. F., Surdam, J., Orinion, E., Slominski-Caster, S., Watson, P., Lerman, C., Tonin, P., Lenoir, G., Serova, O., & Narod, S. (1997). A descriptive study of BRCA1 testing and reactions to disclosure of test results. *Cancer*, 79(11), 2219–2228.

Maher, E. L. (1982). Anomic aspects of recovery from cancer. *Soc Sci Med*, 16(8), 907–912.

Maunsell, E., Brisson, J., & Deschenes, L. (1992). Psychological distress after initial treatment of breast cancer. Assessment of potential risk factors. *Cancer*, 70(1), 120–125.

McCaul, K. D., Branstetter, A. D., Schroeder, D. M., & Glasgow, R. E. (1996). What is the relationship between breast cancer risk and mammography screening? A meta-analytic review. *Health Psychol*, 15(6), 423–429.

McCaul, K. D., Sandgren, A. K., King, B., O'Donnell, S., Branstetter, A., & Foreman, G. (1999). Coping and adjustment to breast cancer. *Psychooncology*, 8(3), 230–236.

Meyerowitz, B. E. (1980). Psychosocial correlates of breast cancer and its treatments. *Psychol Bull*, 87(1), 108–131.

MMWR (1996). Trends in Cancer Screening—United States 1987 and 1992. *MMWR*, 45, 57–61.

Morrow, M., & Harris, J. R. (2000). Local management of invasive breast cancer. In J. R. Harris, M. E. Lippman, M. Morrow, & C. K. Osborne (Eds.), *Diseases of the breast*, 2nd ed. (pp. 515–560). Philadelphia: Lippincott Williams & Wilkins.

National Breast Cancer Coalition (2000). *Department of Defense Breast Cancer Research Program Surpasses $1 billion.* Available: *http://www.natlbcc.org/bin/index.htm.*

National Cancer Institute (1999a). *Breast cancer risk assessment tool.* Available: http://cancernet.nci.nih.gov/clinpdq/risk/Estimating_Breast_Cancer_Risk.html#1.

National Cancer Institute (1999b). *Estimated U.S. prevalence counts.* Available: *http://www-dccps.ims.nci.nih.gov/SRAB/Prevalence/index.html.*

National Institutes of Health Consensus Development Panel (1997). National Institutes of Health Consensus Development Conference Statement: Breast Cancer Screening for Women Ages 40–49, January 21–23, 1997. National Institutes of Health Consensus Development Panel. *J Natl Cancer Inst*, 89(14), 1015–1026.

Nayfield, S. G., Karp, J. E., Ford, L. G., Dorr, F. A., & Kramer, B. S. (1991). Potential role of tamoxifen in prevention of breast cancer. *J Natl Cancer Inst*, 83(20), 1450–1459.

Newman, B., Millikan, R. C., & King, M. C. (1997). Genetic epidemiology of breast and ovarian cancers. *Epidemiol Rev*, 19(1), 69–79.

Northouse, L. L. (1981). Mastectomy patients and the fear of cancer recurrence. *Cancer Nurs*, 4(3), 213–220.

Northouse, L. L. (1992). Psychological impact of the diagnosis of breast cancer on the patient and her family. *J Am Med Womens Assoc*, 47(5), 161–164.

Offit, K. (1998). *Clinical cancer genetics.* New York: Oxford University Press.

Orel, S. G., Reynolds, C., Schnall, M. D., Solin, L. J., Fraker, D. L., & Sullivan, D. C. (1997). Breast carcinoma: MR imaging before re-excisional biopsy. *Radiology*, 205(2), 429–436.

Page, D. L., & Jensen, R. A. (1996). Ductal carcinoma in situ of the breast: Understanding the misunderstood stepchild [editorial; comment]. *JAMA*, 275(12), 948–949.

Parkin, D. M., P. Pisani, J. F., & Ferlay, J. (1999). Global cancer statistics. *CA Cancer J Clin*, 49, 33–64.

Pasacreta, J. V. (1997). Depressive phenomena, physical symptom distress, and functional status among women with breast cancer. *Nurs Res*, 46(4), 214–221.

Pike, M. C. (1987). Age-related factors in cancers of the breast, ovary, and endometrium. *J Chronic Dis*, 40 (Suppl 2), 59S–69S.

Pike, M. C., Krailo, M. D., Henderson, B. E., Casagrande, J. T., & Hoel, D. G. (1983). 'Hormonal' risk factors, 'breast tissue age' and the age-incidence of breast cancer. *Nature*, *303*(5920), 767–770.

Pisano, E. D., Earp, J., Schell, M., Vokaty, K., & Denham, A. (1998). Screening behavior of women after a false-positive mammogram. *Radiology*, *208*(1), 245–249.

Polinsky, M. L. (1994). Functional status of long-term breast cancer survivors: Demonstrating chronicity [published erratum appears in *Health Soc Work* 1994 Nov; 19(4):297]. *Health Soc Work*, *19*(3), 165–173.

Ries, L., Eisner, M., Kosary, C., Hankey, B., Miller, B., Clegg, L., & Edwards, B. (2000a). *SEER cancer statistics review, 1973–1997*. Bethesda, MD: National Cancer Institute.

Ries, L. A., Wingo, P. A., Miller, D. S., Howe, H. L., Weir, H. K., Rosenberg, H. M., Vernon, S. W., Cronin, K., & Edwards, B. K. (2000b). The annual report to the nation on the status of cancer, 1973–1997, with a special section on colorectal cancer. *Cancer*, *88*(10), 2398–2424.

Rockhill, B., & Colditz, G. A. (1999). Making sense of breast cancer risk. *Semin Breast Dis, 2*(4), 272–279.

Rockhill, B., Kawachi, I., & Colditz, G. A. (2000). Individual risk prediction and population-wide disease prevention. *Epidemiol Rev, 22*(1), 176–180.

Rockhill, B., Weinberg, C. R., & Newman, B. (1998). Population attributable fraction estimation for established breast cancer risk factors: Considering the issues of high prevalence and unmodifiability. *Am J Epidemiol, 147*(9), 826–833.

Rosenquist, C. J., & Lindfors, K. K. (1998). Screening mammography beginning at age 40 years: A reappraisal of cost-effectiveness. *Cancer, 82*(11), 2235–2240.

Rowland, J. H., & Massie, M. J. (2000). Psychosocial issues and interventions. In J. R. Harris, M. E. Lippman, M. Morrow, & C. K. Osborne (Eds.), *Diseases of the breast*, 2nd ed. (pp. 1009–1031). Philadelphia: Lippincott Williams & Wilkins.

Samarel, N., Fawcett, J., & Tulman, L. (1997). Effect of support groups with coaching on adaptation to early stage breast cancer. *Res Nurs Health, 20*(1), 15–26.

Scaf-Klomp, W., Sanderman, R., van de Wiel, H. B., Otter, R., & van den Heuvel, W. J. (1997). Distressed or relieved? Psychological side effects of breast cancer screening in The Netherlands. *J Epidemiol Community Health, 51*(6), 705–710.

Schover, L. R. (1997). *Sexuality and fertility after cancer*. New York: Wiley.

Schwartz, L. M., Woloshin, S., Sox, H. C., Fischhoff, B., & Welch, H. G. (2000). US women's attitudes to false positive mammography results and detection of ductal carcinoma in situ: Cross sectional survey. *BMJ, 320* (7250), 1635–1640.

Shapiro, S., Coleman, E. A., Broeders, M., Codd, M., de Koning, H., Fracheboud, J., Moss, S., Paci, E., Stachenko, S., & Ballard-Barbash, R. (1998). Breast cancer screening programmes in 22 countries: Current policies, administration and guidelines. International Breast Cancer Screening Network (IBSN) and the European Network of Pilot Projects for Breast Cancer Screening. *Int J Epidemiol, 27*(5), 735–742.

Smigel, K. (1995). Breast cancer death rates decline for white women [news]. *J Natl Cancer Inst, 87*(3), 173.

Smith, R. (1995). Epidemiology of breast cancer. In D. Kopans & E. Mendelsen (Eds.), *Syllabus: A categorical course in breast imaging*. Chicago: Radiological Society of North America.

Smith, R. A. (1999). Risk-based screening for breast cancer: Is there a practical strategy? *Semin Breast Dis, 2*(4), 280–291.

Spiegel, D. (1997). Psychosocial aspects of breast cancer treatment. *Semin Oncol, 24*(1 Suppl 1), S1-36–S31-47.

Spiegel, D., Bloom, J. R., Kraemer, H. C., & Gottheil, E. (1989). Effect of psychosocial treatment on survival of patients with metastatic breast cancer. *Lancet, 2*(8668), 888–891.

Spiegel, D., Morrow, G. R., Classen, C., Raubertas, R., Stott, P. B., Mudaliar, N., Pierce, H. I., Flynn, P. J., Heard, L., & Riggs, G. (1999). Group psychotherapy for recently diagnosed breast cancer patients: A multicenter feasibility study. *Psychooncology, 8*(6), 482–493.

Stabiner, K. (1997). *To dance with the devil*. New York: Delacorte Press.

Stanton, A. L., & Snider, P. R. (1993). Coping with a breast cancer diagnosis: A prospective study. *Health Psychol, 12*(1), 16–23.

Steggles, S., Lightfoot, N., & Sellick, S. M. (1998). Psychological distress associated with organized breast cancer screening. *Cancer Prev Control, 2*(5), 213–220.

Struewing, J. P., Abeliovich, D., Peretz, T., Avishai, N., Kaback, M. M., Collins, F. S., & Brody, L. C. (1995). The carrier frequency of the BRCA1 185delAG mutation is approximately 1 percent in Ashkenazi Jewish individuals [published erratum appears in *Nat Genet* 1996 Jan; 12(1):110]. *Nat Genet, 11*(2), 198–200.

Struewing, J. P., Hartge, P., Wacholder, S., Baker, S. M., Berlin, M., McAdams, M., Timmerman, M. M., Brody, L. C., & Tucker, M. A. (1997). The risk of cancer associated with specific mutations of BRCA1 and BRCA2 among Ashkenazi Jews. *N Engl J Med, 336*(20), 1401–1408.

Sutton, S., Saidi, G., Bickler, G., & Hunter, J. (1995). Does routine screening for breast cancer raise anxiety? Results from a three wave prospective study in England. *J Epidemiol Community Health, 49*(4), 413–418.

Tabar, L., Dean, P. B., Duffy, S. W., & Chen, H. H. (2000). A new era in the diagnosis of breast cancer. *Surg Oncol Clin N Am, 9*(2), 233–277.

Tabar, L., Fagerberg, C. J., Gad, A., Baldetorp, L., Holmberg, L. H., Grontoft, O., Ljungquist, U., Lundstrom, B., Manson, J. C., Eklund, G., *et al.* (1985). Reduction in mortality from breast cancer after mass screening with mammography. Randomised trial from the Breast Cancer Screening Working Group of the Swedish National Board of Health and Welfare. *Lancet*, *1*(8433), 829–832.

Watson, M., Lloyd, S., Davidson, J., Meyer, L., Eeles, R., Ebbs, S., & Murday, V. (1999). The impact of genetic counselling on risk perception and mental health in women with a family history of breast cancer. *Br J Cancer*, *79*(5-6), 868–874.

Weinstein, M. C., Siegel, J. E., Gold, M. R., Kamlet, M. S., & Russell, L. B. (1996). Recommendations of the Panel on Cost-effectiveness in Health and Medicine. *JAMA*, *276*(15), 1253–1258.

White, E., Lee, C. Y., & Kristal, A. R. (1990). Evaluation of the increase in breast cancer incidence in relation to mammography use. *J Natl Cancer Inst*, *82*(19), 1546–1552.

Zhang, S., Hunter, D. J., Forman, M. R., Rosner, B. A., Speizer, F. E., Colditz, G. A., Manson, J. E., Hankinson, S. E., & Willett, W. C. (1999). Dietary carotenoids and vitamins A, C, and E and risk of breast cancer. *J Natl Cancer Inst*, *91*(6), 547–556.

19

Menopause

NANCY E. AVIS, SYBIL CRAWFORD,
and CATHERINE B. JOHANNES

INTRODUCTION

According to popular view and many experts, the menopause, or "change of life," is thought to represent a major cultural, psychological, and physiological milestone for women during the middle years. It signifies the end of reproduction and is a prominent biological marker for an aging process in cultures that extol youthfulness. Menopause has been viewed through the ages as a sign of sin and decay, psychological loss, and more recently as a deficiency disease (Kaufert & McKinlay, 1985; McCrea, 1983). It is often assumed that menopause is inevitably accompanied (to a greater or lesser extent) by hot flushes, sweats, prolonged menstrual irregularities, vaginal dryness, and a host of other "symptoms," including depression, irritability, weight gain, insomnia, dizziness, and loss of interest in sex.

Much of this perception is derived from early research based on clinical samples of women who sought treatment for menopause-related problems. In the 1980s several large community-based studies were begun. Results from these studies have provided much needed scientific data on menopause among more representative samples and have often dispelled some of these perceptions.

During the last decade, the interest in menopause skyrocketed. Certainly much of this newfound interest was due to the current baby-boom generation of women who were beginning to approach menopause. This large cohort of women grew up asserting more control over their reproductive lives and encouraged frank and open discussions of previously taboo topics. Furthermore, with the increased attention to and promotion of hormone replacement therapy (HRT), menopausal women are faced with making a decision that could ultimately affect the rest of their lives. In the past, menopause was something one had little control over and required little active involvement. Now, with menopause increasingly implicated as a risk factor for subsequent disease, and numerous options available for preventing these diseases, menopause has become a time requiring active decision-making by women.

Menopause occurs at a time when women are also experiencing other life changes and responsibilities associated with aging. Children are getting older and may be leaving, or returning home. Parents are aging and may cause increased worry or caretaking responsibility.

NANCY E. AVIS • Department of Public Health Sciences, Wake Forest University School of Medicine, Winston-Salem, North Carolina 27157.   SYBIL CRAWFORD • University of Massachusetts Medical School, Worcester, Massachusetts, 01655.   CATHERINE B. JOHANNES • Epidemiology Division, Ingenix Pharmaceutical Services, Newton, MA 02462.

Handbook of Women's Sexual and Reproductive Health, edited by Wingood and DiClemente. Kluwer Academic / Plenum Publishers, New York, 2002.

For some women this may be a time of increased independence and positive growth. It is often difficult to disentangle the effects of menopause per se from other events associated with mid-age or aging. This chapter reviews the epidemiology of menopause, menopausal symptoms, long-term consequences of menopause, and indications for hormone replacement therapy. The chapter concludes with health policy implications and suggestions for future research.

EPIDEMIOLOGY

Biological Aging

At birth, the ovaries contain approximately 500,000 oocytes. Only 400 to 500 of these oocytes will ever fully ripen and be released during menstruation. The oocyte and surrounding cells, called follicles, produce the hormones estrogen and progesterone. The normal menstrual cycle is regulated through repetitive changes in hypothalamic–pituitary–ovarian hormonal secretion (Steger & Peluso, 1987). Ovarian steroids (estrogen and progesterone) and peptides (inhibins A and B) provide negative feedback to gonadotropins (follicle stimulating hormone (FSH) and luteinizing hormone (LH)). At the beginning of the menstrual cycle, the pituitary releases FSH, which targets the ovaries and causes follicles to develop. Typically, one follicle begins to mature and releases increasing amounts of estrogen. Inhibin levels also increase during this time, and the uterine lining, the endometrium, begins to thicken. The follicle eventually grows large enough and, triggered by a mid-cycle surge of LH and FSH, ruptures, releasing the ovum (ovulation). The ruptured follicle forms the corpus luteum and under the influence of LH produces estrogen and progesterone. These high circulating levels of estrogen and progesterone, and increased inhibin levels inhibit the release of FSH. If fertilization does not occur, the corpus luteum degenerates and thus stops producing estrogen and progesterone. With the decline in these two hormones, FSH is no longer inhibited and be-

gins to rise again, the endometrium breaks down, and the menstrual cycle begins anew.

Menopause is a gradual process that begins long before a woman notices changes in her menstrual cycles. Beginning in her thirties, a woman has an increasing number of anovulatory cycles (without ovulation) as the number of ovarian follicles declines. Women are generally unaware of these anovulatory cycles. Beginning around age 40, gradual changes in hormone levels occur, prior to overt changes in menstrual cyclicity (Metcalf & Livesey, 1985; World Health Organization, 1996). FSH levels gradually increase, and there is evidence of an age-related decline in the sensitivity of the hypothalamic–pituitary axis to negative feedback by the ovarian steroid hormones (Lenton, Sexton, Lee, & Cooke, 1988; Metcalf, 1988). A linear decline in the number of follicles occurs until about age 40 (Burger, 1996). Following the first break in menstrual cycle regularity, usually considered the onset of the perimenopause, rising FSH levels lead to an increase in the recruitment of ovarian primordial follicles (Faddy, Gosden, Gougeon, Richardson, & Nelson, 1992), which in turn depletes follicular reserves (Richardson, Senikas, & Nelson, 1987). Beginning around age 40 and as women approach age 50, there is a sharp drop in the number of ovarian follicles (Burger, 1996; Faddy *et al.*, 1992; Richardson *et al.*, 1987). Ovarian hormone production slows, and more and more cycles become anovulatory. Levels of inhibin B, an indicator of the number of follicles, fall, and FSH levels increase further because of lack of suppression by inhibin B (Burger *et al.*, 1998; Klein, Illingworth, Groome, McNeilly, Battaglia, & Soules, 1996). Later in the transition when the menstrual cycle becomes irregular and cycle intervals become longer, the follicles become unresponsive to gonadotropins, resulting in a drop in estrogen and progesterone levels (Burger *et al.*, 1998; Sowers & La Pietra, 1995). FSH levels increase even further in an attempt to stimulate the follicles. Eventually the follicles do not respond and menstruation stops altogether. Natural menopause is due to the exhaustion of remaining follicles. Without follicles the postmenopausal ovary can no longer produce the ovarian steroids and peptides. Hormone levels stabilize approximately one to two years after the final menstrual period, with elevated levels of gonadotropins and low levels of ovarian steroids.

It is important to point out that following menopause, estrogen production does not stop altogether. While the ovary accounts for more than 90% of total body production of estradiol, the most potent naturally occurring estrogen, other forms of estrogen, such as estrone are produced by other glands such as the adrenal and by peripheral conversion of circulating hormones, such as testosterone. Peripheral aromatization (conversion) of androgens in tissues such as blood, liver, and adipose tissue continue to provide a source of estrone to postmenopausal women.

Menopause Defined

A variety of indicators have been used to define menopause status, including age, menstrual bleeding patterns, and levels of reproductive hormones. Early studies employed chronologic age as an indicator of natural menopause (Bungay, Vessey, & McPherson, 1980; Rostosky & Travis, 1996; Sowers & La Pietra, 1995). However, because of variability in the age at final menstrual period (McKinlay, Brambilla, & Posner, 1992), chronologic age is an unsatisfactory proxy variable for postmenopausal status.

Later epidemiological studies base definitions of menopause status on reported menstrual bleeding patterns and gynecological surgery. The standard epidemiological definition of natural menopause is twelve consecutive months of amenorrhea in the absence of surgery or other cause (e.g., pregnancy, radiation therapy) that would terminate menstruation. This definition has been employed in European studies since the 1950s (Magursky, Mesko, & Sokolik, 1975) and was suggested by Treloar (1974) on the basis of his prospective study of normal menstrual patterns. Two working group meetings of the World Health Organization (WHO, 1981, 1996) also recommended use of

this definition. Note that the point at which a woman experiences her final menstrual period (FMP) can only be determined retrospectively.

Perimenopause has been defined to begin with the onset of endocrinologic and menstrual changes just prior to the FMP (Metcalf, 1988; Treloar, 1974, 1981; WHO, 1981, 1996) and is characterized by variability in hormone concentrations (Reame, Kelche, Beitins, Yu, Zawacki, & Padmanabhan, 1996). Some researchers include the first year after the FMP as part of the perimenopausal period (Metcalf, 1988; WHO, 1981, 1996), due to continuing fluctuations in reproductive hormones until one-to-two years after the FMP (Burger, 1996). No standard definition of perimenopause exists, however (Brambilla, McKinlay, & Johannes, 1994; Greendale & Sowers, 1997), making cross-study comparisons of this important transition difficult.

Levels of reproductive hormones, particularly follicle-stimulating hormone (FSH), also have been used to classify women with respect to menopause status. A cutoff of 35–40 IU/l for FSH is often employed in both clinical practice and in research studies as indicative of postmenopausal status (Goldenberg, Grodin, Rodbard, & Ross, 1973; Wilson & Foster, 1992). A cutoff of 10–20 IU/l has also been taken as indicating perimenopause (Cooper & Baird, 1995). Values of hormones, however, vary widely both within and across women during perimenopause (Burger, 1994a, b, 1996). Moreover, hormone concentrations also change as a function of chronologic age (Burger, 1994a; Reame et al., 1996). Consequently, although average values of hormone levels exhibit general trends during the perimenopause, no single cutoff value—particularly for use with a single serum sample—is likely to yield an accurate classification of menopause status for an individual woman (Stellato, Crawford, McKinlay, & Longcope, 1998).

In any discussion of menopause, it is crucial to distinguish between natural and surgical or induced menopause. The latter has been defined by the WHO (1981, 1996) as the cessation of menses due to removal of the uterus and at most one ovary, or removal of both ovaries with or without removal of the uterus. Surgically menopausal women differ in a number of respects from other women, including lower age, greater access to health care, and lower general levels of health (Johannes & Avis, 1996; McKinlay, 1994; McKinlay, Brambilla, Avis, & McKinlay, 1991; Sowers & La Pietra, 1995). Their menopausal experiences may differ from those of other women for these reasons, and also because of differences in rapidity and timing of changes in reproductive hormone concentrations (Bush, 1990; Sowers & La Pietra, 1995). Consequently, surgically menopausal women are often treated as a separate stratum in study design and analyses (McKinlay, 1994). In describing the menopause experience, this chapter refers to the experience of natural menopause.

Factors Related to Age of Menopause

Most studies using appropriate methodology—that is, not relying on recall of the date of the FMP or a woman's self-categorization— have found a median age at the FMP of 50–52 years (McKinlay, 1996; McKinlay, Bifano, & McKinlay, 1985). Eighty percent of women experience their FMP between ages 44–55 (Treloar, 1974).

There is wide variability among women in the age at natural menopause (McKinlay *et al.*, 1992). It is hypothesized that menopause occurs after sufficient depletion of oocytes (Gosden, 1985; Whelan, Sandler, McConnaughey, & Weinberg, 1990), beginning with a sharp drop in the number of ovarian follicles in the last decade before FMP (Burger, 1996; Faddy *et al.*, 1992). Menstrual functioning also requires a level of estrogen sufficient for endometrial growth. Thus, factors that delay or suppress ovulation—such as multiple pregnancies—or affect the synthesis or metabolism of estrogen might delay the onset of menopause.

The most well-established and consistently noted factor related to age of menopause is cigarette smoking. On average, smokers reach menopause one to two years earlier than do nonsmokers (Adena & Gallagher, 1982; Brambilla & McKinlay, 1989; Bromberger, Matthews, Kuller, Wing, Meilhan, & Plantinga, 1997; Cramer, Harlow, Xu, Fraer, & Barbieri, 1995a; Everson, Sandler, Wilcox, Schreinemachers, Shore, & Weinberg, 1986; Jick & Porter, 1977; Kaufman & Sloane, 1980; McKinlay *et al.*, 1985; Torgerson, Avenell, Russell, & Reid, 1994; Willett *et al.*, 1983). Findings regarding a dose–response relationship are not as consistent across studies, with some results suggesting a lower age at FMP with higher levels of smoking (Cramer *et al.*, 1995a; Torgerson *et al.*, 1994; Willett *et al.*, 1983) while others indicate that any level of smoking may be sufficient (Brambilla *et al.*, 1989; McKinlay *et al.*, 1985). One recent study noted an earlier age at menopause for passive smokers (Everson *et al.*, 1986). Smoking appears to have an impact on both oocytes and estrogen levels. Carbon monoxide and polycyclic aromatic hydrocarbons in smoke may destroy oocytes (Baron, LaVecchia, & Levi, 1990; Cramer *et al.*, 1995a). In addition, alkaloid components of smoke, including nicotine, may interfere with estrogen synthesis (Barbieri, McShane, & Ryan, 1986; Baron *et al.*, 1990). Smoking also may affect estradiol metabolism, leading to greater formation of less active estrogens (Baron *et al.*, 1990; Michnovicz, Hershcopf, Naganuma, Bradlow, & Fishman, 1986).

Menopause has been found to occur later in heavier women (Hoel, Wakabayashi, & Pike, 1983; MacMahon & Worcester, 1966; Sherman, Wallace, Bean, & Schlabaugh, 1981; Stanford, Hartage, Brinton, Hoover, & Brookmeyer, 1987; Willett *et al.*, 1983), women with higher income and education (Brambilla & McKinley, 1989; Cramer *et al.*, 1995a; McKinlay *et al.*, 1992; Stanford *et al.*, 1987; Torgerson *et al.*, 1994), and ever-married women (Cramer *et al.*, 1995a; Cramer, Xu, & Harlow, 1995b; McKinlay *et al.*, 1985; McKinlay, Jefferys, & Thompson, 1972; Stanford *et al.*, 1987). These associations may be due in part to confounding with factors such as smoking or parity. Compared with Caucasians, menopause may occur earlier in African-Americans (Bromberger *et al.*, 1997; Stanford *et al.*, 1987) and later in Asians (Avis, Kaufert, Locke, McKinlay, & Vass, 1993).

With respect to reproductive and menstrual history, some findings suggest that nulliparous women have an earlier menopause than parous women (Cramer *et al.*, 1995a,b; Stanford *et al.*, 1987; Torgerson *et al.*, 1994; Whelan *et al.*, 1990; Willett *et al.*, 1983). There is some evidence of a "dose–response" relationship with number of children or age at first birth (Cramer *et al.*, 1995a; Stanford *et al.*, 1987; Torgerson *et al.*, 1994; Whelan *et al.*, 1990). Results regarding use of hormone replacement therapy or oral contraception are mixed (Stanford *et al.*, 1987; Treloar, 1981), although other studies have found no relationship (Brambilla & McKinlay 1989; Cramer *et al.*, 1995a,b). With few exceptions (Cramer *et al.*, 1995b), age at menarche has not been significantly associated with age at menopause (Cramer, 1995a; McKinlay *et al.*, 1972; Stanford *et al.*, 1987; Whelan *et al.*, 1990; Willett *et al.*, 1983). Women with short menstrual cycles during their twenties and thirties—and thus, faster depletion of oocytes—may experience menopause earlier (Cramer *et al.*, 1995b; Whelan *et al.*, 1990).

With the exception of smoking, results of studies are often inconsistent, due in part to differences in populations studied, definitions of menopause status, methods of data collection, and data analysis. As previously mentioned, studies using retrospective data on age at reproductive events or age at FMP are particularly subject to biased or inaccurate recall (Bean, Leeper, Wallace, Sherman, & Jagger, 1979; McKinlay *et al.*, 1972; Paganini-Hill, Krailo, & Pike, 1984).

SYMPTOMS ASSOCIATED WITH MENOPAUSE

It is often assumed that menopause is inevitably accompanied (to a greater or lesser extent) by hot flushes, sweats, prolonged menstrual irregularities, vaginal dryness and a host of other "symptoms," including depression, irritability, weight gain, insomnia, and dizziness. Earlier analyses of primarily cross-sectional data in Caucasian populations have provided evidence that these signs and symptoms of menopause are far from universal (Greene & Cooke, 1976, 1980; McKinlay & Jefferys, 1974; Neugarten & Kraines, 1965). These same studies have also suggested that with the exception of hot flushes and accompanying sweats, other supposed menopausal symptoms are not directly related to this physiological change.

The following is a review of the primary symptoms thought to be associated with menopause through the impact of hormonal changes on the central nervous system: vasomotor symptoms (hot flashes/flushes and night sweats), depression and mood changes, sleep disturbances, and memory problems.

Vasomotor Symptoms

Vasomotor symptoms (hot flashes/flushes and night sweats) are the primary symptoms associated with menopause. Estimates of the incidence of hot flashes from population studies in the United States and worldwide have ranged from 24% to 93% (Kronenberg, 1990). Some discrepancies in the prevalence of hot flash reporting reflect inconsistencies in research methodology, as well as study populations. Age ranges and menopause status of women studied differ; some studies are based on patient samples while others on general population samples; and the specific symptom questions and the frame also differ. However, even within study or controlling for methodology, a high degree of variability of symptom reporting is found among women, thus suggesting considerable individual variation in symptom experience.

While cross-sectional studies often report the highest prevalence of hot flashes postmenopause, there are sparse longitudinal data on the age and menopause status at which hot flashes begin. McKinlay *et al.* (1992) report data from the Massachusetts Women's Health Study (MWHS), on the relationship of hot flashes to the menopause transition. The MWHS is a large prospective study of women transitioning through the menopause. McKinlay *et al.* (1992) found that hot flash reporting peaked just prior to the point where menopause is defined. These findings contradict the widely held health clinical impression that hot flashes begin to increase after last menstrual period. McKinlay *et al.* (1992) also report that hot flashes were related to the duration of the perimenopausal period—women who had a longer perimenopause were more likely to report hot flashes. Women who abruptly went into menopause, with little or no perimenopausal transition, reported fewer hot flashes.

Some women report never experiencing hot flashes, while others report experiencing hot flashes throughout the day. There are no good population data on the distribution of hot flash frequency across women. Data from the MWHS show that 19% of postmenopausal women report having never experienced a hot flash, and of those who experienced hot flashes, only 19% said they were very bothersome. The most bothersome symptom experienced was menstrual flow problems. While only 13% of women reported this symptom, 53% of those who did, reported this symptom as very bothersome. From the high variability among women of hot flashes experienced, it is clear that factors other than hormonal changes affect this symptom experience.

Except for findings about estrogen levels, there are limited data on factors that may predispose women to hot flashes. Thin women may have more hot flashes because they have higher levels of sex hormone binding globulin and their circulating estrogen is less biologically active. Factors thought to be related to symptomatology include sociocultural (Beyenne, 1986; Kaufert, 1982; Lock, 1986), psychological (Avis & McKinlay, 1991; Hunter, 1992; Swartzman, Edelberg, & Kemmann, 1990), reproductive (Beyenne, 1986), and dietary (Beyenne, 1986), as well as hormonal changes (Kronenberg, 1990).

Although hot flashes are the most common complaint associated with menopause for women in the United States and most Western cultures, this is not true elsewhere. The rate of hot flash reporting varies widely between and within cultures. Researchers have studied Japa-

nese, Mayan, and Rajput women in India and find they report far lower rates of hot flashes than their Western counterparts. Many factors may be involved ranging from reproductive history, diet, and exercise to social, cultural, and attitudinal variables. A study comparing symptom reporting in three distinct population groups of women (United States, Canada, and Japan), all aged 45–55 at the time of survey found symptom reporting in the Japanese women was generally low across all menopausal status categories (Avis *et al.*, 1993). The percentage of Japanese women reporting hot flashes or night sweats was considerably lower (14.7%) than it was for the Canadian (36%) or U.S. women (38%). This finding is further supported by research from the Study of Women's Health Across the Nation (SWAN). In this large, multiethnic, multirace study of women ages 40–55, Chinese and Japanese women were significantly less likely to report vasomotor symptoms than their Caucasian, African-American, and Hispanic counterparts (Avis, Stellato, Crawford, Bromberger, Ganz, Cain, & Kagawa-Singer, 2001).

Whether the low incidence of vasomotor symptoms reflects cultural, psychological, or physiological differences, or some combination of all three, requires further examination. Japanese women may not perceive these heat changes as remarkable and/or they may experience them at a much lower rate, possibly due to the much lower fat content in their diets. Another hypothesis is that the low rate of hot flash reporting among Japanese women may be due to phytoestrogens in their diet (Aldercreutz, Hamalaiven, Gorbach, & Grodin, 1992).

There is also evidence that psychological factors influence menopausal symptoms. Laboratory studies have shown increased reporting of hot flashes during stress (Swartzman *et al.*, 1990). Other evidence for a psychological component to hot flashes comes from the results of clinical trials of estrogen replacement therapy (ERT). Studies of ERT's effectiveness that include a placebo control have often found a significant placebo effect on symptom reduction (e.g., Clayden, Bell, & Pollard, 1974; Coope,

Thomson, & Poller, 1975; Poller, Thomson, & Coope, 1980). Other studies have shown that premenopausal attitudes towards menopause are predictive of menopausal symptomatology (Avis & McKinlay, 1991; Hunter, 1992; Matthews, 1992). Avis, Crawford, and McKinlay (1997) also found increased hot flash reporting among women with more psychological and physical symptoms *prior* to menopause and those with lower education.

Depression and Mood

Numerous cross-sectional studies have examined the association between menopause status and mood. Most of these studies do not find a relation between menopause status and depression or dysphoric or negative mood, using such measures as the CES-D (Kaufert, Guilbert, & Hassard, 1988; McKinlay, McKinlay, & Brambilla, 1987; Porter, Penney, Russell, Russell, & Templeton, 1996; Woods & Mitchell, 1997), a psychiatric interview (Gath *et al.*, 1987; Hallstrom & Samuelsson, 1985), dysphoric mood (Dennerstein, Smith, Morse, Burger, Green, Hooper, & Ryan, 1993), negative affect (Dennerstein, Smith, & Morse, 1994), nervousness and mood lability (Holte & Mikkelsen, 1991), anxiety/fears (Hunter, Battersby, & Whitehead, 1986), psychological symptoms (Kuh, Wadsworth, & Hardy, 1997; Porter *et al.*, 1996), and individual symptoms of irritability, anxiety, and/or depression (Ballinger, 1976; Cawood & Bancroft, 1996). On the other hand, several studies have found a relation between menopause status and mood, mostly in the perimenopause (Avis *et al.*, 1993; Ballinger, 1975; Collins & Landgren, 1995; Hunter *et al.*, 1986). These studies, however, generally have not controlled for vasomotor symptoms. The one study that did control for symptoms found that the association disappeared when vasomotor symptoms were included in the model (Collins & Landgren, 1995).

While the majority of studies in this area have been cross-sectional, several prospective or longitudinal studies have been conducted (Avis, Brambilla, McKinlay, & Vass, 1994; Hallstrom

& Samuelsson, 1985; Holte, 1992; Hunter, 1990; Kaufert, Guilbert, & Tate, 1992; Kuh *et al.*, 1997; Matthews *et al.*, 1990; Woods & Mitchell, 1996). Each of these studies analyzes their longitudinal data somewhat differently. To summarize, findings show that onset of menopause is not related to increased rates of depressive symptoms (Kaufert *et al.*, 1992; Woods & Mitchell, 1996) or mental disorder (Hallstrom & Samuelsson, 1985), postmenopausal women do not show higher rates of anxiety or depression compared to when they were premenopausal (Holte, 1992), and postmenopausal women do not differ in anxiety or depression from premenopausal women (Matthews *et al.*, 1990).

One study, that included women during the perimenopause, followed a nationally representative sample of British women born in 1946 (Kuh *et al.*, 1997). This paper reports results of surveys completed by over 1200 women when they were 36 years of age and again when they were 47 years (Kuh *et al.*, 1997). Psychological symptoms at age 47 were unrelated to natural menopause status, except for a slight rise in irritability among perimenopausal women. However, women who had had a hysterectomy or were on HRT reported significantly more psychological symptoms. They further found that psychological symptoms at age 47 were strongly related to current family life and work stress, anxiety, depression, and health problems at age 36.

Two exceptions to these findings are reported by Avis *et al.* (1994) and Hunter (1990). Using data from the Massachusetts Women's Health Study, Avis *et al.* (1994), addressed the effect of change in menopause status on depression as measured by the CES-D scale, while controlling for prior depression. To study change in menopause status, a menopause transition variable was created that took into account a woman's menopausal status at the two time-points (27 months apart) at which depression was measured (referred to as T_1 and T_2). Across all menopause statuses, those women who were classified as depressed at T_1 had higher rates of depression at T_2. For women who were not depressed at T_1, the rate of depression at T_2 increased slightly as women moved from pre–pre to pre–peri, and was highest for women who remained perimenopausal for at least 27 months. The rate of depression began to decrease as women moved from peri- to post-menopause, and was lowest for those women who were postmenopausal for at least 27 months. Controlling for premenopausal depression, there was still a slight increase in depression among the peri–peri women.

In further analyses of the MWHS data, Avis *et al.* (1994) examined whether this increased rate of depression among the peri–peri women could be attributed to symptoms associated with menopause (i.e., hot flashes, night sweats, and menstrual problems). When menopausal symptoms were added to the regression model, it became a significant predictor of T_2 depression, and menopausal transition was no longer statistically significant. Over all menopause transition categories, those women who reported experiencing hot flashes, night sweats, and/or menstrual problems consistently showed higher rates of depression.

Hunter (1990) reports follow-up data on 36 women who were initially premenopausal and became peri- or postmenopausal three years later. While she found that the women reported significantly more depressed mood at follow-up, she did not have a comparison group to control for age and she did not control for vasomotor symptoms in analysis. There was no change in anxiety. She found no evidence of an increase in psychiatric caseness as defined by the General Health Questionnaire.

In summary, it thus appears that from longitudinal studies there is no evidence that onset of perimenopause leads to increased depression. One study that examined length of the perimenopause (Avis *et al.*, 1994) did find a small increase in depression associated with a long perimenopause, which was not significant when vasomotor symptoms were included in the model.

While there is no evidence that menopause is associated with increased mood disturbance on a population level, an unanswered question is whether some women may be more vulnerable to mood effects of hormonal changes. Several researchers have proposed that while menopause does not cause mood disturbances in all women, there may be a subgroup of women at higher risk for depression or other mood changes (Brace & McCauley, 1997; Charney, 1996; Steiner, 1992). It has been suggested that women with a history of PMS have an increased sensitivity to hormone changes (Bancroft & Backstrom, 1985) and that women with previous affective disorders that are cyclic or associated with reproductive events are at higher risk (Pearlstein, Rosen, & Stone, 1997). While the postpartum period is not always associated with depression, women with previous depression, a history of premenstrual dysphoric disorder, or a history of bipolar disorder are at increased risk for postpartum depression (Blehar & Oren, 1995). However, it is premature to conclude that this pattern is related to a hormonal imbalance. Other factors that may be related are coping style or a greater sensitivity to symptoms. Further, since most studies involve retrospective reporting of reproductive and psychiatric history, there is the inherent problem of selective recall among women experiencing problems at the time of the study.

Sleep

Sleep disturbances are often thought to be associated with menopause. However, the degree to which sleep disturbances are directly related to hormonal changes or are secondary to hot flashes and night sweats has not been established. Episodes of wakening and insomnia are known to occur in association with hot flashes and women with severe vasomotor symptoms are at risk for sleep disturbances. A study published by Erlik and colleagues (1981) found a significant correlation between hot flashes and waking episodes, both of which were reduced by estrogen therapy.

Shaver and colleagues (1988) objectively measured sleep patterns in a community-based sample of 82 women aged 40–59 recruited without regard to sleep quality. Women were classified by menopause status. Few differences in sleep variables were found overall by menopause stages. However, peri- and postmeno-pausal women who were experiencing hot flashes tended to spend more time in bed, have a lower mean sleep efficiency index, and have greater rapid eye movement latency than asymptomatic women.

In a subsequent study, Shaver and colleagues (1991) compared subjective and objective reports of sleep quality. Interestingly, they found that less than half of women reporting poor sleep showed poor sleep on objective measures. They found that women who self-reported poor sleep, but showed no objective indicators of poor sleep had the highest ratings of psychological distress and somatic symptoms. Women having *both* subjective and objective poor sleep had the highest mean menopausal symptom score, but this was only statistically significant from the subgroup classified with good sleep by both criteria. Data published by Hunter in 1992 show that sleep disturbances are more common in women who do not exercise regularly, have histories of emotional problems before the menopause, and who are in poor health.

In a 1993 review, Regestein (1993) concludes that sleep disturbances increase around menopause, but menopausal status itself explains only a small part of this increase.

Memory

Like sleep disturbances, memory complaints have also been thought to be associated with menopause (Anderson, Hamburger, Liu & Rebar, 1987; Malleson, 1953; Kopera, 1973). The effect of menopausal hormonal changes on memory, however, has not been well studied and there are no data showing that menopause is associated with changes in memory or cognitive function. Most studies in this area have looked at the effect of estrogen replacement therapy (ERT) on cognitive functioning. Despite this lack of evidence, several mechanisms have been proposed to explain the possible effect of estrogen replacement on cognitive functioning. Estrogen might influence the concentration of certain neurotransmitters (Luine, Park, Joh, Reis, & McEwen, 1980), induce anatomical changes in the nerve cells in the ventro-medial hypothalamus (McEwen, 1991), improve carotid artery blood flow (Gangar, Vyas, Whitehead, Crook, Meire, & Campbell, 1991), or improve depressed mood (Aylward, 1973).

Research on the effect of postmenopausal estrogen replacement on cognitive functioning, has reported contradictory results. Some studies showed improved memory among women taking ERT (Campbell & Whitehead, 1977; Fedor-Freybergh, 1977; Sherwin, 1988), while other studies show no effect at all (Barrett-Connor & Kritz-Silverstein, 1993; Ditkoff, Crary, Cristo, & Lobo, 1991; Rauramo, Langerspetz, Engblom, & Punnonen, 1975; Vanhulle & Demol, 1976). Except for Barrett-Connor and Kritz-Silverstein (1993), these studies generally have small sample sizes and limited tests of cognitive function. Further, most studies have been conducted with recently postmenopausal women and have not separated the effect of estrogen on cognitive function from its effect on symptom relief (particularly sleep). To date, there have not been good studies on the effect of naturally occurring hormonal changes during menopause and their relation to memory or of the effect of ERT on cognitive function separate from its effect on dysphoric mood and somatic symptoms (Barrett-Connor & Kritz-Silverstein, 1993). A recent review of this research concluded that while there are plausible biological mechanisms that might account for a beneficial effect of estrogen therapy on cognition, the studies conducted in women have substantial methodologic problems and have produced conflicting results (Yaffe, Sawaya, Lieberburg, & Grady, 1998). Any research on the effect of menopause on cognitive function must consider the role of night sweats and subsequent sleep disturbances on cognitive function.

LONG-TERM CHANGES FOLLOWING MENOPAUSE

The hormonal changes accompanying menopause are thought to impact other bodily systems, in particular the musculoskeletal, cardiovascular, and urogenital systems. Changes in these systems are thought to precipitate increases in heart disease, diabetes, hypertension, osteoporosis, urinary incontinence, and autoimmune disease (Bjorntorp, 1988). It is currently unknown, however, to what extent changes in these systems are directly associated with reductions in estrogen, aging, or concurrent behavioral changes.

Musculoskeletal

Osteoporosis, a condition characterized by loss of bone mass resulting in increased porosity, brittleness and fragility of bone, is one of the leading causes of morbidity and mortality in the elderly (Riggs & Melton, 1986, 1992). The vertebra is one of the most common sites of bone loss leading to curvature of the spine, loss of height, and pain (Riggs & Melton, 1986). In the United States, 25 million people are afflicted with osteoporosis, 80% of whom are women. The most serious consequence of osteoporosis is the increased risk for a bone fracture, especially in the hip. The relationship between osteoporosis and fracture, however, is still debated (U.S. Congress & Office of Technology Assessment, 1992). Bone mass in older women is a function of two major factors: peak amount of bone mass and rate of bone loss (Heaney, Gallagher, Johnson, Neer, Parfitt, & Whedon, 1982). Peak bone mass is determined to a large extent by genetic inheritance (Pollitzer & Anderson, 1989) and other factors such as diet and physical activity (Kanders, Dempster, & Lindsay, 1988). Hormonal status exerts it greatest effect on rate of bone loss.

Women lose about 50% of their trabecular bone and 30% of their cortical bone mass over their lifetime, about half of which is lost during the 10 years after menopause (Riggs *et al.*, 1986, 1992). The most rapid bone loss in White females occurs around the time of menopause. Approximately one quarter to one third of a woman's lifetime bone loss from the spine occurs during the early menopausal period. Estrogen appears to protect bone and stimulate calcium absorption while FSH is thought to interfere with parathormone which prevents loss of calcium in the urine and helps transport calcium.

Although there is an acceleration of bone loss with the cessation of menses, it is unclear when menopausal bone loss begins. Further, different bone sites may vary in their rate of bone loss (Sowers & McKinlay, 1995). Data from the MWHS show that bone loss is easily detectable in the late perimenopause and is equally rapid in the 12 months before and after the last menstrual period. This finding is consistent with other studies of late perimenopausal women (Pouilles, Tremollieres, & Ribot, 1993; Sowers, Clark, Hollis, Wallace, & Jannausch, 1992).

It is important to point out that most of the studies in this area have been conducted on White women. Existing data suggest that African-American women are at lower risk for hip and spinal fractures than White women. Some studies suggest that African-American women may not experience the same postmenopausal bone loss as White women (Krolner & Pors, 1982; Mazess, 1982; Ruegsegger, Dambacher, Ruegsegger, Fischer, & Anliker, 1984). A recent prospective study of African-American and White women found a higher average bone mass in younger African-American women and a slower rate of bone loss in the early menopausal period in African-American women as compared to White women. The rate of bone loss in women more than five years postmenopausal did not differ (Luckey, Wallenstein, Lapinski, & Meier, 1996).

Cardiovascular

Cardiovascular diseases (CVD) are the leading cause of death among women in the United States, claiming twice as many lives annually as all forms of cancer combined (American Heart Association, 1998). Mortality rates of CVD increase in women increase sharply with age, with the largest apparent increase occurring around the age of 50, coinciding with the time of menopause (Stampfer, Colditz, Willett, Mason, Rosner, & Speizer, 1991). Although CVD mortality rates are higher for men than for women at all ages, this gender gap appears to narrow after the age of menopause. This has led to speculation that declining estrogen levels associated with menopause result in an increased risk of CVD (Eaker, Chesbro, Sacks, Wenger, Whisnant, & Winston, 1993; Gorodeski 1994). Evidence for this widely held notion derives from comparison of age-specific disease rates in men and women; numerous observational studies of exogenous postmenopausal estrogen replacement therapy (Barrett-Connor & Goodman-Gruen, 1995; Bush *et al.*, 1987; Grady *et al.*, 1992; Grodstein & Stampfer, 1995; Stampfer *et al.*, 1991); and studies of menopause in relation to blood pressure, lipids, and other cardiovascular risk factors.

A closer examination of age-specific CVD mortality rates in men and women does not support the assumption that the apparent narrowing of the gender gap around age 50 is due to declining ovarian function associated with menopause. If this were true, the rate of increase in deaths, or slope of the line as plotted on a log scale, would be steeper in women over the age of 50 compared with that for younger women. There is no such sharp increase in the CVD mortality rate for women at the time of menopause, in contrast to plots of mortality rates for breast cancer, a disease exhibiting a clear menopause-related increase (Bush, 1990; Stampfer, Colditz, & Willet, 1990; McKinlay, Crawford, McKinlay, & Stellato, 1994). The reduced sex difference in mortality appears to be more a result of declining mortality rates in men rather than increasing rates in women.

While natural menopause does not appear to be associated with a dramatic increase in the risk of CVD, surgical menopause (hysterectomy with bilateral oophorectomy) at a young age approximately doubles the risk of coronary heart disease for women who do not take estrogen replacement therapy (Colditz, Willett, Stampfer, Rosner, Speizer, & Hennekens, 1987). These women experience an abrupt decline in estrogen levels as opposed to the gradual decline seen with natural menopause.

Results of epidemiological studies relating natural menopause to CVD risk are inconsistent, and interpretation is hampered by methodological difficulties. In general, studies that have carefully controlled for age and cigarette smoking have found little association of natural menopause with increased CVD risk (Crawford & Johannes, 1999). Increases in total and LDL-cholesterol levels and small decreases in HDL have been noted, even after adjustment for age and smoking (Matthews, Meilhan, Kuller, Kelsey, Caggiula, & Wing, 1989). Lipid studies have shown that total cholesterol and LDL-cholesterol levels increase more rapidly in women during the 15 years around the menopause than during the same period in men (Brown, Hutchinson, Morrisett, Boerwinkle, Davis, & Gotto, 1993; Matthews *et al.*, 1989). The evidence of a substantial effect of endogenous estrogens on lipid levels, however, is lacking. In several studies no consistent change has been found between changes in endogenous estrogen levels and changes in lipids and lipoproteins among women traversing the menopause (Cauley, Gutai, Kuller, & Powell, 1990; Kuller, Gutai, Meilahn, Matthews, & Plantinga, 1990; Longcope, Crawford, & McKinlay, 1996). Estrogens do exhibit direct favorable effects on arterial wall function and blood flow, thus declining levels could facilitate the development of atherosclerosis and impaired blood flow (Lobo, Pickar, Wild, Walsh, & Hirvonen, 1994), but appear to have no effect on blood pressure (Crawford & McKinlay, 1999).

Natural menopause may have some gradual effect on cardiovascular risk. The current body of evidence does not support an abrupt increase in CVD risk at the time of menopause. Other important risk factors for CVD such as smoking, diabetes, diet, and obesity have a stronger impact on CVD risk in aging women.

Urogenital

Urinary Incontinence

Urinary symptoms, including incontinence, have often been thought to be part of the menopausal syndrome. The belief is that because bladder and urethral tissue are estrogen sensitive, there is a causal relationship between estrogen deficiency and incontinence. However, it is difficult to determine whether urinary changes are a direct result of estrogen deficiency or are part of the general aging process (Versi,

1990). In a study of 600 working women aged 35–60 years of age, Osborne (1976) did not find an increase in stress incontinence at menopause. In a study of 10,000 women, Thomas and colleagues (1980) did not find an increase in prevalence of urinary incontinence in women aged 45–60. Neither Hording and colleagues (1986) nor Hagstad and Janson (1986) found an increase in incontinence between age matched pre- and postmenopausal women.

Studies of the effect of ERT on urinary incontinence have yielded mixed results (Versi, 1990). While uncontrolled trials have shown subjective improvement (Versi & Cardozo, 1988), results of placebo controlled trials are not as favorable. Neither Fantl and colleagues (1988) nor Versi and Cardozo (1988) found significant effects of ERT in postmenopausal women with stress incontinence.

Sexual Functioning

It is generally recognized that sexual behavior changes with age. In particular, frequency of sexual activity declines with age (Kinsey, Pomeroy, Martin, & Gebhard, 1948, 1953; Laumann, Gagnon, Michael, & Michaels, 1994; Pfeiffer, Verwoerdt, & Davis, 1972). Reasons for this decline among women include loss of or lack of a partner, partner's sexual problems, health changes, and physiological changes due to changing hormonal levels (Avis *et al.*, 2000). The impact of menopause on declines in sexual functioning is of particular interest because of decreases in ovarian hormones at this time (which may be directly or indirectly related to aspects of sexual functioning) and because menopause can be viewed as a marker in the aging process. There is much debate, however, over the relative impact of menopause on sexual functioning. Much of the research in this area is based on patient-based samples, or women who are having sexual problems. Furthermore, changes in ovarian hormones often lead to vasomotor symptoms, sleep disruption, and possibly mood changes. All of these factors may also impact sexual functioning. Thus, any attempt to understand the role of menopause *per se* on

sexual functioning needs to take into account these factors.

In general, sexual functioning is studied in terms of satisfaction, frequency of activity (intercourse, masturbation, orgasm), desire (including interest and sexual thoughts or fantasies), arousal, attitudes toward sexuality, and difficulties such as pain during intercourse and problems reaching orgasm. These reflect the characterization of sexual functioning in terms of libido and potency (Davidson, 1985; Iddenden, 1987). Libido includes sexual interest, desire, drive, motivation, and pleasure. Potency is the physiologically measurable event during sexual arousal/activity—the sexual response (Masters & Johnson, 1966). While postmenopausal declines in ovarian hormone production and reproductive atrophy may increase the incidence of dyspareunia and vaginal dryness (potency), it is less clear how menopause affects sexual interest or libido (Davidson, 1985).

Research among general populations of women does not show clear associations between menopause and declines in sexual functioning. While some studies have found lower sexual interest among peri- or postmenopausal women as compared to premenopausal women (Cawood & Bancroft, 1996; Dennerstein *et al.*, 1994; Hallstrom, 1977; Hunter *et al.*, 1986), other studies have not found an association between menopause status and sexual desire (Køster & Garde, 1993), frequency of sexual activity (Dennerstein, Dudley, Hopper, & Burger, 1997; Hawton, Gath, & Day, 1994), or general sexual dysfunction (Osborn, Hawton, & Gath, 1988). In general, satisfaction with one's sexual relationship has not been found to be related to menopause or age (Avis *et al.*, 2000; Hawton *et al.*, 1994; Hunter *et al.*, 1986). There are at least three possible explanations for this: (1) frequency of activity is not related to satisfaction; (2) people accommodate to the age-related declines that occur; and/or (3) people's expectation with respect to sexual activity or desire declines with age.

The Massachusetts Women's Health Study, one of the most comprehensive community-based studies of women transitioning through the menopause, found that menopause status was significantly related to lower sexual desire, a belief that interest in sexual activity declines with age, and women's reports of decreased arousal compared to when in their forties (Avis *et al.*, 2000). Menopause status was unrelated to frequency of sexual intercourse, satisfaction with one's sexual relationship, difficulty reaching orgasm, and pain during or after intercourse in either unadjusted or multiple regression analyses.

Taken as a whole, these studies suggest that menopause may have an impact on some aspects of sexual functioning, but not others. Some inconsistencies in findings can be explained by the wide variation in the specific sexual functioning questions that are asked, the time frame used (e.g., past month, past year, etc.), whether women without partners are included in analyses, and nature of the study sample. Further, many of these studies only look at univariate associations and do not adjust for other variables in the analyses that may be related to sexual functioning (e.g., age, partner problems, and health).

Psychosocial and aging factors are often reported as more important determinants than ovarian function of sexual functioning among mid-aged women (Hagstad, 1988; Hawton *et al.*, 1994; Køster & Garde, 1993; Leiblum, Bachmann, Kemmann, Colburn, & Swartzman, 1983). Some of these factors include the availability of a partner (Køster & Garde, 1993; Leiblum *et al.*, 1983; Pfeiffer *et al.*, 1972), previous sexual behavior and enjoyment (Christensen & Gagnon, 1965; Pfeiffer *et al.*, 1972), the marital relationship (Bachmann *et al.*, 1985; Cawood & Bancroft, 1996; Clark & Wallin, 1965; Hawton *et al.*, 1994), mental health (Avis *et al.*, 2000; Dennerstein *et al.*, 1994; Hawton *et al.*, 1994), general physical health (Avis *et al.*, 2000; Hunter, 1990; Køster & Garde, 1993), stress (Hunter, 1990), expectations (Køster & Garde, 1993), and male partner problems (Pfeiffer *et al.*, 1972).

In the Massachusetts Women's Health Study, Avis *et al.* (2000) found that health was a significant variable related to all aspects of sexual functioning. Depression and greater psychological symptoms were related to lower satisfaction, frequency, and desire. Interestingly, smoking was related to less desire and lower frequency of sexual intercourse. This finding is consistent with results reported by Greendale and colleagues (1996) and are consistent with other research on the negative effects of smoking on sex steroid levels (Johnston, Hui, Witt, Appledorn, Baker, & Longcope, 1985; Michnovitz & Bradlow, 1990).

While only a few studies have examined sexual functioning and hormones, they consistently do not find a relation between estradiol level and sexual functioning (Avis *et al.*, 2000; Bachmann, Leiblum, Kemmann, Colburn, Swartzman, & Shelden, 1984; Bachmann *et al.*, 1985; Cawood *et al.*, 1996; Dennerstein *et al.*, 1997; Leiblum *et al.*, 1983; McCoy & Davidson, 1985). Some of these studies, however, look at frequency of sexual intercourse (Leiblum *et al.*, 1983; McCoy & Davidson, 1985), which may be a poor indicator of sexual functioning for women, since frequency of activity is often determined more by the male partner. The one exception to these negative findings was a study by Cutler and colleagues (Cutler, Garcia, & McCoy, 1987) who found that a subset of perimenopausal women with especially low estradiol levels (<35 mg/pl) had reduced coital frequency. However, their outcome was frequency of intercourse.

On the other hand, studies that have looked at other aspects of sexual functioning such as desire or interest also do not find an association with hormone levels (Avis *et al.*, 2000; Bachmann *et al.*, 1984, 1985; Cawood *et al.*, 1996; Dennerstein *et al.*, 1997). In the MWHS, pain was the only aspect of sexual functioning that was related to E_2. Others have also found that lowered estrogen levels have been associated with vaginal dryness (Dennerstein *et al.*, 1997; Hutton, Jacobs, & James, 1979; Morrel, Dixen, Carter, & Davidson, 1984; Sarrel, 1987).

In general, these studies suggest that elevated estrogen levels are not an important factor in libido or potency, but are related to levels of vaginal lubrication. Thus, while hormone levels affect vaginal dryness and dyspareunia, they do not appear directly related to sexual drive or interest.

A number of researchers have argued that androgens, and not estrogens, are the relevant hormone in relation to sexual functioning. Investigators have found that androgens maintain sexual interest after surgical menopause, while estrogens do not (Sherwin, 1991; Sherwin & Gelfand, 1987). Most of this work has been conducted among women who have an oophorectomy and are given supraphysiologic levels of the hormone.

Only a few studies have examined the relation between natural androgens and sexual functioning (Cawood *et al.*, 1996; Dennerstein *et al.*, 1997; McCoy et al, 1985) and none of these studies has found an association. In fact, Dennerstein *et al.* (1997) found only weak evidence for androgen involvement (FAI with libido), but in a negative direction. A review by Campbell and Udry (1994) concluded that while some amount of T is important to maintain sexual motivation, there is no evidence that within the normal range of T, there is an association between T and libido.

It is important to point out that most studies of the impact of menopause on sexual functioning are conducted among women who are newly postmenopausal. It is possible that the effects of declines in ovarian functioning do not impact sexual functioning until later. We have very little data on sexual functioning among the general population of women in their sixties and seventies.

HORMONE REPLACEMENT THERAPY AND ALTERNATIVES

Hormone replacement therapy is currently touted as an antidote to these long-term consequences of menopause/aging. In evaluating the effectiveness of hormone therapy in preventing disease and disability, it is necessary to consider the two primary types of hormone therapy: estrogen alone (ERT) or estrogen combined with a progestin (combined therapy or

HRT). Estrogen alone gained widespread use in the mid-1960s when it was promoted aggressively by pharmaceutical companies and by books such as Wilson's *Feminine Forever*. In the mid-1970s, however, three studies showed that estrogen considerably increased a woman's risk for endometrial cancer (Mack *et al.*, 1976; Smith, Prentice, Thompson, & Hermann, 1975; Ziel & Finkle, 1975). Based on these findings, unopposed estrogen is generally not recommended for women who still have a uterus. In response to these studies, the pharmaceutical companies began searching for a way to counter this effect of estrogen. The combination of estrogen and progestin prevents an excess of estrogen from building up in the endometrium and reduces a woman's risk of endometrial cancer.

Indications for and against HRT

The strongest evidence for a preventive effect of HRT is found for osteoporosis (Ettinger, Genant, & Cann, 1985; Genant, Baylink, & Gallagher, 1989; Grady *et al.*, 1992; Lindsay & Cosman, 1990; Lindsay, Hart, Forrest, & Baird, 1980). However, while research suggests that estrogen use can retard bone loss, once estrogen replacement stops, the bone loss resumes (Lindsay, Hart, Maclean, Clark, Kraszewski, & Garwood, 1978). Further, recent evidence suggests that even estrogen use up to 10 years postmenopause and then discontinued provides little benefit for women 75 years and older, who have the highest risk of fracture (Cauley, Seeley, Ensrud, Ettinger, Black, & Cummings, 1995; Felson, Zhang, Hannan, Kiel, Wilson, & Anderson, 1993). Studies have also shown that beginning hormone therapy later in life may provide almost as much protection against osteoporotic fracture as lifelong therapy started at menopause (Ettinger & Grady, 1994; Schneider, Barrett-Connor, & Morton, 1997).

Studies of estrogen replacement therapy have consistently shown reduced risk of CVD among users (Grady *et al.*, 1992; Grodstein & Stampfler, 1995; Stampfer & Colditz, 1991), with greatest benefits for current users (Reis *et al.*, 1994; Williams, Adams, Herrington, & Clarkson, 1992; Williams, Adams, & Klopfenstein, 1990). Most research has focused on intermediate outcomes rather than actual disease. Exogenous estrogens result in favorable changes in lipids and lipoproteins, because of the suppression of hepatic lipase activity (PEPI Writing Group, 1995; Rijpkema, Van der Sanden, & Ruijs, 1990; Tikkanen, Nikkilae, Kuusi, & Sipinen, 1982; Walsh, Schiff, Rosner, Greenberg, Ravnikar, & Sacks, 1991). Estrogen is also associated with improved blood flow and vascular reactivity and vasomotion (Barrett-Connor & Bush, 1991; Rosano, Sarrel, Poole-Wilson, & Collins, 1993; Williams *et al.*, 1992), as well as a beneficial decrease in coagulation factors fibrinogen and plasminogen (Lobo *et al.*, 1994; Koh, Mincemoyer, & Bui, 1997; PEPI Writing Group, 1995).

A number of studies, however, have noted detrimental effects of exogenous estrogen, including increased triglycerides (Barrett-Connor & Bush, 1991; PEPI Writing Group, 1995; Rijpkema *et al.*, 1990; Williams *et al.*, 1992), increased clotting Factors VII and X and a decrease in antithrombin III (Lobo *et al.*, 1994; PEPI Writing Group, 1995), and increased venous thromboembolism, pulmonary embolism, and deep vein thrombosis (Grodstein *et al.*, 1996; Hulley, Grady, *et al.*, 1998; Jick, Derby, Myers, Vasilakis, & Newton, 1997).

Many of the studies are observational and thus subject to selection bias in that women who take estrogen are healthier than women who do not (Barrett-Connor, 1996; Barrett-Connor *et al.*, 1991; Derby, Hume, Barbour, McPhillips, Lasater, & Carleton, 1993; Johannes, Crawford, Posner, & McKinlay, 1994; Matthews, Kuller, Wing, Meilhan, & Plantinga, 1996; McKinlay, 1994; Rossouw, 1999), resulting in an overestimate of the benefits of estrogen therapy (Sotelo & Johnson, 1997). Moreover, it is difficult to translate the impact of estrogen on intermediate outcomes into the impact on clinical outcomes (Rossouw, 1999). Ongoing clinical trials will provide answers to this question. The first of these to be published, the Heart and Estrogen/Progestin Study, found

no effect of estrogen replacement therapy on coronary heart disease events among women with established coronary disease (Hulley *et al.*, 1998).

One of the primary potential risks associated with long-term use of HRT is breast cancer, which is clearly a hormonally mediated disease (Howe & Rohan, 1993). Breast cancer risk is modified by markers of hormonal status such as age of menarche, pregnancy, and age of menopause affecting risk (Howe & Rohan, 1993). Early menopause, particularly if it involves surgical removal of both ovaries greatly reduces risk (Trichopoulos, MacMahon, & Cole, 1972). Because of the well-recognized role of hormonal factors in breast cancer, there is considerable concern over the effect of exogenous hormone use in increasing a woman's risk for breast cancer, yet this remains a controversial issue. Meta-analyses of the relation between estrogen use and breast cancer have shown conflicting results. Two of these analyses concluded that there was no risk (Armstrong, 1988; Dupont & Page, 1991), while two others concluded that there was a small increased risk (Sillero-Arenas, Delgado-Rodriguez, Rodigues-Canteras, Bueno-Cavanillas, & Galvez-Vargas, 1992; Steinberg *et al.*, 1991). The studies reported in these meta-analyses are limited, however, in that most of the women studied had used estrogen for less than 10 years, some had poor study design, and dosages have changed over time. The most recent and comprehensive metaanalysis concluded that the risk of breast cancer increases in relation to the increasing duration of use in current or recent users of HRT but not in past users. The effects of HRT are more adverse in thinner than heavier women, the breast cancers diagnosed in women who use HRT are less advanced clinically than those diagnosed in never users, and progestins do not reduce increased risk associated with estrogens (Collaborative Group on Hormonal Factors in Breast Cancer, 1997). Although, the data were insufficient to adequately determine whether a combined estrogen–progestin regiment increased risk beyond that associated with estrogen alone.

Until recently, studies primarily looked at

the effect of estrogen alone. However, a recent study reported by Schairer and colleagues (2000), is the first large study to compare risk of breast cancer associated with an estrogen–progestin regimen with that associated with estrogen alone. This study found that the estrogen–progestin regimen increases breast cancer beyond that associated with estrogen alone. Not only was the overall relative risk of breast cancer greater for those on an estrogen–progestin regimen, but the relative risk for each year of use increased more for combined therapy.

Alternatives to HRT

Alternatives to HRT include both other medications and lifestyle changes. As potential alternatives to estrogen replacement therapy, a new class of compounds called selective estrogen receptor modulators (SERMS) are being developed. SERMS may be thought of as "designer estrogens," compounds that are tailored to possess estrogen agonist-like actions on bone tissues and serum lipids while displaying estrogen antagonist properties in the breast and uterus. Tamoxifen, the first SERM in clinical use, seems to block estrogenic effects in breast tissue, but evidence is accumulating that it may stimulate uterine tissue, increasing the risk of hyperplasia and endometrial cancer. Raloxifene, a newer SERM, is thought to have favorable effects on bone density and blood lipids while blocking estrogen receptors in the breast as well as the uterus. Recent data, however, suggest that while raloxifene has some effect on lipids, this is less than estrogens and that raloxifene also increases hot flashes (Walsh *et al.*, 1998). SERMS are very new therapies at this time. Their actual impact on lipids and long-term cardioprotective effects are unknown (Rifkind & Rossouw, 1998).

Other antiresorptive therapies such as bisphosphonates (e.g., alendronate, etidronate) have shown some degree of effectiveness for preventing and treating osteoporosis (Liberman *et al.*, 1995). While these therapies do not provide any cardiovascular benefit, they also do not appear to increase the risk of cancer. Long-term effects of alendronate are not yet known.

Many of the benefits of HRT can be achieved through other much safer means. Lifestyle changes such as smoking cessation, weight reduction, and exercise are effective alternatives to HRT for reducing risk of coronary heart disease (Manson *et al.*, 1992) and may be beneficial in preventing osteoporosis (Dalsky, 1987; Sinaki, 1989), although systematic evidence is lacking on this issue. Dietary supplementation with calcium and vitamin D has been shown to reduce bone loss (Chapuy *et al.*, 1992; Dawson-Hughes, Gerard, Krall, & Harris, 1997), as has weight-bearing exercise (Nelson, Fiatarone, Morganti, Trice, Greenberg, & Evans, 1994). Calcitonin and alendronate provide newer therapeutic options to reduce bone loss.

Nondrug or "natural" remedies such as dong quai, foods containing high levels of phytoestrogens (e.g., soy), and acupuncture have gained in popularity, particularly for the treatment of hot flashes. Unfortunately, we lack good scientific data based on randomized clinical trials on the effectiveness of these alternatives. In one randomized trial, Hirata and colleagues (1997) found no evidence that dong quai was significantly more effective in reducing hot flashes than placebo. Murkies and colleagues (1995) found some evidence for the effectiveness of soy flour, but Baird and colleagues (1995) did not. Wyon and colleagues (1995) reported some evidence for the effectiveness of acupuncture in reducing hot flashes. There are numerous studies on these alternatives currently underway. We are likely to see more research in this area in the coming years.

HEALTH POLICY IMPLICATIONS

Over 40 million women will enter their forties and fifties in the next two decades. The overwhelming majority of women now experience menopause and can expect to live approximately 30 years (or half of their adult life) beyond this event. The management and treatment of peri- and postmenopause potentially have enormous implications for the medical care system and the pharmaceutical industry. Already, numerous hospitals and clinics are developing Menopause Clinics to capture women at this point in time. Some refer to this aggressive marketing of menopause as the medicalization of essentially a normal physiological event.

While women are drawn to the benefits of hormone replacement therapy, they are also concerned about its potential risks and negative side effects. Industry is quite actively searching for palatable alternatives to the treatment for hot flashes and the long-term effects of bone loss. Numerous randomized clinical trials are already underway to study the effectiveness of these approaches. How alternatives are marketed and covered by insurance companies will have long-range implications.

New research will also begin having an impact on medical practice. For example, many clinicians have firmly believed that HRT has cardiovascular benefits. However, recent research is clearly calling into question this belief. It is worth noting that while the FDA has approved HRT for the treatment of menopausal symptoms and osteoporosis, the effectiveness of HRT for cardiovascular disease has not been approved. Research is also questioning the timing of administering HRT for the prevention of osteoporosis. It now appears that administration at the time of menopause is less critical than later in life at the time a woman is most likely to have a fracture. And new research suggesting an increased risk of breast cancer with combined therapy is raising questions about potential risks.

SUMMARY AND CONCLUSIONS

This chapter reviewed menopause and the long-term changes following menopause. It is apparent from this review that the physiological and hormonal changes associated with menopause do not affect all women the same and that women differ in how they respond to this physiological event. Factors that influence a woman's response are cultural, behavioral, psychosocial, as well as physiological. There is also evidence that women who experience a more difficult time during menstruation have a more difficult menopause. This may reflect a consistent pattern of responding to physiological changes and/or symptoms or reflect an underlying physiological mechanism related to both experiences. While Western societies often hold negative views of menopause, menopausal and postmenopausal women often have more positive views than society as a whole. In fact, following menopause, many women experience a new period of developmental growth and increased energy. How an individual woman responds to menopause is a complex interaction of physiology, her current life circumstances, attitudes/concerns about fertility, the culture in which she lives, and her history of responding to physiological changes/symptoms.

While numerous symptoms are often thought to be associated with menopause, only vasomotor symptoms have been clearly and consistently related to menopause. Such symptoms as mood changes or depression and sleep or memory problems have not been clearly and consistently related to menopause. Though some women do experience sleep difficulty or negative affect at the time of menopause, it has been difficult to disentangle whether this is a direct result of menopause or an indirect effect of vasomotor symptoms. Further, many women do not experience such symptoms at all and we lack a good understanding of factors related to experiencing these symptoms.

Following menopause, women experience musculoskeletal, cardiovascular, and urogenital changes. However, it is currently unknown to what extent changes in these systems are directly associated with the decline in estrogen, aging, or concurrent behavioral changes. The decision regarding how to prevent such changes is a complex one for most women involving weighing various risks and benefits of such possibilities as pharmaceutical intervention, behavioral or lifestyle changes, or various other "alternative" approaches. Unfortunately, we lack good data on the long-term consequences of many of these approaches.

Finally, our current knowledge of the menopausal transition is primarily limited to white women. We know very little about the range of experiences in women of other racial/ethnic backgrounds. Future research needs to study this life transition among women of diverse racial/ethnic groups, determine long-term health changes that are directly attributable to menopause versus those due to aging, and better understand the risks and benefits of hormone replacement therapy and its alternatives.

REFERENCES

Adena, M. A., & Gallagher, H. G. (1982). Cigarette smoking and age at menopause. *Annals of Human Biology, 9*, 121–130.

Adlercreutz, H., Hamalaiven, O., Gorbach, S., & Grodin, B. (1992). Dietary phytoestrogens and the menopause in Japan. *Lancet, 339*, 123–133.

American Heart Association. (1998). *Heart and stroke statistical update.* American Heart Association, Dallas, Texas.

Anderson, E., Hamburger, S., Liu, J. H., & Rebar, R. W. (1987). Characteristics of menopausal women seeking assistance. *American Journal of Obstetrics and Gynecology, 156*, 428–433.

Armstrong, B. K. (1988). Estrogen therapy after the menopause: Boom or bane? *Medical Journal of Australia, 18*, 213–214.

Avis, N. E., Brambilla, D., McKinlay, S. M., & Vass, K. (1994). A longitudinal analysis of the association between menopause and depression: Results from the Massachusetts Women's Health Study. *Annals of Epidemiology, 4*, 214–220.

Avis, N. E., Crawford, S. L., & McKinlay, S. M. (1997). Psychosocial, behavioral, and health factors related to menopause symptomatology. *Women's Health: Research on Gender, Behavior, and Policy, 3*, 103–120

Avis, N. E., Kaufert, P. A., Lock M., McKinlay, S. M., & Vass, K. (1993). The evolution of menopausal symptoms. *Journal of Clinical Endocrinology and Metabolism, 7*, 17–32.

Avis, N. E., & McKinlay, S. M. (1991). A longitudinal analysis of women's attitudes towards the menopause: Results from the Massachusetts Women's Health Study. *Maturitas, 13*, 65–79.

Avis, N. E., Stellato, R., Crawford, S., Johannes, C., & Longcope, C. (2000). Is there an association between menopause status and sexual functioning? *Menopause, 7*, 297–309.

Avis, N. E., Stellato, R., Crawford, S., Bromberger, J., Ganz, P., Cain, V., & Kagawa-Singer, M. (2001). Is there a menopausal syndrome? Menopausal status and symptoms across racial/ethnic groups. *Social Science and Medicine, 52*, 345–356.

Aylward, M. (1973). Plasma trytophan levels and mental depression in postmenopausal subjects: Effects of oral piperazine-oestrone sulphate. *International Research Communications Systems Medical Science, 1*, 30–34.

Bachmann, G. A., Leiblum, S. R., Kemmann, E., Colburn, D. W., Swartzmann, L., & Shelden, R. (1984). Sexual expression and its determinants in the post-menopausal woman. *Maturitas, 6*, 19–29.

Bachmann, G. A., Leiblum, S. R., Sandler, B., Ainsley, W., Narcessian, R., Shelden, R., & Hymans, H. N. (1985). Correlates of sexual desire in post-menopausal women. *Maturitas, 7*, 211–216.

Baird, D., Umbach, D., Landsdell, L., Hughes, C. L., Setchell, K. D., Weinberg, C. R., Haney, A. F., Wilcox, A. J., & Mclachlan, J. A. (1995). Dietary intervention study to assess estrogenicity of dietary soy among postmenopausal women. *Journal of Clinical Endocrinology and Metabolism, 80*, 1685–1690.

Ballinger, C. B. (1975). Psychiatric morbidity and the menopause: Screening of general population sample. *British Medical Journal, 3*, 344–346.

Ballinger, C. B. (1976). Psychiatric morbidity and the menopause: Clinical features. *British Medical Journal, 1*, 1183–1185.

Bancroft, J., & Bachstrom, T. (1985). Premenstrual syndrome: A review. *Clinical Endocrinology, 22*, 313–336.

Barbieri, R. L., McShane, P. M., & Ryan, K. J. (1986). Constituents of cigarette smoke inhibit human granulosa cell aromatase. *Fertility and Sterility, 46*, 232–236.

Baron, J. A., LaVecchia, C., & Levi, F. (1990). The antiestrogenic effect of cigarette smoking in women. *American Journal of Obstetrics and Gynecology, 162*, 502–514.

Barrett-Connor, E. (1996). The menopause, hormone replacement, and cardiovascular disease: The epidemiologic evidence. *Maturitas, 23*, 227–234.

Barrett-Connor, E., & Bush, T. L. (1991). Estrogen and coronary heart disease in women. *Journal of American Medical Association, 265*, 1861–1867.

Barrett-Connor, E., & Goodman-Gruen, D. (1995). Prospective study of endogenous sex hormones and fatal cardiovascular disease in postmenopausal women. *British Medical Journal, 311*, 1193–1196.

Barrett-Connor, E., & Kritz-Silverstein, D. (1993). Estrogen replacement therapy and cognitive function in older women. *Journal of the American Medical Association, 20*, 2637–2641.

Bean, J. A., Leeper, J. D., Wallace, R. B., Sherman, B. M., & Jagger, H. (1979). Variations in the reporting of menstrual histories. *American Journal of Epidemiology, 109*, 181–185.

Beyenne, Y. (1986). Cultural significance and physiological manifestations of menopause: A biocultural analysis. *Cultural, Medicine and Psychiatry, 10*, 47–71.

Bjorntorp, V. A. (1988). The associations between obesity, adipose tissue. Distribution and disease. *Acta Medica Scandinavica, Supplement, 723*, 121–134.

Blehar, M. C., & Oren, D. A. (1995). Women's increased vulnerable to mood disorders: Integrating psychobiology and epidemiology. *Depression, 3*, 3–12.

Brace, M., & McCauley, E. (1997). Oestrogens and psychological well-being. *Annals of Medicine, 29*, 283–290.

Brambilla, D. J., & McKinlay, S. M. (1989). A prospective study of factors affecting age at menopause. *Journal of Clinical Epidemiology, 42*, 1031–1039.

Brambilla, D. J., McKinlay, S. M., & Johannes, C. B. (1994). Defining the perimenopause for application in epidemiologic investigations. *American Journal of Epidemiology, 140*, 1091–1095.

Bromberger, J. T., Matthews, K. A., Kuller, L. H., Wing, R. R., Meilhan, E. N., & Plantinga, P. (1997). Prospective study of the determinants of age at menopause. *American Journal of Epidemiology, 145*, 124–133.

Brown, S. A., Hutchinson, R., Morrisett, J., Boerwinkle, E., Davis, C. E., & Gotto, A. M. (1993). Plasma lipid, lipoprotein cholesterol and apoprotein distributions in selected US communities. *Arteriosclerosis and Thrombosis, 13*, 1139–1158.

Bungay, G. T., Vessey, M. P., & McPherson, C. K. (1980). Study of symptoms in middle life with special reference to the menopause. *British Medical Journal, 281*, 181–183.

Burger, H. G. (1994a). The menopause: When is it all over or is it? *Australian and New Zealand Journal of Obstetrics and Gynaecology, 34*, 293–295.

Burger, H. G. (1994b). Diagnostic role of follicle-stimulating hormone (FSH) measurements during the menopausal transition—an analysis of FSH, oestradiol and inhibin. *European Journal of Endocrinology, 130*, 38–42.

Burger, H. G. (1996). The endocrinology of the menopause. *Maturitas, 23*, 129–136.

Burger, H. G., Cahir, N., Robertson, D. M., Groome, N. P., Dudley, E., Green, A., & Dennerstein, L. (1998). Serum inhibins A and B fall differentially as FSH rises in perimenopausal women. *Clinical Endocrinology, 48*, 809–813.

Bush, T. L. (1990). The epidemiology of cardiovascular disease in postmenopausal women. *Annals of the New York Academy of Sciences, 592*, 263–271.

Bush, T. L., Barrett-Connor, E., Cowan, L. D., Criqui, M. H., Wallace, R. B., Suchindran, C. M., Tyroler, H. A., & Rifkind, B. M. (1987). Cardiovascular mortality and noncontraceptive use of estrogen in women: Results from the Lipid Research Clinics Program Follow-up Study. *Circulation, 75*, 1102–1109.

Campbell, B., & Udry, J. (1994). Implications of hormonal influences on sexual behavior for demographic models of reproduction. *Annals of the New York Academy of Science, 706*, 117–127.

Campbell, S., & Whitehead, M. (1977). Oestrogen therapy and the menopausal syndrome. *Clinical Obstetrics and Gynaecology, 4*, 31–47.

Cauley, J. A., Gutai, J. P., Kuller, L. H., & Powell, J. G. (1990). The relation of endogenous sex steroid hormone concentrations to serum lipid and lipoprotein levels in postmenopausal women. *American Journal of Epidemiology, 132*, 884–894.

Cauley, J., Seeley, D., Ensrud, K., Ettinger, B., Black, D., & Cummings, S. R. (1995). Estrogen replacement therapy and fractures in older women. Study of osteoporotic fractures research group. *Annals of Internal Medicine, 122*, 9–16.

Cawood, E. H. H., & Bancroft, J. (1996). Steroid hormones, the menopause, sexuality and well-being of women. *Psychological Medicine, 26*, 925–936.

Charney, D. A. (1996). The psychoendocrinology of menopause in cross-cultural perspective. *Transcultural Psychiatry Research Review, 33*, 413–434.

Chapuy, M., Arlot, M., Duboeuf, F., Brun, J., Crouzet, B., Arnaud, S., Delmas, P. D., & Meunier, P. J. (1992). Vitamin D3 and calcium to prevent hip fractures in the elderly woman. *New England Journal of Medicine, 327*, 505–512.

Christensen, C. V., & Gagnon, J. H. (1965). Sexual behavior in a group of older women. *Journal of Gerontology, 20*, 351–356.

Clark, A. L., & Wallin, P. (1965). Women's sexual responsiveness and the duration and quality of their marriage. *American Journal of Sociology, 71*, 187–196.

Clayden, J. R., Bell, J. W., & Pollard, P. (1974). Menopausal flushing: Double-blind trial of a non-hormonal medication. *British Medical Journal, 1*, 409–412.

Colditz, G. A., Willett, W. C., Stampfer, M. J, Rosner B., Speizer, F. E., & Hennekens, C. H. (1987). Menopause and risk of coronary heart disease in women. *New England Journal of Medicine, 316*, 1105–1110.

Collaborative Group on Hormonal Factors in Breast Cancer (1997). Breast cancer and hormone replacement therapy: Collaborative reanalysis of data from 51 epidemiologic studies of 52,705 women with breast cancer and 108,411 women without breast cancer. *Lancet, 350*, 1047–1059.

Collins, A., & Landgren, B. M. (1995). Reproductive health, use of estrogen and experience of symptoms in perimenopausal women: A population-based study. *Maturitas, 20*, 101–111.

Coope, J., Thomson, J. M., & Poller, L. (1975). Effects of "natural oestrogen" replacement therapy on menopausal symptoms and blood clotting. *British Medical Journal, 4*, 139–143.

Cooper, G. S., & Baird, D. D. (1995). The use of questionnaire data to classify peri- and premenopausal status. *Epidemiology, 6*, 625–628.

Cramer, D. W., Harlow, B. L., Xu, H., Fraer, C., & Barbieri, R. (1995a) Cross-sectional and case-controlled analyses of the association between smoking and early menopause. *Maturitas, 22*, 79–87.

Cramer, D. W., Xu, H., & Harlow, B. L. (1995b) Does "incessant" ovulation increase risk for early menopause? *American Journal of Obstetrics and Gynecology, 172*, 568–573.

Crawford, S. L., & Johannes, C. B. (1999). The epidemiology of cardiovascular disease in postmenopausal women. In Therapeutic Controversy. Hormone Replacement Therapy—Where Are We Going? *Journal of Clinical Endocrinology and Metabolism, 84*, 1803–1806.

Cutler, W., Garcia, C., & McCoy, N. (1987). Perimenopausal sexuality. *Archives of Sexual Behavior, 16*(3), 225–234.

Dalsky, G. J. (1987). Exercise: Its effects on bone mineral content. *Clinical Obstetrics and Gynecology, 30*, 820–832.

Davidson, J. (1985). Sexual behavior and its relationship to ovarian hormones in the menopause. *Maturitas, 7*, 193–201.

Dawson-Hughes, B., Gerard, E., Krall, E., & Harris, S. (1997). Effects of calcium and vitamin D supplementation on bone density in men and women 65 years of age or older. *New England Journal of Medicine, 337*, 670–676.

Dennerstein, L., Dudley, E., Hopper, J., & Burger, H. (1997). Sexuality, hormones and the menopausal transition. *Maturitas, 26*, 83–93.

Dennerstein, L., Smith, A. M. A., & Morse, C. (1994). Psychological well-being, mid-life and the menopause. *Maturitas, 20*, 1–11.

Dennerstein, L., Smith, A. M. A., Morse, C., Burger, H., Green, A., Hopper, J., & Ryan, M. (1993). Menopausal symptoms in Australian women. *Medical Journal of Australia, 159*, 232–236.

Derby, C. A., Hume, A. L., Barbour, M. M., McPhillips, J. B., Lasater, T. M., & Carleton, R. A. (1993). Correlates of postmenopausal estrogen use and trends through the 1980s in two southeastern New England communities. *American Journal of Epidemiology, 137*, 1125–1135.

Ditkoff, E. C., Crary, W. G., Cristo, M., & Lobo, R. A. (1991). Estrogen improves psychological function in asymptomatic postmenopausal women. *Obstetrics and Gynecology, 78*, 991–995.

Dupont, W. D., & Page, D. L. (1991). Menopausal estrogen replacement therapy and breast cancer. *Archives of Internal Medicine, 151*, 67–72.

Eaker, E. D., Chesbro, J. H., Sacks, F. M., Wenger, N. K., Whisnant, J. P., & Winston, M. (1993). Cardiovascular disease in women. *Circulation, 88*, 1999–2009.

Erlik, Y., Tataryn, I. V., Meldrum, D. R., Lomax, P., Bajorek, J. G., & Judd, H. L. (1981). Association of waking episodes with menopausal hot flushes. *Journal of the American Medical Association, 245*(17), 1741–1744.

Ettinger, B., Genant, H. K., & Cann, C. E. (1985). Long-term estrogen replacement therapy prevents bone loss and fractures. *Annals of Internal Medicine, 102*(3), 319–324.

Ettinger, B., & Grady, D. (1994). Maximizing the benefit of estrogen therapy for prevention of osteoporosis. *Menopause, 1*, 19–24.

Everson, R. B., Sandler, D. P., Wilcox, A. J., Schreinemachers, D., Shore, D. L., & Weinberg, C. (1986). Effect of passive exposure to smoking on age at natural menopause. *British Medical Journal, 293*, 792.

Faddy, M. J., Gosden, R. G., Gougeon, A., Richardson, S. J., & Nelson, J. F. (1992). Accelerated disappearance of ovarian follicles in mid-life: Implications for forecasting menopause. *Human Reproduction, 7*(10), 1342–1346.

Fantl, J. A., Wyman, J. F., Anderson, R. L., Matt, D. W., & Bump, D. C. (1988). Postmenopausal urinary incontinence: Comparison between non-estrogen supplemented and estrogen-supplemented women. *Obstetrics and Gynecology, 71*, 823–828.

Fedor-Freybergh, P. (1977). The influence of oestrogen on the well-being and mental performance in climacteric and postmenopausal women. *Acta Obstetrica et Gynecologica Scandinavica, 64*, 5–69.

Felson, D. T., Zhang, Y., Hannan, M. T., Kiel, D. P., Wilson, P. W., & Anderson, J. J. (1993) The effect of postmenopausal estrogen therapy on bone density in elderly women. *New England Journal of Medicine, 329*(16), 1141–1146.

Gangar, K. F., Vyas, S., Whitehead, M., Crook, D., Meire, H., & Campbell, S. (1991). Pulsatility index in internal carotid artery in relation to transdermal oestradiol and time since menopause. *Lancet, 338*, 839–842.

Gath, D., Osborn, M., Bungay, G., Ilse, S., Day, A., Bond, A., & Passingham, C. (1987). Psychiatric disorder and gynaecological symptoms in middle aged women: A community survey. *British Medical Journal, 294*, 213–218.

Genant, H. K., Baylink, D. J., & Gallagher, J. C. (1989). Estrogens in the prevention of osteoporosis in postmenopausal women. *American Journal of Obstetrics and Gynecology, 16*, 1842–1846.

Goldenberg, R. L., Grodin, J. M., Rodbard, D., & Ross, G. T. (1973). Gonadotropins in women with amenorrhea. *American Journal of Obstetrics and Gynecology, 116*, 1003–1012.

Gorodeski, G. I. (1994). Impact of the menopause on the epidemiology and risk factors of coronary artery heart disease in women. *Experimental Gerontology, 29*, 357–375.

Gosden, R. G. (1985). *Biology of menopause: The causes and consequences of ovarian aging.* London: Academic Press.

Grady, D., Rubin, S. M., Petitti, D. B., Fox, C. S., Black, D., Ettinger, B., Ernster, V. L., & Cummings, S. R. (1992). Hormone therapy to prevent disease and prolong life in postmenopausal women. *Annals of Internal Medicine, 117*, 1016–1037.

Greene, J. G., & Cooke, D. J. (1976). A factor analytic study of climacteric symptoms. *Journal of Psychosomatic Research, 40*, 425–430.

Greene, J. G., & Cooke, D. J. (1980). Life stress and symptoms at the climacterium. *British Journal of Psychiatry, 136*, 486–491.

Greendale, G., Hogan, P., Shumaker, S., for the PEPI Investigators. (1996). Sexual functioning in postmenopausal women: The Postmenopausal Estrogen/Progestin Interventions (PEPI) Trial. *Journal of Women's Health, 5*, 445–458.

Greendale, G. A., & Sowers, M. (1997). The menopause transition. *Endocrinology and Metabolism Clinics of North America, 26*(2), 261–277.

Grodstein, F., & Stampfer, M. (1995). The epidemiology of coronary heart disease and estrogen replacement in postmenopausal women. *Progress in Cardiovascular Diseases*, *38*, 199–210.

Grodstein, F., Stampfer, M. J., Manson, J. A., Colditz, G. A., Willett, W. C., Rosner, B., Speizer, F. E., & Hennekens, C. H. (1996). Postmenopausal estrogen and progestin use and the risk of cardiovascular disease. *New England Journal of Medicine*, *335*, 453–461.

Hagstad, A. (1988). Gynecology and sexuality in middle-aged women. *Women Health*, *13*, 57–80.

Hagstad, A., & Janson, P. O. (1986). The epidemiology of climacteric symptoms. *Acta Obstetrica et Gynecologica Scandinavica, Supplement*, *134*, 59–65.

Hallstrom, T. (1977). Sexuality in the climacteric. *Clinics in Obstetrics and Gynecology*, *4*, 227–239.

Hallstrom, T., & Samuelsson, S. (1985). Mental health in the climacteric: The longitudinal study of women in Gothenburg. *Acta Obstetrica et Gynecologica Scandinavica, Supplement*, *130*, 13–18.

Hawton, K., Gath, D., & Day, A. (1994). Sexual function in a community sample of middle-aged women with partners: Effects of age, marital, socioeconomic, psychiatric, gynecological, and menopausal factors. *Archives of Sexual Behavior*, *23*(4), 375–395.

Heaney, R. P., Gallagher, J. C., Johnson, C. C., Neer, R., Parfitt, A. M., & Whedon, G. D. (1982). Calcium nutrition and bone health in the elderly. *American Journal of Clinical Nutrition*, *36*, 986–1013.

Hirata, J. D., Swiersz, L. M., Zell, B., Small, R., & Ettinger, B. (1997). Does dong quai have estrogenic effects in postmenopausal women? A double-blind, placebo-controlled trial. *Fertility and Sterility*, *68*, 981–986.

Hoel, D. G., Wakabayashi, T., & Pike, M. (1983). Secular trends in the distribution of the breast cancer risk factors—menarche, first birth, menopause, and weight—in Hiroshima and Nagasake, Japan. *American Journal of Epidemiology*, *11*, 78–89.

Holte, A. (1992). Influences of natural menopause on health complaints: A prospective study of healthy Norwegian women. *Maturitas*, *14*, 127–141.

Holte, A., & Mikkelsen, A. (1991). Psychosocial determinants of climacteric complaints. *Maturitas*, *13*, 205–215.

Hording, U., Pedersen, K. H., Sidenius, K., & Hedegaard, L. (1986). Urinary incontinence in 45-year-old women. An epidemiologic survey. *Scandanavian Journal of Urology and Nephrology*, *20*, 183–186

Howe, G. R., & Rohan, T. E. (1993). The epidemiology of breast cancer in women. In J. Lorrain (Ed.), *Comprehensive management of menopause* (pp. 39–51). New York: Springer-Verlag.

Hulley, S., Grady, D., Bush, T., Furberg, C., Herrington, D., Riggs, B. L., & Vittinghoff, E. (1998). Randomized trial of estrogen plus progestin for secondary prevention of coronary heart disease in postmenopausal women. *Journal of American Medical Association*, *280*, 605–613.

Hunter, M. S. (1990). Somatic experience of the menopause: A prospective study. *Psychosomatic Medicine*, *52*, 357–367.

Hunter, M. (1992). The South-East England longitudinal study of the climacteric and postmenopause. *Maturitas*, *14*, 117–126.

Hunter, M., Battersby, R., & Whitehead, M. (1986). Relationships between psychological symptoms, somatic complaints and menopausal status. *Maturitas*, *8*, 217–228.

Hutton, J. D., Jacobs, H. C., & James, V. H. T. (1979). Steroid endocrinology after the menopause—a review. *Journal of the Royal Society of Medicine*, *72*, 835–841.

Iddenden, D. A. (1987). Sexuality during the menopause. *Medical Clinics of North America*, *71*, 87–94.

Jick, H., Derby, L. E., Myers, M. W., Vasilakis, C., & Newton, K. M. (1997). Risk of hospital admission for idiopathic venous thromboembolism among users of postmenopausal estrogens. *Lancet*, *348*, 981–983.

Jick, H., & Porter, J. (1977). Relation between smoking and age of natural menopause. *Lancet*, *1*, 1354–1355.

Johannes, C. B., Crawford, S. L., Posner, J. G., & McKinlay, S. M. (1994). Longitudinal patterns and correlates of hormone replacement therapy use in middle-aged women. *American Journal of Epidemiology*, *140*, 439–452.

Johannes, C. B., & Avis, N. E. (1996). The short-term health consequences of hysterectomy. *Journal of Women's Health*, *5*, 278.

Johnston, C. C., Hui, S. L., Witt, R. M., Appledorn, R., Baker, R. S., & Longcope, C. (1985). Early menopausal changes in bone mass and sex steroids. *Journal of Clinical Endocrinology and Metabolism*, *61*, 905–911.

Kanders, B., Dempster, D. W., & Lindsay, R. (1988). Interaction of calcium nutrition and physical activity on bone mass in young women. *Journal of Bone Mineral Research*, *3*(2), 145–149.

Kaufert, P. A. (1982). Anthropology and the menopause: The development of a theoretical framework. *Maturitas*, *4*, 181–193.

Kaufert, P. A., Gilbert, P., & Hassard, T. (1988). Researching the symptoms of menopause: An exercise in methodology. *Maturitas*, *10*, 117–131.

Kaufert, P. A., Gilbert, P., & Tate, R. (1992). The Manitoba Project: A reexamination of the link between menopause and depression. *Maturitas*, *14*, 143–155.

Kaufert, P. A., & McKinlay, S. M. (1985). Estrogen replacement therapy: The production of medical knowledge and the emergence of policy. In E. Lewin & V. Olesen (Eds.), *Women, health and healing: Toward a new perspective* (pp. 113–138). New York: Tavistock.

Kaufman, D. W., & Sloane, D. (1980). Cigarette smoking and age at natural menopause. *American Journal of Public Health*, *70*, 420–422

Kinsey, A. C., Pomeroy, W. B., & Martin, C. W. (1948). *Sexual behavior in the human male*. Philadelphia: W. B. Saunders.

Kinsey, A. C., Pomeroy, W. B., Martin, C. W., & Gebhard,

P. H. (1953). *Sexual behavior in the human female.* Philadelphia: W. B. Saunders.

Klein, N. A., Illingworth, P. J., Groome, N. P., McNeilly, A. S., Battaglia, D. E., & Soules, M. R. (1996). Decreased inhibin B secretion is associated with the monotropic FSH rise in older, ovulatory women: A study of serum and follicular fluid levels of dimeric inhibin A and B in spontaneous menstrual cycles. *Journal of Clinical Endocrinology and Metabolism, 81,* 2742–2745.

Koh, K. K., Mincemoyer, R., & Bui, M. N. (1997). Effects of hormone-replacement therapy on fibrinolysis in postmenopausal women. *New England Journal of Medicine, 336,* 683–690.

Kopera, H. (1973). Estrogens and psychic functions. *Frontiers Hormone Research, 2,* 118–133.

Køster, A., & Garde, K. (1993). Sexual desire and menopausal development. A prospective study of Danish women born in 1936. *Maturitas, 16,* 49–60.

Krolner, B., & Pors, N. S. (1982). Bone and mineral content of the lumber spine in normal and osteoporotic women: Cross-sectional and longitudinal studies. *Clinical Science, 62,* 329–336.

Kronenberg, F. (1990). Hot flashes: Epidemiology and physiology. *Annals of the New York Academy of Sciences, 592,* 52–86.

Kuh, D. L., Wadsworth, M., & Hardy, R. (1997). Women's health in midlife: The influence of the menopause, social factors and health in earlier life. *British Journal of Obstetrics and Gynaecology, 104,* 923–933.

Kuller, L. H., Gutai, J. P., Meilhan, E. N., Matthews, K. A., & Plantinga, P. (1990). Relationship of endogenous sex steroid hormones to lipids and apoproteins in postmenopausal women. *Arteriosclerosis, 10,* 1058–1066.

Laumann, E. O., Gagnon, J. H., Michael, R. T., & Michaels, S. (1994). *The social organization of sexuality: Sexual practices in the United States* (pp. 77–147, 351–375). Chicago: University of Chicago Press.

Leiblum, S., Bachmann, G., Kemmann, E., Colburn, D., & Swartzman, L. (1983). Vaginal atrophy in the postmenopausal woman. The importance of sexual activity and hormones. *Journal of American Medical Association, 249,* 2195–2198.

Lenton, E. A., Sexton, L., Lee, S., & Cooke, I. D. (1988). Progressive changes in LH and FSH and LH:FSH ratio in women throughout reproductive life. *Maturitas, 10,* 35–43.

Liberman, U. A., Weiss, S. R., Bröll, J., Minne, H. W., Quan, H., Bell, N. H., Rodriguez Portales, J., Downs, R. W. Jr., Dequeker, J., & Favus, M. (1995). Effect of oral Alendronate on bone mineral density and the incidence of fracture in postmenopausal osteoporosis. *New England Journal of Medicine, 333,* 1437–1443.

Lindsay, R., & Cosman, F. (1990). Estrogen in prevention and treatment of osteoporosis. *Annals of the New York Academy of Sciences, 592,* 326–333.

Lindsay, R., Hart, D. M., McLean, A., Clark, A. C., Kraszewski, A., & Garwood, J. (1978). Bone response to termination of estrogen treatment. *Lancet, I,* 1325–1327.

Lindsay, R., Hart, D. M., Forrest, C., & Baird, C. (1980). Prevention of spinal osteoporosis in oophorectomized women. *Lancet, 2,* 1151–1154.

Lobo, R. A., Pickar, J. H., Wild, R. A., Walsh, B., & Hirvonen, E. (1994). Metabolic impact of adding medroxyprogesterone acetate to conjugated estrogen therapy in postmenopausal women. *Obstetrics and Gynecology, 84,* 987–995.

Lock, M. (1986). Ambiguities of aging: Japanese experience and perceptions of menopause. *Culture, Medicine, and Psychiatry, 10,* 23–46.

Longcope, C., Crawford, S., & McKinlay, S. (1996). Endogenous estrogens: Relationships between estrone, estradiol, non-protein bound estradiol, and hot flashes and lipids. *Menopause, 3,* 77–84.

Luckey, M. M., Wallenstein, S., Lapinski, R., & Meier, D. E. (1996). A prospective study of bone loss in African-American and white women—a clinical research center study. *Journal of Clinical Endocrinology and Metabolism, 81*(8), 2948–2956.

Luine, V. N., Park, D., Joh, T., Reis, D., & McEwen, B. (1980). Immuno-chemical demonstration of increased choline acetyltransferase concentration in rat preoptic area after estradiol administration. *Brain Research, 191,* 273–277.

Mack, T. M., Pike, M. C., Henderson, M. E., Pfeffer, R. I., Gerkins, V. R., Arthur, M., & Brown, S. E. (1976). Estrogens and endometrial cancer in a retirement community. *New England Journal of Medicine, 294,* 1262–1267.

MacMahon, B., & Worcester, J. (1966). Age at menopause: United States 1960–1962. *US Vital & Health Statistics, II, 19,* 1–19.

Magursky, V., Mesko, M., & Sokolik, L. (1975). Age at menopause and onset of the climacteric in women of Martin District. *International Journal of Fertility, 20,* 17–23.

Malleson, J. (1953). An endocrine factor in certain affective disorders. *Lancet, 2,* 158–164.

Manson, J., Tosteson, H., Satterfield, S., Herbert, P., O'Connor, G. T., Baring, J. E., & Hennekens, C. H. (1992). The primary prevention of myocardial infarction. *New England Journal of Medicine, 326,* 1406–1416.

Masters, W. H., & Johnson, V. E. (1966). *Human sexual response.* Boston: Little Brown.

Matthews, K. A. (1992). Myths and realities of the menopause. *Psychosomatic Medicine, 54,* 1–9.

Matthews, K. A., Kuller, L. H., Wing, R. R., Meilhan, E. N., & Plantinga, P. (1996). Prior to use of estrogen replacement therapy, are users healthier than nonusers? *American Journal of Epidemiology, 143,* 971–978.

Matthews, K. A., Meilhan, E. N., Kuller, L. H., Kelsey, S.

F., Caggiula, A. W., & Wing, R. R. (1989). Menopause and risk factors for coronary heart disease. *New England Journal of Medicine, 321,* 641–646.

Matthews, K. A., Wing, R. R., Kuller, L. H., Meilhan, E N., Kelsey, S. F., Costello, E. J., & Caggiula, A. W. (1990). Influences of natural menopause on psychological characteristics and symptoms of middle-aged healthy women. *Journal of Consulting and Clinical Psychology, 58,* 345–351.

Mazess, R. B. (1982). On aging bone mass. *Clinical Orthopedics and Related Research, 165,* 239–252.

McCrea, F. (1983). The politics of menopause: The discovery of a deficiency disease. *Social Problems, 31,* 111–123.

McCoy, N. L., & Davidson, J. M. (1985). A longitudinal study of the effects of menopause on sexuality. *Maturitas, 7,* 203–210.

McEwen, J. B. (1991). Steroid hormones are multifunctional messengers to the brain. *Trends in Endocrinology Metabolism, 2,* 62–67.

McKinlay, J. B., Crawford, S., McKinlay, S. M., & Stellato, D. E. (1994). On the reported gender difference in coronary heart disease: An illustration of the social construction of epidemiologic rates. In S. M. Czajkowski, D. R. Hill, & T. B. Clarkson (Eds.), *Women, behavior, and cardiovascular disease* (pp. 223–252). National Institutes of Health Publications No. 94-339.

McKinlay, J. B., McKinlay, S. M., & Brambilla, D. (1987). The relative contributions of endocrine changes and social circumstances to depression in mid-aged women. *Journal of Health and Social Behavior, 28,* 345–363.

McKinlay, S. M. (1994). Issues in design, measurement, and analysis for menopause research. *Experimental Gerontology, 29,* 479–493.

McKinlay, S. M. (1996). The normal menopause transition: An overview. *Maturitas, 23,* 137–145.

McKinlay, S. M., Bifano, N. L., & McKinlay, J. B. (1985). Smoking and age at menopause in women. *Annals of Internal Medicine, 103,* 350–356.

McKinlay, S. M., Brambilla, D. J., Avis, N. E., & McKinlay, J. B. (1991). Women's experience of the menopause. *Current Obstetrics and Gynecology, 1,* 3–7.

McKinlay, S. M., Brambilla, D. J., & Posner, J. G. (1992). The normal menopause transition. *American Journal of Human Biology, 4,* 37–46.

McKinlay, S. M., & Jefferys, M. (1974). The menopausal syndrome. *British Journal of Preventive Social Medicine, 28,* 108–115.

McKinlay, S. M., Jefferys, M., & Thompson, B. (1972). An investigation of the age at menopause. *Journal of Biosocial Science, 4,* 161–173.

Metcalf, M. G. (1988). The approach of menopause: A New Zealand study. *New Zealand Medical Journal, 101,* 103–106.

Metcalf, M. G., & Livesey, J. H. (1985). Gonadotrophin excretion in fertile women: Effect of age and the onset of the menopausal transition. *Journal of Endocrinology, 105,* 357–362.

Michnovicz, J. J., & Bradlow, H. L. (1990). Dietary and pharmacological control of estradiol metabolism in humans. *Annals of the New York Academy of Sciences, 595,* 291–299.

Michnovicz, J. J., Hershcopf, R. J., Naganuma, H., Bradlow, H. L., & Fishman, J. (1986). Increased 2-hydroxylation of estradiol as a possible mechanism for the anti-estrogenic effect of cigarette smoking. *New England Journal of Medicine, 315,* 1305–1309.

Morrel, M. J., Dixen, J. M., Carter, C. S., & Davidson, J. M. (1984). The influences of age and cycling status on sexual arousability in women. *American Journal of Obstetrics and Gynecology, 148,* 66–71.

Murkies, A. L., Lombard, C., Strauss, B. J., Wilcox, G., Burger, H. G., & Morton, M. S. (1995). Dietary flour supplementation decreases post-menopausal hot flushes: Effect of soy and wheat. *Maturitas, 21,* 189–195.

Nelson, M. E., Fiatarone, M. A., Morganti, C. M., Trice, I., Greenberg, R. A., & Evans, W. J. (1994). Effects of high-intensity strength training on multiple risk factors for osteoporotic fractures. A randomized controlled trial. *Journal of the American Medical Society, 272,* 1909–1914.

Neugarten, B. L., & Kraines, R. J. (1965). "Menopausal symptoms" in women of various ages. *Psychosomatic Medicine, 27*(3), 266–273.

Osborne, J. L. (1976). Postmenopausal changes in micturition habits and in urine flow and urethral pressure studies. In S. Campbell (Ed.), *The management of the menopause and postmenopausal years.* Lancaster: MTP Publications.

Osborn, M., Hawton, K., & Gath, D. (1988). Sexual dysfunction among middle aged women in the community. *British Medical Journal, 296,* 959–962.

Paganini-Hill, A., Krailo, M. D., & Pike, M. C. (1984). Age at natural menopause and breast cancer: The effect of errors in recall. *American Journal of Epidemiology, 119,* 81–85.

Pearlstein, M. D., Rosen, K., & Stone, A. B. (1997). Mood disorders and menopause. *Endocrinology and Metabolism Clinics of North America, 26,* 279–294.

PEPI Writing Group (1995). Effects of estrogen or estrogen/progestin regimens on heart disease risk factors in postmenopausal women: The Postmenopausal Estrogen/Progestin Intervention. *Journal of the American Medical Association, 273,* 199–208.

Pfeiffer, E., Verwoerdt, A., & Davis, G. (1972). Sexual behavior in middle life. *American Journal of Psychiatry, 128,* 1262–1267.

Poller, L., Thomson, J. M., & Coope, J. (1980). A double-blind cross-over study of piperazine oestrone sulphate and placebo with coagulation studies. *British Journal of Obstetrics and Gynaecology, 87,* 718–725.

Pollitzer, W. S. & Anderson, J. J. B. (1989). Ethnic and genetic differences in bone mass: A review with a hereditary v. environmental perspective. *American Journal of Clinical Nutrition, 50*(6), 1244, 1259.

Porter, M., Penney, G. C., Russell, D., Russell, E., & Templeton, A (1996). A population based survey of women's experience of the menopause. *British Journal of Obstetrics and Gynaecology, 103,* 1025–1028.

Pouilles, J. M., Tremollieres, F., & Ribot, C. (1993). The effects of menopause on longitudinal bone loss from the spine. *Calcified Tissue International, 52,* 340–343.

Rauramo, L., Langerspetz, K., Engblom, P., & Punnonen, R. (1975). The effects of castration and peroral estrogen therapy on some psychological functions. *Frontiers in Hormone Research, 8,* 133–151.

Reame, N. E., Kelche, R. P., Beitins, I. Z., Yu, M. Y., Zawacki, C. M., & Padmanabhan, V. (1996). Age effects of follicle-stimulating hormone and pulsatile luteinizing hormone secretion across the menstrual cycle of women. *Journal of Clinical Endocrinology and Metabolism, 81,* 1512–1518.

Regestein, Q. R. (1993). Menopausal aspects of sleep disturbance. In J. Lorrain (Ed.), *Comprehensive management of menopause* (pp. 358–366). New York: Springer-Verlag.

Reis, S. E., Gloth, S. T., Blumenthal, R. S., Resar, J. R., Zacur, H. A., Gerstenblith, G., & Brinker, J. A. (1994). Ethinyl estradiol acutely attenuates abnormal coronary vasomotor responses to acetylcholine in postmenopausal women. *Circulation, 89,* 52–60.

Richardson, S. J., Senikas, V., & Nelson, J. F. (1987). Follicular depletion during the menopausal transition: Evidence for accelerated loss and ultimate exhaustion. *Journal of Clinical Endocrinology and Metabolism, 65,* 1231–1237.

Rifkind, B. M., & Rossouw, J. E. (1998). Of designer drugs, magic bullets, and gold standards. *Journal of the American Medical Association, 279,* 1483–1491.

Riggs, B. L., & Melton, L. J. (1986). Involutional osteoporosis. *New England Journal of Medicine, 314,* 1676–1686.

Riggs, B. L., & Melton, L. J. (1992). The prevention and treatment of osteoporosis. *New England Journal of Medicine, 327,* 620–627.

Rijpkema, A. H. M., Van der Sanden, A. A., & Ruijs, A. H. C. (1990). Effects of postmenopausal and oestrogen-progestogen replacement therapy on serum lipids and lipoproteins: A review. *Maturitas, 12,* 259–285.

Rosano, G. M. C., Sarrel, P. M., Poole-Wilson, P. A., & Collins, P. (1993). Beneficial effect of oestrogen on exercise-induced myocardial ischaemia in women with coronary artery disease. *Lancet, 342,* 133–136.

Rossouw, J. E. (1999). Does estrogen have a role in the prevention of cardiovascular disease? In Therapeutic Controversy. Hormone Replacement Therapy—Where Are We Going? *Journal of Clinical Endocrinology and Metabolism, 84,* 1806–1810.

Rostosky, S. S., & Travis, C. B. (1996). Menopause research and the dominance of the biomedical model 1984–1994. *Psychology Women Quarterly, 20,* 285–312.

Ruegsegger, P., Dambacher, M. A., Ruegsegger, E., Fischer, J. A., & Anliker, M. (1984). Bone loss in premenopausal women. *Journal of Bone and Joint Surgery, 66a,* 1015–1023.

Sarrel, P. M. (1987). Sexuality in the middle years. *Obstetrics and Gynecology Clinics of North America, 14,* 49–62.

Schairer, C., Lubin, J., Troisi, R., Sturgeon, S., Brinton, L., & Hoover, R. (2000). Menopausal estrogen and estrogen-progestin replacement therapy and breast cancer risk. *Journal of the American Medical Association, 283*(4), 485–491.

Schneider, D., Barrett-Connor, E., & Morton, D. (1997). Timing of postmenopausal estrogen for optimal bone mineral density. The Rancho Bernardo Study. *Journal of the American Medical Association, 277,* 543–547.

Shaver, J., Giblin, E., Lentz, M., & Lee, K. (1988). Sleep patterns and stability in perimenopausal women. *Sleep, 11,* 556–561.

Shaver, J. L., Giblin, E., & Paulsen, V. (1991). Sleep quality subtypes in midlife women. *Sleep, 14,* 18–23.

Sherman, B., Wallace, R., Bean, J., & Schlabaugh, L. (1981). Relationship of body weight to menarcheal and menopausal age: Implications for breast cancer risk. *Journal of Clinical Endocrinology and Metabolism, 52,* 488–493.

Sherwin, B. (1988). Estrogen and/or androgen replacement therapy and cognitive functioning in surgically menopausal women. *Psychoneuroendocrinology, 13,* 345–357.

Sherwin, B. (1991). The impact of different doses of estrogen and progestin on mood and sexual functioning in postmenopausal women. *Journal of Clinical Endocrinology and Metabolism, 72,* 336–343.

Sherwin, B., & Gelfand, G. (1987). The role of androgens in the maintenance of sexual functioning in oophorectomized women. *Psychosomatic Medicine, 49,* 397–409

Sillero-Arenas, M., Delgado-Rodriguez, M., Rodigues-Canteras, R., Bueno-Cavanillas, A., & Galvez-Vargas, R. (1992). Menopausal hormone replacement therapy and breast cancer: A meta-analysis. *Obstetrics and Gynecology, 79,* 286–294.

Sinaki, M. (1989). Exercise and osteoporosis. *Archives of Physical and Medical Rehabilitation, 70,* 220–229.

Smith, D. C., Prentice, R., Thompson, D. J., & Hermann, W. L. (1975). Association of extrogenous estrogen and endometrial carcinoma. *New England Journal of Medicine, 293*(23), 1164–1167.

Sotelo, M., & Johnson, S. (1997). The effects of hormone replacement therapy on coronary heart disease. *Endocrinology and Metabolism Clinics of North America, 26,* 313–328.

Sowers, M. R., Clark, M. K., Hollis, B., Wallace, R. B., & Jannausch, M. (1992). Radial bone mineral density in pre- and post-perimenopausal women: A prospective study of rates and risk factors for loss. *Journal of Bone and Mineral Research, 7,* 647–657.

Sowers, M. R., La Pietra, M. T. (1995). Menopause: Its epidemiology and potential association with chronic diseases. *Epidemiologic Reviews, 17,* 287–302.

Stampfer, M. J., & Colditz, G. A. (1991). Estrogen replacement therapy and coronary heart disease: A quantitative assessment of the epidemiologic evidence. *Preventive Medicine, 20,* 47–63.

Stampfer, M. J., Colditz, G. A., & Willett, W. C. (1990).

Menopause and heart disease. *Annals of the New York Academy of Sciences, 592*, 193–204.

Stampfer, M. J., Colditz, G. A., Willett, W. C., Mason, J. E., Rosner, B., & Speizer, F. E. (1991). Postmenopausal estrogen therapy and cardiovascular disease. *New England Journal of Medicine, 325*, 756–762.

Stanford, J. L., Hartge, P., Brinton, L. A., Hoover, R. N., & Brookmeyer, R. (1987). Factors influencing the age at natural menopause. *Journal of Chronic Disease, 409*, 995–1002.

Steger, R. W., & Peluso, J. J. (1987). Sex hormones in the aging female. *Endocrinology and Metabolism Clinics of North America, 16*, 1027–1033.

Steiner, M. (1992). Female-specific mood disorder. *Clinical Obstetrics and Gynecology, 35*, 599–611.

Steinberg, K. K., Thacker, S. B., Smith, S. J., Stroup, D. F., Zack, M. M., Flanders, W. D., & Berkelman, R. L. (1991). A meta-analysis of the effect of estrogen replacement therapy on the risk of breast cancer. *Journal of the American Medical Association, 265*, 1985–1989.

Stellato, R., Crawford, S., McKinlay, S., & Longcope, C. (1998). Can follicular stimulating hormone be used to define menopause? *Endocrine Practice, 4*, 137–141.

Swartzman, L. C., Edelberg, R., & Kemmann, E. (1990). The menopausal hot flush: Symptom reports and concomitant physiological changes. *Journal of Behavioral Medicine, 13*(1), 15–31.

Thomas, T. M., Plymat, K. R., Blannin, J., & Meade, T. W. (1980). Prevalence of urinary incontinence. *British Medical Journal, 281*, 1243–1245.

Tikkanen, M. J., Nikkilae, A., Kuusi. T., & Sipinen, S. (1982). High density lipoprotein2 and hepatic lipase: Reciprocal changes produced by estrogen and norgestrel. *Journal of Clinical Endocrinology and Metabolism, 54*, 1113–1117.

Torgerson, D. J., Avenell, A., Russell, I. T., & Reid, D. M. (1994). Factors associated with onset of menopause in women aged 45–49. *Maturitas, 19*, 83–92.

Treloar, A. E. (1974). Menarche, menopause and intervening fecundability. *Human Biology, 46*, 89–107.

Treloar, A. E. (1981). Menstrual cyclicity and the premenopause. *Maturitas, 3*, 249–264.

Trichopoulos, D., MacMahon, B., & Cole, P. (1972). Menopause breast cancer risk. *Journal of the National Cancer Institute, 48*, 605–613.

U.S. Congress & Office of Technology Assessment (1992). *Policy issues in the prevention and treatment of osteoporosis.* Washington, DC: U.S. Government Printing Office.

Vanhulle, G., & Demol, R. (1976). A double-blind study into the influence of estriol on a number of psychological tests in post-menopausal women. In P. A. van Keep, R. B. Greenblatt, & M. Albeux-Fernet (Eds.), *Consensus on menopausal women research* (pp. 94–99). Lancaster, England: MTP Press.

Versi, E. (1990). Incontinence in the climacteric. *Clinical Obstetrics and Gynecology, 33*(2), 392.

Versi, E., & Cardozo, L. D. (1988). Oestrogens and lower urinary tract function. In J. W. W. Studd, & M. I.

Whitehead (Eds.), *The menopause* (pp. 76–84). Oxford: Blackwell Scientific.

Walsh, B. W., Kuller, L. H., Wild, R. A., Paul, S., Farmer, M., Lawrence, J. B., Shah, A. S., & Anderson, P. W. (1998). Effects of raloxifene on serum lipids and coagulation factors in healthy postmenopausal women. *Journal of the American Medical Association, 279*, 1445–1451.

Walsh, B. W., Schiff, I., Rosner, B., Greenberg, L., Ravnikar, V., & Sacks, F. M. (1991). Effects of postmenopausal estrogen replacement on the concentrations and metabolism of plasma lipoproteins. *New England Journal of Medicine, 325*, 1196–1204.

Whelan, E. A., Sandler, D. P., McConnaughey, R., & Weinberg, C. R. (1990). Menstrual and reproductive characteristics and age at natural menopause. *American Journal of Epidemiology, 131*(4), 625–632.

Willett, W., Stampfer, M. J., Bain, C., Lipnick, R., Speizer, F. E., Rosner, B., Cramer, D., & Hennekens, C. H. (1983). Cigarette smoking, relative weight, and menopause. *American Journal of Epidemiology, 117*, 651–658.

Williams, J. K., Adams, M. R., Herrington, D. M., & Clarkson, T. B. (1992). Short-term administration of estrogen, and vascular responses of atherosclerotic coronary arteries. *Journal of the American College of Cardiology, 20*, 452–457.

Williams, J. K., Adams, M. R., & Klopfenstein, H. S. (1990). Estrogen modulates responses of atherosclerotic coronary arteries. *Circulation, 81*, 1680–1687.

Wilson, J. D., & Foster, D. W. (1992). *Williams textbook of endocrinology*, 8th ed. Philadelphia: W. B. Saunders.

Woods, N. F., & Mitchell, E. S. (1996). Patterns of depressed mood in midlife women: Observations from the Seattle Midlife Women's Health Study. *Researching in Nursing and Health, 19*, 111–123.

Woods, N. F., & Mitchell, E. S. (1997). Pathways to depressed mood for midlife women: Observations from the Seattle Midlife Women's Health Study. *Researching in Nursing and Health, 20*, 119–129.

World Health Organization Scientific Group (1981). *Research on the menopause.* WHO Technical Services Report Series 670. Geneva: World Health Organization.

World Health Organization Scientific Group (1996). *Research on the menopause in the 1990s.* WHO Technical Services Report Series No. 866. Geneva: World Health Organization.

Wyon, Y., Lindgren, R., Lundeberg, T., & Hammar, M. (1995). Effects of acupuncture on climacteric vasomotor symptoms, quality of life, and urinary excretion of neuropeptides among postmenopausal women. *Menopause, 2*, 3–12.

Yaffe, K., Sawaya, G., Lieberburg, I., & Grady, D. (1998). Estrogen therapy in postmenopausal women: Effects on cognitive function and dementia. *Journal of the American Medical Association, 279*, 688–695.

Ziel, H. K., & Finkle, W. D. (1975). Increased risk of endometrial carcinoma among users of conjugated estrogens. *New England Journal of Medicine, 293*(23), 1167–1170.

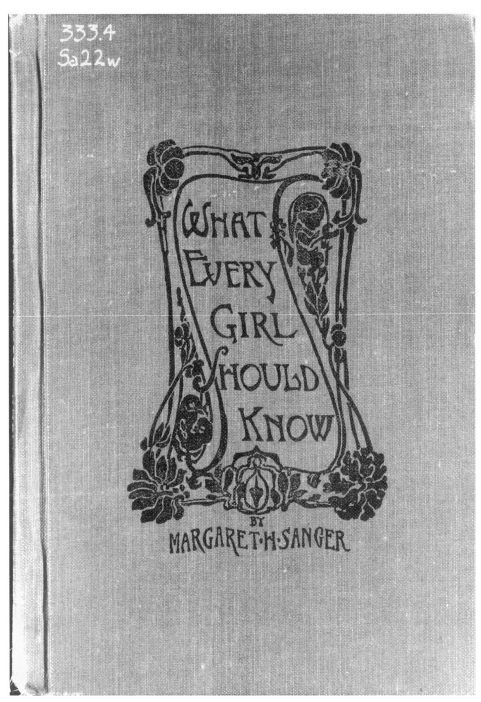

Cover of *What Every Girl Should Know*, by Margaret Sanger, 1916 (KI-LIB: 333.4 Sa22w). (Reproduced with permission of the Kinsey Institute for Research in Sex, Gender, and Reproduction.) In 1912, Margaret H. Sanger began publishing a newspaper column, "What Every Girl Should Know" which provided information about birth control and sexually transmitted infections. Her explicit articles on syphilis drew the attention of government censors and the column was banned in 1913. The following week, the newspaper ran an empty box in place of Sanger's column. The headline read, "What Every Girl Should Know—Nothing! By order of the U.S. Post Office."

III

Technological and Ethical Issues in Women's Sexual and Reproductive Health

20

Contraceptive Technology

ANNE FOSTER-ROSALES and FELICIA H. STEWART

INTRODUCTION: THE EVOLUTION OF CONTRACEPTIVE TECHNOLOGY IN THE UNITED STATES

Contraception is not a modern concept; from ancient times to the present day, human beings have sought to control their fertility. Withdrawal, coitus interruptus for the purpose of avoiding pregnancy, is mentioned in Genesis, and historians, anthropologists, and archeologists describe a wide variety of strategies, including botanical preparations and barriers used for their antifertility effects, in virtually every culture studied. Many societies noted the connection between sexual intercourse and pregnancy, and also identified menarche as a marker for the beginning of a woman's fertility. Sperm were first described in 1677 by Leeuwenhoek, one of the most significant discoveries made possible by his work developing microscopy (Robertson, 1990). It was not until 1930, however, that the mid-cycle timing of ovulation and predictive basal body temperature patterns were discovered; these made fertility awareness (rhythm) methods possible.

ANNE FOSTER-ROSALES and FELICIA H. STEWART • Department of Obstetrics, Gynecology, and Reproductive Sciences, University of California, San Francisco, California 94143-0744.

Handbook of Women's Sexual and Reproductive Health, edited by Wingood and DiClemente. Kluwer Academic / Plenum Publishers, New York, 2002.

Modern hormonal methods were not feasible until the 1950's when chemists extracted synthetic hormones from plant sources. Although researchers had used natural hormone extracts for several decades and understood some of their critical fertility roles, they could not be used for treatment because extraction methods were so cumbersome and expensive. In 1954, synthetic progestin hormone was first used to treat menstrual and fertility problems by Dr. Edward Tyler in Los Angeles, and two synthetic progestins were made commercially available in 1957. The first birth control pill, Enovid, was approved by the U.S. Food and Drug Administration (FDA) in 1960 (Robertson, 1990). Even in 1960, however, the development of an optimal dose and regimen was constrained: it was not possible then to measure the hormonal level in a woman's blood accurately so researchers simply had to "guess" about an appropriate dose for the first pills. As laboratory methods improved, and clinical experience and research accumulated over the next 40 years, hormone doses used for birth control products declined steadily, and today's pills contain about one third as much estrogen and one half to one quarter as much progestin as the first pills.

Many social influences, as well as political and legal constraints, have affected—and still affect—the availability of family planning methods to women and their partners all over the world. The United States has been no exception.

In the United States, federal and state laws, and policies imposed through regulation, have been the subjects of political conflict for both contraception and abortion. Historically, harsh legal restrictions against providing contraceptive services prevailed in federal and state law for almost a century. In 1873, the federal Comstock law, sponsored by Anthony Comstock and his Society for the Suppression of Vice, banned interstate commerce involving contraceptive devices and information. State "Comstock" laws were also widespread, severe and enduring; Massachusetts law made dissemination of birth control information a crime punishable by jail (Hatcher *et al.*, 1998). Providing birth control to an unmarried woman continued to be illegal in some states until the 1970s when the last of the Comstock laws was repealed (Hatcher *et al.*, 1998).

Then, and now, the principal voices and funding for the political minority that opposes legal abortion also opposes laws and policies that would increase access to contraceptive methods. Because public opinion in the United States overwhelmingly supports access to contraception, however, contemporary political efforts to restrict access have been somewhat more indirect, and somewhat less successful than has been the case for abortion. Nevertheless, the impact of anticontraception efforts has been significant. In both the private and public sector, investment in the field has been constrained, and those working in the field have found limited support. Access to contraceptive services and products has been limited, especially in the private sector, and the pharmaceutical industry has been hesitant to participate actively in the field.

Even though women in the United States today have a variety of effective, safe contraceptives from which to choose, for financial and practical reasons, access to services, and to the full range of options, is limited, especially for women who are poor. Many health insurance plans do not cover contraception, require substantial co-pays, or cover only some of the FDA approved methods. Women who want to consider long acting, highly effective methods such

as intrauterine devices (IUDs) or implants often encounter such limitations and they create financial pressures that may affect women's decisions. Public funding of contraceptive services for poor women also is inadequate. The federal Medicaid program provides comprehensive coverage for family planning, but assistance for low-income women who are uninsured and not eligible for Medicaid is sufficient to serve only about half of those in need (Alan Guttmacher Institute, 2000).

Federal funding for low-income women through the Title X program has not kept pace with inflation and has been a battleground for political conflict.

As a matter of public health policy, it is especially ironic that public programs remain underfunded and that health plan regulations continue to discourage use of effective contraceptive options. Unlike many other accepted preventive health measures, contraception is not merely a cost-effective health service, but actually saves health care dollars by preventing unintended pregnancy (Trussell *et al.*, 1995). Pregnancy is so costly that the highly effective methods are among the most cost effective options available even though the initial expenditure required for them is higher than that for less efficacious methods.

Legislative efforts to address contraceptive exclusion in health plans have been successful in several states, and in federal legislation regulating health plans offered to federal employees. These Contraceptive Equity laws require that health plans include coverage for contraceptive services, prescriptions and devices on a par with whatever their coverage is for other services, medications and devices; in other words, contraceptives cannot be singled out for "exclusion."

As is the case for public funding of services, public sector investment in contraceptive research and development has been severely constrained. Federal funding for contraceptive development research, principally through the National Institute of Health (NIH) and the Agency for International Development (AID), increased during the 1970s and 1980s, but was cut in the 1990s and has not since kept up with the inflation in costs for medical research. Considering that almost all women (and men) need and use contraception at some time during their lives, the level of research funding for this field is very small compared to that allocated for issues such as heart disease and cancer, which affect many fewer individuals. Continuing political strife over congressional appropriations for contraception is one reason for the disparity; another is the longstanding shortfall in investment for women's health issues in general. The perceived threat of political conflict, along with product liability concerns, have been serious barriers to private sector investment by pharmaceutical companies in the field. The result has been limited investment in research and development for contraceptive products and lengthy delays in bringing new products to the U.S. market, even when they have been successfully introduced in other countries.

The aura of controversy along with inadequate funding, have deprived this field of appropriate recognition as an integral part of women's health. Family planning issues often are marginalized in health professional school curricula and in the organization of training programs. New graduates may complete their training with little or no education about or experience with family planning, and those who chose to work in the field as researchers or educators do so knowing that their area of interest is not a likely route for professional success.

Despite, or perhaps because of, these adverse circumstances, the field is responsible for some of the most significant and creative advances in health care in the last 40 years. Family planning is acknowledged as one of the 10 most important public health advances of the last century (MMWR, 1999) because of its crucial role in reducing maternal and infant mortality and morbidity. Family planning leaders (then called birth control pioneers) created new strategies and organizations so that women themselves could act to change health care. They also developed the idea of self-care or peer-care: women providing services directly to other women. In 1916, Margaret Sanger and her sister, Ethel Byrne, opened the first United States birth control clinic in Brooklyn, New York, for which they were jailed. Toward the end of her life, Margaret Sanger subsequently played a vital role in finding scientists to develop the contraceptive pill (Hatcher *et al.*, 1998) and securing funding support for this effort.

The linked concepts of informed consent, full disclosure to patients, and participation of the patient in decision making were also developed in the family planning field. The first legislative description of required information for informed consent was written—at the insistence of family planning and women's health activists—for consent prior to surgical sterilization. The first FDA-mandated patient information brochure was developed in response to concerns about possible dangers and side effects with birth control pills. These innovations, now widely adopted in other fields of medicine, fundamentally changed the relationship between clinicians and patients.

PATTERNS OF CONTRACEPTIVE USE IN THE UNITED STATES

Who Needs Contraception and What Do Women Use?

Approximately 60 million U.S. women are in their childbearing years (aged 15–44). One third do not need contraception because they are sterile, pregnant, postpartum or trying to become pregnant, or because they are abstinent. Approximately 90% of the remaining women "at risk for unintended pregnancy" use a method of contraception (see Table 1). The remaining "nonusers" include women who are at risk, but have not yet begun using contraception, those who do not wish to do so because of religious beliefs, and women "in between" methods. A large majority of nonusers have used contraception in the past and/or will do so in the future. As might be expected, however, nonusers account for a substantial proportion of all unintended pregnancies, about half. The other half occur among women *who are using a method* at the time pregnancy occurs: either the

TABLE 1. Contraceptive
Methods Used by U.S. Women

Method	No. of users (in millions)	% of users
Tubal sterilization	10.727	27.7
Pill	10.410	26.9
Male condom	7.889	20.4
Vasectomy	4.215	10.9
Withdrawal	1.178	3.0
Injectable	1.146	3.0
Periodic abstinence	.883	2.3
Diaphragm	.720	1.9
Other	.670	1.8
Implant (Norplant)	.515	1.3
IUD	.310	0.8
Total	38.663	100.0

Source. Alan Guttmacher Institute and National Center for Health Statistics (1998).

method has failed, or pregnancy has occurred because it was not used correctly or consistently (Hatcher, Pluhar, Zieman, Nelson, Darney, & Watt, 1999).

For a typical U.S. couple, achieving family planning goals over a lifetime is a daunting task. The typical woman undergoes menarche at about age 13, and is potentially fertile for more than a decade before she reaches the average age of first marriage. This interval is also a high-risk time for sexually transmitted diseases (STDs), so protection against both pregnancy and infection need to be considered. After a very few years of childbearing—with contraception needed primarily for spacing between approximately two pregnancies—the couple then faces at least two more decades before the woman can expect menopause at age 51. During her 36 fertile years, the average woman will have only 4 years when pregnancy might be a welcome outcome. Maintaining perfectly correct and consistent contraceptive use for such a long time is extremely difficult, and contraceptive failures occur for some couples even despite perfect use. Based on the experience of women reported in the 1982 National Survey of Family Growth, a typical woman must expect 0.81 contraceptive failures during her lifetime, which

translates to nearly one unintended birth or abortion for each U.S. woman.

Several factors influence method choices including availability and cost as well as personal factors such as health history, age, and previous experience. In 1995, the most popular choices among U.S. couples were sterilization surgery (14.9 million), oral contraceptive pills (10.4 million), and male condoms (7.9 million) (see Tables 1 and 2). Among younger women, injectables were the next most commonly used option (1.6 million users overall) (Hatcher, 1998).

Couples in the U.S. are much more likely to rely on surgical sterilization and less likely to use the IUD than are couples in other comparable countries (see Figure 1) (Spinelli, Talamanca, & Lauria, 2000). A similarly wide discrepancy between methods chosen by female physicians in the United States compared to methods used by the general population has also been reported (see Figure 2) (Frank, 1999). This discrepancy is not logical since the IUD provides long-lasting, easy to use contraceptive protection that is comparable or superior to that of sterilization, and the IUD has the advantages of lower cost and reversibility. Health plan coverage limitations are one reason for the difference. Many providers in the United States, however, lack training for IUD insertion, and do not offer the method in their practices.

TABLE 2. Percentage of U.S.
Contraceptive Users Relying on
Sterilization

Age group	Percentage of U.S. contraceptive users relying on tubal sterilization in 1995
15–19	0
20–24	4
25–29	17
30–34	29
35–39	41
40–44	50
All contraceptive users	28

Source. Westhoff *et al.* (2000). Tubal sterilization: focus on the U.S. experience.

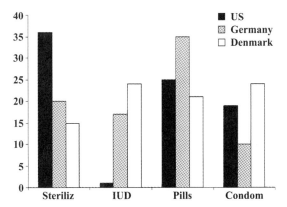

FIGURE 1. Contraceptive choices in the United States, Germany, and Denmark. (Spinelli *et al.*, 2000, Patterns of contraceptive use in five European countries. European Study Group on Infertility and Subfecundity.)

Contraceptive Effectiveness and Failure

Research to determine contraceptive effectiveness actually measures "failures"—the number of women who become pregnant while using a specific method. It would be misleading, however, to create an "effectiveness" rate (such as "99% effective") by subtracting the percent failures from 100% because not all the women would have become pregnant during the study even if they had used no method at all. In other words, the method is responsible for only some of the "success" in a study: some of the women would not have become pregnant no matter what method they were using (or no method). There is no simple way to measure

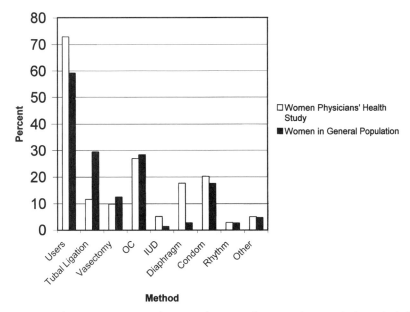

FIGURE 2. Percent of contraceptive users and percent of contraceptive users using a particular method. OC = oral contraceptive; IUD = intrauterine device. When more than one method was listed, classification is by the one most effective for preventing pregnancy (Frank, 1999, Contraceptive use by female physicians in the United States.)

effectiveness in research and the likelihood of pregnancy varies considerably for different groups. The likelihood of pregnancy (called fecundity) depends on age, frequency of intercourse, and personal health history of both the woman and her partner. The impact of such factors cannot be measured directly, so there is no reliable way to determine the proportion of pregnancies truly prevented by a method.

Describing contraceptive effectiveness accurately and honestly has one more complication. As might be expected, subjects in a study who are able to use the method "perfectly" have a lower failure rate than do subjects who are not correct and consistent users. For some methods such as implants, IUDs, and surgical sterilization, this difference is quite small—correct and consistent use is not difficult for users; for other methods, however, the gap is wider. That is why "perfect use" failure rates for condoms, barrier methods such as the diaphragm, and for pills are significantly lower than failure rates for "typical" users. Typical use failure rates reflect how effective a method is for an average person who may not always use it consistently and correctly. Failure rates for perfect use and for typical use are shown in Table 3.

Cost of Contraceptives

Contraception saves health care dollars because it prevents unintended pregnancies. Pregnancy is expensive whether the outcome is full term delivery or spontaneous or induced abortion. Figure 3 shows the five-year health care costs for using no method—the cost of health care for pregnancies that would occur—and for use of 15 available methods (Trussell, Koenig, Stewart, & Darroch, 1997). The total for each method includes the cost of the method itself, the cost of treatment for medical complications, and the cost of medical care for unintended pregnancies that occur because of method failure among typical users. All 15 methods are less expensive than using no method. Furthermore, some methods that seem inexpensive are actually not thrifty because their higher failure rates mean more unin-

tended pregnancies. The most cost-effective methods are intrauterine devices, vasectomy, implants (Norplant), and injectable contraception (Depo-Provera).

Mechanisms of Action: How Do Contraceptives Work?

A series of critical steps are required to establish pregnancy successfully (American College of Obstetricians and Gynecologists [ACOG], 1998):

- Normal maturation of sperm and egg
- Release of sperm (ejaculation)
- Release of egg (ovulation)
- Transport of sperm through the vagina, cervix, uterus, and fallopian tubes
- Final sperm maturation (capacitation) to prepare for fertilization
- Fusion of sperm with egg and normal steps in fertilization
- Transport of fertilized egg from the fallopian tube to the uterus
- Normal cell division of the fertilized egg to form a blastocyst
- Normal development of the uterine lining for implantation
- Implantation of the blastocyst into the lining of the uterus
- Maintenance of normal hormone levels to stabilize the uterine lining until implantation is completed and the placenta begins producing hormones

Pregnancy is defined by the National Institutes of Health/Food and Drug Administration (OPRR, 1983) and by ACOG (Hughes, 1972) as beginning with implantation, which occurs approximately seven days after fertilization. The level of pregnancy hormone is high enough for pregnancy tests to detect within a few days after implantation. Many pregnancies, however, are lost through spontaneous abortion during the first few weeks. If this occurs prior to implantation, or during the following week, the woman is unlikely to suspect that she has been pregnant. She may have no symptoms or signs at all, or she may have a menstrual period

TABLE 3. Percentage of Women Experiencing an Unintended Pregnancy during the First Year of Typical Use and the First Year of Perfect Use of Contraception and the Percentage Continuing Use at the End of the First Year: United States

Method (1)	Percentage of women experiencing unintended pregnancy within the first year of use		Percentage of women continuing use at one year (4)
	Typical use (2)	Perfect use (3)	
Chance	85	85	
Spermicides	26	6	40
Periodic abstinence	25		63
Calendar		9	
Ovulation method		3	
Symptothermal		2	
Postovulation		1	
Cap			
Parous women	40	26	42
Nulliparous women	20	9	56
Sponge			
Parous women	40	20	42
Nulliparous women	20	9	56
Diaphragm	20	6	56
Withdrawal	19	4	
Condom			
Female (Reality)	21	5	56
Male	14	3	61
Pill	5		71
Progestin only		0.5	
Combined		0.1	
IUD			
Progesterone T	2.0	1.5	81
Copper T 380A	0.8	0.6	78
LNg20	0.1	0.1	81
Depo-Provera	0.3	0.3	70
Norplant and Norplant-2	0.05	0.05	88
Female sterilization	0.5	0.5	100
Male sterilization	0.15	0.10	100

Source. Contraception Technology (1998).

that is a little abnormal in timing, and perhaps slightly heavier than usual.

Contraceptives prevent pregnancy by interfering with one or more of the critical steps. Condoms prevent semen from being released in the vagina, so sperm are not present to fertilize an egg. Vaginal barrier methods and spermicides kill sperm before they have a chance to travel through the cervical canal to enter the uterus (Stewart, Guest, Stewart, & Hatcher, 1987). Hormonal methods, including emergency contraceptive pills, have multiple actions that together result in their high effectiveness. Oral contraceptives, emergency contraceptives, and injectables primarily work by preventing ovulation. They also interfere with sperm transport through the cervix by causing the cervical mucous to be thick and sticky. Progestin-only minipills and implants also can suppress ovulation, but are less consistent in doing so. Their effectiveness relies more heavily on alterations in cervical mucous, and may also result from other hormone effects on the steps necessary for fertilization (ACOG, 1998).

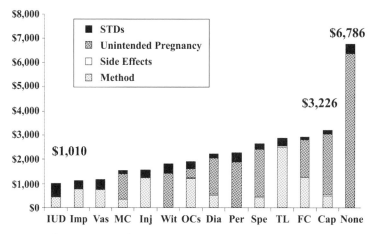

FIGURE 3. Total costs of contraception at five years. (Trussell *et al.*, 1997, Medical care cost savings from adolescent contraceptive use.)

Hormonal method users also have a reduced monthly growth of the endometrium (uterine lining) and a change in fallopian tube contractions. Potentially these could interfere with transport of the blastocyst through the fallopian tube to the uterus or with implantation. Whether or not these postfertilization effects actually do contribute to hormonal method efficacy, however, is not known. Once pregnancy occurs, none of these hormonal methods can interrupt it or cause an abortion (ACOG, 1998).

Intrauterine devices, used either for ongoing contraception or for emergency contraception, also work by inhibiting fertilization. The presence of an IUD in the uterine cavity causes the uterine lining to release white blood cells and alters the composition of fluid in the uterine lining. Copper from the copper IUD contributes to these effects. Progestin-releasing IUDs have the additional effect of causing cervical mucous to be thick and sticky, thus blocking sperm passage through the cervix. These changes are toxic to sperm and interfere with sperm motility. Sperm are not able to travel to the fallopian tubes, and fertilization is prevented. The presence of an IUD may also interfere with implantation of a fertilized egg, should fertilization occur, because the lining of the uterus is altered (Speroff & Darney, 1996).

The rare woman who becomes pregnant using an IUD should have it removed as soon as possible if the string is visible, and an IUD should not be inserted if the woman is (or might be) already pregnant. The presence of an IUD increases the risk of spontaneous abortion in these situations (Speroff & Darney, 1996).

The primary mechanism of action for all contraceptives involves steps *before* fertilization. For women who have religious concerns about the possibility of a postfertilization effect, however, it is important to be forthright. Additional effects of hormonal methods and IUDs potentially could have postfertilization effects by inhibiting implantation. It is important to note that the same is true for the contraceptive effect of breast-feeding (the LAM, lactational amenorrhea method), which depends on the suppression of ovulation as well as a thin uterine lining inhospitable for implantation should fertilization occur (ACOG, 1998).

BARRIER METHODS OF CONTRACEPTION

Barrier methods of birth control include the diaphragm, cervical cap, sponge, spermicide, and male and female condoms. They provide a physical and/or chemical barrier to prevent fertilization by keeping sperm and egg apart, and in the case of spermicides, killing sperm. Condoms enclose the penis in a protective sheath during intercourse and ejaculation. The other barriers are used inside the vagina to cover and block the opening in the cervix (cervical os) that leads to the uterine cavity along with spermicide to kill sperm. Nonoxynol-9, the active ingredient in spermicides available in the United States, is lethal to many organisms, including those that cause gonorrhea, genital herpes, trichomonas, syphilis, and HIV/AIDS. Unfortunately, however, it is a detergent that can cause vaginal irritation and even ulceration, and it disrupts normal bacterial flora in the vagina. Women who use spermicide or condoms lubricated with spermicide have an increased risk for bladder infection and for problems with bacterial vaginosis and vaginal yeast infections (Hatcher *et al.*, 1998). Even more important, some studies of commercial sex workers using spermicide have had worrisome results concerning HIV/AIDS risk. It is possible that vaginal irritation caused by spermicide could increase a woman's susceptibility to acquiring HIV/AIDS (CDC, 2000). If there is any question about potential STD/HIV/AIDS risk, abstinence is the safest choice. Consistent, correct use of latex male condoms greatly reduces risk for bacterial STDs and for HIV/AIDS. It may be best to avoid spermicide products if infection risk is a concern.

The male condom has a lower failure rate than other barrier methods. About half of the women who become pregnant while using barrier methods report that contraceptive failure has occurred in a context of inconsistent or incorrect use. Although condom tears, breaks or slippage do occur in about 2% of uses (Hatcher *et al.*, 1998), the marked difference between the condom's probability of pregnancy during typical use and during perfect use is primarily attributable to inconsistent use. Emergency contraception is an important back-up for condom users in case of a break or inconsistent use.

Vaginal barrier efficacy is affected by whether the woman has experienced childbirth or not. The cervical cap is substantially less

effective for women who have given birth than the diaphragm or female condom. For nulliparous (no previous full-term delivery) women, the female condom, diaphragm, and cervical cap all provide similar contraceptive efficacy. The sponge is also substantially less effective for women who have given birth compared to women who have not, and is somewhat less effective than the diaphragm or cap (Hatcher *et al.*, 1998).

Male Condoms

The male condom is a thin sheath made of latex, natural membrane or polyurethane (plastic) placed over the glans and shaft of the penis during intercourse. Latex condoms are the most widely available, protect against both pregnancy and STDs, and are low in cost. Natural membrane condoms are more porous than latex condoms and are therefore recommended for contraceptive use only and not for protection against STDs. Polyurethane is thinner and stronger than latex and can provide a less constricting fit. Some men find that they enhance sensitivity. Plastic condoms provide effective protection against pregnancy and although research on their effectiveness in preventing STDs is limited, their strength and lack of porosity make use for STD risk reduction reasonable as well. Natural membrane and plastic condoms can be used with all lubricants, whereas latex condoms should not be used with oil-based lubricants or medications, including petroleum jelly. Some condoms are lubricated with the spermicide nonoyynol-9. There is no evidence that these condoms are more effective than condoms without spermicide, and the addition of spermicide may have some disadvantages. Women whose partners use condoms lubricated with spermicide have an increased risk for developing a bladder infection.

Condom use offers several noncontraceptive benefits. Correct and consistent use of male condoms greatly reduces both partners' risks for acquiring HIV/AIDS and STDs. Condoms also reduce long-term risks associated with STDs including infertility (scarred fallopian tubes) and ectopic pregnancy. Condoms are readily available and portable, low in cost (25–50 cents each), encourage male participation in preventing pregnancy and STDs, help some men with erection enhancement, provide proof of protection, and cause no significant medical complications or side effects (Hatcher et al., 1998).

Condom use also has some disadvantages for its users: condoms may reduce sensitivity and spontaneity, cause some men to have problems with maintaining an erection, cause embarrassment, be perceived as a hassle, and can trigger an allergy in men and women who are allergic to latex (Hatcher et al., 1998).

Female Condoms

The Reality Female Condom is a soft, loose-fitting polyurethane sheath that lines the vagina and partially shields the external genital area. Female condoms are 7.8 cm in diameter and 17 cm long; the sheath contains two flexible polyurethane rings. One ring is inserted inside the vagina and serves as an anchor, while the other ring rests outside the vagina, and holds the sheath open. The condom is coated on the inside with a silicone-based lubricant (it does not contain spermicide) and additional lubricant is provided for the woman to use if needed. Polyurethane is less likely to tear than latex and does not deteriorate when exposed to oil-based products. Female and male condoms should not be used together because they can adhere to each other and cause one or both to slip out of position (Hatcher et al., 1998).

Female condoms offer several noncontraceptive benefits: a woman can use them without help from her partner, and they probably prevent HIV/AIDS and STDs, as well as STD related infertility. They are available without a prescription, are portable, provide proof of protection, and their use has no serious medical complications or side effects (Hatcher et al., 1998).

Diaphragm and Cervical Cap

The diaphragm is a dome-shaped rubber cup with a firm, flexible rim. Before it is in-

serted, the inside of the diaphragm is coated with spermicidal cream or jelly. Although the diaphragm does not create a tight seal against the walls of the vagina, it does hold spermicide directly against the cervix to immobilize sperm before they can enter the cervical canal. The diaphragm must be inserted into the vagina before intercourse. It is placed inside the vagina so that the back rim is behind the cervix and the front rim is tucked behind the pubic bone. Once in position, the diaphragm provides contraception for six hours. After that time, or if intercourse is repeated, insertion of additional spermicidal jelly/cream in the vagina is recommended. After intercourse, the diaphragm should be left in place for at least six hours, then removed and washed. If intercourse is anticipated again, it can be reinserted after applying new spermicide. Wearing the diaphragm continually for more than 24 hours is not recommended because of the risk of vaginal infection and Toxic Shock Syndrome (Hatcher et al., 1998; Speroff & Darney, 1996).

Diaphragms are available in four different inner rim styles: flat spring, coil spring, arcing spring, and wide-seal, and range in diameter from 50 to 100 mm. Along with muscle tone, the depth and width of the vagina determine the type and size of the diaphragm that is needed. Fitting requires a visit to a health care provider. Childbirth can change vaginal size, so refitting after full term pregnancy is important. Changes in weight—unless they are very substantial—are not likely to affect diaphragm fit (Hatcher et al., 1998; Speroff & Darney, 1996).

The Prentif Cavity Cervical Cap is a latex cup with a deep dome and a firm round rim, similar to the diaphragm. The cap fits snugly just over the cervix and is held in place by suction. It comes in four sizes and must be fitted by a health care provider. The cap should be filled one-third full with spermicide prior to insertion; it holds spermicide in place against the cervix during intercourse. The cap should be left in place for at least six hours after intercourse and can provide contraception for up to 48 hours no matter how many times intercourse occurs. Additional spermicide is not necessary for repeated intercourse. The cervical cap should not be worn continuously for longer than 48 hours because of vaginal infection risk and toxic shock syndrome risk. Refitting is necessary after childbirth (Hatcher et al., 1998; Speroff & Darney, 1996).

The diaphragm and cervical cap have several noncontraceptive advantages: using them involves no interruption of lovemaking, and they are easy to transport and reuse. There are also some disadvantages: some women and men are allergic to latex or nonoxynol-9 and cannot use vaginal barriers. Women who use barriers have an increased risk of urinary tract infection, Toxic Shock Syndrome, and some women have discomfort or cramps caused by diaphragm rim pressure. Oil-based medications or lubricants including petroleum jelly should not be used with the diaphragm or cervical cap, as these substances cause deterioration of the latex (Hatcher et al., 1998; Speroff & Darney, 1996).

Contraceptive Sponge

The polyurethane Today Sponge acts as a cervical barrier and as a source of spermicide; it contains 1 gram of nonoxynol-9. The sponge has a concave dimple on one side that is designed to fit over the cervix and a polyester/nylon loop on the other side to make removal easier. It can be placed in the vagina up to 24 hours before intercourse. For insertion, the sponge is first moistened with tap water and then inserted so it sits against the cervix. The sponge provides contraceptive protection for up to 24 hours, no matter how many times intercourse occurs. After intercourse, the sponge should be left in place for at least 6 hours before it is removed and discarded. It should not be left in the vagina for more than 24–30 hours because of the risk of vaginal infection and Toxic Shock Syndrome (Hatcher et al., 1998). The contraceptive sponge comes in one size and is available without a prescription.

Sponge advantages include contraceptive protection for up to 24 hours regardless of the frequency of intercourse and easy use. It is not messy, is available over the counter, and does not interrupt lovemaking. Its use does not cause significant medical side effects except for the approximately 4% of users who experience irritation or allergic reactions. In addition, 8% of sponge users have problems with vaginal dryness, soreness or itching, and some women find removal difficult (Speroff & Darney, 1996).

Vaginal Spermicides: Foams, Film, Creams, Suppositories, Gels

Spermicides can be used alone, with barrier method, or along with any other contraceptive method for added protection against pregnancy. They come in many forms including jellies, creams, foams, soluble films, melting suppositories and tablets. The active chemical in products available in the United States is nonoxyol-9, a detergent that destroys the sperm cell membrane. In addition to their sperm-killing effect, spermicidal foams also provide a mechanical barrier to trap sperm in the vagina.

Vaginal gels, cream, and foam deliver 50–150 mg of spermicide. These products are commonly used along with the diaphragm and cervical cap, but can also be used alone. Vaginal contraceptive film has a spermicide concentration of 28% and can be used with the diaphragm or along with a condom. The sheet of film must be inserted close to the cervix at least 15 minutes before intercourse to allow time for the sheet to melt and disperse. Spermicide suppositories provide 2–6 % spermicide and can be used alone or with a condom; waiting 10 to 15 minutes between suppository insertion and intercourse is required to allow time for the suppository to dissolve and disperse. (Hatcher et al., 1998; Speroff & Darney, 1996).

The effectiveness of spermicides depends on proper and consistent use. For the product to be effective it must be placed in the vagina, near the cervix, no more than 1 hour before intercourse.

Advantages of spermicide use include spermicides do not require a prescription, are easy to use, and can provide lubrication during intercourse. However, some people may experience allergy and irritation, find the taste unpleasant, and the product messy. In addition, spermicides are not recommended when there is any concern about infection risk for STD or HIV/AIDS. Using spermicides may cause vaginal irritation and could increase susceptibility to infection. Women who use spermicides have an increased risk for yeast vaginitis, bacterial vaginosis and urinary tract infection (Hatcher et al., 1998).

Emergency Contraception

Emergency contraceptives are methods women can use after unprotected intercourse to prevent pregnancy. Emergency contraception is also an important part of treatment following sexual assault. The three main options are a regimen of combined oral contraceptive pills, in the past, sometimes called "the morning-after-pills," progestin-only minipills, or IUD insertion. In the United States, it is estimated that wider use of emergency contraception could prevent 1.7 million unwanted pregnancies and reduce the annual number of abortions by as much as 800,000 (Speroff & Darney, 1996).

Emergency Contraceptive Pills (ECPs)

Combined oral contraceptive pills taken within 72 hours of intercourse can help to prevent pregnancy. Recent research from the Population Council shows that this method is still reasonably effective up to five days after unprotected intercourse (Ellertson et al., 2000). The regimen is an initial dose of 100–120 micrograms of ethinyl estradiol combined with 0.50–0.75 milligrams of levonorgestrel taken as soon as possible after intercourse and a second identical dose 12 hours after the first. The progestin only regimen is 20 progestin-only pills, containing levonorgestrel, taken as soon as possible within 72 hours after unprotected sex and a second dose taken 12 hours later. The progestin-only regimen causes less nausea than the com-

bined regimen.* Plan B, marketed specifically for emergency contraception, contains two 0.75-mg levonorgestrel tablets (Hatcher et al., 2000). Table 3 shows the correct emergency contraception dosing for various brands of pills (Stewart & Trussell, 2000).

ECPs act by delaying or preventing ovulation so no egg is available for fertilization. They may also interfere with the transport of sperm or ova and alter the endometrium to impair implantation. After a single combined ECP treatment, reported pregnancy rates range from 0.5 to 2.5 per 100 women treated. Emergency contraceptive pills do not protect against future pregnancy, STD/HIV, and are not recommended for long-term contraception (Hatcher et al., 1998).

If a woman wishes to take oral contraceptives for birth control, she can continue taking the pills after the emergency treatment. When combined OCs are used as EC, a significant number of women may experience nausea and up to a quarter may vomit. This can be prevented or reduced by providing antinausea medicine. If the woman is unknowingly pregnant at the time she uses ECPs or if pregnancy occurs despite their use, the pregnancy will not be disrupted or affected. As ECPs act prior to implantation, they do not cause abortion (Hatcher et al., 1998).

IUDs for Emergency Contraception

Copper-releasing intrauterine devices are another highly effective option for emergency contraception. This method is nearly 100% effective in preventing pregnancy with a pregnancy rate of only 0.1%. An IUD can be used up to five days after intercourse and thus may be an option for women who cannot or do not take ECPs in time for them to be effective. Women wishing to use the IUD for continued contraception can leave the IUD in place in the uterus

*WHO. Randomised controlled trial of levonorgestrel versus the Yuzpe regimen of combined oral contraceptives for emergency contraception. Task Force on Postovulatory Methods of Fertility Regulation. Lancet, (1998), 352 (9126), 428–433.

for up to 10 years. This method is not a good choice for women with multiple partners or those who have been sexually assaulted, as it does not protect against STD/HIV (Hatcher *et al.*, 1998; Speroff & Darney, 1996). Progestin-releasing IUDs are not a recommended option for emergency treatment.

HORMONAL METHODS

Combined Oral Contraceptives

Oral contraceptive pills available in the United States contain the synthetic estrogen ethinyl estradiol and one of several different progestins. The low, daily use of synthetic hormones suppresses the ovarian cycle, so ovulation does not occur. In addition, cervical mucus remains thick and acts to impede sperm travel, and the uterine lining does not thicken as it would during a natural cycle. For optimal contraceptive efficacy, pills should be taken daily at around the same time. Among perfect users only about one woman in one thousand becomes pregnant within the first year of use (Table 1). Among typical users, however, the failure rate is 5%. This difference in effectiveness is caused by incorrect and inconsistent pill taking (Hatcher *et al.*, 1998; Speroff & Darney, 1996).

Combined oral contraceptive pills have many non-contraceptive benefits. Using pills helps protect against endometrial cancer, ovarian cancer, benign breast disease, pelvic inflammatory disease, ectopic pregnancy, and anemia. In addition, menstrual cramping and bleeding are reduced, as are premenstrual symptoms, acne; sexual enjoyment may be enhanced by reducing fear of pregnancy and not interrupting lovemaking. Women can also use the combined pill to have more control over the timing of their periods (Hatcher *et al.*, 1998; Speroff & Darney, 1996).

OCs also have disadvantages. They do not protect against sexually transmitted infections, must be taken on a daily basis, may cause nausea or headaches especially during the first sev-

eral cycles, and may effect mood and decrease libido. Serious medical complaints are rare; the most serious is the risk of cardiovascular disease. Women who are over 35 and smoke, have liver disease, advanced diabetes, certain vascular disorders (pulmonary embolism, deep vein thrombosis), certain cancers (breast), or suspect pregnancy should avoid taking oral contraceptives (Hatcher *et al.*, 1998; Speroff & Darney, 1996).

Progestin-Only Pills

Progestin-only pills, commonly called minipills, do not contain estrogen. Their contraceptive effectiveness depends on a combination of factors: the continuous level of progestin prevents ovulation in up to 40% of users, cervical mucus remains thick and sticky, normal development of the corpus luteum (ovarian cyst that forms after ovulation) is disrupted, and the uterine lining is thin and unfavorable for pregnancy. Unlike combined OCs, minipills do not totally suppress natural hormone production, and the woman's natural hormone cycle continues to determine menses (Hatcher *et al.*, 1998; Speroff & Darney, 1996). Among typical users 5% of women become pregnant within the first year of use (Table 1). Like combined OC pills, the minipill is only effective when taken consistently; however, there is little margin of error with minipills. The probability of pregnancy greatly increases if only one or two pills are missed (Hatcher *et al.*, 1998).

Using minipills for contraception has several advantages. They offer contraceptive protection almost as good as that of combined pills when used correctly. They are easy to take and do not interrupt lovemaking. Women who are not able to take estrogen may be able to take the minipill. Their use decreases premenstrual symptoms and their users have fewer side effects than do women using combined pills. Disadvantages for minipill use include unpredictable bleeding patterns, such as spotting. The minipill may be associated with side effects commonly experienced with hormonal supplements, such as headaches, nausea, breast tenderness, and mood changes. As with all progestin methods, there is also a higher risk for ectopic pregnancy with the minipill than with the regular combined pill, in the rare event that pregnancy occurs during use (Hatcher *et al.*, 1998).

Contraceptive Implants: Norplant

Norplant is a subdermal implant system that releases the progestin. The system consists of six Silastic rods that contain levonorgestrel, implanted just under a woman's skin. The hormone is gradually released from the rods into the bloodstream, and results in thickened cervical mucous, as well as a thin endometrium. Ovulation is suppressed less commonly, and therefore bone density remains the same due to relatively normal circulating estrogen levels. The rods have been shown to be effective for seven years of continuous use. They can be removed when the woman desires pregnancy or if problems arise. After removal, fertility is restored within days. The Norplant contraceptive effect is similar to the minipill with the same risks and contraindications, plus those associated with insertion and removal. Norplant, however, is significantly more effective than other hormone contraceptive options because it does not require the woman to do anything on a daily basis to maintain contraceptive protection. Users of Norplant experience a low 0.09% failure rate during the first year of use. In addition, the Norplant system is less expensive than a five-year supply of oral contraceptives. Highly effective one- and two-implant systems may soon be available (Hatcher *et al.*, 1998; Speroff & Darney, 1996).

Implant disadvantages include side effects typical for progestin methods, such as breast tenderness, headaches, and irregular spotting. If not placed correctly, removal of implants can be difficult. For this reason, it is recommended that the implants be placed and removed by experienced practitioners, such as in high-volume family planning clinics or academic centers. Overall, users of this method report very high satisfaction rates (Speroff & Darney, 1996).

Contraceptive Injectables: Depo-Provera, Lunelle

Depo-Provera is a progestin-only injectable contraceptive provided in a dose of 150 mg of medroxy progesterone acetate (DMPA) intramuscularly every three months. Unlike Norplant, Depo-Provera users have high levels of progestin which inhibit follicle stimulating hormone (FSH) and luteinizing hormone (LH) and in turn inhibit ovulation. There is also a thickening of cervical mucus and reduction in the activity of cilia in the fallopian tube. These mechanisms act together to prevent fertilization. Depo-Provera is an extremely effective contraceptive option. In the first year of use, the probability of failure is only 0.3% and approximately 70% of women continue use of the method after one year (Table 3) (Hatcher *et al.*, 1998).

There are many advantages to Depo-Provera. Women who cannot take estrogen may be able to use this method of contraception. Many Depo-Provera users develop a very thin uterine lining, which eliminates menstrual periods after several months of use. This amenorrhea is considered by many women to be an advantage. The method is an effective contraceptive that does not require daily action on the part of the woman except a "shot" every three months. The method is easy to administer and does not interrupt lovemaking. The contraceptive action is reversible once the effect wears off and the method does not cause a loss of fertility. Depo-Provera is a method that is growing in popularity in many countries, including the United States (Hatcher *et al.*, 1998; Speroff & Darney, 1996).

A disadvantage of Depo-Provera is that, unlike other methods, it cannot be immediately discontinued. After stopping the injections, women may have up to 6–12 months delay in return of fertility. Some women find it cumbersome to get injections every 12 weeks. The most common side effect is spotting, which may be a nuisance, but is not dangerous. Other possible side effects of Depo-Provera include weight gain, depression, breast tenderness, and menstrual irregularities. In addition, high-density lipoprotein (HDL) cholesterol levels fall in women using the method. Some women may exhibit an allergic reaction to the method. Long-term users of Depo-Provera develop decreased bone density. However, the bone density is regained when ovulation is resumed (Hatcher et al., 1998; Speroff & Darney, 1996).

Lunelle is a monthly estrogen-progestin injection that combines 25 mg of medroxyprogesterone acetate with 5 mg of estradiol cypionate. Like combined oral contraceptives, Lunelle prevents pregnancy by preventing ovulation. Women using Lunelle have less spotting and irregular bleeding and a lower likelihood of side effects than combined oral contraceptive users. Among more than 700 women using the product in a 60-week clinical trial, no unintended pregnancies were observed, confirming high contraceptive efficacy (Kaunitz, Garceau, & Cromie, 1999). Most women in the study experienced regular monthly periods, and no serious events were observed. The return of ovulation after three monthly injections was documented as early as 63 days after the third injection, which is much sooner than with Depo Provera (Newton, 1996). Women do not have to worry about daily pill taking with Lunelle, and lovemaking is not interrupted.

INTRAUTERINE DEVICES (IUDS)

Three IUDs are currently available in the United States: the Copper-T 380 (Paraguard), the Progesterone T (Progestasert), and the levonorgestrel IUD, Mirena. Copper IUDs release small amounts of copper, which alter the biochemical environment in the uterine lining. In addition, copper alters the cervical mucus and endometrial secretions, and increases prostaglandin production. The IUD is made of polyethylene, the horizontal arms of the T-shaped device are coated with a sleeve of copper, and the vertical portion has copper wire wound around it. There is a loop of polyethylene string at the bottom of the T. There is no measurable increase in copper serum levels and the device is approved for up to 10 years of use. It is the most commonly used IUD in the United States at this time (Hatcher et al., 1998; Speroff & Darney, 1996).

The Progesterone T (Progestasert) IUD releases 65 mg of progesterone daily and is approved for one year of contraception. The progestin thickens cervical mucus, creating a barrier to sperm penetration and survival. Blood progestin levels are not increased, however, so potential progestin side effects, such as headaches are not common. The IUD is made of ethylene vinyl acetate copolymer and the vertical stem contains the progesterone. Strings are attached at the base of the T (Hatcher et al., 1998; Speroff & Darney, 1996).

The Mirena Levonorgestrel IUD releases 20 micrograms of levonorgestrel daily and is currently approved for five years of use; studies to determine long-term effectiveness are continuing and have shown good effectiveness for seven years. The IUD is made of polyethylene, and the vertical stem holds a silastic cylinder, which releases the levonorgestrel. This method of contraception produces serum levels of levonorgestrel about half those of Norplant. Thus, ovulation may be partially inhibited, but the primary effects are local and the low dose of hormone minimizes the systemic hormonal effects. This method reduces menstrual cramps as well as uterine bleeding and, after an initial interval of less predictable bleeding, may lead to fewer total bleeding days, or amenorrhea. Although not approved specifically for this use, the Mirena IUD may provide an option for progestin treatment during hormone replacement therapy in postmenopausal women and may also be an effective treatment for abnormal uterine bleeding.

The effectiveness of the IUD is dependent on many factors. The IUD is more likely to prevent pregnancy if it is coated with copper or a progestin, has a large surface area, is inserted all the way to the top of the uterus and the user checks the strings regularly. Among typical users in the first year, the failure rate for the CuT380A (copper T) is 0.8% and for the Progesterone T is 2.0% (Table 3). Among typical users in the first year, the failure rate of the levonorgestrel IUD is 0.1%; over seven years, the cumulative probability of pregnancy is only 1.1%. The failure rates for women using these IUDs are lower than failure rates for tubal ligation. Currently the levonorgestrel IUD is the most effective method of reversible contraception available (Hatcher *et al.*, 1998, 2000; Speroff & Darney, 1996).

The presence of an intrauterine device produces an intrauterine environment that is hostile to sperm so sperm are not able to travel to the fallopian tubes and fertilization does not occur. The IUD does not affect ovulation. The uterine lining is also affected and becomes less favorable for implantation. Following removal of the IUD, the normal intrauterine environment is restored and pregnancy is achieved at normal rates despite duration of IUD use, no matter how long an IUD is used (Hatcher *et al.*, 1998; Speroff & Darney, 1996).

Women who have not had a child are not encouraged to use IUDs because they do not protect against STDs and can increase the risk of PID during the first few weeks following insertion. Between 2–10% of women with an IUD experience spontaneous expulsions within the first year of use with higher rates for nulliparous women. Some women experience cramping and bleeding after insertion of the IUD, and others complain of increased vaginal discharge while wearing the device. Finally, IUDs must be obtained, inserted, and removed by a physician. The IUD confers several advantages: women who cannot use hormonal methods can use the copper IUD for contraception; the IUD does not interfere with lactation; progestin IUDs decrease menstrual blood loss, and relieve painful menstrual periods; the levonorgestrel IUD is an effective treatment for heavy periods and may reduce the risk of developing pelvic inflammatory disease (PID); and the IUD causes no systemic side effects and is easy to use. Those ideal candidates for an IUD include women who are in a mutually monogamous relationship, want a reversible long-term contraceptive, and have had at least one child. The IUD is an excellent option for women with serious medical conditions (such as pulmonary hypertension) for whom pregnancy and delivery could be potentially life-threatening.

FERTILITY AWARENESS METHODS

Fertility awareness methods rely on identifying the beginning and end of a woman's fertile time during the menstrual cycle. To determine the start of the fertile time, women can observe cervical secretions, changes in the cervix and use a calendar calculation. Cervical secretions change along with the menstrual cycle: they are scant after menses, appear sticky and thick during the first week of the cycle, become clear and stretchy around mid-cycle to facilitate sperm travel, and dry up to form a cervical plug around ovulation.

As ovulation approaches, the cervix becomes wider and softer and lifts higher in the vagina. It returns to a lower position after ovulation and becomes more firm and closed. To determine the end of the fertile time, women can use the indicators mentioned above, as well as monitor the change in their basal (resting) body temperature, which rises around the time of ovulation. The most fertile time begins about five days before ovulation and ends the day after ovulation. The couple should abstain from intercourse or use the barrier or spermicide methods for several days longer than the fertile time to decrease the chance of pregnancy. The calendar calculation method was developed in the 1930s and determines which days a woman is fertile based on her previous menstrual cycles.

Among typical users of the fertility awareness methods, about one in four women experience an unintended pregnancy during the first year of use because it is difficult to predict exactly when the time of ovulation occurs, and because some couples find it difficult to abstain during the fertile period. An advantage of this method is that for close to half of the cycle no additional contraceptive has to be used, but couples have to abstain or use another form of contraception during the fertile time. The failure rates for fertility awareness methods are higher than many other contraceptive methods (Hatcher *et al.*, 1998; Speroff & Darney, 1996).

OTHER METHODS

Lactational Amenorrhea

Lactation, or breast-feeding, causes hormonal changes, which delay the return of ovulation. During the first six months following birth, women who are fully breast-feeding (i.e., using no supplementary food for the baby) and have not experienced their first postpartum menses are very unlikely to become pregnant; studies find six-month pregnancy rates of 0.5% to 1.5% (Hatcher *et al.*, 1998). While pregnancy rates during lactational amenorrhea compare favorably with other methods of contraception, adding another method would provide even greater contraceptive efficacy. After six months of breast-feeding, the chance of pregnancy steadily increases and another contraceptive, one without estrogen, is necessary for continued protection. Also, many women are not able to adhere to exclusive breast-feeding; when breast-feeding is supplemented with formula and/or more than 5 hours passes between breast-feedings, the risk of ovulation, and therefore pregnancy, increases (Speroff & Darney, 1996).

Withdrawal

Withdrawal, or coitus interruptus, prevents fertilization by preventing the sperm and egg from coming into contact. When the male partner feels that ejaculation is imminent, he withdraws his penis from the vagina and external genitalia. Among typical users, the probability of pregnancy during the first year is about 4% with perfect use but 19% with typical use. Withdrawal has several advantages: it costs nothing, is available in all situations, and involves no other device. However, the rate of preg-

nancy among typical users is high compared to other contraceptives. Reasons for failure may be a lack of self-control, difficulty predicting ejaculation by the male, and the possibility of pre-ejaculatory fluid in the urethra containing sperm. In addition, interruption of intercourse may diminish pleasure. Finally, withdrawal does not provide effective protection against STDs (Hatcher *et al.*, 1998).

Douching

Douching refers to washing out the vagina with a special "cleaning" product or water. In the United States, vaginal douching is practiced by about one third of women over 18 years of age, with the greatest frequency found among non-white women and women of lower socioeconomic status. Many women incorrectly believe douching is needed to "clean" the vagina. Washing the outer genital region with water during a shower is all that is necessary to maintain hygiene under normal conditions. Douche products often contain chemicals that irritate the vagina. Women who douche have an increased risk for pelvic inflammatory disease and ectopic pregnancy (Goldman & Hatch, 2000). Any abnormal vaginal secretions or unpleasant odor should be evaluated by a clinician, not treated with douching, as these may be symptoms of an infection. Douching is not a reliable method of contraception.

STERILIZATION

Since 1970, more than one million sterilizations have been performed annually in the United States. Nearly 15 million women rely on sterilization as their contraceptive method: 11 million rely on female sterilization and four million on their male partners' vasectomy. Sterilization for women involves mechanically blocking the fallopian tubes to prevent the sperm and egg from uniting. Vasectomy is the male sterilization operation that blocks the vas deferens to prevent the passage of sperm into the ejaculated seminal fluid (Hatcher *et al.*, 1998; Speroff & Darney, 1996).

Female Sterilization

Female sterilization is a safe procedure with low fatality rates between 1 and 2 per 100,000. The procedure is permanent and involves ligation, mechanical occlusion with clips or rings, or electrocoagulation of the fallopian tubes. The fallopian tubes are usually approached through the abdomen via a minilaparotomy incision or laparoscopy. The risk of pregnancy following female sterilization is much lower than barrier contraceptive methods but somewhat higher than that for long-term methods such as Mirena and Copper-T IUDs and Norplant. The Collaborative Review of Sterilization (CREST) study found a first-year probability of pregnancy of 5.5 for every 1000 sterilization operations and a 10-year cumulative probability of 18.5 pregnancies for every 1000 operations (Peterson, Xia, Wilcox, Tylor, & Trussell, 1999). There are many potential reasons for sterilization failure including pregnancy at the time of surgery, surgical error (which accounts for 30–50% of failure), and equipment or device failure. Ligation via tying and cutting and silastic rings are the techniques with the lowest failure rates (Speroff & Darney, 1996).

The majority of women who undergo the procedure in the United States are over 30 years of age (Table 3). Because most couples have children before the end of their reproductive lifespan, they look toward sterilization as a permanent and effective long-term contraceptive procedure. Women are more likely to regret their decision if they are young, have a change in marital status, have recently given birth or are low-income. For these reasons, an IUD or contraceptive implants, such as Norplant may be appropriate alternatives, as they are long-acting reversible methods. Sterilization does not protect against STD/HIV, therefore condom use must be considered whenever STD risk is a consideration.

Vasectomy

Vasectomy is a very effective contraceptive method with a probability of pregnancy of about 0.1% in the first year. The operation is simple and can be done under local anesthesia in a doctor's office. The no-scalpel technique has even lower complications rates than classical surgical methods, which involve a small incision in the scrotum. Complications are rare, but include infection, bruising, and blood clots in the scrotum. It is import to note that a vasectomy does not cause erectile dysfunctions, a common fear among men. Advantages of a vasectomy include potential for increased enjoyment of sexual activity for both partners and decreased fear of pregnancy. It provides an opportunity for the male partner to take on an important contraceptive role, relieving the woman of this responsibility. No supplies or clinic visits are needed once the sperm count is documented to be zero. Vasectomy failure can result from spontaneous recanalization of the vas deferens, division or occlusion of the wrong structure during surgery, and a congenital duplication of the vas deferens that went unnoticed during the procedure. As with female sterilization, vasectomy does not protect against STD/HIV, and condom use should be considered when STD risk is a concern (Hatcher *et al.*, 1998; Speroff & Darney, 1996).

Male versus Female Sterilization

Female sterilization is appropriate for women who are certain that they do not wish to have more children and need a reliable contraceptive method. The procedure offers permanence, high effectiveness, lack of significant long-term side effects, no need for partner compliance or interruption of lovemaking, privacy of choice and nothing to buy or remember for contraception. But, since sterilization is intended to be permanent and reversal is difficult and expensive, later regret is possible (Hatcher *et al.*, 1998).

Vasectomy offers permanence, high effectiveness, removal of contraceptive burden from the woman, no long-term side effects, high acceptability, and no interruption of lovemaking. Vasectomy is cheaper and is safer than female tubal occlusion and offers a quicker recovery. Neither female nor male sterilization protects against STDs, and both require special training and supplies.

CHOOSING A CONTRACEPTIVE METHOD: WHAT IS THE BEST CHOICE?

The best contraceptive method for a particular woman or man is the method that she or he will use consistently and correctly: no one contraceptive is perfect for everyone. For example, a woman may wish to use oral contraceptives, but if she frequently forgets her pills, and wants a highly effective method, she may wish to consider a long-acting method, such as Depo-Provera, an IUD, or Norplant. If pregnancy prevention is imperative, then less effective methods, such as withdrawal, fertility awareness methods, and the diaphragm or cervical cap may be less attractive to the woman and her partner.

FUTURE CONTRACEPTIVE METHODS

Thorough counseling and careful health screening will allow the woman and her clinician to determine what methods are safest and most compatible with her needs and preferences. For many couples, preventing STDs and HIV is an extremely important priority along with pregnancy prevention; in this situation "double protection" or a dual method use is essential. When a woman uses her method consistently and correctly, and when her male partner does the same with condoms, pregnancy prevention is maximized and STD/HIV transmission is less likely.

The future of contraceptive technology is promising. Contraceptive research continues on a variety of male and female methods. Several new female contraceptive methods are on the horizon: Nuvaring vaginal ring, EVRA contraceptive patch, Norplant II, and Implanon implants. Male hormonal contraceptives in the form of implants, injectables or pills have undergone years of testing and may be available within the next decade. Research also continues on contraceptive vaccines, on nonsurgical methods for permanent sterilization, such as the STOP_intratubal device, and on vaginal microbicides, which have the potential to combine pregnancy prevention and STD/HIV prevention in the same product.

Vaginal rings are silastic loops that contain either progestin or both progestin and estrogen. The Nuvaring contains etonogestrel (120 mg/day) on one side and ethinyl estradiol (15 mg/day) on the other side. The vaginal ring is inserted into the upper vagina and worn for three weeks and removed for one week to allow for menstruation. The mechanism of action is similar to the combined oral pill, although the ring allows for a sustained release of hormone. Due to the sustained release system along with the lower dose of estrogen, the vaginal ring is less likely to cause side effects (such as nausea) than birth control pills. The vaginal ring is worn continuously, but can be removed for a few hours daily or during intercourse if the woman prefers. A primary benefit of the vaginal ring is that women do not have to be burdened with daily dosing. The ring has been shown to be safe for the vaginal tissue and is effective with a low pregnancy rate of 0.3–1.5% (Newton, 1996).

The contraceptive patch, EVRA, is a 20-cm^2 patch that contains estrogen (25 mg/day) and progestin (250 mg/day). The hormones are released over one week like with the vaginal ring. FDA approval is anticipated in the future (Newton, 1996).

Norplant II works just like the original Norplant, however, consists of just two levonorgestrel-containing rods instead of six. The change to two rods will allow for easier, faster, and less painful insertion and removal of the device. It is approved for three years of use but not currently marketed in the United States. The Implanon rod is a single-rod implant containing the progestin etonorgestrel; it is placed using a self-contained disposable insertion device. The rod is made out of ethylene vinyl acetate and releases etonorgestrel at a rate of 60 mg/day. It is highly effective for three years with a low 0.05% pregnancy rate in the first year of use. Like the currently available implants, these devices work by inhibiting ovulation and thickening cervical mucus to prevent sperm transport. Implant users can expect decreased menstrual cramping and bleeding, but estrogen production is sufficient to maintain bone density. Since new implants require fewer rods, insertion and removal should be simpler than for a six-rod device (Newton, 1996).

CONCLUSION

Contraception is one of the most important public health advances of the last century. However, development of and access to effective methods has required continuing political and legislative struggle. Contraception plays a vital role in preserving women's health and is a cost-effective preventive health service. There is no single "perfect" contraceptive, but there are a variety of methods that are safe and effective when used correctly and consistently. Dual-method use to include condoms is of particular importance in maximizing pregnancy prevention, as well as, prevention of sexually transmitted infections and HIV. A number of new methods are on the horizon, however, continuing research is needed to develop even better and safer methods.

REFERENCES

Alan Guttmacher Institute. (2000). *Fulfilling the promise: Public policy and US family planning clinics*. New York: Author.

American College of Obstetricians and Gynecologists.

(1998). Statement on contraceptive methods. Washington, DC: Author.

CDC (2000). From the Centers of Disease Control and Prevention. CDC statement on study results of product containing nonoxynol-9. *JAMA, 284*, 1376.

Ellertson, C., Webb, A., Blanchard, K., Bigrigg, A., Haskell, S., Evans, M., Ferden, S., Leadbetter, C., Spears, A., Johnstone, K., Shochet, T., & Trussell, J. Three simplifications of the Yuzpe regimen of emergency contraception: Results of a randomized, controlled trial in five centers (manuscript).

Frank, E. (1999). Contraceptive use by female physicians in the United States. *Obstetrics and Gynecology, 94*, 666–671.

Goldman, M., & Hatch, M. (2000). *Women and health*. San Diego, CA: Academic Press.

Hatcher, R. A., Pluhar, E., Ziemann, M., Nelson, A., Darney P., Watt A. P., & Hatcher P. (2000). *Managing contraception*. Tiger, GA: Bridging the Gap.

Hatcher, R. A., Pluhar, E., Zieman, M., Nelson, A., Darney, P., & Watt, A. P. (1999). *A personal guide to managing contraception for women & men*. Edition for the year 2000. Decatur, GA: Bridging the Gap Communications.

Hatcher, R. A., Trussell, J., Stewart, F., Cates, W., Stewart, G., Guest, F., & Kowal, D. (1998). *Contraceptive technology*, 17th ed. New York: Ardent Media.

Hatcher, R. A., Stewart, F., *et al.* (1998). *Contraceptive Technology*, 17th ed. New York: Ardent Media.

Hughes, E. (1972). *Obstetric-gynecologic terminology*. Philadelphia: American College of Obstetricians and Gynecologists.

Kaunitz, A. M., Garceau, R. J., & Cromie, M. A. (1999). Comparative safety, efficacy, and cycle control of Lunelle monthly contraceptive injection (medroxyprogesterone acetate and estradiol cypionate injectable suspension) and Ortho-Novum 7/7/7 oral contraceptive (norethindrone/ethinyl estradiol triphasic). *Contraception, 60*, 179–187.

MMWR (1999). Ten great public health achievements—United States, 1900–1999. *Morbidity and Mortality Weekly Report, 48*, 241–243.

Newton, J. (1996). New hormonal methods of contraception. *Bailliere's Clinical Obstetrics and Gynaecology, 10*, 87–101.

OPRR (1983). Protection of human subjects: Code of Federal Regulations. Author.

Peterson, H. B., Xia, Z., Wilcox, L. S., Tylor, L. R., & Trussell, J. (1999). Pregnancy after tubal sterilization with bipolar electrocoagulation. US Collaborative Review of Sterilization Working Group. *Obstetrics and Gynecology, 94*, 163–167.

Piccinino, L. J., & Mosher, W. D. (1998). Trends in contraceptive use in the United States: 1982–1995. *Family Planning Perspectives, 30*(1), 4–10, 46.

Robertson, W. H. (1990). *An illustrated history of contraception*. CITY, NJ: Parthenon.

Speroff, L., & Darney, P. (1996). *A clinical guide for contraception*, 2nd ed. Baltimore: Williams and Wilkins.

Spinelli, A., Talamanca, I. F., & Lauria, L. (2000). Patterns of contraceptive use in 5 European countries. European Study Group on Infertility and Subfecundity. *American Journal of Public Health, 90*, 1403–1408.

Stewart, F., Guest, F., Stewart, G., & Hatcher, R. (1987). *Understanding your body: Every woman's guide to gynecology and health*. New York: Bantam Books.

Stewart, F., & Trussell, J. (2000). Prevention of pregnancy resulting from rape: A neglected preventive health measure. *American Journal of Preventive Medicine, 19*, 228–229.

Trussell, J., Koenig, J., Stewart, F., & Darroch, J. E. (1997). Medical care cost savings from adolescent contraceptive use. *Family Planning Perspectives, 29*, 248–255.

Trussell, J., Leveque, J. A., Koenig, J. D., London, R., Borden, S., Henneberry, J., La Guardia, K. D., Stewart, F., Wilson, T. G., & Wysocki, S. (1995). The economic value of contraception: A comparison of 15 methods. *American Journal of Public Health, 85*, 494–503.

Westhoff, C., & Davis, A. (2000). Tubal sterilization focus on the U.S. experience. *Fertility and Sterility, 73*(5), 913–922.

21

Reproductive Health Technology and Genetic Counseling

JOAN H. MARKS and MARY H. MILLER

INTRODUCTION

In the fifty years from 1956 to 2006 the field of human genetics will have moved from the numbering of the 46 human chromosomes to the expected mapping of the approximately 35,000 human genes. This explosion of knowledge about genetic aspects of human health has been coupled with similar strides in reproductive technologies to overcome infertility or other barriers to the birth of healthy children. The need for the medical community to communicate this information in a useful way to those who may benefit from it has led to the growth of the profession of genetic counseling.

The goal of this chapter will be to describe the latest developments in reproductive technology. These include the appropriate genetic screening of couples before or after conception; assisted reproductive technologies for couples experiencing infertility or genetic risks; screening of the fetus; prenatal diagnosis; decision-making around affected pregnancies; and issues of termination, adoption, and continuing affected pregnancies. Moreover, we will attempt to point out the social, psychological, and public health aspects that permeate the increasing utilization of these technologies in our society.

GENETIC COUNSELING AND REPRODUCTION

The ability to reproduce has been considered a mark of physical maturity and sexual competence. In recent years, however, fertility has become a major medical problem for increasing numbers of people. Greater efforts to assist couples to reach their reproductive potential has also led to greater understanding of the psychosocial implications of parenthood, as well as of the inability to reproduce. Obstetrical data which demonstrate that women under age 30 have easier, less complicated pregnancies have placed pressure on women who wish to extend their reproductive years well into their forties. The resulting problems which these "older" mothers face have increased our understanding of the psychological needs which both men and women of any age experience in their drive to produce healthy biological children.

Genetic counseling begins with a recognition that a specific risk exists for a couple and their pregnancy above the baseline 2–3% risk

JOAN H. MARKS • Human Genetics Program, Sarah Lawrence College, Bronxville, New York 10708. MARY H. MILLER • St. Vincent's Hospital, New York, New York 10010.

Handbook of Women's Sexual and Reproductive Health, edited by Wingood and DiClemente. Kluwer Academic / Plenum Publishers, New York, 2002.

for a baby to be born with a birth defect or mental retardation. Pregnancy involves the transmission of parental genes to the baby. Some of these genes may be altered, and therefore nonworking. The genetic background of the developing fetus interacts with the prenatal ("before birth") environment, which may include the mother's diet, use of prescription or non-prescription drugs, exposure to chemicals, radiation, or infections, and underlying health conditions such as diabetes or seizures. Any of these situations can be teratogenic, that is, increase the risk for the birth of a baby with a birth defect or mental retardation. Maternal age is a risk factor for chromosomal abnormalities. Thus a woman's risk for the birth of a baby with an abnormal number of chromosomes increases with her age (Figure 1).

Recognition of these increased risks is generally made by primary care practitioners, such as obstetricians, nurse midwives, pediatricians, and internists. Although some practitioners prefer to handle many aspects of genetic counseling themselves, the increasing complexity of genetic information and testing options

and the recognition of the extensive contact and support couples may require in this process have resulted in increased referrals to genetic counselors. A genetic counselor is a trained and certified health professional who has usually received a master's degree in a specialized program that emphasizes both understanding of the latest information in human genetics, and the psychosocial aspects of conveying this information to couples in what may be a time of crisis. The goal of genetic counseling is to empower the couple to make the best decisions for their particular situation by providing the information and support they need (National Society of Genetic Counselors [NSGC], 1983). It is in its nondirective methods that genetic counseling differs markedly from the direct advice that most often characterizes the medical practitioner's approach.

Prenatal genetic counseling involves, at a minimum, the accurate assessment of genetic risk faced by an actual or intended pregnancy for a given couple; the description of the risks, benefits, and limitations of any genetic screening or testing that addresses their situation; and

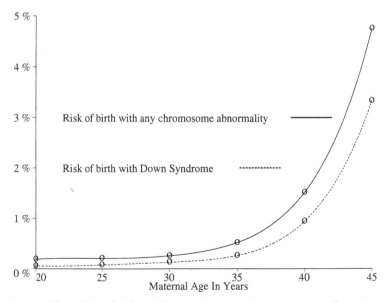

FIGURE 1. Percent risk for the birth of a baby with Down syndrome or with any chromosome abnormality vs. increasing maternal age. Adapted from data in Johnson & Miller (1992); used with permission.

the exploration of their concerns, priorities, values, and circumstances that clarify their decision-making. If testing is chosen, the genetic counselor will oversee the process, choose an appropriate lab, and ensure that adequate samples are obtained from the appropriate family members and are properly transported. Often a counselor advocates for clients for insurance coverage of necessary tests. The counselor will summarize the genetic counseling session in writing for the referring practitioner and will be involved with the referring practitioner in communicating any test results to the clients, providing psychosocial support, discussing the impact of the results, exploring decision-making, and providing any necessary referrals. The counselor serves as the couple's advocate in all these areas, including the right to choose not to pursue testing.

PREGNANCY RISKS

Every pregnancy has a minimum 2–3% risk for the birth of a child with mental retardation or a birth defect requiring medical attention. At the rate of 3.5–4.0 million births per year in the United States, this involves over 150,000 affected births a year. Some pregnancies may be at greater risk for certain conditions because of age, ethnicity, family history, consanguinity (blood relatedness), or medical history. Most will be referred for counseling by a medical practitioner, but with increasing exposure of the general public to genetic information, however, more couples will be self-referred. Some will come for pre-conception counseling while most will be pregnant.

Most current prenatal diagnosis has developed from the ability to sample fetal cells by amniocentesis and determine the chromosome pattern or karyotype. The karyotype of a normal male 46, XY is depicted in Figure 2a. This was first successfully accomplished in 1966. Subsequently it has become possible, given a known risk, to test fetal cells for specific mutations in the DNA of certain genes. Amniotic fluid can also be tested directly for infectious organisms

or for substances associated with a risk of birth defects. The growth of genetic counseling has paralleled these technological advances. Many conditions occur, however, for which testing is not available.

The benefits of prenatal genetic diagnosis include providing risk information to couples who would not consider a pregnancy otherwise, and, most often, reassuring at-risk couples when test results are normal. The benefits of learning about an abnormal condition early in pregnancy include time to prepare psychologically for the birth of the baby and to plan the optimal delivery and care. For some couples, termination may be an option and diagnostic information can often, but not always, be provided within the time limits for legal termination. A couple may also decide testing is not appropriate for them. The burden of prenatal diagnosis is making the decision whether or not to use this technology. Rapp (1999) examined the social impact and cultural meaning of prenatal diagnosis in *Testing Women, Testing the Fetus*.

Age Risks in Pregnancy

A chance error in dividing the 23 pairs of chromosomes to form sex cells occurs more often (95%) in forming the egg than in forming the sperm, and occurs more frequently when a woman is older. Down syndrome, caused by inheriting three number 21 chromosomes vs. the usual two, is the most common of these disorders, occurring approximately once in 800 births. Down syndrome, or trisomy 21 (Figure 2b), results in moderate to severe mental retardation. Individuals with Down syndrome have increased risk for congenital heart defects and, later in life, leukemia and Alzheimer's disease. Other abnormalities of the numbered chromosomes, trisomy 18 and trisomy 13, are less common than trisomy 21 but more severe: affected infants are profoundly mentally retarded and have multiple physical defects such that most do not live more than a year, and many die within weeks of birth. Current public health policy in the United States is to offer testing to

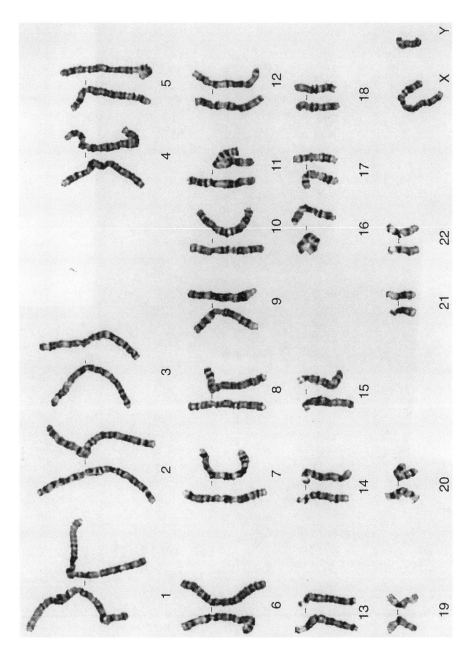

a

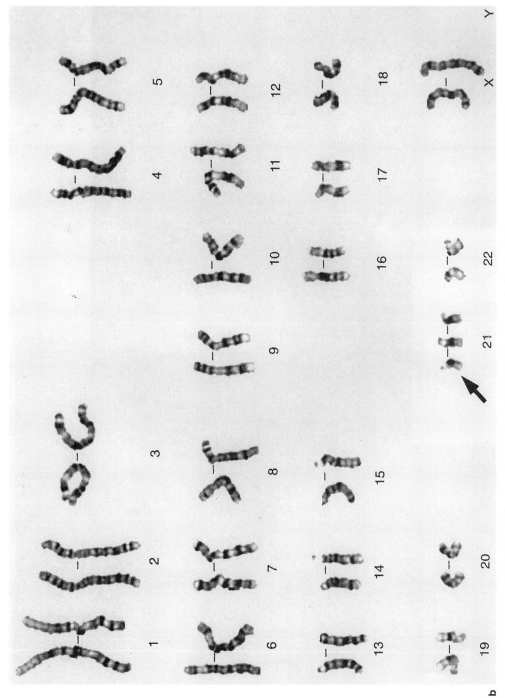

FIGURE 2 a) Karyotype of a normal male: 46,XY. b) Karyotype of a female with Down syndrome: 47,XX,+21.

a woman who is 35 or older at the time of delivery to diagnose chromosome problems. Thirty-five was selected as a cutoff because the risk for Down syndrome is roughly equal to the risk of complications from the diagnostic tests. It is always the woman's decision whether or not to pursue testing.

Because the risk of trisomy is never zero, even in a young woman, various screening tests have been developed to refine the risk of younger women. If screening indicates that a woman's risk is greater than or equal to that of a 35-year-old woman, she is also offered counseling and diagnostic testing for her pregnancy. These screening and diagnostic tests will be discussed in some detail below, but it is important to recognize that the cut-off levels are determined by public health policies that vary from country to country based on the perceived costs and benefits (Heckerling & Verp, 1994).

Risks Associated with Ethnicity

A second simple way to screen for genetic risk is to review the couple's ethnic back-ground. Every ethnic group has certain inherited diseases that occur more frequently in that population than in others. All these disorders are inherited as autosomal recessive diseases, that is, both parents are healthy carriers of the same altered gene. Figure 3 shows the one in four risk for each pregnancy to be affected if both parents carry the same altered gene. The original gene mutation may have occurred many generations ago, and spread through many descendants in that ethnic group. The group is characterized as having a certain carrier frequency for that disease gene, the statistical risk that an individual of that ethnic background will carry the altered gene. The Northern European population, for instance, has a 4% risk of carrying an altered cystic fibrosis gene. Other conditions for which screening is currently recommended include Tay-Sachs disease in the Eastern European Jewish and French Canadian populations; Canavan's disease and cystic fibrosis in the Eastern European Jewish population; sickle cell disease and related hemoglobin disorders in African, Italian, and Greek populations; and several different hemo-

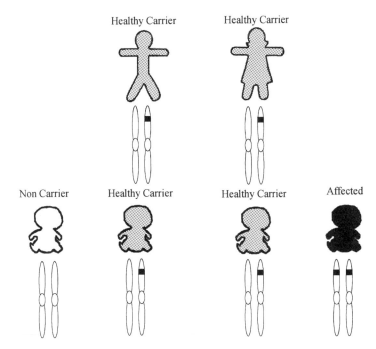

FIGURE 3. Autosomal recessive inheritance: two parents who are healthy carriers of the same altered gene have a 1-in-4 chance with each pregnancy of having a child who inherits both altered genes and is affected with the inherited disease.

globin disorders in the Asian and South-East Asian populations. The list will necessarily become longer as more disease genes are identified and as sensitive, specific tests are developed for them. Education of the public in a way that empowers, rather than stigmatizes, populations will be as important as gene discovery and test development.

Genetic Risks from Family History

A family history taken by a primary care practitioner is another simple way to screen for genetic disorders. While autosomal recessive disorders can be found in siblings but not usually in multiple generations, other patterns of genetic inheritance, such as autosomal dominant, X-linked, and mitochondrial, have been observed from generation to generation. Other disorders which show family clustering are polygenic (influenced by a number of genes), or multifactorial (combining a genetic predisposition with environmental influences). Such conditions include congenital hip dislocation, adult onset diabetes, and schizophrenia. Although prenatal testing is not available for these conditions as it increasingly is for single gene defects, familial clusters can be identified and recurrence risks estimated.

Even if testing is not available for a given condition, a discussion of inheritance patterns, risks, and alternatives may be very informative for a couple who may not have an accurate understanding of their actual risks. For most single gene disorders the maximum risk is 50%, which, of course, means an equal chance that a child would not be affected. Couples may have family myths which distort their understanding of who is at risk, such as believing someone with a close physical resemblance to an affected family member has a higher risk of the condition than other family members. Genetic counselors are skilled in eliciting family dynamics and can educate other family members as well as those originally referred.

Risks of Consanguinity

Family relationships can present a genetic risk in terms of consanguinity. Couples who are first cousins should be offered genetic counseling about their additional 1–3% risk over the general population risk of 2–3% for birth defects or mental retardation. However, the risk of genetic disorders rises steeply with incestuous relationships. Father–daughter and brother–sister conceptions carry a 30–40% risk of a child with a birth defect or mental retardation. Public health workers who are in contact with vulnerable populations need to be aware of the high risk posed for these conceptions in terms of both genetic and social outcomes. Only three states, Alabama, Mississippi, and South Dakota—do not provide public funding for termination of incestuous pregnancies (National Abortion & Reproductive Rights Action League [NARAL], 1999).

Risks Related to Medical History or Exposures

A primary care practitioner should also be alert to reproductive risks based on medical history or teratogenic exposures. While 10–15% of all recognized conceptions end in miscarriages, repeated miscarriages may signal a genetic problem. Although 95% of such cases will be due to medical, rather than genetic, causes, couples are often relieved if an explanation can be provided for their losses and testing can be offered for their pregnancies. A pregnancy may be at risk because of a woman's health status, such as insulin-dependent diabetes, lupus, seizure disorders, or radiation or chemotherapy for cancer, which increase the risk for pregnancy loss and certain birth defects. A woman may be concerned about her exposure to teratogenic chemicals, infections, prescription drugs, street drugs, or alcohol. A genetic counselor can access the latest information and offer any appropriate testing, but testing is not available for every risk factor.

To summarize, couples or individual women may be referred for genetic counseling based on the woman's age, the couple's ethnic background, a family history of health conditions, consanguinity, or medical history. The genetic counselor reviews all these aspects in detail with a couple, and may be able to offer them specific testing such as parental carrier testing, chorionic villus sampling (CVS), amniocentesis, or ultrasound. It is the woman's decision whether to pursue or decline any testing. But what if the couple has had difficulty conceiving, or if, because of genetic risk, the father or the mother wishes his or her sex cells to be replaced by a donor's cells? These challenges can often be met by assisted reproductive technologies, abbreviated ART.

INFERTILITY AND ASSISTED REPRODUCTIVE TECHNOLOGIES

In the United States, the percentage of infertile women increased from 8.4% in the 1982 and 1988 cycles of the National Survey of Family Growth to 10.2% in the 1995 cycle. Thus in 1995, approximately 6.2 million women nationally were infertile (Goldman, Missmer, Barbieri, 1996). Infertility is often defined as the inability to conceive after twelve months of unprotected sexual intercourse. Twelve months is derived from the biological and clinical observations that about 90% of noncontracepting couples of normal fertility will conceive within a year. Infertility can be further classified as primary or secondary. Primary infertility is defined as a couple who has attempted, but has never achieved, conception. Secondary infertility arises after having conceived at least once, regardless of the outcome, but being unable to conceive subsequently. A number of etiologic factors have been associated with infertility, including women's body mass index (i.e., being obese or being slightly underweight); menstrual cycle characteristics (i.e., having a shorter cycle [< 27 days], longer duration of flow [> 8 days], dysmenorrhea); having a history of STDs; and engaging in lifestyle factors such as smoking, coffee drinking, and alcohol use (Goldman, Missmer, Barbieri, 1996).

Infertility can be a great burden psychologically and socially. Both partners can feel diminished when they are not able to produce children, but women in particular have been socialized to expect that they will parent at least two children. Confronting infertility, they ex-

perience feelings of bereavement and depression (Hunt & Monach, 1997) for their loss of expected children. They may feel stigmatized by their failure to achieve a social and cultural goal. They may also suffer learned helplessness (Syme, 1997) from years of infertility treatment. In many marriages, blame is placed by one partner on the other, for either infertility or for the birth of a child with a birth defect. The stress of these negative feelings can easily result in serious problems in a relationship or in divorce. When a child is born with a genetic defect, blaming one's partner can not only damage the marriage but it can seriously interfere with the parents' ability to care for the child. The genetic components of reproductive fitness, therefore, should be viewed in the context of the psychological issues discussed above.

The simplest form of ART is artificial insemination, where a sperm sample is introduced directly to the cervix or the uterus at the ideal time for conception. The sperm may be from the woman's partner or from a donor. Artificial insemination is a method of dealing with infertility from low sperm count. Sperm banking may be chosen if a woman's partner is to undergo cancer therapy. Sperm from a screened donor may be used if the woman's partner has genetic risks. Women who are choosing a donor may wish to consult with a genetic counselor to be sure that screening of the sperm donor addresses any risks associated with their ethnic background or family history and is complete in its examination of the donor's medical history.

Since 1978, when Louise Brown was born as the first "test tube baby," couples have turned to *in vitro* fertilization and embryo transfer to overcome infertility. After extensive preparation with hormones, egg cells are removed from the ovary by laparoscopic surgery and fertilized in lab dishes with sperm from the partner or donor. After the fertilized eggs have demonstrated their competency by dividing into a cluster of eight or more cells, they are implanted into the woman's uterus, or into the uterus of a surrogate if the egg donor has uterine conditions such as malformations or hysterectomy that prevent her from carrying the pregnancy. Frequently, several embryos are transferred to increase the likelihood of successful pregnancy, which runs 8–20% per cycle. Modifications of the basic technique continue to be developed to increase the success rate. A donor egg can be used in these procedures, if a woman has a functional uterus but is not able to ovulate, or if she carries a genetic risk. If a woman faces an increased risk of premature menopause because of cancer therapy, she may attempt egg- or ovary-preserving techniques of ART before treatment is initiated.

Many times, couples and their physicians focus on overcoming the infertility and do not address genetic risks to the pregnancy until after a pregnancy has been established. If a couple has had comprehensive counseling about their risks, however, they may choose pre-implantation genetic testing. In this test one or two cells are removed from each 8–16 cell embryo. If the couple has a risk for a child with Tay-Sachs disease, for example, the DNA of the Tay-Sachs gene is copied millions of times by polymerase chain reaction and examined for mutations. On the basis of this test, only embryos shown to be free of known Tay-Sachs mutations would be implanted.

SCREENING PREGNANCIES FOR DOWN SYNDROME

All pregnancies are at some risk for Down syndrome. Although the risk increases with a woman's age, 70% of infants with Down syndrome are born to women under 35, simply because they have more babies. This fact has motivated efforts to devise screening tests to detect a sub-population of young women who are at higher risk. If a woman is found to be at increased risk by a screening test, she can be offered a diagnostic test such as chorionic villus sampling or amniocentesis.

The most widespread of these screening tests is known as the maternal serum triple screen, or sometimes "the AFP test," after its first component. The test, performed between 15 and 21 weeks of pregnancy, measures three substances in the mother's blood which are made by the fetus and/or the placenta: alpha-fetoprotein (AFP), human chorionic gonadotropin, and estriol. If the dating of the pregnancy is accurate, the concentration of these substances, coupled with the woman's age, has a statistical correlation with a woman's risk for carrying a fetus with trisomy 21 or trisomy 18. The parameters of the test are set so that 5% of women are "screen positive," or considered to be at increased risk for Down syndrome. Most women who are screen positive will turn out to have normal pregnancies, but the screen positive population includes many affected pregnancies. The detection rate is 60% in women under 35 and 70% in women 35 and over. The public health value of this test is such that in 1994, the American College of Obstetricians and Gynecologists recommended that it be offered to all pregnant women under 35.

A woman who has a screen positive result should receive genetic counseling about her options for diagnostic testing of the pregnancy by amniocentesis. A screening test does not need to be perfect to be useful, and the triple screen is not perfect. Efforts continue to increase the detection rate or to lower the false positive rate by adding or substituting other compounds. At the same time, there has been an effort to move this type of screening earlier into the first trimester (first 13 weeks) of pregnancy. There are several advantages associated with earlier testing. Since most women will have healthy pregnancies, most will be reassured earlier in the pregnancy, compared to the current screening test. Those who screen positive have the option of an earlier diagnostic test, CVS. If the fetus is affected, they have the advantage of making their decisions when the pregnancy may still be private. If they choose to terminate the pregnancy, the techniques are simpler and safer. In addition, early termination is considered to be less psychologically traumatic.

The first trimester screen with the best results so far is a combination of biochemical measurement of two pregnancy-related substances in the mother's blood—the free beta form of human chorionic gonadotropin and pregnancy-associated plasma protein A—and an ultrasound measurement of the thickness of the skin at the nape of the fetus' neck, a measurement called nuchal translucency. Although the sensitivity of this test depends largely on the skill and training of the ultrasonographer, there is hope that it will soon become a major tool in pregnancy screening. The triple screen blood test will always be necessary for women who initiate their prenatal care too late for first trimester screening. The AFP component of the triple screen will also retain its usefulness as a screen for neural tube defects such as spina bifida, an opening in the spine exposing the spinal cord, which occurs about once every 1,000 births.

PRENATAL DIAGNOSTIC TESTING

Amniocentesis

Amniocentesis is a technique of sampling fetal cells in the amniotic fluid to determine the fetal karyotype and perform any indicated DNA testing. The procedure is performed beginning at 15 weeks after the first day of the last menstrual period. Under ultrasound guidance a needle is directed through the woman's abdominal wall and into the amniotic sac. Two to three tablespoons (20cc) of amniotic fluid, which contains skin cells and other cells shed by the fetus, are withdrawn into a syringe for subsequent analysis of the fetal cells. The level of AFP in the fluid is also measured. During pregnancy some AFP crosses the placenta to the maternal circulation and is measured in the triple screen discussed above. In some birth defects, including spina bifida, the AFP level in the amniotic fluid is much higher than normal and provides a 96% detection rate for such birth defects. Karyotype analysis is over 99% accurate. Specific DNA testing is also highly accurate. AFP results are available within a few days; karyotype analysis and DNA results can take up to two weeks.

Amniocentesis can thus address age-related risks for chromosomal problems, some specific genetic risks based on family history, and some birth defects associated with maternal health conditions or teratogen exposures. It cannot address all causes of birth defects and mental retardation. Normal results on amniocentesis studies can reduce the risk of birth defects or mental retardation to the 2–3% general population risk. Amniocentesis also has a risk itself for causing miscarriage. The risk for miscarriage is most often quoted at 0.5% above the background risk of a miscarriage, which varies with the woman's age and health status. Balancing the risk of the procedure with the usefulness of the diagnostic information is a very personal decision, and different couples make different choices.

Chorionic Villus Sampling (CVS)

CVS is a technique of sampling the chorionic villi to determine fetal karyotype and perform any indicated DNA testing. Chorionic villi are part of the placenta and arise from the same progenitor cells as the fetus. This test can be performed beginning at 10 weeks after the first day of the last menstrual period. Under ultrasound guidance a small sample of placental villi are removed through a thin tube passed through the cervix to the placenta or through a needle positioned in the placenta from the abdominal surface. The karyotype analysis and DNA studies have the same accuracy as amniocentesis results, but are often available within ten days. Direct AFP testing is not part of CVS analysis, but maternal serum AFP can be measured after 15 weeks of pregnancy. CVS also has the same limitations as amniocentesis in that it cannot address all causes of birth defects and mental retardation. National risk figures for miscarriages associated with CVS performed at 10 weeks or later are 1% above the background risk of miscarriage. Experienced centers are reporting lower risks, and the figures may be adjusted downward in time. However, it is critical for the couple to consider this risk in deciding whether this test is the best choice for them.

Ultrasound

Fetal imaging by ultrasound, or low energy sound waves, has different goals at different stages of pregnancy. In terms of detecting birth defects, a detailed study of fetal anatomy at 18–20 weeks of pregnancy is able to detect many anomalies such as structural abnormalities in the skull, brain, spine, heart and other organs, and many other features such as cleft lip, incomplete development of the diaphragm, obstruction of the urinary tract, etc. The detection rate varies with the type of anomaly, but there are many birth defects, such as blindness or deafness, that cannot be detected by ultrasound.

A particular finding, such as a heart defect, may have different causes, and further chromosomal or genetic testing by amniocentesis may clarify the etiology. However, it is not always possible to determine a specific cause or to give a detailed prognosis for a fetus. Parents may make decisions to continue or terminate a pregnancy based on the finding of a particular defect without knowing its cause. On the other hand, normal findings on ultrasound examination can be very reassuring, particularly if a couple has had a previous child with a birth defect detectable by ultrasound. Normal ultrasound findings also indicate a lower risk of chromosomal abnormalities such as Down syndrome. This cannot guarantee the birth of a perfectly healthy baby, however. Ultrasound studies as performed in the United States have not been shown to pose a risk to the fetus.

ABORTION

Abortion Types and Prevalence

Abortion was legalized in the United States with the 1973 Supreme Court decision of *Roe v. Wade*, which protects a woman's decision to terminate a pregnancy for any reason during the first trimester (within 13 weeks from the first day of the last menstrual period). After that point and before fetal viability, states can regulate abortion procedures in view of the mother's health. Once a fetus is viable, states can regulate or prohibit abortions unless the procedure is judged to be medically necessary to preserve the health or life of the mother. Statistics from the Centers for Disease Control (CDC) for 1996 indicate that 314 pregnancies were terminated for every 1000 carried to term (Koonin et al., 1999). The fact that 54% of terminations occurred by seven weeks gestation and 88% by 13 weeks suggests that most were carried out for personal, rather than medical reasons. Indeed, only 4% of abortions were obtained at 16–20 weeks, and 1.5% at 21 weeks or later. Not all later terminations are for medical indications, since the survey points out that younger women, who may have had more denial of their pregnancies or difficulty accessing services, are disproportionately represented in the later terminations. However, an Alan Guttmacher Institute (AGI) survey of abortion patients regarding their reasons for choosing termination found that 3% were concerned that the fetus had a health problem (cited in AGI, 1997). Overall, legal induced abortion remains a relatively safe procedure with less than one death per 100,000 procedures (Koonin et al., 1999). The mortality rate varies with the type of procedure and increases with the length of the pregnancy (Gans Epner, Jonas, & Seckinger, 1998), as discussed below.

States differ in the point at which they begin to restrict abortions, on their use of public funds to pay for abortions, insurance coverage, restrictions on minors, mandated counseling with or without delays for the procedure, and restrictions on "partial birth abortions," a variant of dilation and evacuation. These regulations are subject to change as legislatures respond to various pressures. The AGI and NARAL websites provide the most current information (AGI, 1999; NARAL, 1999).

Suction Curettage

Relatively few terminations following prenatal diagnosis are likely to occur before 12 weeks, when suction curettage is the most common technique for removal of the products of conception. Suction curettage accounted for 99% of early terminations in 1996 (Koonin *et al.*, 1999). At this early stage of pregnancy, dilation of the cervix or sharp curettage is seldom needed.

Dilation and Evacuation

Most genetic terminations occur after 12 weeks, when dilation and evacuation (D&E) is performed. The cervix is dilated with laminaria, which slowly swell upon contact with the moisture in the cervix. The patient receives sedation and local anesthesia and instruments are introduced through the dilated cervix to remove fetal and placental tissue, followed by curettage. Rare complications can include retained products of conception, hemorrhage, infection or perforation of the uterus. Overall mortality for D&E is 3.7 deaths per 100,000 procedures vs. 0.2 deaths per 100,000 procedures for early suction abortions (Gans Epner *et al.*, 1998). A disadvantage of D&E is that it may preclude a fetal autopsy in cases where a definitive diagnosis has not been given for a malformation.

Labor Induction

If a fetal autopsy will provide important information or if the pregnancy has progressed beyond 16 weeks gestation, the abortion may be performed by labor induction. If the fetus could be viable, the heart is stopped by an injection of drugs, and the amniotic fluid may be replaced by hypertonic saline. Spontaneous labor follows or is induced by hormones, resulting in the delivery of an intact dead fetus. In addition to the possibility of autopsy information, some couples may find a psychological advantage in seeing and holding the baby. The CDC (Koonin *et al.*, 1999) reported that 2% of second trimester (13–28 weeks of pregnancy) terminations in 1996 were by instillation (induction) or 0.4% of all abortions. The AGI analysis of 1992 data (AGI, 1997) determined that 86% of all late abortions (after 20 weeks) were performed by D&E, with most of the remainder by induction.

The overall mortality rate for abortion by induction is 7.1 deaths per 100,000 procedures.

Other Techniques

In rare circumstances, an abortion may be performed by hysterectomy or by hysterotomy, a procedure similar to cesarean section. Abortion by any technique has a higher risk later in pregnancy, but is not likely to be statistically greater than the risk of maternal death from childbirth, 6.7 deaths per 100,000 deliveries (Gans Epner *et al.*, 1998).

ABORTION AND SOCIAL VALUES

Here we will briefly consider some of the values and social factors that have polarized debate on pregnancy termination. Although on a personal level, individual decisions are very complex (an AGI survey [1997] found an average of four reasons contributed to a decision to terminate a pregnancy), on a political level there has been a movement into two camps: pro-choice and pro-life. The pro-choice sentiment, as exemplified by organizations such as NARAL and Planned Parenthood Federation of America, is that a woman should have control over her body and her reproductive life. Considering the health risks of pregnancy, labor, and delivery, which pose a greater risk to a woman's health than most types of abortion, the United States Supreme Court concurred with this view to some extent in its decision that states could not prohibit abortions performed to preserve the woman's health or life. However the Court has also recognized the state's interest in the rights of the fetus, particularly after the point of viability, defined by the Court as "the capacity for meaningful life outside the mother's womb, albeit with artificial aid." Although the Supreme Court recognized that the point of viability would change with advances in neonatal care, the decision of viability would always be a medical, not a legislative, one (Gans Epner *et al.*, 1998).

The pro-life position is based on the assertion that human life must be protected and that it begins at the moment of conception. The pro-life position is often associated with the philosophical or religious position that human life is sacred, and that the sanctity of life is more important than the quality of life. Indeed, not only are the ethical values complex (Hemminki, Santalahti, & Louhiala, 1997), but religions may differ in the acceptability of prenatal diagnosis and abortion (AGI, 1997; Fineman & Gordis, 1982; Hirsch, 1996). Even when abortion is permissible, it is always a very serious decision.

Clearly, there are many factors that impact a woman's decision about whether to carry or terminate an affected pregnancy. At the most general level it is the legal environment she finds herself in at the time of diagnosis. Does her state permit termination at this point? Are services available and affordable? Then a host of personal factors must be weighed, including her religious and ethical values, and social pressures, such as the wishes of her partner and the family and friends who provide her social support. Financial considerations may play a part in the decision if a parent will have to stay home to provide long-term care for the child. States that provide financial incentives for the adoption of handicapped children do not automatically extend stipends to birth parents. If a woman chooses to carry the pregnancy, what resources will be available to meet the needs of the child? How will the birth of the child or the decision to terminate the pregnancy affect her relationship with her partner and any other children?

STRATEGIES FOR INFORMED DECISION-MAKING

Many couples approach prenatal diagnosis with a clear idea of what choice they would make in the event of negative findings. A theoretical decision about a hypothetical situation may differ from an actual decision, but it is a useful part of the process of making an informed decision about testing. Frequently a

counselor will ask a couple, without making presumptions, what "bad news" would mean to them. This is an opportunity for the couple to articulate their values, concerns, and motivations. Some couples may hesitate to enter this imaginative territory, stating that they want to think positively, but confronting the question encourages them to accept the fact that they could be in a position of having to deal with deciding whether to end a wanted pregnancy. Discussing what they perceive to be their options may also help a couple decide whether or not to undertake a diagnostic procedure with a risk of miscarriage. If a couple feels that they could not terminate a pregnancy under any circumstances, they may not choose to put the pregnancy at risk for prenatal diagnosis by CVS or amniocentesis. However, they may still choose to accept the risk if they feel it is outweighed by the opportunity to have information that allows them to prepare for the birth of the child. Some couples realize that for them the most useful aspect of prenatal diagnosis is ending the uncertainty they have endured when a risk exists.

A particularly difficult situation may arise when a previous child or other family member has been affected with a birth defect or genetic disease. Not only may the recurrence risk be as high as 25–50%, but the condition has been personalized for the couple. They may consider a decision to abort an affected pregnancy as a rejection of the affected family member. At the same time, the family may be hard-pressed to deal with further strain. Couples who have chosen adoption for an affected child frequently state that they would choose prenatal diagnosis and termination of affected future pregnancies (Finnegan, 1993).

When making a decision about prenatal diagnosis, it may be enough for a couple to decide "Is this information useful for us to have at this point of pregnancy?" If the answer is "yes" they may choose prenatal diagnosis, knowing that they may be in a position of making a decision about "bad news" in a results session. If their fetus is diagnosed with an abnormality, it is important to review the diagnostic information, its accuracy, the prognosis, and all their options before making any decision. They need to know that their options include abortion, raising the child, and choosing adoption for the child. They should review up-to-date literature on the condition and may choose to contact national support organizations for the particular disability, meet children and perhaps adults with the condition, visit families raising such children, contact families that have chosen adoption, and check the schools and resources available in their area. A couple may not need all this information to feel comfortable with their decision. If they are having difficulty making a decision, the counselor may guide them in the use of structured scenarios in which they tune in to their emotional responses to each choice. This exercise may help to clarify the most significant factors involved in choosing the least painful course of action.

Every choice will be a difficult choice and will involve grieving for the loss of the expected healthy child. As in grieving a death, there are stages of mourning this loss that can include denial, anger, bargaining and depression before reaching acceptance (Kubler-Ross, 1969). In addition to mourning the loss of the hoped-for child, the couple will often have issues of sorrow, guilt and possibly blame in confronting the reality of an affected child, regardless of their decision for the pregnancy. They may feel isolated in their misfortune. There is seldom a satisfactory answer to "Why us?". Statistical probabilities are not very comforting if your pregnancy is the affected one.

PSYCHOLOGICAL CONSEQUENCES OF DECISIONS

Choosing to Terminate a Pregnancy after Prenatal Diagnosis

Emotions after genetic termination are likely to differ from those after a procedure based on personal choice. The pregnancy has been accepted, and is often wanted, perhaps

deeply so. Also, the pregnancy is usually further along, and the woman may have bonded with her pregnancy. The abortion procedure itself may resemble labor and delivery more than early procedures. All of these features may deepen the sense of loss. Long-term psychological repercussions of terminating a pregnancy because of diagnosed abnormalities are not very different from the emotional response to a late miscarriage or early death of a newborn (Salversen, Oyen, Schmidt, Malt, & Eik-Nes, 1997). Both types of events are severe stressors comparable to the acute response to a diagnosis of breast cancer or to rape. In Salversen's study (1997), 14% of women reported significantly increased intrusive thoughts about the loss one year after the event.

The fact that a couple may be convinced that abortion is the right choice for them does not mean that it is not a painful decision. Dates such as the baby's due date, or the anniversary of the confirmation of the pregnancy or of the prenatal diagnosis may be especially difficult as couples are reminded of their hopes for the pregnancy and of their loss. Couples may draw closer to support each other, but particularly if feelings of guilt and blame persist, they may drift farther apart. Minnick & Delp (1999) describe the emotions of parents who made the decision to abort in *A Time to Decide, a Time to Heal*.

Choosing Adoption for a Child with a Birth Defect or Mental Retardation

Psychological repercussions for parents who choose to place a baby with a birth defect for adoption often focus on guilt that they cannot raise a child with disabilities with unconditional love while another family can. The feelings of the birth parents are not resolved with the placement, and they need time for mourning and healing. Adoption may be chosen following prenatal diagnosis, but most often the birth of the affected child is unexpected. Adoption may be chosen relatively quickly and the baby may not go home with the birth parents. Sometimes the decision and often the arrange-

Vignette 1

Rose wrote eloquently about her experience with an abnormal prenatal diagnosis after she became pregnant for the third time at the age of forty. She and her husband had previously decided to terminate any chromosomally abnormal pregnancy, so making a decision when they learned that their baby had Down syndrome was not emotionally difficult. What was more wrenching than they ever imagined was having to face and accept responsibility for that decision. Much of the unexpected emotional impact of their situation came from their tentative or provisional attitude toward the pregnancy while they awaited the amniocentesis results. By denying the importance of the pregnancy to themselves, they were unprepared for the force of the blow of the diagnosis. Because they had kept the pregnancy private from all but a few close friends and their two daughters, they felt more alone and unsupported in their grief.

The diagnosis made Rose feel singled out, ashamed, embarrassed, freakish, abandoned, and the abortion experience itself was very isolating. It was helpful to have friends and family acknowledge her loss and her grief and to have her emotions validated in a support group. Her comments on her children's responses show the impact of this event on the family unit. Although Rose and her husband drew closer together through this experience, she acknowledged that at the bottom, grief is very lonely. In time she realized that she could accept her loss, though she would never forget it.

ments take longer, and the parents, or their surrogates, may continue to visit the baby in the hospital or the baby may go home with the birth parents or to a foster family before the adoption is arranged. It is not unusual for the parents to hope for the baby's death or even to fantasize about killing the baby, as the baby's death would end their dilemma about raising the child (Finnegan, 1993). Often birth parents are surprised to learn that there are waiting lists of families ready to adopt children with birth defects or mental retardation. In dealing with their feelings of guilt or inadequacy, birth parents must realize that adoptive parents do not feel responsible for causing the child's problem as the birth parents usually do. Also, adoptive parents are able to choose a child. They may be willing to raise a child with a disfiguring or limiting birth defect as long as the child has normal intelligence; they may be willing to raise a child with mental retardation as long as the child "looks okay." It is important for the birth family to have a choice also—to raise the child or to choose adoption. Finnegan's book *Shattered Dreams—Lonely Choices* (1993) describes the adoption decision and its repercussions for 20 birth families. The National Adoption Information Clearinghouse (NAIC) website provides a factsheet on adopting a child with a birth defect.

Choosing to Raise a Child with a Birth Defect or Mental Retardation

At one time, children born with a serious birth defect or mental retardation were routinely institutionalized. Some parents nevertheless chose to raise their children themselves, and it became clear that these children progressed much more than their institutionalized peers. Now, the pendulum has swung back to the point that when a child is born with a disability, the expectation is that the parents will take it home and raise it. Many parents do this, includ-

Vignette 2

Sharlene and her husband William had four children ages 5 to 12. William worked in construction, while Sharlene was a homemaker. Finances were tight and William repeatedly urged Sharlene to terminate her fifth, unexpected pregnancy, but as a fundamentalist Christian she felt she could not. She stopped speaking to her husband about her pregnancy and just said she was "going out" when she had a clinic visit. About three months into her pregnancy she was diagnosed with insulin-dependent diabetes, and the clinic started to monitor her pregnancy with detailed ultrasound for the birth defects associated with this condition. Unfortunately, when she was 20 weeks pregnant a sonogram revealed sacral agenesis, a condition in which the lower part of the spinal column does not develop properly. Although intelligence is not affected, there may be limited motion or paralysis of the legs and abnormalities of the urogenital system.

Sharlene cried when she was told the outlook. Her religious convictions were such that she never considered abortion as an option, but she focused her prayers on a miracle, saying "God can do anything." Convinced that her faith would result in a normal birth and fearing her husband's reaction to news of the birth defect, she did not tell him about the baby's problem. She did not go to the tertiary care hospital for the cesarean section scheduled because the baby's legs were fixed in a flexed position, and underwent an emergency cesarean section at her local hospital. Her son was transferred to the intensive care unit of the tertiary hospital where she visited him after her recovery. Her son's needs were such that she could not take him home, even if the home environment had been receptive, and after a few weeks in intensive care he was transferred to a step-down facility where he receives physical therapy. He is now six months old and Sharlene visits him regularly, bringing her older children. Her husband has not seen his son. Social workers at the facility are working with the family in the hope that the baby can go home. Other choices are guardianship or a family care home where legal custody remains with the parents, foster care, and adoption. Sharlene and her family are being given the time and the support to arrive at the best decision for their family.

ing some parents who received the diagnosis prenatally. The decision to raise the child may be easier for parents who learn the diagnosis after the child's birth, where the focus is on a unique individual who has a particular disability, whereas with prenatal diagnosis the focus is more on the disabling condition in the abstract. If the diagnosis comes at birth, however, the parents must deal with feelings of shock, grief, guilt, and isolation in the vulnerable and emotionally tumultuous post-partum period. They may also reject the infant at first as they contemplate the changes in their family life and their capacity to deal with the child's problems.

Raising a child with a disability can bring great joy and reward to the birth family, and it has the benefit of fulfilling social expectations. It also presents real strains on the parents individually, on their relationship, and on their other children (Dyson, 1997). Divorce is not uncommon. One study has shown that among children placed in foster care because of abuse, children with a birth abnormality are represented at twice their incidence in the general population (Needell & Barth, 1998). Perspectives from parents raising children with disabilities are described in *Ordinary Families, Special Children* (Seligman & Darling, 1997).

Vignette 3

Dorothy and her husband Omar spent long hours working together in Omar's restaurant, but Dorothy's schedule was flexible to allow her time with their four-year-old daughter, Sally. The couple had always planned on two children, and with things going well in the restaurant, they conceived again. The pregnancy was uneventful until detailed ultrasound at 18 weeks showed the baby had a serious heart defect. Dorothy and Omar were counseled that 30% of structural heart defects were associated with chromosomal abnormalities. Fortunately, amniocentesis revealed normal chromosomes, but they were very worried about the severity of the heart defect. They learned that the baby would not survive without either a heart transplant or a series of three major surgeries to correct the pattern of blood flow in her heart. Some couples would have chosen abortion, but Dorothy and Omar never hesitated in their decision to give the baby the best chance they could. Obstetrical care was transferred to the specialist hospital where the surgery would take place and plans were made to induce labor before the due date. The baby, Kate, was safely delivered and the first round of surgery, performed a day after her birth, went well. Kate went home two weeks later with around-the-clock professional nursing care.

Dorothy stopped working with Omar at the restaurant so she could be more involved in the care of their daughter. Other family members volunteered to help in her place. Omar and Dorothy found it difficult to give Sally the attention she demanded with the family focus on the needs of the newborn, and she acted out in nursery school. Dorothy talked to the teachers about what was going on at home, and tried to devote time alone with Sally. In spite of the added stress on their lives, the couple are convinced they made the right decision. They are focused on having Kate in optimal condition for the next stage of surgery when she is five months old. They are aware that the overall death rate for the complete series of surgeries is 50%, but they also know there is a good prognosis for survivors. The open communication in their marriage and their strong religious faith have helped them support each other through difficult moments. Dorothy said "I couldn't live with myself if we didn't give this little girl the best chance that we could."

ETHICAL ISSUES

Nondirectiveness

The misuses of genetics in the first half of the twentieth century have affected the way genetic counseling is practiced today. In the past, the concepts of genetics were distorted and turned to the service of public policy in the eugenics movement. Anxiety over high reproductive rates among the socially disadvantaged led to passage of sterilization laws in many states to restrict the reproduction of the men-

tally retarded. Stereotypes about the genetic desirability of different ethnic groups led to racial exclusion laws in immigration policies. Eugenic ideals also produced the concept of racial purity which was adopted by the Nazi movement in Germany. The horror of the Holocaust convinced geneticists that decisions involving genetic information should not be made by public policy but should be made by the individuals involved. The genetics professionals who provide and explain this information are trained not to let their personal beliefs influence the decisions made by their clients.

This policy, nondirectiveness, is one of the core ethical values of genetic counseling (NSGC, 1992). Decisions about conceiving a pregnancy in the face of genetic risk, seeking prenatal diagnosis, or continuing a pregnancy known to be affected with a genetic condition are intensely personal. Those who are familiar with the customary medical model of seeking advice and direction from a medical expert may expect to be guided in these decisions and ask "What would you do?" Cultural groups with a strong tradition of authority and less focus on individual autonomy may feel ill-prepared to make a decision. Input from spiritual advisors, respected figures, and family may be sought, but the personal biases of the genetic counselor should never intrude. Debate continues in the profession (Kessler, 1992) about what subtle behaviors may be directive and whether a counselor can ever be certain she is being nondirective without an independent review of a session. However, the specialized training of genetic counselors helps them to acknowledge and keep separate their personal opinions while they help to clarify the values, needs, and goals of their clients in the decision-making process.

Public Health Policy

Although decisions are personal, public health policies such as the maternal age at which chromosome testing should be offered are based on cost/benefit analysis that presumes a certain uptake of testing, termination of affected pregnancies, and costs of testing versus costs of care for affected children (Heckerling & Verp, 1994). It is a valid goal of public policy to prevent serious genetic disorders in the population (Harper, 1998), provided that decisions are made by individual families and counseling is non-directive. Prenatal screening and testing have reduced the birth frequency of Down syndrome in many populations (Harper, 1998). However, in some circles criticism has been raised that it is discriminatory for health policies to permit termination for genetically affected fetuses later in pregnancy than abortion

of fetuses with no apparent disabilities (Glover & Glover, 1996).

Will genetic testing alter the frequency of mutant genes in the population? For autosomal recessive conditions like Tay-Sachs disease or cystic fibrosis, this is very unlikely. Most of the altered genes are distributed in the healthy carrier population, rather than in the rare affected individuals. Genetic testing has reduced the incidence of some dominantly inherited genetic diseases (Harper, 1998) but some of these conditions, such as achondroplasia, a dwarfing condition, are due primarily to new mutations, rather than to passing on pre-existing ones. Conversely, effective therapies for genetic diseases will likely increase the frequency of the disease genes in the population. It is always important to clarify the primary aim of a screening program. If the goal is to help individual families by giving them a choice, a secondary benefit may also be a reduction in the frequency of the disorder. A goal of eliminating the disorder does not leave room for personal choice.

Sex Selection

The question of using genetic information for sex selection has been an ethically troubling one for the genetics community. Few genetics professionals would support testing solely to determine the sex of the child with termination of the unwanted gender, although this is antithetical to the right of a woman to make her own reproductive decisions. (Sex selection in cases where there is a serious X-linked condition, where half of males would be predicted to be affected and no females would be affected, has general support.) It is a fact that some cultures have a strong preference for male children. In China and India the male to female sex ratio has been markedly skewed by prenatal diagnosis and sex selection (Pennings, 1996). In the United States and other Western countries the demand has been more for "family balancing," achieving a child of the unrepresented sex (Belkin, 1999). The market has responded to these concerns with preconceptual sex selection, where sperm can be separated by various techniques into predominantly X-bearing (female producing) or Y-bearing (male producing) populations. The techniques are 80–90% successful in producing girls and 70–80% successful in producing boys. Although sperm separation cannot guarantee a particular sex, both parents and medical professionals find it less ethically troubling than amniocentesis and abortion. Belkin (1999) describes the personal experiences of couples making this choice. Guidelines have been proposed for the conditions where sex selection would be morally acceptable (Pennings, 1996).

Attention has been focused on sex selection as an example of use of reproductive technology for other than medical or therapeutic reasons. Will parents select for I.Q. or athletic ability? Most desired traits are not dependent on a single chromosome or single gene, and selection technology is not available. What is clear from the commercialization of sex selection is that many parents will choose to use available technology in their efforts to achieve the child they want.

CONCLUSIONS

The field of genetics and advances in reproductive technologies have combined to give couples unprecedented information and control over their reproductive lives. Control, however, means that there is a burden of choice that previous generations did not face. Couples may be counseled about their reproductive risks related to age, ethnicity, consanguinity, and family and medical history, and about the services such as assisted reproductive technologies, CVS, amniocentesis, ultrasound, and screening tests which can address their risks. Their burden is to choose whether or not to pursue any of the options available to them, and the decision is theirs alone. The central tenets of genetic counseling are to be nondirective in providing information and to advocate for the woman's choice about testing and in decisions regarding

affected pregnancies, whether they involve termination, adoption, or raising the child.

There are areas such as sex selection by testing and abortion that are ethically troubling for genetics professionals, but market forces are responding to the desires of parents with preconception techniques of sex selection. Open discussion of the social and ethical implications of these reproductive health technologies by the public and the profession will be necessary to shape public policy.

Where are these technologies headed? The pressure from parents is to provide earlier diagnostic information without the risk of invasive techniques. It is now possible to recover rare fetal cells circulating in the mother's bloodstream. The goal is to provide accurate diagnosis of genetic and chromosomal disorders from these fetal cells (Cheung, Goldberg, & Kan, 1996).

Ethical issues will become even more complex. Should prenatal diagnosis be performed for adult onset diseases, such as a hereditary predisposition to breast and ovarian cancers? If fewer children are born with birth defects, will those who are born suffer more or less discrimination? If parents choose to bear affected children, will their medical costs continue to be covered by insurance? How will genetic information about families and individuals be kept confidential? The answers to these questions will affect us all.

REFERENCES

Alan Guttmacher Institute. (1997). Issues in brief—the limitations of U. S. statistics on abortion. Available: www.agi-usa.org/pubs/ib14.html

Alan Guttmacher Institute. (1999, August). The status of major abortion-related laws and policies in the states. Available:www.agi-usa.org/pubs/ib13.html

Belkin, L. (1999, July 25). Getting the girl. *The New York Times Magazine*, pp. 26–31, 38, 54–55.

Cheung, M. C., Goldberg, J. D., & Kan, Y. W. (1996). Prenatal diagnosis of sickle cell anemia and thalassaemia by analysis of fetal cells in maternal blood. *Nature Genetics, 14,* 264–268.

Dyson, L. L. (1997). Fathers and mothers of school-age

children with developmental disabilities: Parental stress, family functioning, and social supports. *American Journal of Mental Retardation, 102*, 267–279.

Fineman, R. M., & Gordis, D. M. (1982). Occasional essay: Jewish perspective on prenatal diagnosis and selective abortion of affected fetuses, including some comparison with prevailing Catholic beliefs. *American Journal of Medical Genetics, 12*, 355–360.

Finnegan, J. (1993). *Shattered dreams—lonely choices: Birthparents of babies with disabilities talk about adoption.* Westport, CT: Bergin & Garvey.

Gans Epner, J. E., Jonas, H. S., & Seckinger, D. L. (1998). Late-term abortion. *Journal of the American Medical Association, 280*, 724–729.

Goldman, M. B., Missmer S. A., & Barbieri, R. L., (1996). Infertility. In M. B. Goldman, & M. C. Hatch (Eds.), *Women & health* (pp. 196–214). Boston: Academic Press.

Glover, N. M., & Glover, S. J. (1996). Ethical and legal issues regarding selective abortion of fetuses with Down syndrome. *Mental Retardation, 34*, 207–214.

Harper, P. S. (1998). Genetic counselling: Population aspects. In *Practical genetic counselling*, 5th ed. (pp. 315–326). Boston: Butterworth Heinemann.

Heckerling, P. S., & Verp, M. S. (1994). A cost-effectiveness analysis of amniocentesis and chorionic villus sampling for prenatal genetic testing. *Medical Care, 32*, 863–880.

Hemminki, E., Santalahti, P., & Louhiala, P. (1997). Ethical considerations in regulating the start of life. *Perspectives in Biology & Medicine, 40*, 586–591.

Hirsch, J. F. (1996). Medical abortion: Ethics, laws and religious points of view. *Child's Nervous System, 12*, 507–614.

Hunt, J., & Monach, J. H. (1997). Beyond the bereavement model: The significance of depression for infertility counseling. *Human Reproduction, 12*(Suppl. 11), 188–194.

Johnson, M. P., & Miller, O. J. (1992). Cytogenetics. In M. I. Evans (Ed.), *Reproductive risks and prenatal diagnosis* (pp. 237–249). Norwalk, CT: Appleton & Lange.

Kessler, S. (1992). Psychological aspects of genetic counseling. VII. Thoughts on directiveness. *Journal of Genetic Counseling, 1*, 9–17.

Koonin, L. M., Strauss, L. T., Chrisman, C. E., Montalbano, M. S., Bartlett, L. A., & Smith, J. C. (1999, July). Abortion surveillance—United States, 1996. *Morbidity & Mortality Weekly Reports—Surveillance Summaries* [On-line serial], 48(SS04). Available: www.cdc.gov/

Kubler-Ross, E. (1969). *On death and dying.* New York: Collier Books.

Minnick, M. S., & Delp, K. J. (Eds.) (1999). *A time to decide, a time to heal*, 4th ed. St. Johns, MI: Pineapple Press.

National Abortion & Reproductive Rights Action League. (1999). Who decides? A state-by-state review of abortion and reproductive rights. Available: www.naral.org/publications/whod/html

National Adoption Information Clearinghouse. Adopting children with developmental disabilities. Available: www.calib.com/naic/factsheets

National Society of Genetic Counselors (1983). What is a genetic counselor? Available: www.nsgc.org/what_is.html

National Society of Genetic Counselors (1992). Code of ethics. Available: www.nsgc.org/Taking_a_Stand.html

Needell, B., & Barth, R. P. (1998). Infants entering foster care compared to other infants using birth status indicators. *Child Abuse & Neglect, 22*, 1179–1187.

Pennings, G. (1996). Ethics of sex selection for family balancing: Family balancing as a morally acceptable application of sex selection. *Human Reproduction, 11*, 2339–2345.

Rapp, R. (1999). *Testing women, testing the fetus: The social impact of amniocentesis in America.* New York: Routledge.

Salversen, K. A., Oyen, L., Schmidt, N., Malt, U. F., & Eik-Nes, S. H. (1997). Comparison of long-term psychological responses of women after pregnancy termination due to fetal anomalies and after perinatal loss. *Ultrasound in Obstetrics & Gynecology, 9*, 80–85.

Seligman, M., & Darling, R. B. (1997). *Ordinary families, special children: A systems approach to childhood disability*, 2nd ed. New York: Guilford Press.

Syme, G. B. (1997). Facing the unacceptable: The emotional response to infertility. *Human Reproduction, 12*(Suppl. 11), 183–187.

22

Legal and Ethical Issues Impacting Women's Sexual and Reproductive Health

SANA LOUE

INTRODUCTION

Numerous ethical and legal issues arise in the context of women's sexual and reproductive health. An in-depth discussion of all such issues is not possible in the context of a single chapter. Consequently, this chapter focuses on a number of highly visible issues, including those arising in the context of the physician–patient relationship, the HIV epidemic, participation in research, and coerced reproductive interventions.

It must be stated from the outset that one's conclusions with respect to the ethical issues posed in particular situations may differ depending on one's ethical perspective or system of analysis. The first portion of this chapter, then, provides brief explanations of several of the most frequently relied upon approaches to the ethical assessment of situations. Additionally, an assessment of a particular dilemma from legal and ethical perspectives may yield varying

conclusions. It cannot be assumed that because a legal obligation to perform an act or refrain from performing an act exists, that a corresponding ethical obligation exists, and vice versa. Consequently, this discussion, wherever possible, distinguishes between legal and ethical precepts.

APPROACHES TO ETHICAL ANALYSIS

Principlism

Central to principle-based theory is the existence of governing principles that enunciate obligations (Beauchamp & Childress, 1994.) The term "principlism" is often used to refer to four standard principles said to be derived from the Nuremberg Code, and further elucidated by the Helsinki Declarations. Principlism is, in essence, the overriding approach utilized in the United States. These principles are respect for autonomy, nonmaleficence, beneficence, and justice (Beauchamp & Childress, 1994).

Respect for autonomy encompasses the concept of informed consent. In turn, informed consent requires capacity, voluntariness, dis-

SANA LOUE • Department of Epidemiology and Biostatistics, Case Western Reserve University School of Medicine, Cleveland, Ohio 44109-1998.

Handbook of Women's Sexual and Reproductive Health, edited by Wingood and DiClemente. Kluwer Academic / Plenum Publishers, New York, 2002.

closure of information, and understanding. Capacity, or the lack of it, is often determined by reference to one of three standards: (1) the ability to state a preference; (2) the ability to understand information and one's own situation; and (3) the ability to utilize information to make a life decision (Appelbaum & Grisso, 1988; Appelbaum, Lidz, & Meisel, 1987). Voluntariness refers to the individual's ability to consent or refuse a treatment or procedure or participation without coercion, duress, or manipulation (Beauchamp & Childress, 1994).

The concept of disclosure focuses on the provision of information to the patient or research participant. Ethically, the health care provider must disclose the facts that the patient or research participant would consider important in deciding whether to consent or to withhold consent, information that the health care provider believes is material, the recommendation of the health care provider, the purpose of the consent, and the scope of the consent, if given (Beauchamp & Childress, 1994). Legally, additional information may be required. For instance, legally a physician may be required to disclose personal interests that may affect his or her judgment, whether or not those interests are related to the patient's health (*Moore v. Regents of the University of California*, 1990).

Understanding is related to the disclosure of information in a way that can be understood. Studies have shown, for instance, that information provided to prospective participants in research studies is often written at a level above the participants' educational level (Hammerschmidt & Keane, 1992; Meade & Howser, 1992) and often includes unfamiliar words, long words, and long sentences (Rivera, Reed, & Menius, 1992). Understanding may also be impeded in situations where the patient or research participant comprehends the information but refuses to accept the information. For instance, a patient may refuse to consent to an HIV test where she intellectually understands what behaviors may subject an individual to an increased risk of transmission, but believes that such a test is unnecessary for her because she is not ill and she believes that HIV-infected persons must look and feel sick.

Nonmaleficence refers to the obligation to refrain from harming others. Conversely, the principle of beneficence "refers to a moral obligation to act for the benefit of others" (Beauchamp & Childress, 1994). This must be distinguished from benevolence, which refers to the character trait of one who acts for the benefit of others. Although some beneficent acts may be admirable, they are not necessarily obligatory, such as the donation of blood or of an organ to another. The principle of justice refers to the distribution of the benefits and burdens, e.g., of health care and of research. How those benefits and burdens should be distributed is the subject of intense and ongoing debate.

The principlistic approach has been criticized on a number of grounds. First, the principles themselves can be in conflict in specific situations and they provide little or no guidance in resolving such conflicts. For instance, the principle of autonomy would suggest that a woman has the right to decide whether or not to participate in a clinical trial for a new drug designed to reduce transmission of a sexually transmitted disease, based upon receipt of all information material to that decision-making process. Beneficence, however, would argue that she should not be permitted to participate because of the unknown and unknowable risks to any future unborn children. Second, principlism does not have a systematic theory as its foundation (Green, 1990). Third, various critics have argued that principlism is too individualistic, rights-focused, and rationalistic and is exceedingly narrow in its understanding of various religious and cultural frameworks (Clouser & Gert, 1990; DuBose, Hamel, & O'Connell, 1994).

Casuistry

Casuistry refers to a case-based system of ethical analysis (Jonsen, 1995). Situations are examined based on typification, relationships to maxims, and certitude (Artnak, 1995). Typification refers to a comparison of the case at hand with the caregiver's past experiences, and identification of the similarities and differences between the instant case and those that preceded it. Relationships to maxims refers to reliance on "rules of thumb," that consider the characteristics of the situation at hand. Certitude refers to the certainty of the outcome in relationship to all of the alternative courses of action that are available. In essence, casuistry represents a "bottom-up" approach to the development of knowledge rather than a "top-down" approach, as is perceived to be the case with principlism.

Communitarianism

Communitarianism is premised on several themes: the need for a shared philosophical understanding with respect to communal goals and the communal good, the need to integrate what is now fragmented ethical thought, and the need to develop "intersubjective bonds that are mutually constitutive of [individuals'] identities" (Kuczewski, 1997). Unlike principlism, which focuses on the rights of the individual, communitarianism examines communal values and relationships and attempts to ascertain which are present and which are absent. Sandel (1982) has explained the communitarian perspective:

> In so far as our constitutive self-understandings comprehend a wider subject than the individual alone, whether a family or tribe or city or class or nation of people, to this extent they define a community in the constitutive sense. And what marks such a community is not merely a spirit of benevolence, or the presence of communitarian values, or even certain "shared final ends" alone, but a common vocabulary of discourse and a background of implicit practices and understandings.

Where communitarianism emphasizes the need for a common vocabulary and shared understanding, casuistry rejects such a foundation, arguing that it is the "breakdown of tradition [that] forces reexamination of particular instances of action and a return to concrete practical reasoning ..." (Kuczewski, 1982; see Jonsen, 1980).

Feminist Ethics

Feminist ethics encompasses various perspectives. One of the foremost is that of the "ethics of caring." This ethic derives from empirical observations which found that men tend to resolve situations utilizing an ethic of rights, with an emphasis on fairness, while women tend to rely on an ethic of caring that focuses on needs, care, and the prevention of harm (Gilligan, 1982). Feminist ethics rejects the cognitive emphasis of other approaches to ethical analysis and emphasizes the moral role of the emotions. The detachment inherent in the cognitive approaches is criticized precisely because it fails to recognize the attachment inherent in relationships. Sichel (1991) has termed this perspective "feminine" ethics, as distinct from "feminist" ethics:

> "Feminine" at present refers to the search for women's unique voice and most often, the advocacy of an ethics of care that includes nurturance, care, compassion, and networks of communications. "Feminist" refers to those theorists, whether liberal or radical or other orientation, who argue against patriarchal dominations, for equal rights, a just and fair distribution of scarce resources, etc.

Tong (1996), however, has argued that a care-oriented ethic is not in and of itself neglectful of issues relating to gender inequity. Rather, an ethics of relationships and nurturance should encourage all human beings to care for each other and facilitate women's liberation from oppressive systems and structures (Manning, 1992). Such feminists have been termed "cultural feminists" (West, 1988).

There are several feminist approaches to bioethics in addition to those of the cultural feminists. Liberal feminists assert that women are restrained from entrance and success in the "public world" as a result of various legal and customary obstacles. Men and women can be equals only after women are afforded the same educational and occupational opportunities as men (Friedan, 1974).

Marxist feminists claim that capitalism, not merely the larger society as claimed by the liberal feminists, is responsible for the oppression of women. The replacement of the capitalist structure with one that is socialist will allow women and men to be economic equals, facilitating the development of political equality (Barrett, 1980). Radical feminists attribute women's subordination to their reproductive roles and responsibilities and to "the institutionalization of compulsory heterosexuality" rather than to economic, educational, or occupational inequality (Rich, 1980). Psychoanalytic feminists also focus on sexuality and roles, maintaining that systems of dual parenting and careers are needed so that children are not routinized to images of a working father and a nurturing mother (Mitchell, 1974).

Although distinct, each of these theories focuses on "a methodology of feminist thought" (Tong, 1997). Sherwin (1992) has observed that "I believe we must expect and welcome a certain degree of ambivalence and disagreement within feminist theorizing. Contemporary feminism cannot be reduced to a single, comprehensive, totalizing theory." Feminist theory has consequently been criticized as being underdeveloped, too contextual and hostile to principles, and overly confined to the private sphere of relationships (Beauchamp & Childress, 1994).

Utilitarianism

The theory of utilitarianism is premised on the idea of utility: that the "aggregate welfare is the ultimate standard of right and wrong" (Reiman, 1988). The "right" course of action is determined by summing the "good" consequences and the "bad" consequences to welfare that may result from each alternative course of action and selecting that course of action that appears to maximize the "good" consequences to welfare. How to measure gains and losses to welfare, however, is far from simple and, to a great degree, depends on which values are most important and how they are to be weighed. For instance, the maximization of good can be premised on the value of happiness, i.e., whichever course of action produces the greatest degree of happiness, or it can refer to the maximization of goods valued by rational persons.

The role of rules in utilitarianism is somewhat controversial. Some utilitarians ("act utilitarians") would argue that rules provide a rough guide, but do not require adherence where the greatest good in a particular circumstance may result from breach of the rule. Others emphasize the importance of the rule in maximizing the "good" consequences, as demonstrated by one utilitarian in discussing the importance of truth telling in the context of the physician–patient relationship:

> The good, which may be done by deception in a few cases, is almost as nothing, compared with the evil which it does in many, when the prospect of its doing good was just as promising as it was in those in which it succeeded. And when we add to this the evil which would result from a general adoption of a system of deception, the importance of a strict adherence to the truth in our intercourse with the sick, even on the ground of expediency, becomes incalculably great (Hooker, 1849).

Utilitarianism has been criticized on several grounds. Beauchamp and Childress (1994) have argued that utilitarianism appears to permit blatantly immoral acts where such acts would maximize utility. Donagan (1968) has asserted that utilitarianism fails to distinguish between those actions that are morally obligatory and those that are performed based on personal ideals and are above and beyond the call of moral obligation.

LEGAL AND ETHICAL ISSUES

Many, if not all, of the issues discussed below involve challenges to the legal principle of individual bodily integrity:

> No right is held more sacred, or is more carefully guarded, by the common law, than the right of every individual to the possession and control of his own person, free from all restraint or interference of others, unless by clear and unquestionable authority of the law (*Cruzan v. Director*, Missouri Department of Health, 1990).

Concomitantly, they also involve significant ethical issues, such as the limits of individual autonomy and to whom the obligations of beneficence and nonmaleficence are owed. These challenges can be seen in physicians' failure to include their female patients in determinations affecting their own health; in legislative and judicial pronouncements that subordinate the health interests of women to those of the fetus through mandated, unwanted procedures and treatments; and in the exclusion of women from biomedical research for fear of the potential consequences to their potential offspring.

Physician–Patient Relations

Numerous issues arise in the course of a woman's relationship with her physician, including the extent to which the woman's confidences will be preserved and the extent to which the physician's counseling is directive or nondirective in relation to HIV testing and reproductive choice. From a principlistic framework, the manner in which these issues are resolved reflects directly the extent to which a woman's autonomy is respected by the physician.

HIV testing may carry with it significant risks, depending on the political and legal climate in which it is to occur. In some jurisdictions, physicians may be permitted or compelled by statute or by case law to warn the sexual partner and/or needlesharing partner of their HIV-infected patient that he or she may have been exposed to HIV (see *Tarasoff v. Regents of the University of California*, 1976), despite the patient's objection to this disclosure. The physician's advisory to the sexual or needlesharing partner may, however, place the woman at increased risk of violence (Gielen, Fogarty, O'Campo, Anderson, Keller, & Faden, 2000). Conversely, the physician could be potentially liable to the partner if he or she fails to disclose the woman's HIV status to the partner and that individual becomes HIV-infected as a result. Depending upon the law of the particular jurisdiction, the physician may wish to consider whether disclosure to the partner is permissive

or mandatory, the potential risk to the partner, the identifiability of the partner, and the risk to the woman of disclosure.

The Public Health Service has from the earliest days of the HIV epidemic encouraged prenatal HIV antibody testing and counseling:

> Identifying pregnant women with HIV infection as early in pregnancy as possible is important for ensuring appropriate medical care for these women; for planning medical care for their infants; and for providing counseling on family planning, future pregnancies, and the risk of sexual transmission of HIV to others (United States Public Health Service, 1988: 75).

The importance of HIV testing during pregnancy has become, perhaps, even greater since the development of effective treatment to reduce the risk of vertical transmission of HIV (Brenner & Wainberg, 2000).

There remains, however, the danger that health professionals may subtly pressure HIV-positive women to abort in order to avoid even a minimal risk that their cihld will be born HIV-infected and may not provide information to the patient that is sufficient to make a truly informed choice:

> [The] compelling state interest in fetal survival seems to evaporate when the mother and/or fetus have been exposed to HIV. When HIV infections become a factor in the abortion decision, the state's duty to defend potential life shifts to the interest of protecting society from the possibility of another person living with AIDS.... The abandonment of the fight to protect the lives of HIV-positive babies cannot be divorced from the moral judgements passed on anyone who tests positive (Franke, 1989: 209).

A recent study with 69 women found, for instance, that less than half felt that their physicians provided them with adequate counseling about birth control and safer sex, while almost half of the women indicated that information about AZT would affect their future reproductive choices (Duggan *et al.*, 1999).

Participation in Biomedical Research

During the initial years of the HIV epidemic, women's ability to participate in clinical trials was extremely limited. This was problematic because access to high-quality HIV care and potential access to new therapies was most likely through participation in clinical trials (Pham, Freeman, & Kohn, 1992). Cotton and colleagues (1991) found, for instance, that only 6.7% of the participants in the AIDS Clinical Trials Group (ACTG) sponsored by the National Institute for Allergy and Infectious Disease (NIAID) were women. Access to participation was further restricted by requiring that prospective participants produce evidence of a negative pregnancy test and adequate contraception (Faden, Kass, & McGraw, 1996), by excluding women of childbearing potential (Korvick, 1993), by excluding injection drug users, and/or by requiring that trial participants be followed for their medical care by a private physician (Faden, Kass, & McGraw, 1996).

Although the number of adult female participants in clinical trials has since increased, the majority are participants in clinical trials relating to vertical transmission. Clinical trials not involving vertical transmission have often required, as indicated, that women present the results of a negative pregnancy and proof that they are using an adequate form of contraception (Faden, Kass, & McGraw, 1996). Within a principlistic view, it would appear that the principles of beneficence (maximizing good) and nonmaleficence (avoiding doing harm) have been maximized in relation to the principles of respect for autonomy and justice. Respect for autonomy would demand that a woman be permitted to decide for herself whether to become pregnant; justice would assure a more equal distribution of the benefits and the burdens of the research to females as well as to males. In striking this balance, it also appears that the interests of the fetus have been delineated as separate from and in conflict with those of the mother (Arras, 1990).

A utilitarian view might argue against women's exclusion because the maximization of good may well be achieved as the result of participation in a successful clinical trial, e.g., the reduction of HIV-related symptoms resulting in improved quality of life and independent

functioning, an increase in generalizable knowledge regarding the disease and its treatment. Under a feminist paradigm, the reliance on women's reproductive role as a basis for their exclusion from participation perpetuates their subordination within existing infrastructures and systems and encourages reference to the male as the universalized norm. As DeBruin (1994) notes,

> [O]ur society does not conceive of men in terms of gender; it conceives of them gender-neutrally, as persons. Thus, men's identity and experience serve, in effect, as the characterization or standard of what it is to be a person. This is true only of men's identity and experience; it is not true of women's.

Legal efforts have been made to address existing inequities, including the passage and enactment by Congress of the NIH Revitalization Act of 1993, which mandates the increased inclusion of women and minorities in clinical studies, and the revision by the National Institutes of Health (NIH) and the Food and Drug Administration (FDA) of policies relating to the inclusion of women in clinical studies. Sherwin (1994a, 1994b) has argued that such distinctions based on race and sex are themselves problematic within a traditional ethics framework, which opposes the use of race and sex as criteria for the distribution of research benefits and burdens. Under a feminist approach, however, this emphasis may be not only relevant and acceptable, but in specific circumstances may be desirable in order to counteract the oppression and neglect endured by women and minorities within the framework of medical research.

Despite federal regulatory requirements that research participants be equitably selected (see 45 CFR section 46.111(3); 21 CFR section 56.111(3), 1998), women have been excluded from participation in biomedical research based on both scientific and ethical concerns: (1) that homogeneity, which is necessary to maximize the available data and minimize difficulties associated with statistical analysis, would be compromised; (2) that federal regulations require the exclusion of women in certain circumstances; (3) that the inclusion of women increases potential liability due to potential harm to a potential fetus and thereby decreases the funds available directly to research and discourages sponsors of research; and (4) that researchers who believe it is morally wrong to include pregnant or potentially pregnant women should not be forced to conduct research in a manner that is contrary to their beliefs (Merton, 1996). The one notable exception has been the inclusion of women in contraceptive research, which is directly related to men's interest in controlling production of children. Contraceptive research may permit men to have sexual pleasure without the production of children; research on infertility, pregnancy, and childbirth has allowed men to assert more control over the production of perfect children and over an aspect of women's lives over which they previously held less power (Rosser, 1989).

Each of these arguments is subject to refutation. First, research has indicated that drug metabolism and dose–response differ between men and women (Hamilton & Parry, 1983; Raskin, 1974). Consequently, it cannot be assumed that the results of clinical trials involving men are generalizable to women (Council on Ethical and Judicial Affairs, 1991). Second, the concept of homogeneity is a relative one that depends on our state of knowledge with respect to a specific health problem or population at a specific point in time (Levine, 1978). For instance, research involving diabetes must distinguish between types of diabetes.

Although FDA regulations rendered it more difficult to include pregnant and potentially pregnant women in research, their participation was not completely prohibited. Legal liability for harm to the fetus resulting from parental participation is a possibility not only as a result of maternal participation, but also due to paternal transmission of adverse effects as a result of exposures in the context of a research protocol. Indeed, civil liability against a researcher for harm to offspring has been sought only where the research participants were misinformed or not informed at all about the nature of the drug to be administered (*Mink v. University of Chicago*, 1978; *Wetherill v. Uni-*

versity of Chicago, 1983). Additionally, liability may be even greater where women and/or their children are injured due to reliance on medications marketed for their use but tested only on men.

The National Research Act of 1974 provides that

> No individual shall be required to perform or assist in the performance of any part of a health service program or research activity funded in whole or in part [by the Department of Health and Human Services] if his performance or assistance in the performance of such part of such program or activity would be contrary to his religious beliefs or moral convictions.

However, the usurpation of a woman's right to decide whether or not to participate in research in favor of the "rights" of her potential child is violative of respect for autonomy within the principlistic framework and perpetuates the oppression and subordination of women within the feminist paradigm. Roberts (1991) has argued that

> The right to bear children goes to the heart of what it is to be human. The value we place on individuals determines whether we see them as entitled to perpetuate themselves in their children. Denying someone the right to bear children—or punishing her for exercising that right—deprives her of a basic part of her humanity.

Coerced Reproductive Interventions

Numerous judicial decisions, often based on the application of specific state statutes, have forced women to undergo unwanted interventions during the course of their pregnancies. Cesarean sections have been judicially ordered and performed in situations involving placenta previa, failed progress of labor, and placental abruption (*Jefferson v. Griffin Spaulding County Hospital Authority*, 1995; Kolder, Gallagher, & Parsons, 1987). Maternal blood transfusions have been ordered to control life-threatening hemorrhage (*In re* Jamaica Hospital, 1985). Some courts, however, have refused to allow such a drastic intrusion by the state into the right to refuse medical treatment, despite the state's interest in family unity or a potentially increased risk to the fetus (*Fosmire v. Nicoleau*, 1990; *In re* Doe, 1994).

By 1992, at least 167 women had been arrested and charged with criminal offenses due to their use of drugs during pregnancy or other prenatal risk (Chavkin, 1991; Moss, 1991; Strickland & Whicker, 1992). Legislators in at least nine states have attempted to expand child abuse statutes to encompass prenatal substance abuse (Sherman, 1992). As of 1994, Florida, Illinois, Indiana, Minnesota, Nevada, Oklahoma, Rhode Island, and Utah included drug exposure in utero in their child abuse and neglect laws (Roberts, 1990). The 1989 conviction of Jennifer Jones by the state of Florida was a highly publicized instance of this type of prosecution. Jones was convicted based on the alleged transplacental passage of a cocaine derivative immediately after birth. Notably, the state did not prosecute any individuals for the provision of the drug to Jones (Chavkin & Kandall, 1990; Garcia, 1990). Prosecutors of another woman charged with prenatal substance abuse attempted to strengthen their case against her by demonstrating that

> she paid no attention to the nutritional value of the food she ate,... she simply picked the foods that tasted good to her without considering whether they were good for her unborn child. (Johnson, 1986)

Despite the apparent success of legal actions to coerce unwanted reproductive interventions, it is not at all clear that these are ethically justifiable. Under a principlistic analysis, coerced interventions violate the principle of respect for autonomy by violating the bodily integrity of persons who are mentally competent and have not provided consent. The pregnant woman and the physician are both obligated to ensure the well-being of and prevent harm to the fetus, although the extent of that obligation may vary depending on a number of factors, including the age of the fetus. The disproportionate utilization of coerced interventions in situations involving minority women indicates that the principle of justice may also be violated (Kolder, Gallagher, & Parsons, 1987; Roberts, 1991).

Strong (1997) has argued that a modified casuistic approach is most appropriate in assessing the ethical justifiability of a coerced intervention in a given situation. Strong asserts that the acceptability of an intervention increases as both the degree of harm that it would prevent to the fetus increases and the likelihood that it would succeed in preventing harm increases. Conversely, where the risk to the woman's life or health is increased by the proposed intervention, the justifiability of the intervention decreases. Additional factors to be considered in each situation in analyzing the justifiability of the (non)intervention include the consequences to other family members, the potential burden on the community, the need to protect the fetus's life, and the need to protect the physician's integrity.

A radical feminist approach would decry the coercive nature of the intervention, arguing that it is indicative of women's subordination as a function of their reproductive roles. The approach of cultural feminists may be more closely aligned with that of casusists. Where the proposed intervention is likely to prevent significant harm to the fetus and would entail no increased risk to the mother, the ethic of care may support the intervention.

Several other views have been advanced in an attempt to resolve such situations. The American Medical Association (1990) has asserted that court-ordered treatment may be justified ethically if the intervention (1) does not pose a risk or poses an insignificant risk to the woman's health; (2) entails minimal invasion of the woman's bodily integrity; and (3) would clearly prevent substantial and irreversible harm. Clearly, a cesarean is an extreme invasion of the woman's bodily integrity and may, depending upon the specific circumstances, pose a significant risk to the woman's health. The Committee on Bioethics of the American Academy of Pediatrics (1988) finds court-ordered treatment ethically justifiable where (1) the intervention poses little risk to the woman; (2) the intervention is appropriate and there is a high likelihood that it will be effective; and (3) there is a substantial likelihood that the fetus will suffer irrevocable harm without the intervention.

CONCLUSION

Women's sexual health raises numerous ethical and legal issues in addition to those addressed here. These include issues related to abortion, physician-assisted suicide and euthanasia, genetic engineering, surrogate motherhood, and the allocation of health resources, to name but a few. It is impossible to address each of these in the confines of one chapter. What is clear, though, is that the examination of all such issues requires an analysis from multiple, differing perspectives; that a legal analysis may yield a different result than will an ethical analysis; and that the resulting conclusions may vary, not only as a result of the perspective applied but also as a function of time and place.

REFERENCES

American Academy of Pediatrics, Committee on Bioethics (1988). Fetal therapy: Ethical considerations. *Pediatrics, 821,* 898–899.

American Medical Association, Board of Trustees (1990). Legal interventions during pregnancy: Court-ordered medical treatments and legal penalties for potentially harmful behavior by pregnant women. *Journal of the American Medical Association, 264,* 2663–2670.

Appelbaum, P. S., & Grisso, T. (1988). Assessing patients' capacities to consent to treatment. *New England Journal of Medicine, 319,* 1635–1638.

Appelbaum, P. S., Lidz, C. W., & Meisel, A. (1987). *Informed consent: Legal theory and clinical practice.* New York: Oxford University Press.

Arras, J. (1990). AIDS and reproductive decisions: Having children in fear and trembling. *Milbank Quarterly, 68,* 353–381.

Artnak, K. E. (1995). A comparison of principle-based and case-based approaches to ethical analysis. *HEC Forum, 7,* 339–352.

Barrett, M. (1980). *Women's oppression today.* London, England: Verso.

Beauchamp, T. L., & Childress, J. F. (1994). *Principles of biomedical ethics,* 4th ed. New York: Oxford University Press.

Brenner, B. G., & Wainberg, M. A. (2000). The role of antiretrovirals and drug resistance in vertical trans-

mission of HIV-1 infection. *Annals of the New York Academy of Sciences, 918,* 9–15.

Chavkin, W. (1991). Mandatory treatment for drug use during pregnancy. *Journal of the American Medical Association, 266,* 1556–1561.

Chavkin, W., & Kandall, S. (1990). Between a rock and a hard place: Perinatal drug abuse. *Pediatrics, 85,* 223–225.

Clouser, D., & Gert, B. (1990). A critique of principlism. *Journal of Medicine and Philosophy, 15,* 219–236.

Cotton, D. J., Feinberg, J., & Finkelstein, D. M. (1991). Participation of women in a multicenter HIV clinical trials program in the United States. Presented at the Seventh International Conference on AIDS [abstract no. Tu.D.114].

Council on Ethical and Judicial Affairs, American Medical Association (1991). Gender disparities in clinical decision making. *Journal of the American Medical Association, 266,* 559–562.

Cruzan v. Director, Missouri Department of Health (1990). 497 U.S. 261, quoting *Urban Pacific Railroad Company v. Botsford* (1891). 141 U.S. 150, 251 (refusal to compel submission to medical examination).

DeBruin, D. (1994). Justice and the inclusion of women in clinical studies: A conceptual framework. In Institute of Medicine, *Report of the Committee on the Legal and Ethical Issues Relating to the Inclusion of Women in Clinical Research, vol. 2* (pp. 127–150). Washington, DC: National Academy Press.

Donagan, A. (1968). Is there a credible form of utilitarianism? In M. Bayles (Ed.), *Contemporary utilitarianism* (pp. 187–202). Garden City, NY: Doubleday.

DuBose, E., Hamel, R., & O'Connell, L. J. (1994). *A matter of principles? Ferment in U.S. bioethics.* Valley Forge, PA: Trinity Press International.

Duggan, J., Walerius, H., Purohit, A., Khuder, S., Bowles, M., Carter, S., Kosy, M., Locher, A., O'Neill, K., Gray, A., & Chakraborty, J. (1999). Reproductive issues in HIV-seropositive women: A survey regarding counseling, contraception, safer sex, and pregnancy choices. *Journal of the Association of Nurses in AIDS Care, 10,* 84–92.

Faden, R., Kass, N., & McGraw, D. (1996). Women as vessels and vectors: Lessons from the HIV epidemic. In S. M. Wolf (Ed.), *Feminism and bioethics: Beyond reproduction* (pp. 252–281). New York: Oxford University Press.

Fosmire v. Nicoleau (1990). 75 N.Y.2d 218, 551 N.Y.S.2d 876.

Franke, K. (1989). Turning issues upside down. In I. Rieder & P. Ruppelt (Eds.), *Matters of life and death: Women speak out about AIDS.* London: Virago.

Friedan, B. (1974). *The feminine mystique.* New York: Dell.

Garcia, S. A. (1990). Birth penalty: Societal response to perinatal chemical dependence. *Journal of Clinical Ethics, 1,* 135–140.

Gielen, A. C., Fogarty, L., O'Campo, P. Anderson, J., Keller, J., & Faden, R. (2000). Women living with HIV: Disclosure, violence, and social support. *Journal of Urban Health*, 77, 480–491.

Gilligan, C. (1982). *In a different voice*. Cambridge, MA: Harvard University Press.

Green, R. (1990). Method in bioethics: A troubled assessment. *The Journal of Medicine and Philosophy*, 15, 188–189.

Hamilton, J., & Parry, B. (1983). Sex-related differences in clinical drug response: Implications for women's health. *Journal of the American Medical Women's Association*, 38, 126–132.

Hammerschmidt, D. E., & Keane, M. A. (1992). Institutional review board (IRB) review lacks impact on readability of consent forms for research. *American Journal of the Medical Sciences*, 304, 348–351.

Hooker, W. (1849). *Physician and patient*. New York: Baker and Scribner.

In re Doe. (1994). 260 Ill. App. 3d 392, 632 N.E.2d 326 (Ill. App. Ct.).

In re Jamaica Hospital. (1985). 128 Misc. 2d 1006, 491 N.Y.S.2d 898 (N.Y. Sup. Ct.)

Jefferson v. Griffin Spaulding County Hospital Authority (1995). 274 S.E.2d 457.

Johnson, D. E. (1986). Shared interests: Promoting healthy births without sacrificing women's liberty. *Hastings Law Journal*, 43, 569–614.

Jonsen, A. R. (1980). Can an ethicist be a consultant? In V. Abernethy (Ed.), *Frontiers in medical ethics* (pp. 157–171). Cambridge: Ballinger.

Jonsen, A. R. (1995). Casuistry: An alternative or complement to principles? *Kennedy Institute of Ethics Journal*, 5, 237–251.

Kolder, V. E. B., Gallagher, J., & Parsons, M. T. (1987). Court-ordered obstetrical interventions. *New England Journal of Medicine*, 316, 1192–1196.

Korvick, J. A. (1993, June 6–11). Women's participation in AIDS Clinical Trial Group (ACTG) trials in the USA—Enough or still too few? Presented at the Ninth International Conference on AIDS, Berlin.

Kuczewski, M. G. (1997). *Fragmentation and consensus: Communitarian and casuist bioethics*. Washington, DC: Georgetown University Press.

Levine, R. J. (1978). Appropriate guidelines for the selection of human subjects for participation in biomedical and behavioral research. In the National Commission for the Protection of Human Subjects of Biomedical and Behavioral Research, Department of Health, Education, and Welfare. *The Belmont Report: Ethical principles and guidelines for the protection of human subjects of research* (Appendix I, 4-1 to 4-103). Washington, DC: U.S. Government Printing Office [Pub. No. (OS) 78-0013].

Manning, R. C. (1992). *Speaking from the heart: A feminist perspective on ethics*. Lanham, MD: Rowman & Littlefield.

Meade, C. D., & Howser, D. M. (1992). Consent forms: How to determine and improve their readability. *Oncology Nursing Forum*, 19, 1523–1528.

Merton, V. (1996). Ethical obstacles to the participation of women in biomedical research. In S. M. Wolf (Ed.), *Feminism and bioethics: Beyond reproduction* (pp. 216–251). New York: Oxford University Press.

Merton, V. (1993). The exclusion of pregnant, pregnable, and once-pregnable people (a.k.a. women) from biomedical research. *American Journal of Law & Medicine*, 19, 369–451.

Mink v. University of Chicago (1978). 460 F. Supp. 713 (N.D. Ill.).

Mitchell, J. (1974). *Psychoanalysis and feminism*. New York: Pantheon.

Moore v. Regents of the University of California, 793 P.2d 479 (Cal. 1990).

Moore R. D., Hidalgo J., Sugland B. W., & Chaisson R. E. (1991). Zidovudine and the natural history of the acquired immunodeficiency syndrome. *New England Journal of Medicine*, 324, 1412–1416.

Moss, K. L. (1991). Forced drug or alcohol treatment for pregnant and postpartum women: Part of the solution or part of the problem? *New England Journal of Criminal and Civil Confinement*, 17, 1–16.

National Institutes of Health Revitalization Act of 1993, Pub.L. 103-43.

National Research Act of 1974. 42 United States Code section 300a-7(d)(1974 & Supp. 193).

Pham, H., Freeman, P., & Kohn, N. (1992). *Understanding the second epidemic: The status of research on women and AIDS in the United States*. Washington, DC: Center for Women Policy Studies.

Raskin, A. (1974). Age-sex differences in response to antidepressant drugs. *Journal of Nervous and Mental Diseases*, 159, 120–130.

Reiman, J. (1988). Utilitarianism and the informed consent requirement (or: should utilitarians be allowed on medical research ethical review boards?). In B. A. Brody (Ed.), *Moral theory and moral judgments in medical ethics* (pp. 41–51). Boston: Kluwer Academic.

Rich, A. (1980). Compulsory heterosexuality and lesbian existence. *Signs*, 5, 631–660.

Rivera, R., Reed, J. S., & Menius, D. (1992). Evaluating the readability of informed consent forms used in contraceptive clinical trials. *International Journal of Gynecology and Obstetrics*, 38, 227–230.

Roberts, D. (1990, April). Drug addicted women who have babies. *Trial*, 56–61.

Roberts, D. E. (1991, May). Punishing drug addicts who have babies: Women of color, equality, and the right of privacy. *Harvard Law Review*, 104, 1419–1482.

Rosser, S. V. (1989). Re-visioning clinical research: Gender and the ethics of experimental design. *Hypatia*, 4, 125–139.

Ryan White Comprehensive AIDS Resources Emergency (CARE) Act of 1990, Pub. L. No. 101-381.

Sandel, M. (1982). *Liberalism and the limits of justice*. Cambridge: Cambridge University Press.

Sherman, R. (1992, Feb. 24). Split rulings for fetal abuse cases. *National Law Journal*, 3.

Sherwin, S. (1992). *No longer patient: Feminist ethics and health care*. Philadelphia: Temple University Press.

Sherwin, S. (1994a). Women in clinical studies: A feminist view. *Cambridge Quarterly of Health Care Ethics*, 3, 533–538.

Sherwin, S. (1994b). Women in clinical studies: A feminist view. In A. Mastroianni, R. Faden, & D. Federman (Eds.), *Ethical and legal issues of including women in clinical studies, vol. 2* (pp. 11–17). Washington, DC: National Academy Press.

Sichel, B. A. (1991). Different strains and strands: Feminist contributions to ethical theory. *Newsletters on Feminism and Philosophy*, 90, 86–92.

Strickland, R. A., & Whicker, M. L. (1992, Aug.). Fetal endangerment versus fetal welfare: Discretion of prosecutors in determining criminal liability and intent. Presented at the meeting of the American Political Science Association. Chicago.

Strong, C. (1997). *Ethics in reproductive and perinatal medicine: A new framework*. New Haven, CT: Yale University Press.

Tarasoff v. Regents of the University of California. (1976). 551 P.2d 334.

Todd, A. D. (1983). *Intimate adversaries: Cultural conflict between doctors and women patients*. Philadelphia: University of Pennsylvania Press.

Tong, R. (1996). Feminist approaches to bioethics. In S. M. Wolf (Ed.), *Feminism & bioethics: Beyond reproduction* (pp. 67–94). New York: Oxford University Press.

United States Public Health Service. (1988). Public Health Service guidelines for counseling and antibody testing to prevent HIV infection and AIDS. *New York State Journal of Medicine*, 88, 74–76.

West, R. C. (1988). Jurisprudence and gender. *University of Chicago Law Review*, 55, 1–72.

Wetherill v. University of Chicago (1983). 570 F. Supp. 1124 (N.D. Ill.).

21 Code of Federal Regulations, section 46.111 (1998).

45 Code of Federal Regulations, section 46.111 (1998).

23

Women's Sexual and Reproductive Health

Theory, Research, and Practice

RALPH J. DICLEMENTE and GINA M. WINGOOD

INTRODUCTION

Recent advances in women's health have been encouraging (Goldman & Hatch, 2000; Alexander & LaRosa, 1994; Blechman & Brownell, 1998). Major strides have been made in a myriad of health-related areas. One domain that has experienced marked advances in early detection of disease, prevention, and treatment is women's sexual and reproductive health. The chapters in this book describe promising advances in the field of women's sexual and reproductive health: screening, prevention, and treatment, both primary and secondary, both biomedical and psychological. Notwithstanding these advances, complex research challenges and significant sociopolitical hurdles remain to be surmounted. This chapter, unlike its predecessors, attempts to highlight key areas of research and discern fruitful directions for building a science of women's sexual and reproductive health.

It is beyond the scope of this chapter to reiterate the richness of diversity or depth of information captured and articulated so skillfully in previous chapters. It is useful, however, to understand our successes and, as important, to identify and confront existing challenges. By doing so, we hope to bring into sharper focus those areas that hold considerable promise for enhancing women's sexual and reproductive health and, as such, warrant vigorous exploration. Only by understanding the past, its successes and its failures, and gazing toward the future, its opportunities and its challenges, can we move forward with unwavering determination to capitalize on history and create a field that contributes more fully to the enhancement of women's sexual and reproductive health.

Women's Sexual and Reproductive Health: Building a Field from an Interdisciplinary Perspective

Advances in the field of women's sexual and reproductive health are attributable, to a large extent, to the heterogeneity of disciplines that are actively involved in prevention, early detection and treatment research. Diversity is a research strength that facilitates advances by transcending disciplinary boundaries. These advances have been most readily made with

RALPH J. DICLEMENTE and GINA M. WINGOOD • Department of Behavioral Sciences and Health Education, Rollins School of Public Health, Emory University, Atlanta, Georgia 30322.

Handbook of Women's Sexual and Reproductive Health, edited by Wingood and DiClemente. Kluwer Academic / Plenum Publishers, New York, 2002.

true interdisciplinary approaches that involve not just scientists and practitioners addressing a particular research question from a social and behavioral science perspective, a biomedical or epidemiological perspective, or a legal or a ethical perspective, but from the active involvement of all relevant disciplines in an effort to integrate the disciplines to further the development of the field of women's sexual and reproductive health.

The breadth of disciplines involved in women's sexual and reproductive health, as judged by the diversity of contributors to the Handbook, may lead eventually to a rapid convergence of the field of women's sexual and reproductive health. Understanding the complexity, isolating, and quantifying the influences that affect women's sexual and reproductive decision making and behavior is clearly formidable. Changing behavior is unquestionably a formidable challenge, influenced through the complex, reciprocal determinism of individuals' physiological processes, cognitions, and emotional responses; their behavior; the environment; and interpersonal, social, economic, and psychological influences within a cultural context that is superimposed over traditions, values, and patterns of social organization. Such a complex process is not likely to be understood in simplistic, unidimensional, or linear terms. Thus, the interdisciplinary nature of the field is critical to developing a coherent, integrated body of empirical data that acknowledges and accommodates the myriad of genetic, physiological, intrapersonal, interpersonal, social system, and cultural forces. Continued integration and collaboration between researchers and practitioners in the behavioral and social sciences, with clinicians, policy analysts, epidemiologists and biostatisticians, ethicists, legal scholars, and advocates and activists represents the best opportunity to develop a coherent, effective, and interdisciplinary approach to developing the field of women's sexual and reproductive health.

The field of women's sexual and reproductive health can be characterized as showing promise. While certainly requiring a convergence of theory to guide and interpret data, significant methodologic challenges also remain for the field of women's sexual and reproductive health in order to generate an adequate knowledge base. There is, for instance, an urgent need for the development of data collection instruments (i.e., surveys and interviews) that are validated on women and that are culturally and ethnically sensitive. These challenges are inherent in all fields of research but may be particularly great in a field that attempts to address the complexity of influences that impact women's sexual and reproductive health.

More rigorous research that is dedicated to women's sexual and reproductive health is urgently needed. Theoretically driven, methodologically sound, evidence-based research in women's sexual and reproductive health, when rigorously evaluated, offers the greatest promise for contributing to our understanding of how best to enhance the adoption of health-promoting behaviors. Greater specificity will be necessary to more effectively tailor interventions to different populations, taking into account their sexual orientation, ethnicity, and developmental level as well as the setting and social environment in which programs are implemented. For the field of women's sexual and reproductive health to progress more rapidly, however, a comprehensive and coordinated infrastructure to conceptualize, stimulate, and support the continuum of research necessary to impact the continuing and emerging health threats that confront women is of critical importance.

Women's Sexual and Reproductive Health Needs to Target Multiple Levels of Causality

Historically, women's health has been largely viewed as an individual-level phenomenon. More recently, scientists and practitioners have begun to recognize that a host of environmental, sociocontextual, political, and structural influences significantly impact women's sexual and reproductive health. Researchers and practitioners alike are increasingly acknowledging the importance of social contextualism; the need to understand a woman's decision making and behavior within "their" social reality, and intervene not only on the individual level, but address community level as well as broader structural-level changes.

Interventions at the community level represent one important strategy designed to promote women's health by providing women with information and skills to change behavior through naturally occurring channels of influence in the community. Simultaneously, interventions at the community level provide a supportive environment that encourages the adoption and maintenance of health-promoting behavior. Changing community norms also reinforces and maintains the practice of health-promoting behaviors.

Community-level interventions may enhance women's sexual and reproductive health in a number of ways. First, they may foster the adoption of specific health promoting practices and behaviors among women engaged in risky behaviors. Second, they may help sustain newly acquired health-promoting behaviors and, hopefully, solidify these changes. Third, community-level interventions may also serve to amplify individual-level program effects over extended time periods reducing the potential for relapse to high-risk behaviors. And, finally, community-level interventions may foster an atmosphere that discourages the initial adoption of health-damaging behaviors.

While community-level intervention programs represent one area for increased research, it is crucial that broader structural changes take place to ensure that women are empowered and enabled to make the desired changes in behavior. These must include changes in laws, public, and health policy that exert considerable influence on the context and circumstances in which sexual and reproductive decision making and behavior takes place. Therefore, future research will need to examine in greater detail the effects of social, cultural, institutional, political and economic forces as they promote or reinforce risky sexual and reproductive behavior. By understanding these broader, pervasive influences,

it may be possible to develop community-level interventions, initiate policy changes, design institutionally based programs and promote the development of broader, macrolevel societal changes that hold the promise of accessing many more women and constructing a social environment that supports women's adoption and maintenance of health-promoting behaviors.

In Search of New and Promising Theoretical Orientations

The diversity of theoretical approaches in women's sexual and reproductive health is a reflection of this nascent field. Theoretical approaches from a broad spectrum of disciplines have been utilized. The scales of evidence suggest that these theories have been effective at promoting the sexual and reproductive health of women. However effective our current array of theories, it would be premature to foreclose on the utility of other, as of yet, untested theories. In particular, we are beginning to recognize the need for theories that focus on women in society; that permit an understanding of women's sexual and reproductive decision making and behavior within the social and political realities of their environment. Theoretical frameworks that attempt to understand the complex interaction among women's economic, social, political, psychological, and physical health are necessary. Thus, other theoretical models may prove useful and should be empirically tested. Diversity in terms of theory selection needs to be embraced and, indeed, encouraged. As the focus of intervention research shifts from individual-level to broader community-level and structural-level interventions, a different array of theories may be sought to help guide these interventions.

Measurement of Cost Effectiveness in Women's Sexual and Reproductive Health Research

The increasing emphasis on cost containment, the emergence of the managed care environment, and the disproportionate increase in the cost of health care versus other expenditures over the past decade has prompted examining cost-effectiveness as one criterion for evaluating health promotion programs. In our current fiscal environment, it becomes imperative that we not only evaluate program efficacy in terms of impact (e.g., changes in behavior, attitudes, norms, knowledge) and outcomes (e.g., changes in morbidity, mortality, quality of life) but also assess cost-effectiveness. Such information is vitally important to program planners, policymakers, and other persons involved in the design and implementation of health promotion and treatment programs who are responsible for the judicious allocation of limited financial resources.

Health scientists and program planners need to become familiar with the theory and methods used to conduct cost-effectiveness studies (Gold *et al.*, 1996; Haddix *et al.*, 1996). While an interdisciplinary perspective is the hallmark of women's sexual and reproductive health, one area that is underdeveloped is the science of economic evaluation. As women's sexual and reproductive health matures as a field and more interventions are shown to be effective in reducing risk behavior, encouraging early detection of disease, and enhancing treatment outcomes, it will become increasingly important to establish the cost-effectiveness of these interventions.

Looking Forward: Future Directions for Women's Sexual and Reproductive Health

This Handbook is an interdisciplinary forum highlighting the interplay among diverse social, psychological, and environmental influences on women's sexual and reproductive health. Additionally, the Handbook describes promising developments in theory, design, evaluation, and the development of interventions and implementation methods used in women's sexual and reproductive health across a spectrum of risk behaviors and health conditions. It has sought to provide a life-span perspective that addresses a range of sexual and reproductive health conditions. Clearly, the field of women's sexual and reproductive health

is growing in depth and breadth as new theoretical models and innovative health promotion strategies are identified and as societal, health care, and regulatory influences have increased the focus on examining the cost-effectiveness of health promotion programs. The trajectory of advances suggests that in the foreseeable future the field of women's sexual and reproductive health will continue to rapidly expand.

Future sexual and reproductive health promotion interventions must be developed and evaluated on an ongoing basis to monitor programmatic efficacy; not only by measuring statistically significant changes in risk behaviors or incidence of disease, or longevity, but other meaningful changes as well, such as changes in women's quality of life. Programs must also be modified according to evaluation feedback further refining health-promoting interventions and strengthening their potential to effectively promote behavior change and enhance recovery. Equally important as program development, there is a need for effective program technology transfer. Programs which are evaluated and identified as effective should be widely disseminated through diverse channels and adequate training and program materials should be provided to encourage the adoption and appropriate use of these programs. Further, to increase the comprehension and perhaps effectiveness of health promotion programs, they must be developed to address different levels of causation and tailored to be relevant and sensitive to the intended population.

To successfully confront the challenges of women's sexual and reproductive health, innovative program design, rigorous evaluation, rapid dissemination of effective health promotion interventions, and the adoption and integration of research into ongoing, sustainable programs that permit wide and unfettered access must remain a public health priority. As we look forward, we should recognize that future generations will look back and reflect on our efforts. Let the future historians remark upon our inspiration, our willingness to commit both fiscal and human resources, and our unwavering dedication to enhancing women's sexual and reproductive health.

ACKNOWLEDGMENTS. This chapter was supported, in part, by grants from the National Institutes of Health, National Institute of Mental Health (R01 MH61210, R01 MH54412, R01 MH61210).

REFERENCES

Alexander, L. L., & LaRosa, J. H. (1994). *New dimensions in women's health*. Boston: Jones and Bartlett.

Blechman, E. A., & Brownell, K. D. (Eds.). (1998). *Behavioral medicine and women*. New York: Guilford Press.

Gold, M. R., Siegel, J. E., Russell, L. B., & Weinstein, M. C. (Eds.). (1996). *Cost-effectiveness in health and medicine*. New York: Oxford University Press.

Goldman, M. B., & Hatch, M. C. (Eds.). (2000). *Women & health*. New York: Academic Press.

Haddix, A. C., Teutsch, S. M., Shaffer, P. A., & Dunet, D. O. (Eds.). (1996). *Prevention effectiveness: A guide to decision analysis and economic evaluation*. New York: Oxford University Press.

Index

Self-esteem (*cont.*)
  and childhood sexual abuse, 202
Self-examination, of breasts, 353
Self-medication, and drug abuse, 141, 143, 145
Self-mutilation, and childhood sexual abuse, 202
Sensate focus technique, 319, 320
Sex education, *see also* Prevention measures
  peer-led sex education, 271
  sexual-risk targeted programs, 37–38, 114
Sex selection, ethical issues, 434–435
Sex and the Single Girl (Brown), 15
Sex therapy, 318–323
  biofeedback, 319
  clinically directed masturbation, 320
  coital alignment technique, 320
  for female arousal disorders (FAD), 319–320, 322–323
  medication treatments, 322–323
  orgasm consistency training, 319
  for orgasmic disorders, 320, 323
  script modification, 319
  sensate focus technique, 319, 320
  for sexual desire disorders, 318–319, 322
  for sexual pain disorders, 321–322
  vasoactive drugs, 319–320
Sexism
  in gender-role socialization, 75–76
  and stereotyping, 74
Sexual abuse, 76–77, 195–211
  and adolescent behavior problems, 76
  and alcohol abuse, 160, 202, 204
  and body image, 180
  case example, 195–196
  circumstances of, 197
  consent issues, 199
  criteria for establishment of, 199
  definitions of, 197–198, 199
  and drug abuse, 141, 143–144, 202, 204
  dynamics of, 201–202
  forms of, 197, 199
  gender differences, 76
  health care provider recognition of, 206–207, 210
  and high-risk sexual behaviors, 76, 203–204
  and HIV/AIDS, 204–205
  and interpersonal problems, 203
  legal interventions, 198
  in males, 204
  NHSLS findings, 52–53
  and pelvic pain, chronic, 221
  personal perception of, 199–200
  physical health effects, 202
  prevalence of, 76, 197
  prevention programs, 207–208
  and psychiatric disorders, 160–161, 202, 204
  and racial/ethnic minorities, 76–77, 205–206
  research, history of, 198
  and revictimization, 201–202

Sexual abuse (*cont.*)
  sexual assault, 200
  and sexual dissatisfaction, 203
  and sexual dysfunction, 160, 203–204, 309
  treatment of, 208–209
Sexual arousal
  and alcohol abuse, 158–159
  and estrogen, 322
  in pregnancy, 314–315
  and psychoactive drug use, 140
  and testosterone, 311–312
Sexual arousal disorders: *see* Female sexual arousal
  disorder (FSAD)
Sexual assault
  acquaintance rape, 200
  and alcohol abuse, 160–161
  consequences of, 161
  and drug use, 144
  NHSLS findings, 52–53
  rape, definition of, 200
  underreporting of, 200
Sexual attitudes
  NHSLS findings, 65–68
  recreational orientation, 68
  relational orientation, 67–68
  traditional orientation, 65, 67
Sexual attraction, NHSLS findings, 50–51
Sexual aversion disorder (SAD), 305
  and childhood sexual trauma, 309
  features of, 305
  medication treatment, 319
  as panic reaction, 305
  psychological factors, 309
Sexual behavior, *see also* First sexual experience; High-risk sexual behaviors
  adolescents, 23, 24, 29, 31, 233–234
  components of, 266
  and self-efficacy, 266
Sexual Behavior in the Human Female (Kinsey), 14
Sexual desire, sociocultural aspects, 44
Sexual desire disorders
  hypoactive sexual desire disorder (HSD), 304–305
  medication treatment, 322
  and pregnancy/breastfeeding, 315
  psychological factors, 309
  sex therapy for, 318–319
  sexual aversion disorder (SAD), 305
Sexual dysfunction, 303–324
  age factors, 311
  and alcohol abuse, 159–160, 169
  antidepressant effects, 313–314
  and childhood sexual abuse, 160, 203–204, 309
  and depression, 309
  and drug abuse, 142
  DSM-IV classification limitations, 307–308
  DSM-IV criteria, 304
  family influences, 309

About the Editors

Gina M. Wingood, Sc.D., MPH is an Assistant Professor in the Department of Behavioral Sciences and Health Education at Emory University, Rollins School of Public Health. Dr. Wingood received her MPH in Maternal and Child Health from the University of California, Berkeley and her Sc.D. from the Harvard University School of Public Health in Health and Social Behavior. Dr. Wingood's research interest is in primary and secondary HIV prevention for women. Dr. Wingood has published numerous articles on effective HIV prevention interventions for women. She has also written extensively on the impact of such social factors as social inequalities, the mass media, gender roles, rape, domestic violence, dating violence, and childhood sexual abuse as exposures that increase women's vulnerability towards STDs, including HIV. Dr. Wingood's work has appeared in numerous public health journals including *JAMA*, *American Journal of Public Health*, *Pediatrics*, *American Journal of Preventive Medicine*, and *Women's Health*.

Ralph J. DiClemente, Ph.D. is Charles Howard Candler Professor of Public Health and Associate Director, Emory/Atlanta Center for AIDS Research. He holds concurrent appointments as Professor in the School of Medicine, the Department of Pediatrics, in the Division of Infectious Diseases, Epidemiology, and Immunology, and the Department of Medicine, in the Division of Infectious Diseases, and the Department of Psychiatry. He was most recently, Chair, Department of Behavioral Sciences and Health Education at the Rollins School of Public Health, Emory University. Dr. DiClemente was trained as a Health Psychologist at the University of California San Francisco where he received his Ph.D. in 1984 after completing an MSPH in Behavioral Sciences at the Harvard School of Public Health and his undergraduate degree at the City University of New York.

ISBN 0-306-46651-1

90000